Clinical Skills in Child Health Practice

Clinical Skills in Child Health Practice

Edited by

Janet Kelsey

MSc BSc PGCEA Dip Ed (Adv) RSCN RGN RNT
Lecturer in Nursing Child Health
Programme Lead BSc Child Health Nursing
and Teaching Fellow
Faculty of Health and Social Work
University of Plymouth
Plymouth, UK

Gillian McEwing

MSc DipN RSCN RGN RNT
Lecturer in Nursing, Child Health &
Teaching Fellow
Faculty of Health and Social Work
University of Plymouth
Plymouth, UK

SAUNDERS
ELSEVIER

Edinburgh London New York Oxford Philadelphia St Louis Sydney Toronto 2008

CHURCHILL
LIVINGSTONE
ELSEVIER

An imprint of Elsevier Limited

978-0-443-10340-7
Reprinted 2008

British Library Cataloguing in Publication Data
A catalogue record for this book is available from the British Library

Library of Congress Cataloging in Publication Data
A catalog record for this book is available from the Library of Congress

The publisher's policy is to use **paper manufactured from sustainable forests**

Printed in China

Commissioning Editor: Ninette Premdas
Development Editor: Sheila Black
Project Manager: Andrew Palfreyman
Design Direction: Stewart Larking
Illustrations Manager: Kirsteen Wright
Illustrator: Cactus

Dedication

This first edition of *Clinical Skills in Child Health Practice* is dedicated to our parents, partners and children for their support and their faith in our ability to succeed in this venture.

Contents

Contributors

Marion Aylott BSc MA PGCertEd RGN RM RSCN
Lecturer
School of Nursing & Midwifery
University of Southampton
Southampton, UK

Jacqueline S. Baker BSc HV JB RN RM CN5400 5NB904 ENBR23
Senior Nurse
Neonatal Unit
Maelor Hospital
Wrexham, UK

Lucy Bray RN BA Hons MSC
Senior Research Nurse
Medicines for Children Local Research Network
Cheshire, Merseyside and North Wales
Royal Liverpool Children's NHS Trust
Liverpool, UK

Maria Bennallick MSc BSc (Hons) CertEd RN
Knowledge Spa
Faculty of Health and Social Work
Treliske Hospital
Royal Cornwall Hospitals Trust
Truro, UK

Neil Bloxham RGN RSCN ENB415
Charge Nurse/Clinical Educator
Children's High Dependency Unit
Derriford Hospital
Devon, UK

Eileen P. Brennan MSc RSCN RN1 RN8
Nurse Consultant
Renal Unit
Great Ormond Street Hospital
London, UK

Matthew Carey DipHE Nursing (Child)
Staff Nurse Derriford Hospital
Devon, UK

Julie A. Chambers BSc (Hons) TP SRN RSCN SCM DNC
Community Children's Nursing Sister
Pound Lane Health Centre
Down Lisburn Trust
Down Patrick
Co. Down, UK

Margaret A. Chambers MSc BSc (Hons) PGDipEd RSCN DPSN RGN RNT
Lecturer in Child Health Nursing & Teaching Fellow
Faculty of Health and Social Work
University of Plymouth
Plymouth, UK

Sonya E. Clarke MSc BSc (Hons) PGCE PGCert RN RCN/Dip RGN
Teaching Fellow
School of Nursing and Midwifery
Medical Biology Centre
Queen's University Belfast
Belfast, UK

Doris A.P. Corkin BSc (Hons) PGDip CCN RGN RN ENB904
Teaching Fellow
School of Nursing and Midwifery
Medical Biology Centre
Queen's University Belfast
Belfast, UK

Imelda T. Coyne
Associate Professor
Faculty of Health Sciences
School of Nursing and Midwifery
The University of Dublin
Trinity College
Dublin, Ireland

Sarah Doyle MSc RN (Child)
Advanced Paediatric Nurse Practitioner in Urology
Royal Liverpool Children's NHS Trust
Liverpool, UK

Marie Elen BSc PGCert HE RGN RSCN
Lecturer in Child Health
Faculty of Health and Life Sciences
School of Community Health
Napier University
Edinburgh, UK

Sue Frost CertEd DipN
Education and Development Practitioner
Practice Education Centre
Derriford Hospital
Plymouth, UK

Jackie Gekas CertEd RGN RSCN
Senior Staff Nurse
Deputy Ward Manager
Royal Cornwall Hospital

Laura Gilbert BSc (Hons) PGCLT CertHV DipHE RGN RSCN
Lecturer Child Nursing Department of Health Wellbeing and the Family
Canterbury Christ Church University
Canterbury, UK

Stephen Gill MSc RGN RSCN IHMS
Sleep Study Nurse Children's Unit
Dunedin Public Hospital
Dunedin, New Zealand

E. Alan Glasper Phd BA (Hons) CertEd RSCN RGN ONC RNT
Professor of Children's and Young People's Nursing
University of Southampton
Southampton, UK

Diane Gow MSc BA (Hons) RGN RSCN RCNT RNT
Lecturer in Children's and Young People's Nursing
University of Southampton
Southampton, UK

Louise Holliday BSc (Hons) PGCPE RSCN RGN
Medical Ward
Royal Aberdeen Children's Hospital
Aberdeen, UK

Alison Hough BSc (Hons) PGCE DPSN RSCN RGN
Staff Nurse
Royal Cornwall Hospitals
Truro, UK

Emma V.P. Jasper DipHE (Nursing) RN (Child)
Paediatric Staff Nurse
Whithorse Assessment Unit
Derriford Hospital
Plymouth, UK

Karen Jeffery MSc CertEd (FE) RSCN RGN RCNT RNT
Lecturer in Child Health Nursing & Teaching Fellow
Faculty of Health and Social Work
University of Plymouth
Ereter, UK

Denise Jonas MSc BSc (Hons) RSCN RGN PGCH EPR
Lecturer/Practitioner Child Health
School of Nursing
University of Salford and CMMC NHS Trust
Manchester, UK

Julia Judd MSc RSCN RGN ENB219
Advanced Nurse Practitioner in Paediatric Orthopaedics
Southampton General Hospital
Southampton, UK

Janet Kelsey MSc BSc PGCEA DipEd (Adv) RSCN RGN RNT
Lecturer in Child Health Nursing & Teaching Fellow
Programme Lead BSc Child Health Nursing
Faculty of Health and Social Work
University of Plymouth
Plymouth, UK

Carla Kierulff DipHE Nursing (Child)
Staff Nurse
Medical Ward
Royal Aberdeen Children's Hospital
Aberdeen, UK

Jay Kumar BSc (Hons) DipN RGCN RGN
Clinical Skills Educator
Professional Development Team
Birmingham Children's Hospital NHS Trust
Birmingham, UK

Gilli Lewis BN MA RN PGCHE DipAsthma Care
Clinical Teaching Associate
Children's Hospital Capital and Coast Health
Wellington, New Zealand

Pearl Matthews DipN RGN RSCN
Clinical Governance Co-ordinator & Risk Management Lead
Child Health
Southampton General Hospital
Southampton, UK

Gillian McEwing MSc DipN RSCN RGN RNT
Lecturer in Child Health Nursing & Teaching Fellow
Faculty of Health and Social Work
University of Plymouth
Plymouth, UK

Patricia McNeilly MSc BSc PG CertEd RGN RSCN CCN
School of Nursing & Midwifery
Queen's University Belfast
Belfast, UK

Irene J. McTaggart MSc BA PGDE FABD RGN RSCN RCNT RNT
Professional Head of Child Nursing
School of Nursing and Midwifery
University of Dundee
Dundee, UK

Hermione Montgomery BSc (Hons) RN RSCN RM ITHE
Lead Nurse
Quality of Care
Birmingham Children's Hospital NHS Trust
Birmingham, UK

Philomena Morrow MSc BSc (Hons) RNRM RCNT
Nurse Lecturer
Queen's University Belfast
Belfast, UK

Sharon Nurse BSc (Hons) RN RM RCNT
Midwifery Teaching Fellow
School of Nursing and Midwifery
Queen's University Belfast
Belfast, UK

Colleen O'Neill BSc (Hons) MSc HDip RGN RCN
Lecturer
Dublin City
University School of Nursing
Dublin, Ireland

Kelly Owens BSc (Hons) PFDip RGN RN (Child) ENB405 ENB998
Senior Staff Nurse/Clinical Skills Facilitator
Portsmouth Hospitals NHS Trust and University of Southampton
Southampton, UK

Theresa Pengelly MSc BSc (Hons) PGDipEd RSCN
Senior Lecturer in Child Health
University of Worcester Institute of Health, Social Care & Psychology
Worcester, UK

Jayne Price MSc BSc (Hons) PGDipEd RGN RN (Child)
Senior Teaching Fellow
School of Nursing and Midwifery
Queen's University of Belfast
Belfast, UK

Gillian Prudhoe BA (Hons) PGDipEd SRN RSCN ENB405 ENB415
Lecturer, Child and Young Person Nursing
University of Southampton
Education Centre, St Marys Hospital
Portsmouth, UK

Sara Raftery MSc PGDip (Ed) PGDip (Clinical Practice) RGN RCN RNT
Lecturer
Dublin City University School of Nursing
Dublin, Ireland

Jim Richardson BA RGN RSCN PGCE PhD
Principal Lecturer – Child Health Nursing
School of Care Sciences
University of Glamorgan
Glyntaf, UK

Olga Richardson MEd DipNursing ONC ADESN RGN RMN
Lecturer
School of Nursing and Midwifery
Queen's University Belfast
Belfast, UK

Joyce Robertson MA BPhil MCSP
Neonatal Neurodevelopmental Physiotherapist
Birmingham Children's Hospital
Birmingham, UK

Caroline Sanders BSc (Hons) PgDip RCN
Nurse Consultant Urology/Gynaecology
Royal Liverpool Children's NHS Trust
Liverpool, UK

Rosemary Smith MLitt DipNurs RGN RSCN RNT
Lecturer
School of Nursing and Midwifery
Robert Gordon University
Faculty of Health & Social Care
Aberdeen, UK

Jane Swain MN RGN RM RNT CertEd (FE)
Lecturer
Faculty of Health & Social Work
University of Plymouth
Exeter

Sue Syers MSc BSc (Hons) RGN RSCN
Advanced Paediatric Nurse Practitioner
Whitehorse Assessment Unit
Derriford Hospital
Plymouth, UK

Donald Todd BSc (Hons) DipHEdNurs PGDipHlth Prom
Clinical Nurse Manager
Royal Aberdeen Children's Hospital
Aberdeen, UK

Ruth Trengove BSc (Hons) RGN RSCN
Sister
Paediatric High Dependency Unit
Torquay Hospital
Torquay, UK

Lesley E. Wayne MSc BSc (Hons) DipProff Stud Nurse RGN RSCN
Nurse Practitioner
Minor Injuries Unit
Cumberland Centre
Plymouth, UK

Zoe Wood BSc (Hons) RN/CB
Acute Liaison Nurse for Learning
Disabilities Practice Development
Royal Cornwall Hospital Trust
Truro, UK

Elizabeth Wright MSc RSCN RGN ENB219
Advanced Nurse Practitioner in Paediatric Orthopaedics
Southampton University Hospital Trust
Southampton, UK

Preface

Clinical Skills in Child Health Practice is designed to assist all practitioners involved in delivering practical care to children and young people. Delivering this care involves specialist skills and, as the editors of this book, we are aware that we are in a climate of dynamic change. This book has been written by clinical and academic experts in the field of children's and young people's healthcare practice. The delivery of care requires practitioners to have a sound evidence base and demands the use of high-level skills in a versatile and transferable fashion. The intention of this book is, therefore, to provide the current evidence base underpinning the delivery of care to a high standard and to assist in the development of competent and confident practitioners.

This book aims to provide a step by step guide to the clinical skills required of practitioners in children's and young people's health care. It will draw on the latest evidence-based practice to support the teaching and discussion of issues arising from the provision of the clinical skills for use in this client group. In addition to the book, with its detailed and illustrated procedure boxes, readers are able to access multimedia content on the Evolve website. There is a recognised need for clinical skills teaching, be it in the clinical environment or in the skills laboratory. However, there are many problems associated with learning clinical skills in the practice setting. Many practitioners report feeling anxious when performing new skills and describe how they are unprepared for carrying out clinical procedures. In children's and young people's care there is the additional consideration of the families' involvement in care, and opportunities to learn and practice basic skills are limited as a result of parental participation. We recognised the difficulties in teaching this subject in clinical areas and this resource was created to assist students and lecturers to develop these essential skills.

Each chapter begins with an evidence base for the skill, emphasising the underlying principle and the requirements for safe practice. This is followed by a grid setting out step by step performance of the skill, which includes each individual action and its rationale. Pictures are incorporated to improve clarity. Finally there is a 'Test Your Knowledge' section at the end of each chapter that can be used by either individuals or lecturers to help consolidate learning. In most cases, the questions are either suitable for open-ended discussion or consideration, or may be answered by close examination of the text. However, where specific answers or points are thought to be useful, these are provided at the end of the book. PowerPoint presentations (many containing video clips of procedures) are available for almost all chapters and will enable this book to be used as a teaching resource. These can be presented in skills laboratories to student groups prior to practising the skill or they can be used by individual students in self-directed sessions within the skills laboratories. The book and the PowerPoint presentations can also be utilised in the practice areas to provide the opportunity for individuals to examine practice in their own areas in relation to the current evidence base.

In today's healthcare environment practitioners face many challenges. This book was written to help meet some of these challenges and take advantage of new opportunities to provide care for children and young people. We believe this book will become a fundamental resource for all those working in child healthcare practice. We hope you find this book and its associated website a useful resource and if you have any comments or recommendations please contact us by writing to the publishers.

Janet Kelsey and Gillian McEwing
January 2008

Acknowledgements

Chapter 9

Assessment of blood pressure

The author thanks Clare Richardson, Practice Educator at Great Ormond Street Hospital for her contribution to the practice guideline for measuring blood pressure.

Chapter 10

Neurological assessment

The author expresses many thanks to Gillian McEwing and Janet Kelsey for kindly taking the pictures used in this chapter. Also to Joshia Kelsey and Claire Pound for kindly posing for them.

Chapter 14

Artificial feeding

The author expresses many thanks to Paul Morris, clinical skills technician, School of Nursing and Midwifery, Queen's University Belfast, for photographic support, also Andrea McDougall, paediatric dietician, Royal Belfast Hospital for Sick Children, for having read and commented on an earlier draft.

Chapter 15

Enteral feeding

Nutrition via enteral feeding devices

The author expresses many thanks to Kevin Campbell, clinical skills technician, School of Nursing and Midwifery, Queen's University Belfast, for photographic support.

Chapter 16

Administration of medicines

The authors would like to thank Jeny Mosley, Paediatric Pharmacist, Royal Aberdeen Children's Hospital, for reading and offering comments and additions to this chapter. We are also grateful to Gill McEwing for providing the excellent illustrations.

Chapter 18

The management of procedural pain in children using self-administered Entonox (50% nitrous oxide, 50% oxygen)

The author thanks Central Manchester and Manchester Children's University Hospitals NHS Trust for permission to use the photographs appearing in this chapter and the staff of RMCH outpatients for their valuable participation.

Chapter 25

Safe administration of blood and blood products

The authors thank Mike Williams, Haemotologist, for his advice on writing this chapter.

Chapter 28

Blood glucose monitoring

The author thanks Paul Morris, clinical skills technician, School of Nursing, Queen's University Belfast, for kindly taking the pictures used in this chapter.

Chapter 29

Insulin therapy

The author thanks Paul Morris, clinical skills technician, School of Nursing, Queen's University Belfast, for kindly taking the pictures used in this chapter.

Chapter 33

Assessment and management of wounds in children

The author thanks Mr Philip Belsham, A & E Consultant, Derriford Hospital, Plymouth for his advice and comments on reviewing this chapter.

Chapter 34

Occlusive treatments for childhood eczema and other skin conditions

The author gratefully acknowledges the kindness of Ellie who was willingly bandaged and photographed for this chapter. The author's dermatology knowledge was gathered in this time at the Children's Hospital in Birmingham, so he wishes to thank Dr Celia Moss for the initial opportunities and support, and Drs Malobi Ogboli, Ann Cortmill and Ewa Edwards for their long-term instruction in the care and kindness that children with skin conditions need and deserve. The author also wishes to thank the dermatology nursing team for their dedicated professional example of caring for children.

Chapter 37

Developmentally supportive positioning and handling of neonates

Joyce Robertson would particularly like to thank the parents who generously gave permission for her to include photographs of them and their babies. She would also like to thank Katy Thompson and Liz Wright for help with some of the illustrations and Children's Medical Ventures for permission to illustrate their equipment. She also thanks other friends and colleagues who made suggestions and offered help during the writing of this chapter.

Chapter 42

Skeletal pin site care

The authors thank Rose Davies, Specialist Ilizarov Nurse and Paddy Comiskey, Medical Photographer for their photographic contribution.

Chapter 43

Breaking bad news to parents

This chapter is based on the following article and is reproduced with permission of MA Healthcare Ltd: Price J, McNeilly P, Surgenor M 2006 Breaking bad news to parents: the children's nurse's role. International Journal of Palliative Nursing 12(3):115–120.

The author thanks Paul Morris, clinical skills technician, Anne Scott, Carmel McCloy and David McAtackney from the School of Nursing and Midwifery Queen's University of Belfast for their assistance with the photographs used in this chapter.

Chapter 44

Care of the child after death

The authors thank Eileen Scott RGN RSCN, Ward Manager (Acting), Maynard Sinclair Ward, Ulster Communities and Hospital Trust, for her help and advice on writing this chapter.

Section One
Skills that underpin practice

1 Fundamental skills for children's and young people's nurses

E. Alan Glasper • Diane Gow • Pearl Matthews • Gillian Prudhoe • Jim Richardson

The fundamental concepts that underpin this book are ones that must be taken into account when undertaking any procedure whatsoever. Children, young people and their families demand and expect that all procedures are based on best evidence and informed by local and national policies.

Kindness, dignity and each child's, young person's and family's personal uniqueness

Whenever any procedure is planned and carried out during an episode of nursing practice, the approach of the nurse is crucial in ensuring that the child or young person feels that the experience has been a positive and constructive one. These concepts are fundamental to good practice and are underpinned by the Nursing and Midwifery Council's code of professional conduct (Nursing and Midwifery Council 2002).

Some of the cardinal principles that should be observed in all helping and caring interactions are as follows:

- Kindness. Children and their families are sensitive to the manner and approach of the nurse. A gentle and kindly demeanour is reassuring and helps underpin trust.
- Dignity. This is the right of every child and young person and their families. Dignity involves treating others in a respectful way, honouring personal choice as far as possible and recognising modesty needs. Despite this Rylance (1999), in a study conducted in a large children's hospital, found that dignity and other values such as privacy and confidentiality were inadequately valued by staff.
- Personal uniqueness. Recognising every child and young person as a unique individual with his or her own distinctive personality, needs, context and history makes interaction between the nurse and child satisfying and safe. A part of each person's personal uniqueness includes their beliefs, values and customs that form their cultural orientation.

It is important to stress that the families who use healthcare services should be awarded the same rights as adult patients.

Risk and safety

As many as one in ten patients in hospital may suffer an adverse event during their treatment (Reason 1990). The estimated scale of the problem is worrying, and from all acute sector incidents reported to the National Patient Safety Agency (NPSA) to March 2005 it can be estimated that in acute hospitals in England each year approximately 572 000 incidents will be reported, of which around 840 result in a patient death. Children's nurses need to appreciate that young children are particularly defenceless in the face of error, being almost totally dependent on their caregiver to safeguard them.

Seven steps to patient safety

The NPSA (2004) list seven steps to patient safety:

1. Building a safety culture
2. Leadership
3. Risk management activity
4. Reporting
5. Working with patients and the public
6. Learning the right lessons
7. Implementing solutions.

Compliance with the *Standards for Better Health* (Safety Domain, C1a; Department of Health 2005) is crucial for children's and young people's nurses. The core standard of this policy guideline is unambiguous in stating that healthcare organisations must protect patients from and learn from adverse incidents. In perusing the mantra of Florence Nightingale, who is credited with saying that the nurse must first do the patient no harm, we are reminded of the ethical principle of non-maleficence (Beauchamp & Childress 1979), in which all nurses, but perhaps in particular children's nurses, are mandated to follow procedures and protocols that are designed to reduce the risk of error. Such procedures are invaluable when using clinical skills on sick children.

A child safety incident may be defined as any unintended or unexpected incident(s) that could or did lead to harm for one or more children receiving National Health Service-funded healthcare. In this context an adverse incident can be defined as any healthcare occurrence that has led to an unintended or unexplained harm to a child. Similarly a near miss is defined as an occurrence that may have led to a child being harmed but either the mistake was aborted before harm occurred or no harm actually resulted by chance alone. Children's nurses do not want to place themselves in a position in which they make an actual or a near miss incident. This is why this book has been written to give you guidelines to follow in which the provenance of the material has been carefully scrutinised. The areas in which safety may be compromised include:

- medication delivery
- mismatching children and their treatment
- equipment error
- working beyond limits of competence
- failure or delay in making an accurate diagnosis
- suboptimal handover
- suboptimal continuity of care
- failure to ensure follow-up of investigations
- lack of awareness of local procedures and policies.

Because children's nurses are constantly undertaking procedures it might appear that they are constantly running the gauntlet of risk, and it is for this reason that all incidents should be reported. There is no doubt that doctors and nurses are at the sharp end of safety and are often blamed when it goes badly wrong. In a healthcare world dominated by the need for interprofessional working, without active participation by the whole clinical team the drive to bring about real improvement in child patient safety will be distorted. As qualified children's nurses, by reporting patient safety incidents, and their causes, you can help the National Health Service learn and put the right safeguards in place. This will make your clinical area a safer place for children and their families and for you and for your colleagues. Despite this, we need to recognise that:

We all make errors – irrespective of how much training and experience we possess, or how motivated we are to do it right. (Health and Safety Executive 1999)

The national reporting and learning system

The data that the NSPA receive are analysed and interpreted alongside other sources of data and intelligence. All this helps the NPSA to identify priorities for action and to support work on developing solutions to tackle the problems identified. Children's nurses are predominantly in the front line of practice and as such will benefit from NPSA feedback to local organisations. This will help the organisations and enable them to improve systems and procedures locally, helping protect you and other clinical staff from making mistakes with potentially fatal consequences. One example of the work of the NPSA was related to the use of nasogastric tubes, and in this investigation following the death of a child in Yorkshire they:

- searched the published literature
- obtained data from the National Reporting and Learning System
- gained information and advice from experts
- conducted an informal survey of current practice
- undertook an aggregated root cause analysis.

This led to the issuing of a patient safety alert that was widely distributed among children's units, and they commissioned further research.

So what are you doing in your children's unit to reduce risk and protect yourself, the children and their families? Remember, this should be a safety culture not a blame culture:

- Governance forum at which risk issues are discussed monthly
- Local lead for risk management activities
- Identification of specialty triggers
- Regular review of your adverse event reporting
- Full investigation (root cause analysis) of all red NPSA-graded incidents
- Evidence of lessons learnt and practice change (e.g. nasogastric tube checking and cannula dressings)
- Link to audit programme

Children's nurses need to work in a just culture, not a total absence of blame but an atmosphere of trust in which people are encouraged to provide safety-related information. Irrespective of this all children's nurses need to be clear about where the line is drawn between acceptable and unacceptable behaviours.

Children's nurse have a role to play in helping to make care effective and efficient, and they need to play a role in matching care to best evidence (e.g. why do 30% of children receive excessive antibiotics for ear infections?).

Safeguarding children

The five outcomes of *Every Child Matters* (Department for Education and Skills 2003), which are believed to be essential for every single child and young person in this country and are central to well-being in childhood and later life are:

1. being healthy
2. staying safe
3. enjoying and achieving
4. being able to make a positive contribution
5. being able to achieve economic well-being.

Children's nurses are a key component of the workforce who are empowered to deliver these policy aspirations. Supporting children and families has many possible components, but when children are ill certain parameters of their care become of paramount importance. In particular, with regard to safeguarding (child protection) it must be stressed that when clinical procedures are being undertaken nurses must understand what the risk factors are before proceeding. In recognising that some children may need additional support, nurses will need to assess the child's needs and the ability of the parent or carer to assist before implementing the procedure. In all cases, before and during the procedure nurses must be familiar with the organisational safeguarding policies and the procedures necessary for protecting children in the areas in which they work. All children's nurses should be able to recognise how to identify children at risk, and it is crucial to fully document any concerns you have (Powell & Ireland 2006). If during a procedure a child makes a disclosure do not promise confidentiality. If for example you are working in an assessment unit or emergency department, concerns might arise because there are noticeable discrepancies in the story of how the illness or injury occurred. Additionally, fabricated and induced illness, in which carers claim that their child has an illness when in reality they have actually made up the symptoms, is a rare but nevertheless important consideration of children's nurses (Royal College of Psychiatrists 2007). This is reflected in situations in which carers might, for example, falsely report symptoms, falsify specimens or chart data or perpetrate actual harm to the child. Although the term *Münchausen's by proxy* is no longer used, in any case in which professional children's nurses have concerns about safeguarding issues in a child in their care this should be documented and reported to the relevant agency to ascertain if there have been previous concerns raised.

During a routine procedure in which a children's nurse is using a clinical skill a number of observations might be made, one or all of which might raise concerns and yet may be totally unrelated to the purpose or cause of the admission. The National Society for the Prevention of Cruelty to Children (2007) have indicated that a number of signs may be present in a physically abused child, and these might include one or more of the following. Bruises, black eyes and broken bones are obvious signs of physical abuse, but it is the more subtle signs that nurses should observe for during procedures, particularly when a child may be disrobed. These other signs might include injuries that the child or carer cannot explain or explains unconvincingly or the presence of untreated or inadequately treated injuries and, importantly, injuries to parts of the body where accidents are unlikely, such as thighs, back and abdomen. Additionally, the observant nurse might see signs of bruising that look like hand or finger marks, traces of cigarette burns, human bites or evidence of scalds and burns. If nurses conducting a clinical procedure have concerns about a child's welfare they should discuss them with a manager and/or other senior colleagues as appropriate. If concerns remain it is customary to make a referral to social services with written follow-up within 48 h, *but* remember when information sharing that:

> *There is a balance to strike between sharing enough information to help safeguard children effectively and preserving individuals' privacy.*
> *(Department for Education and Skills 2004)*

Emotional abuse, when a parent or carer behaves in a way that is likely to seriously affect the child's emotional development, is less easy to detect during the brief period of a procedure being undertaken but children's nurses should investigate further, perhaps through a more senior colleague, if, for example, they suspect or notice, especially in a young person, signs of deliberate self-harm. Cooper (2006) indicated that the peak age for the development of self-harm presentation is 15–24 for females, and he has stated that children's nurses should use cognitive strategies in their therapeutic relationships with children and young people who exhibit signs of emotional trauma. In this context nurses should present themselves as persons who can be trusted and who have excellent skills in communication that will be perceived by the child or young person as being supportive and client-focused.

Gaining consent to healthcare from children, young people and their families

Whenever a children's nurse undertakes a clinical procedure it is important that an accurate record of the treatment or care is kept to fulfil and demonstrate that there has been completion of the duty of care to that child. The law relating to consent is of utmost importance, serving as a means of protecting and preserving the rights of patients or clients to decide what is to happen to them, thereby upholding the principle of self-determination. However, in children and young people less than 16 years of age the issues of consent are complicated, and children's nurses must have a good working knowledge of current law and practice. Importantly, in the Gillick case (1985) Lord Fraser, in an epoch-making decision, established that minors under the age of 16 may have the capacity to consent to treatment *if* they can demonstrate sufficient understanding and intelligence to appreciate what is being proposed and its implications. This is referred to as being Gillick-competent (sometimes inaccurately described as being Fraser-competent).

The criteria for testing competence

The children's nurse should establish that the young person should be able to understand in simple terms the nature, purpose and necessity for the proposed treatment; believe the information applies to her or him; and retain the information long enough to make a choice. Importantly, and especially before any procedure, the nurse must ensure that the child is enabled to make a choice free from pressure (Larcher 2005). The function of consent is therefore to ensure that a voluntary, uncoerced decision is made by a sufficiently autonomous person, on the basis of adequate information, to accept or reject some proposed course of action that would affect him or her and therefore by definition is informed (Gillon 2003). Although a child or young person may have the capacity to give consent, for it to be valid it must still be given voluntarily without undue pressure or coercion from parents, carers or a potential sexual partner (Department of Health 2001).

Consent is a process rather than a one-off event, and it is required on every occasion when a children's nurse wishes to initiate a procedure, an examination or a treatment or any other intervention, except in emergencies.

Types of consent

Consent may be expressed verbally or non-verbally, and this is known as implied consent, i.e. when actions speak louder than words (e.g. when patients hold out an arm to have their blood pressure taken).

Written consent merely serves as evidence of consent. If elements of voluntariness, appropriate information and capacity have not been satisfied, a signature on a form will not make the consent valid (Department of Health 2001).

Regarding refusal of treatment, unlike for competent adults an adolescent's right to refuse treatment depends on the circumstances. When a child or young person under 16 is Gillick-competent and refuses treatment, in extreme circumstances such a refusal can be overruled. For refusal of treatment to be genuine and valid it needs to be based on an awareness of the implications, be consistent over time and be compatible with the child's view of her or his best interests (Dimond 2004).

Note that the child's or young person's decision to refuse treatment can be overruled by a person with parental responsibility.

In life-threatening situations, the courts have also stated that when there is doubt it is acceptable to undertake treatment to preserve life or prevent serious damage to health (Department of Health 2001).

When the child or young person lacks capacity to consent, this can be given by any one person with parental responsibility or by the court. Those who may have parental responsibility include the child's parents if they were married to each other at the time of conception or birth or the child's mother, but not the father if they were not married, unless the father has acquired parental responsibility via a court or parental responsibility agreement. For children born since December 2003, the unmarried father acquires parental responsibility if he jointly registers the child's birth with the mother and his name appears on the birth certificate. Additionally, adoptive parents or the child's legally appointed guardian can give consent, as can a local authority designated in a care order for the child or an emergency protection order.

It is also important for children's nurses to be aware that consent given by one person with parental responsibility is valid even if another person with parental responsibility withholds consent. In cases in which there is disagreement regarding non-therapeutic procedures that are in the child's best interests, it is advisable to refer the decision to the courts.

Children's rights in modern healthcare

Any children's nurse attempting to undertake a procedure on a child must appreciate that children's rights are increasingly recognised in the healthcare setting and in wider society. The legal context strengthens this in requiring that the primacy of children's best interest is upheld. The United Nations *Convention on the Rights of the Child* (United Nations 1989), which was ratified by the UK in 1991, has profoundly affected our views of children's rights and is a document every children's nurse should be familiar with. In the context of undertaking clinical procedures children should not simply be passive consumers but have the right that their voice should be heard and heeded.

Accountability

In order to be accountable in their work, children's nurses when undertaking procedures should be able to demonstrate that their decisions and actions are based first on a thorough and careful assessment of need. This will include taking the child's and family's preferences into account as far as is possible, for example allowing the child to have a favourite toy with them during the procedure or allowing them to wear their own pyjamas to theatre. Ideally this leads to joint planning in a spirit of partnership based on the best available evidence so that the nurse is able to provide a firm rationale as to the best choice for the child and family. This process should therefore be available for the critical scrutiny of other interested parties (e.g. other members of the healthcare team). When performing or contemplating performing a clinical procedure, nurses must ensure that this is within their range of competence. If the nurse does not have the necessary experience or expertise a referral to another appropriate professional must be made. In this way nurses can demonstrate their responsibility for professional decision making and care delivery. This is an important aspect of undertaking skilled procedures.

Advocacy

The idea of advocacy is based on the fact that everyone may, on occasion, need the help of someone who can speak on his or her behalf to ensure that his or her best interests are served. In the case of children, parents often advocate for their children (Wheeler 2000). Nurses may also fulfil this function if their professional knowledge and skills give them insights that allow them to discern what is in the child's and family's interests. This is especially pertinent during procedures. Children's nurses' knowledge of the processes and structures of what is often perceived by families to be a complex healthcare system allows them to give information on what would best serve a child and family. Nurses, more than any other healthcare professional, often have prolonged contact with a child and family and this gives them a sense of child and family need beyond the purely physical. Their unique knowledge of the child and family gives them insight into when the family's physical, psychological and spiritual resources are strained and their ability to speak for themselves is limited and weakened. Willard (1996) believes that their intention is benign and intended to be helpful and supportive, and that their contribution is based on their knowledge of the child's and family's needs and wishes.

Caution must be exercised, however, to ensure that the nurse is not stating views that they *think* represent the child's and family's views. Children's nurses are not omnipotent, and advocacy must be built on effective communication with the child and family if paternalistic and potentially damaging actions are to be avoided. If the children's nurse is to truly act as a family advocate the concepts of partnership articulated by Casey (2007) must be integral to the performance of any clinical procedure.

Now test your knowledge

- What are the seven steps that must be taken to ensure patient safety?
- What is the role of the NPSA?
- What is iatrogenic illness?
- What is a root cause analysis?
- Can you calculate a drug safely?
- What are the five key outcomes for children in *Every Child Matters*?
- What safeguarding policy do you have in your workplace?
- What would you do if a child made a disclosure to you?
- What is fabricated and induced illness?
- What factors would you take into consideration when seeking consent from a child?
- How would you treat a child who refuses to participate in a clinical procedure?
- What does being Gillick-competent actually mean?
- Under what circumstances can a child's refusal to participate be overruled?

References

Beauchamp T, Childress J (1979) Principles of biomedical ethics. Oxford University Press, Oxford

Casey A (2007) Partnership model of nursing. In Glasper EA, McEwing G, Richardson J (eds) Oxford handbook of children's and young people's nursing. Oxford University Press, Oxford

Cooper M (2006) Child and adolescent mental health: the nursing response. In Glasper A, Richardson J (eds) A textbook of children's and young people's nursing. Churchill Livingstone, Edinburgh, p 700–719

Department for Education and Skills (2003) Every child matters. HMSO, London

Department for Education and Skills (2004) Every child matters: next steps. HMSO, London

Department of Health (2001) Seeking consent working with children. HMSO, London

Department of Health (2005) Standards for better health. HMSO, London

Dimond B (2004) Consent to treatment in bowel interventions: some legal issues. Nursing Times 100(48):66–69

Gillon R(1986) Philosophical Medical Ethics,Wiley London

Gillon R (2003) Ethics needs principles–four can encompass the rest–and respect for autonomy should be 'first among equals'. Journal of Medical Ethics 29:307–312

Health and Safety Executive (1999) Reducing error and influencing behaviour, HSG48. HSE Books, Sudbury

Larcher V (2005) Consent, competence and confidentiality. British Medical Journal 330:353–356

National Patient Safety Agency (2004) Seven steps to patient safety. An overview guide for NHS staff. NHS, London

National Society for the Prevention of Cruelty to Children (2007) Online. Available: http://www.nspcc.org.uk/helpandadvice/whatchildabuse/physicalabuse/physicalabuse_wda33606.html

Nursing and Midwifery Council (2002) Code of professional conduct. NMC, London

Powell C, Ireland L (2006) Protecting children. The role of the children's nurse. In Glasper A, Richardson J (eds) A textbook of children's and young people's nursing. Churchill Livingstone, Edinburgh, p 297–308

Reason J (1990) Human error. Cambridge University Press, Cambridge

Royal College of Psychiatrists (2007) Online. Available: http//www.rcpsych.ac.uk/publications/recent/recent_publications/FII.pdf

Rylance G (1999) Privacy, dignity, and confidentiality: interview study with structured questionnaire. British Medical Journal 318:301

United Nations (1989) The convention on the rights of the child. Online. Available: http://www.unicef.org/crc/crc.htm

Wheeler P (2000) Is advocacy at the heart of professional practice? Nursing Standard 14(36):39–41

Willard C (1996) The nurse's role as patient advocate: obligation or imposition? Journal of Advanced Nursing 24(1):60–66

Further reading

Cawson P, Wattam C, Brooker S, Kelly G (2000) Child maltreatment in the United Kingdom. NSPCC, London

Corby B (2000) Child abuse: towards a knowledge base. Open University Press, Milton Keynes

Department of Health, Department for Education and Skills (2003) Keeping children safe: the Government's response to the Victoria Climbie Inquiry report and Joint Chief Inspectors' report *Safeguarding Children*. HMSO, London

Department of Health, Home Office, Department for Education and Employment (1999) Working together to safeguard children. HMSO, London

Department of Health, Home Office, Department for Education and Employment (2000) Framework for the assessment of children in need and their families. HMSO, London

Department of Health; Home Office; Department for Education and Skills; Department for Culture, Media and Sport; Office of the Deputy Prime Minister; Lord Chancellor (2003) What to do if you're worried a child is being abused. Department of Health, London

2 Communication

Irene J. McTaggart

Communication is a process of sending, receiving and interpreting information for a range of purposes using a variety of verbal and non-verbal methods (Bosek 2002, McCabe 2004). By its nature communication involves at least two people and is reciprocal, with the sender and receiver exchanging roles throughout the communication process. Understanding must be established, with recognition that an individual's perception is affected by the language used and her or his past experiences and personal characteristics (Bosek 2002).

The art of communication is extremely important in the provision of quality nursing care (van Dulmen 1998). When effective communication occurs, it facilitates the development of therapeutic relationships with both the child and the parents and increases the child's and parents' ability to understand and manage situations in which they find themselves (Thorne et al 2004). The development of strong interpersonal relationships with children and their families thus enhances the development and provision of family-centred care (Attree 2001, McCabe 2004). While (2005) cites poor communication skills as the most frequent cause of complaint in the health service, which mirrors the assertions of Dickson et al (1997). This reinforces the importance of ensuring that communication is approached in a systematic, sensitive manner in an attempt to maximise the potential for developing mutual understanding between all parties concerned. Communication occurs formally and informally, involving listening as well as speaking. It is complex and may be influenced by many factors including the language used, the environment in which the encounter occurs and the time available. Past experiences of and relationships between those involved, cultural influences, the child's developmental stage, the situation and the child's condition will also affect the communication exchange.

Communicating with children and families

Children's nurses have a responsibility to ensure that children in their care and their parents have an understanding of what is happening to the child in relation to health and illness. It is crucial that children have the opportunity to participate in any decision making regarding their condition, treatment and future management, feeling part of the healthcare team as appropriate to their developmental stage (Fleitas 2003). This is supported by Mansson & Dykes (2004), who state that informing children helps them cope with what is happening to them by developing their ability to distinguish between reality and their imagination. The United Nations *Convention on the Rights of the Child* (United Nations 1989) also supports the right of the child to receive information and be involved in decision making, although this must be tempered by the child's level of maturity and ability to make the decision. It may then be a cause of concern when van Dulmen (2004) suggests that child patients are often ignored by doctors, while Hallstrom & Elander (2004) state that health professionals have a duty to augment their patients' ability to participate in their care. They go on to assert that, in making a contribution, children develop a sense of individuality and empowerment. van Dulmen (1998) acknowledges that while it is important to give children information, this type of communication is still mainly targeted towards parents.

It is essential to recognise, however, that parents need to be given the opportunity to participate in effective communication related to their child's condition and management of care together with their role as a parent (Kirk et al 2005). When parents and professionals communicate well they form good interpersonal relationships that encourage collaboration between them. This, however, is influenced by the professionals' ability to concede their power in the relationship and acknowledge the contribution parents can make to the care of their child (Espezel & Canam 2003). Informed parents are also better prepared regarding the situations they encounter in the delivery of healthcare to their child when they are in an unfamiliar environment. This enables them to support and reassure their child more effectively (Tiberius et al 2001) and engage in more effective communication with staff members (Tourigny et al 2005). It is crucial that healthcare professionals recognise that children and parents who are poorly informed are more anxious, and this can be to the detriment of the child's recovery (Mansson & Dykes 2004). It is necessary then to ensure that parents understand the situation as fully as possible while ensuring that their child is also included in discussions regarding the delivery of their care as appropriate to their stage of development. Fleitas (2003) is mindful that the stresses of parenting an ill child can reduce the parents' ability to communicate effectively not only with healthcare workers but also with their child, while decision making may also be problematic to them (Beauchamp & Childress 2001).

If it is accepted that children should be involved in decision making, it is equally important to recognise that they must always be given information regarding any procedures about to be performed in an attempt to reduce their anxiety while increasing the development of trust and cooperation. It is not always the case that children are included in relevant discussion, which then compromises their ability to be active participants in the healthcare experience (Alderson & Montgomery 1996). Parents can appoint themselves as gatekeepers responsible for filtering the information given to their child; this can then be reinforced by healthcare workers who give parents information prior to or instead of giving it to the child. It can also be problematic if the child and parents have different points of view regarding the disclosure of information to each other. Attempts to protect children from the reality of their situation may add to their difficulties, as they preclude children from the opportunity to discuss their concerns, thoughts and fears with protecting and comforting adults. In this way adults achieve the opposite of their goal of making the child's situation easier to cope with (McTaggart 2000). Charlton (1996) suggests that early, sensitive and truthful discussion of the child's diagnosis and prognosis will result in improved psychological adjustment of the child. Young et al (2003) found that younger children wanted more detailed explanations than older children, who wanted basic facts; this may be due to the older child's ability to interpret the information or anticipate any possible consequences of the situation. Parents can impede any interaction between the child and healthcare professional by offering themselves as the prime contributor to the interaction (Tates & Meeuwesen 2000). Children can therefore feel excluded from consultations, and some have indicated that they would prefer an opportunity to see their doctor or nurse on a one-to-one basis when, for example, attending outpatient clinics (McTaggart 2000). Allowing this is, however, no guarantee of meaningful dialogue, as van Dulmen (1998) suggests that children's participation is almost entirely restricted to social conversation and humour while they are considered by medical staff to be able to give but not receive medical information. However, it is necessary to recognise the role parents may take as an advocate for their child and the requirement to ensure they are fully equipped to fulfil this function by assisting them in the difficult task of communicating openly with their child. It is therefore clear that the opportunity to plan any communication exchange is desirable although not always possible. However, the experience of developing good communication skills and therapeutic relationships empowers everyone to cope more efficiently in the absence of such preparation.

Evidence-based communication in practice

It is important to recognise that fear of the unknown significantly increases any anxieties experienced by both children and parents (Mansson & Dykes 2004), therefore communicating efficiently and effectively with children and their parents serves to decrease this unpleasant aspect of healthcare. It is beneficial to approach it, when possible, in an organised way in order to maximise the benefits of any communication exchange.

Planning

There can be many reasons for communicating with children and their parents, ranging from informal social chat to the delivery of bad or difficult news. It may be necessary to obtain information, give information, conduct a patient or parent education programme, discuss alternatives of medical management of the child's condition, obtain consent for surgery or prepare the child and family for discharge. This is not an exhaustive list, therefore it can be clearly identified that such activities are demanding and unique to that particular situation. It is important to note, however, that the experiences of today impact on those of the future and when well-managed contribute to the development of successful relationships between children, parents and healthcare professionals (Fig. 2.1).

Purpose

The purpose of the interaction has to be considered when deciding who should proceed with it. For example, if it is to admit a child to the ward it requires a nurse with the ability to assess the needs of the child and parents in a holistic manner. This should initiate the development of an appropriate plan of care and a therapeutic relationship. Alternatively, if it is to assist a medical diagnosis or obtain consent for surgery a doctor would be the most obvious choice. The breaking of difficult or bad news is an example in which the decision may be more complex and can result in more than one healthcare professional being involved. It could be argued that the team member who has a good relationship with the child and parents, whatever her or his professional role, is a suitable choice together with the individual who has the ability to answer any likely questions in the most appropriate manner. The timing of any communication will be related to its purpose; however, it is certain that children, parents and staff will continue to

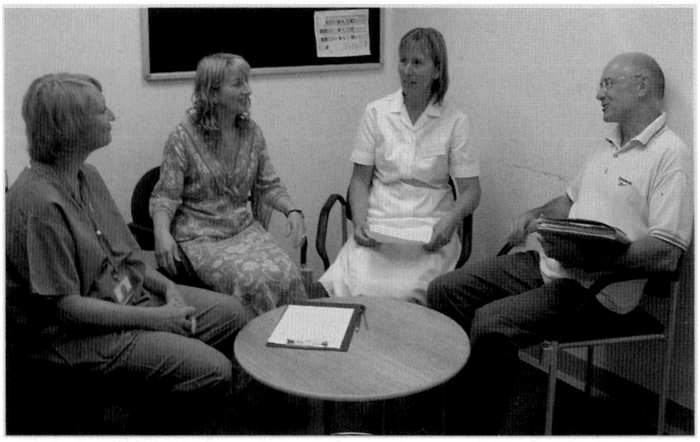

Fig. 2.1 • Good communication helps develop successful relationships between children, parents and healthcare professionals.

communicate throughout the child's healthcare experience. It cannot be assumed that all communication exchanges will be conducted in the same manner, as all situations even with the same family will not be similar.

Prepare yourself

Gather any information you require; this may be from a variety of sources such as nursing and medical notes, other healthcare workers, the child and/or the parents. An attempt should be made to anticipate potential questions that may be asked, and preparation should enable a satisfactory response to be made (Fig. 2.2). If, for example, a child's surgery is cancelled the person informing the child and/or parents should have knowledge of the reasons for the cancellation, the effect any delay may have on the child's condition, and future arrangements to reschedule the surgery. It is important to ascertain the parents' wishes regarding the child's participation in any discussion and the child's desires related to conversations that have taken place and any questions asked in both formal (Fig. 2.3) and informal (Fig. 2.4) settings.

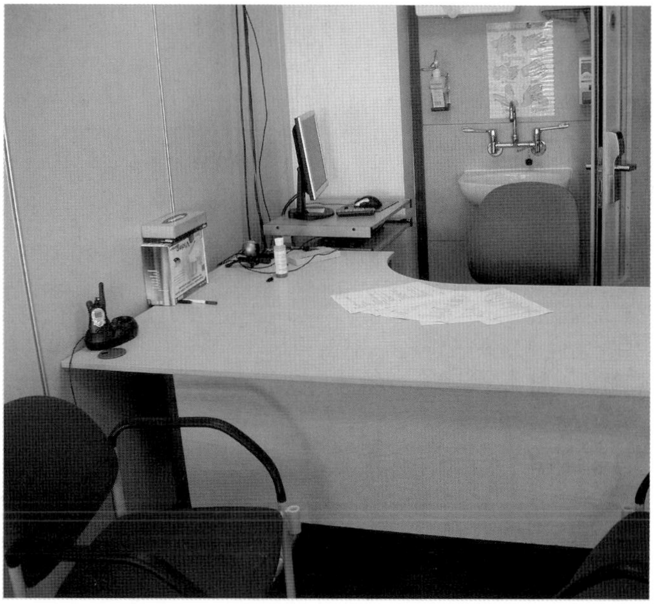

Fig. 2.3 • A formal consultation area.

Environment

A suitable area such as a family room or play area should be selected, with consideration given to the purpose of the interaction. Setting the scene within this environment allows you to ensure maximum comfort for the child and parents while encouraging an atmosphere that may give the child and/or parents confidence to participate in the dialogue, thereby promoting a collaborative relationship (Espezel & Canam 2003). An acceptable level of privacy should be ensured if, for example, you are preparing a child for a procedure; it may be best to take the child to a quiet corner of the play area with some toys and equipment (Fig. 2.5).

Alternatively it may be that discussing options regarding future management of the child's condition requires a quiet room where there is a guarantee of no interruptions. Care should be taken to arrange the furniture in a way that encourages communication rather than obstructing it. Avoid, when possible, sitting behind a large desk with parents and a small child on the other side of it, as this may encourage a paternalistic atmosphere of professional power rather than collaboration. Sufficient seating, including one for the child if present, should be positioned to allow all participants to look towards each other without breaching their personal space or creating a vacuum between any of the parties concerned. Ensure that chairs are not positioned in front of a window with light streaming in, as this results in a person's face being shadowed and his or her facial expressions being difficult to determine while a person sitting opposite has the sun in his or her eyes, again diminishing comfort. Be aware of any constraints within the environment, such as the proximity of others who

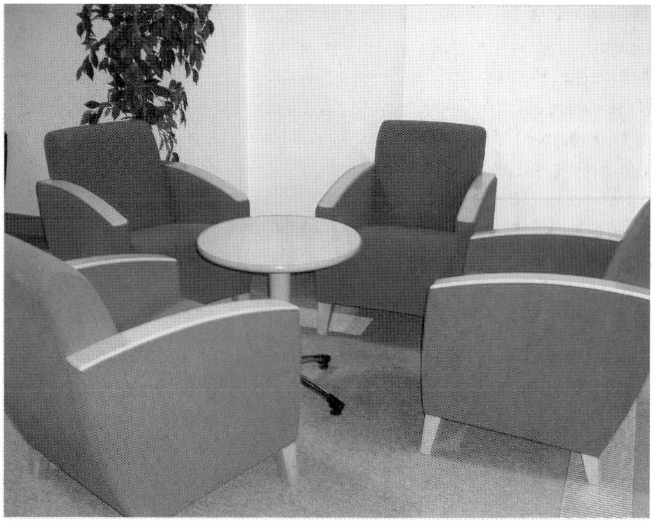

Fig. 2.4 • An informal area for communication.

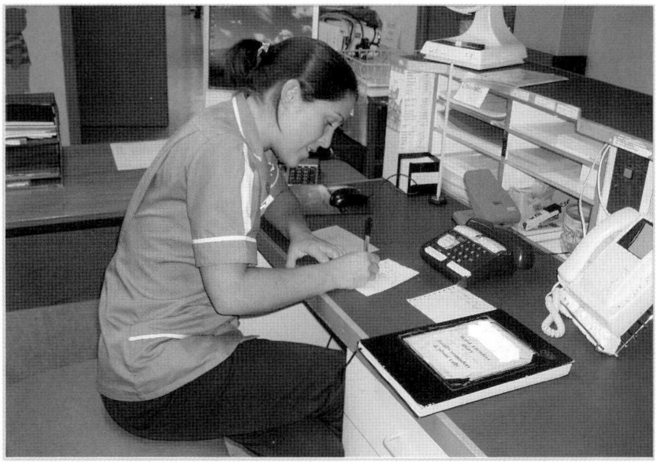

Fig. 2.2 • Preparation is important for successful communication.

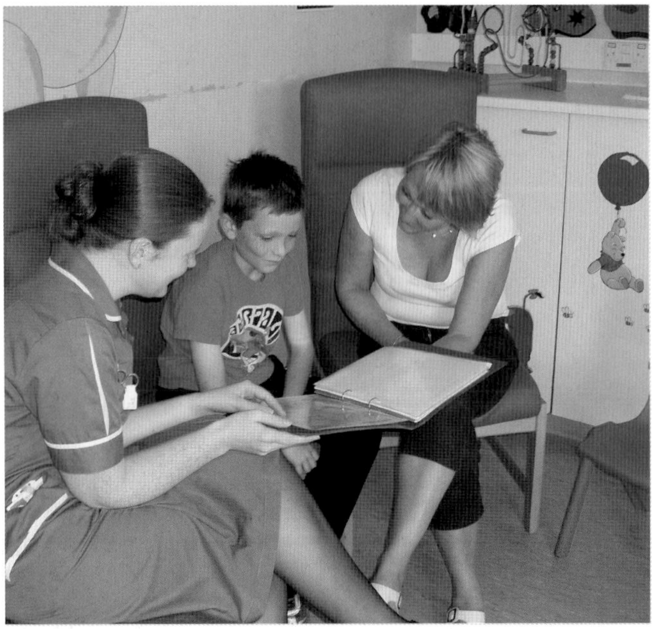

Fig. 2.5 • Preparing a child for a procedure.

may overhear or a glass wall that may cause parents or children to inhibit their non-verbal reactions due to concerns that they may upset a person on other side. This can result in them failing to concentrate on what is being said, thereby reducing the efficacy of the communication. Sufficient time should be allowed to avoid any of the parties involved feeling rushed or reluctant to raise issues of concern.

Conducting the encounter

The healthcare professional should approach the child and parents in an open, friendly and professional manner, speaking to the child first (Fig. 2.6). If they are in a single room the door should be knocked before entering to signal that you are about to enter. Introductions should be made when necessary, and an explanation should be given regarding the purpose of the proposed communication exchange. Invite the appropriate people to the designated area, recognising that it should not be assumed that anyone or everyone at the bedside is to be included in the discussion (Figueroa-Altmann et al 2005). The participants should be asked if they have anything they wish to discuss, together with how much they want or need to know, and this should be taken into account throughout the dialogue. Skilled use of questioning allows comprehensive exploration of the issues concerned. The purpose of the question will determine if it should be open or closed, for example a closed question such as 'Are you feeling better today?' will elicit a yes or no response. 'Would you describe how you are feeling today?' will allow children or parents to express themselves, and with that information you can develop further understanding of their situation. Identifying when to refrain from asking a question is just as important as knowing when to ask it (Christensen & James 2000). If a child or parent seems upset or reluctant to answer it is better to leave it if possible, returning to the subject when she or he is ready, unless it is crucial to obtain information at the time. The use of models such as the Patient/Parent Information and Involvement Assessment Tool can be useful to determine the communication choices of children and their parents (Sobo 2003). Sobo reported that nurses frequently underestimated the communication choices of children and their parents, with only one-third matching the patient–parent self-assessments (p. 261).

Maximising understanding

The use of language suitable to the developmental stage of the child or the requirements of the parents will increase the likelihood of a successful conclusion to the conversation (Fig. 2.7). Medical jargon should be avoided when possible, and if professional terminology is required its meaning should be clarified

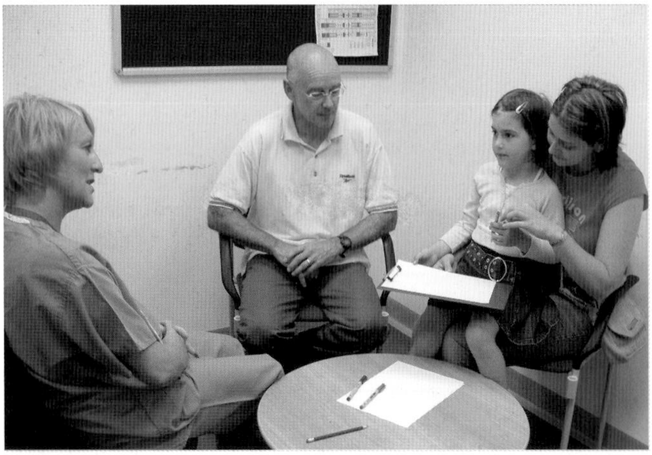

Fig. 2.6 • Speak to the child first.

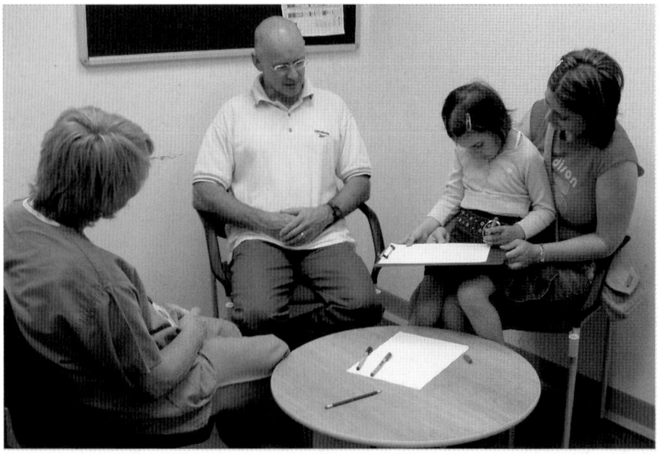

Fig. 2.7 • Use language suitable to the child's developmental stage or the parents' requirements.

by the professional involved (Fleitas 2003). Clear and concise explanations should be given using examples that the recipients of the information can relate to. Be careful not to assume meaning of commonly used language, as this may lead to misunderstandings (Shattell & Hogan 2005).

The use of leaflets, diagrams, toys, medical equipment, X-rays and so on (Fig. 2.8) may increase understanding, as it is easier to remember things that are seen, heard and practised (Bradbury 2000). It may also be helpful to have pen and paper available for others who may wish to take some notes.

Active listening, that is, listening for insight while putting one's own thoughts and feelings aside (Hurd 2005), is essential to ensure that the child's and parents' concerns are established and the overall goal is achieved. Pauses can also be used effectively to fulfil a variety of purposes, such as allowing any of the parties concerned to consider what has been said, formulate a response, identify alternatives to proposed actions or cope with their emotions. It is important, therefore, not to feel compelled to fill the silences but to have the confidence to allow them to bring about their potential benefits. The use of touch can be a powerful tool to provide, for example, comfort, reassurance and acceptance, but it can also be intrusive, so it is essential to relate to the cues of the other person (Fig. 2.9).

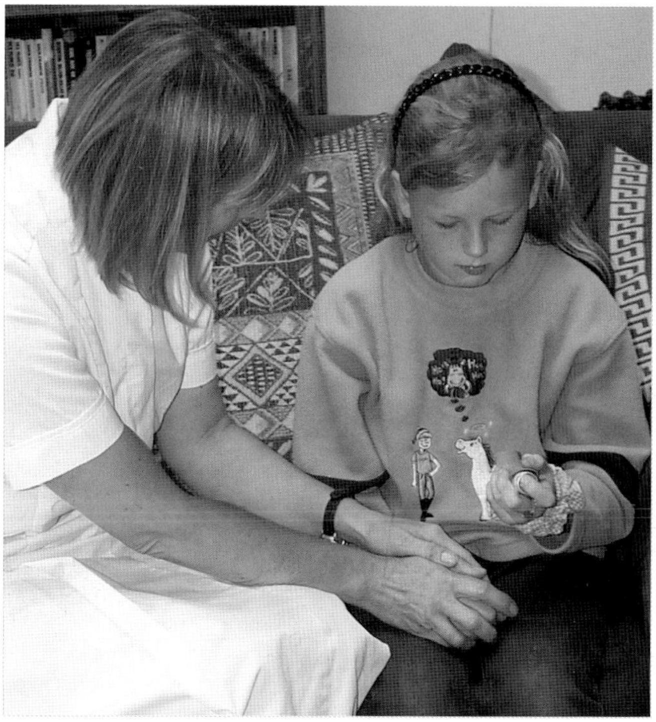

Fig. 2.9 • Communication through touch.

Non-verbal communication

Non-verbal cues include facial expression, eye contact, posture and distracting habits such as playing with a pen or fiddling with your hair (Fig. 2.10). Sitting with an open body posture, leaning towards the other person and using eye contact will elicit more of a response than folded arms and legs, which can be interpreted as an expression of disinterest or defensiveness. Remember that while the healthcare professional is observing the non-verbal responses of the child and parents, they are reciprocating. Respond to both verbal and non-verbal cues,

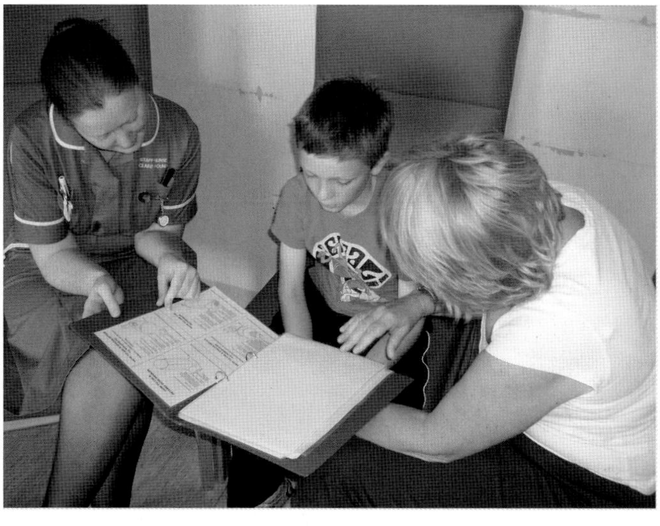

Fig. 2.8 • Diagrams can facilitate understanding.

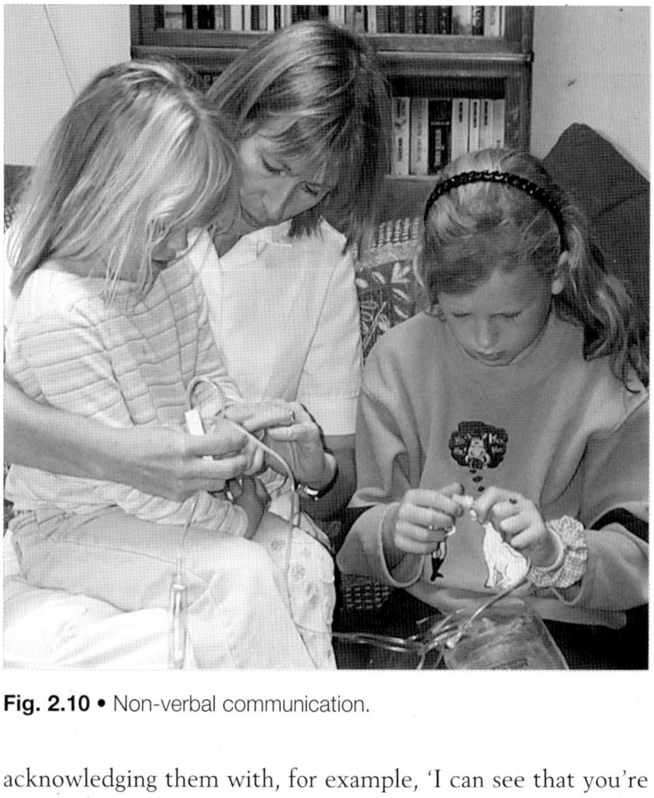

Fig. 2.10 • Non-verbal communication.

acknowledging them with, for example, 'I can see that you're upset; do you want to talk about that?' Perception is influenced not only by what you say but by how it is interpreted by the recipient (Bosek 2002), with effective communication occurring when those in conversation with each other are aware of the impact of their contributions on the other and respond appropriately. Be aware of cultural influences regarding both verbal and non-verbal communication, while avoiding the use of stereotypical behaviours.

Child and parent participation

Children and parents must be given the opportunity to make their concerns known and to ask questions, which should be answered honestly. Remember that it is easy to assume that children are routinely included in any discussion merely because they are in the room (Fig. 2.11; Pengelly 2003). Offer to speak to children separately if they wish to do so (e.g. some children attending a diabetic outpatient clinic may wish to speak to the diabetic specialist nurse on an individual basis).

Healthcare professionals can assist parents empower their child by acquiescing to such requests. Other children may gain confidence from the presence of their parents (Fig. 2.12); they may ask parents to speak on their behalf to either give or gain information, to remember information more accurately or to clarify or reiterate information later (Young et al 2003). Parents can monopolise discussions, thus inhibiting the child's contribution, which may be further compounded by lack of time, for example in an outpatient clinic when extra time is not allocated to allow child participation (van Dulmen 1998). The context of a situation can also affect understanding, as recipients of information may choose to concentrate on positive aspects of the situation, resisting attempts to address serious issues indicating potentially unwelcome but likely future developments.

Summarise

Paraphrasing the discussion is a useful technique to confirm that all parties have the same understanding of the dialogue that has occurred and any further action that has to be taken. During this process all parties should have the opportunity to explain in their words what has been said or agreed, as this may vary from individual to individual; this is more reliable than simply asking if an understanding has been reached.

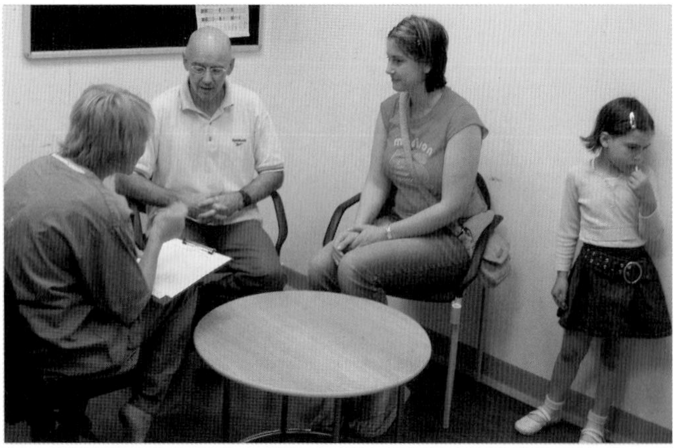

Fig. 2.11 • Do not assume that a child is included in any discussion merely because she or he is in the room.

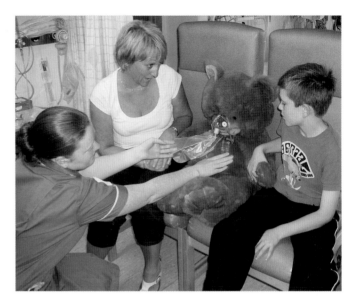

Fig. 2.12 • Children may gain confidence from the presence of their parents.

Make a plan for further discussion as appropriate to the situation, for example for what is to be discussed at the next outpatient appointment or on receipt of medical investigation results. If the child is an in-patient it is preferable to suggest 'later today' than a definite time such as 3 p.m., as unforeseen circumstances can arise to prevent this agreement being kept, resulting in the child or parents feeling let down. Assurances should be given to the child and parents that they do not have to wait until the agreed time if they are anxious or worried.

Recognise that in an emergency situation decision making is often rushed, without the benefit of time. When the situation is stable it should be revisited to allow reflection on any potential consequences to ensure that a suitable level of understanding is achieved and any unresolved issues are dealt with. Children should be given an opportunity to discuss their understanding of events to enable clarification of any misconceptions they may have of their circumstances.

Written guidelines, such as a laminated instruction sheet given to parents being taught how to administer wet wraps, may be helpful. This increases their confidence that they are proceeding correctly, making it a better experience for all concerned.

Conclude

Give the child and parents a further opportunity to raise issues or concerns, thank them for their input, then engage in social discourse to bring the encounter to a close. Record the discussion in all relevant documentation.

Procedures Box 2.1 Communicating with a child and his or her parents

Action
Establish the purpose of the communication, such as assessing the child's condition, gaining written consent or delivering an education package.

Reason *Activities are demanding and unique to that particular situation and when well managed contribute to the development of successful relationships between children, parents and healthcare professionals.*

Action
Identify the best person to meet the purpose.

Reasons *Task performed appropriately.*
Ensures that any legal, ethical or social issues are considered.

Action
Gather required information from, for example, nursing and medical notes, healthcare workers, the child and/or the parents.

Reasons *Healthcare professional are well informed prior to the meeting.*
Promotes the child's and parents' confidence and trust in the healthcare professional.

Action
Anticipate any potential questions.

Reasons *Any required information can be obtained prior to the interaction.*
Enables an informed response, reducing anxiety.

Action
Establish the child's and parents' needs and wishes regarding involvement in discussions.

Reasons *Promotes inclusion of the child and parents as team members in the decision-making process.*
Promotes the autonomy of the child and recognition of parental roles.

Action
Select a suitable area, such as a family room or play area, for the purpose of the interaction.

Reasons *Promotes privacy.*
Encourages an atmosphere that may give the child and/or parents confidence to participate.

Action
Ensure an acceptable level of privacy.

Reason *Prevents inhibition of discussion related to concerns of being overheard.*

Action
Arrange furniture to promote not obstruct participation.

Reason *Allows all participants to look towards each other without breaching personal space.*

Action
Provide sufficient seating, including for the child if present.

Reason *Encourages child involvement and empowerment.*

Action
Ensure that chairs are not positioned in front of a window.

Reason *Allows view of facial expression and minimises discomfort.*

Action
Allow sufficient time.

Reasons *Promotes discussion.*
Avoids any reluctance to raise further issues.

Action
Approach the child and parents in an open, professional manner.

Reason *Promotes a relationship of collaboration.*

Action
Introduce yourself, giving the reason for the communication exchange.

Reason *Allows identification of appropriate participants and prepares them for what is to come.*

Action
Establish the concerns of the participants by use of communication models and skills such as explanations and questions.

Reasons *Allows comprehensive exploration of issues.*
Maximises potential to collect necessary information.
Promotes participation by all present.

Action
Use active listening.

Reason *The child's and parents' concerns are established.*

Action
Give clear, concise explanations, avoiding medical jargon when possible and explaining it clearly when necessary.

Reason *Promotes child and parent understanding and participation.*

Action
Use leaflets, toys, diagrams, medical equipment and X-rays to reinforce verbal information.

Reasons *Increases learning by stimulating senses of hearing, sight and touch.*
Acknowledges the child's developmental stage.

Action
Use pauses effectively; do not feel compelled to fill them.

Reason *Allows consideration of information, formulation of responses, identification of alternatives and coping with emotional responses.*

Action
Observe for non-verbal cues.

Reason *Promotes appropriate responses.*

Action
Be aware of your non-verbal cues.

Reason *Non-verbal cues can affect the other person's perception of both yourself and the current situation.*

Action
Use an open body posture.

Reason *Indicates interest and encourages response.*

Action
Be aware of cultural influences on communication.

Reason *Avoids use of stereotypical behaviours.*

Action
Give opportunities to the child and parents to make their concerns known.

Reasons *Promotes exploration of positive and negative concerns.*
Reduces anxiety.

Procedures Box 2.1 Communicating with a child and his or her parents—cont'd

Action
Answer questions honestly.
Reason *Encourages a relationship of trust.*

Action
Include the child in the discussion; see the child individually if she or he wishes.
Reasons *Avoids the assumption that the child is included simply by being present.*
Reduces the potential of adults dominating the discussion.

Action
Paraphrase discussion.
Reasons *Confirms the understanding of all parties.*
Promotes agreements for further action.
Provides an opportunity to revise decisions.

Action
Plan further discussion as required, with a timescale.
Reason *Promotes collaboration and minimises uncertainty regarding the progress of proposed actions.*

Action
Avoid making agreements that cannot be guaranteed.
Reasons *May reduce the quality of the therapeutic relationship.*
May increase the anxiety of the child and/or parents.

Action
Reflect on emergency communications when a situation has stabilised.
Reason *Allows reflection and clarification of the situation for the child and parents.*

Action
Give written guidelines as required.
Reasons *Reinforces the information given.*
Promotes confidence in the child and/or parents when performing procedures.

Action
Give the child and parents further opportunity to raise issues.
Reason *Promotes a successful conclusion to the discussion.*

Action
Thank the child and parents for their input and engage in social discourse to conclude the discussion.
Reasons *Reinforces the importance of the child's and parents' contribution.*
Continues the therapeutic relationship.

Action
Record the discussion in relevant documentation.
Reasons *Ensures continuity of care.*
Reduces the potential for error or conflicting information being given.

Now test your knowledge

- Critically evaluate how you would communicate with a child and family when admitting the child to a ward for minor surgery. What strategies could you use to establish their anxieties and minimise any effects?
- How would you educate a 6-year-old child about the dietary requirements related to his diabetes mellitus?
- How would you prepare a young mother prior to the immunisation of her first child? Consider the communication skills you could utilise in this situation.

References

Alderson P, Montgomery J (1996) Health care choices: making decisions with children. Institute for Policy Research, London

Attree M (2001) Patients' and relatives' experiences and perspectives of 'good' and 'not so good' quality care. Journal of Advanced Nursing 33:456–466

Beauchamp T, Childress J (2001) Principles of biomedical ethics, 5th edn. Oxford University Press, Oxford

Bosek MSD (2002) Effective communication skills: the key to preventing and resolving ethical situations. JONA's Healthcare Law, Ethics and Regulation 4(4):93–97

Bradbury A (2000) Successful presentation skills. Kogan Page, London

Charlton R (1996) Medical education – addressing the needs of the dying child. Palliative Medicine 10:240–246

Christensen PH, James A (eds) (2000) Research with children: perspectives and practices. Falmer Press, London

Dickson D, Hargie O, Morrow N (1997) Communication skills training for health professionals, 2nd edn. Chapman & Hall, London

van Dulmen AM (1998) Children's contributions to pediatric outpatient encounters. Pediatrics 102(3):563–568

van Dulmen AM (2004) Pediatrician–parent–child communication: problem-related or not? Patient Education and Counselling 52:61–68

Espezel JE, Canam CJ (2003) Parent–nurse interactions: care of the hospitalized child. Journal of Advanced Nursing 44(1):34–41

Figueroa-Altmann AR, Bedrossian L, Steinmiller E et al (2005) Kids care: improving partnerships with children and families. American Journal of Nursing 105(6):72a–72c

Fleitas J (2003) The power of words: examining the linguistic landscape of pediatric nursing. American Journal of Maternal Child Nursing 28(6):384–388

Hallstrom I, Elander G (2004) Decision-making during hospitalization: parents' and children's involvement. Journal of Clinical Nursing 13:367–375

Hurd GM (2005) Communication is key. Total Health 27(5):53–54

Kirk S, Glendinning C, Callery P (2005) Parent or nurse? The experience of being the parent of a technology-dependent child. Journal of Advanced Nursing 51(5):456–464

McCabe C (2004) Nurse–patient communication: an exploration of patients' experiences. Issues in Clinical Nursing 13:41–49

McTaggart IJ (2000) Children and parents' perceptions of the support they receive when the child has a life threatening or life limiting condition. Thesis, University of Stirling

Mansson ME, Dykes AK (2004) Practices for preparing children for clinical examinations and procedures in Swedish pediatric wards. Pediatric Nursing 30(3):182–187

Pengelly T (2003) Communicating with young people with life-threatening conditions [research and commentary]. Paediatric Nursing 15(4):12

Shattell M, Hogan B (2005) Facilitating communication: how to truly understand what patients mean. Journal of Psychosocial Nursing 43(10):29–32

Sobo EJ (2003) Pediatric nurses may misjudge parent communication preferences. Journal of Nursing Care Quality 19(3):253–262

Tates K, Meeuwesen L (2000) 'Let mum have her say': Turn-taking in doctor–parent–child communication. Patient Education and Counseling 40(2):151–162

Thorne S, Con A, McGuiness L et al (2004) Good communication with healthcare providers helped patients with multiple sclerosis cope and adapt. Qualitative Health Research 14:5–22

Tiberius RG, Sackin HD, Tallet S et al (2001) Conversations with parents of medically ill children: a study of interactions between medical students and parents and pediatric residents and parents in the clinical setting. Teaching and Learning in Medicine 13(2):97–109

Tourigny J, Chapados C, Pineault R (2005) Determinants of parental behaviour when children undergo day-care surgery. Journal of Advanced Nursing 52(5):490–497

United Nations (1989) Convention on the rights of the child. UN, Geneva

While A (2005) Taking up the challenge of communication. British Journal of Community Nursing 10(10):484

Young B, Dixon-Woods M, Windridge KC et al (2003) Managing communication with young people who have a potentially life threatening chronic illness: qualitative study of patients and parents. British Medical Journal 326:305

3 Therapeutic play in hospital

Margaret A. Chambers

The importance of play for children in hospital has been recognised for many years (Save the Children Fund 1989). While children's nurses now recognise its importance, it nevertheless often comes low down on their lists when compared with other practical and specialised skills. It may be argued that this is even more apparent since the rise of the hospital play specialist (HPS) and hospital play schemes across the UK, with nurses delegating the play role in favour of ever more technical skills. Play, and particularly therapeutic play, is arguably part of the holistic care of the child and therefore the responsibility of all children's nurses (Chambers 1993).

While this chapter will focus on therapeutic play activities in hospital, it should be noted that children's nurses in any setting can use the techniques of therapeutic play to communicate with children and to identify their fears and misconceptions about hospitals, medical treatment and nursing care. It is through therapeutic play activities that children can rehearse or relive their anxieties and develop coping skills. If we are to accept that the psychosocial care of children is at least as important as their physical care and that the child's emotional well-being contributes to recovery, it is important that children's nurses learn to incorporate therapeutic play activity into their everyday nursing practice.

According to Gilman & Frauman (1987) play is a familiar concept but difficult to define, while Hall & Reet (2000) suggest that much of the literature about play is conceptual rather than empirical and is rooted in sociology and psychology. While this suggests that play has not been well researched, it means rather that theoretical definitions of play are hard to find. Even so, the literature reveals a number of characteristics of what is described as 'normative' play, the everyday, normal play activity of children (Vessey & Mahon 1990), the internal motivation and voluntary activity of the play being two important characteristics of normative play (Bolig 1990).

Early theories saw play simply as a way of getting rid of excess energy (Spencer 1898). Recapitulation theory (Garvey 1977) suggested that play represents ancestral behaviour – children climb and swing in much the same way as our monkey ancestors did, and Piaget (1951) linked play to his cognitive developmental theories. Play should be a source of enjoyment for both the participant and the observer and may be described as any activity that is undertaken for intrinsic pleasure not extrinsic purposes. Play is often described as the natural activity of the child. However, the pleasures of play are universal and not confined to the years of childhood (Fig. 3.1).

Why do children play? Although it has already been suggested that the role of play is largely to have fun, there are many other reasons why play is important to the developing child. Play makes an important contribution to normal growth and development and is a crucial part of children's lives. Children who are deprived of the opportunity to play may fail to grow and develop normally (Harvey & Hales-Tooke 1972).

According to Chambers (2007a) play is therefore essential for:

- physical development, fine and gross motor skills, strength and stamina
- social development, social skills and social behaviours, control of aggression
- moral development, for example learning to take turns, learning to win and lose, learning not to cheat, self-control and consideration for others
- psychological development, such as the development of self-awareness and self-actualisation
- cognitive development
- problem solving
- communication
- normalising the environment
- practising adult behaviours and skills
- language development
- distraction from anxiety-provoking situations
- mastering and making sense of the environment, understanding the world in which the children live and differentiating between what is real and what is not
- having fun.

What is therapeutic play?

Two terms are in common usage: *therapeutic play* and *play therapy*, and these terms are sometimes used interchangeably. This is a particular feature of the North American literature. However, it is important to differentiate between the two terms because in the UK at least they have very different meanings.

Wilson (2000) described play therapy as a dynamic relationship between therapist and child in which the communication medium is play. Landsdown (1996) argues that is it essential to distinguish between play therapy undertaken by a trained psychotherapist and therapeutic play in hospital and

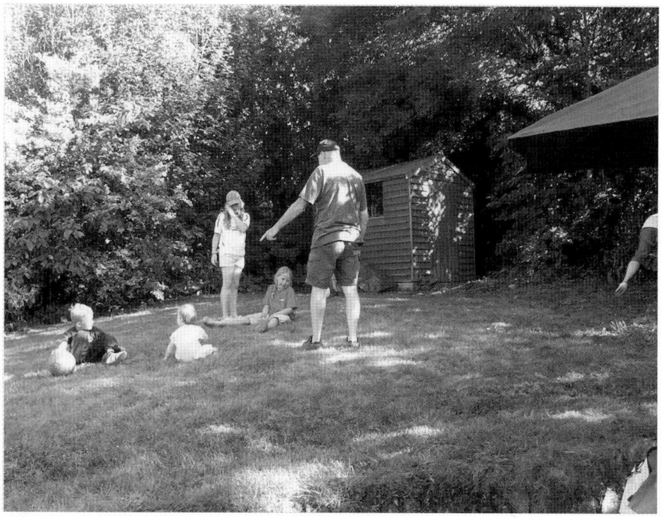

Fig. 3.1 • Children and an adult enjoying play activity.

community settings. Play therapy has been described as a tool for the diagnosis and treatment of emotionally disturbed children (Chambers 2001) and as an approach to helping children explore their problems during psychotherapy or counselling sessions using play (Miles 1981).

Therapeutic play, on the other hand, is the use of play as therapy to help otherwise normal children faced with an environmental threat such as illness or hospitalisation to come to terms with their fears and to master their experiences (Chambers 1993). Therapeutic play is an intervention used to help children to cope or develop their coping skills when they are faced with often overwhelming stress, and it has been defined as a pleasurable activity that contributes to general well-being, especially the mental well-being of the player (Chambers 2001). Because any threat to the child causes stress, therapeutic play activity is not limited to the hospital setting. However, much of the literature relating to therapeutic play focuses on the hospitalised child and medical procedures, and it is therefore sometimes termed *play in hospital* (Bolig 1984, Douglas 1993, Save the Children Fund 1989, Taylor et al 1999).

Bolig (1984) has described the five main functions of play in hospital as:

1. to provide diversion
2. to play out anxieties and problems
3. to restore normal aspects to life
4. to aid understanding of hospital events
5. to communicate fear.

The Save the Children Fund (1989) describe the functions as:

- To aid normality
- To reduce anxiety
- To speed recovery
- To facilitate communication
- To prepare for hospitalisation or medical procedures.

Play in hospital has other benefits too. Hall & Reet (2000) discuss the benefits of play for parents. They argue that seeing the beneficial effects of play on their children allows parents to relax and to manage and cope with the hospital experience.

The evidence base for the value of therapeutic play is both dated and small and, with a few notable exceptions, tends to relate to specific activities – for example preparation for procedures – rather than to therapeutic play per se. Much of what there is has come from North America.

Ethically it may be difficult to produce more up-to-date research because observation clearly demonstrates that therapeutic play *is* an effective medium for communication with hospitalised children and for the reduction of hospital anxiety. A selection of the research is presented here.

Clatworthy (1981) attempted to show that therapeutic play could be used as a treatment for hospital-induced anxiety, using a two-group experimental design. Anxiety was measured on admission and discharge using the Missouri Children's Picture Series (Sine et al 1974). The experimental group of children received therapeutic play for 30 min daily, while the control group did not. The results showed that the experimental group showed no significant rise in their anxiety levels, while the control group demonstrated a significant increase in their anxiety levels on discharge as measured by the Missouri Children's Picture Series. Clatworthy acknowledges the limitations of the study (particularly the lack of instruments to specifically measure hospital anxiety in children) but nevertheless concludes that therapeutic play should be incorporated into the care provided for all hospitalised children.

The best-known British study into therapeutic play was undertaken by Rodin in 1983. One hundred and eleven children took part in the study into the value of play preparation prior to venepuncture and were randomly allocated into three equal groups. Group A children were given medical preparation games before the venepuncture. Group B children were given games that had no medical content, and group C children received no games at all but just stayed with their parents in a waiting area. A behaviour rating scale was devised by the researcher using physical behavioural signs. The results showed that children in group A demonstrated less anxiety during venepuncture than children in the other two groups. The effectiveness of the preparation was increased if the children had also been told about the blood test in advance. Rodin concluded that all children should be given relevant information in a child-friendly way prior to hospitalisation and medical procedures.

Demerest et al (1984) explored a medical play intervention for the reduction of children's anxiety prior to surgery using an experimental design. Twenty-four children undergoing tonsillectomy or adenoidectomy were randomly assigned to one of two experimental groups or to the control group. One experimental group was exposed to a slideshow demonstrating the medical equipment and the procedure that the child would undergo, using a model – another child undergoing the procedure. The second experimental group of children, the in vitro group, was encouraged to undertake medical role play and actively utilise the medical equipment that was shown on the slideshow. The control group was given toys and games to play with. They had no contact with hospital equipment and they did not discuss the surgical procedures they were to undergo. Anxiety levels were measured on admission and 1 week after discharge using the anxiety scale of the Personality Inventory for Children (Wirt et al 1977). The Hospital Fears Rating Scale (Melamed & Siegel 1975) was administered three times: after the intervention, at the onset of surgery and in the recovery room. Results of the study indicate that the in vitro group had significantly lower anxiety levels than either of the other two groups, and that these two groups were not significantly different from each other. The researchers concluded that allowing children to undertake medical play reduced the 'strangeness' of the objects and mitigated the anxiety response by familiarisation with the clinical environment.

Ispa et al (1988) studied the effects of supervised play in a hospital waiting room. Thirty children were observed over a 4-month period by four observers sitting unobtrusively in the waiting area. Half the children were supervised by a play specialist and the other half were not. The results demonstrated that those children who were supported by the play specialist were less likely to exhibit signs of fear and anxiety. While this was a small-scale study and the authors describe 'trends approaching significance', the results are in concordance with those of similar studies (Alcock et al 1985, Hoffman & Flutterman 1971, Williams & Powell 1980).

A study by Pederson (1995) explored the possibility that guided imagery may reduce children's pain and anxiety while undergoing cardiac catheterisation. Twenty-four children took part in the study, in three groups – imagery group, control group and presence group; in the last of these a researcher provided empathetic support. Anxiety was measured using the State–Trait Anxiety Inventory for Children (Spielberger et al 1973) and pain by the children's self-report using a visual analogue scale (McGrath 1987). Behavioural distress was measured using the Observational Scale of Behavioural Distress (Jay et al 1983), and salivary cortisol, normally raised in extreme stress, was measured using salivary cortisol radioimmunoassay (Gunner 1986). The results showed a lack of significance between the groups on behavioural distress, visual analogue pain scale and salivary cortisol and suggest that guided imagery did not reduce pain and distress. Pederson suggests, however, that teaching imagery in advance of the procedure may increase its effectiveness.

Categorisation of therapeutic play

There are a number of ways in which therapeutic play can be categorised, and there is a common misconception that therapeutic play is entirely focused on diversion, preparation and medical play. This chapter and the associated video clip and PowerPoint presentation will also suggest other types of therapeutic play activity, for example bolstering a child's self-esteem and body image and activities to reduce boredom in isolation settings.

Normal play

Normal play has already been discussed as a pleasurable activity that is therapeutic in its own right. All hospital play schemes must make provision for normal play activity. This is essential for keeping children occupied during the long hospital day; it acts as a diversion from the otherwise clinical environment and provides escape from other more stressful forms of therapeutic play. Play and play areas have a normalising effect on the otherwise clinical environment, and seeing their children happily engaged in play has positive effects on the parents, reducing stress and facilitating the development of a therapeutic relationship with health professionals.

Play activities planned for hospitalised children should be both age- and cognitively appropriate and culturally sensitive, and special provision should be made for children with special needs. A sensory room (Fig. 3.2 and Box 3.1) should be provided for those children whose disabilities prevent them from accessing other forms of play activity, but this may not be exclusively their territory. Children may, for example, enjoy having their daily physiotherapy sessions in the sensory room, which provides a calm environment for such procedures.

Whenever possible, children should access the play area or play room (Fig. 3.3), where their play can be supervised

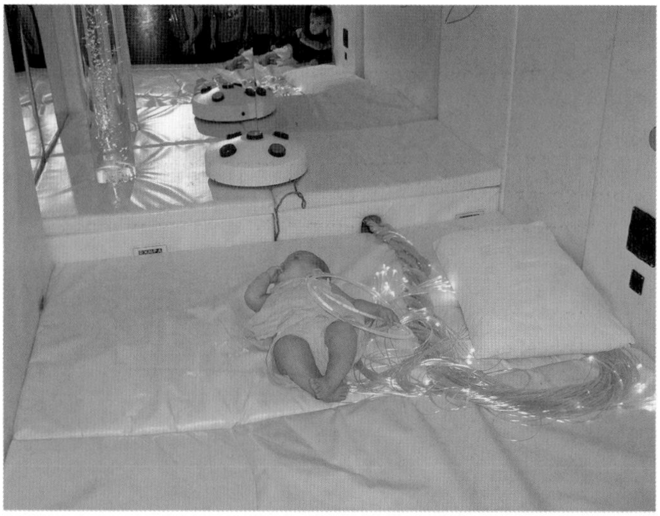

Fig. 3.2 • A sensory room.

Box 3.1. The sensory room

- Soft play area
- Interesting and varied lighting effects
- Bubble tubes
- Atmospheric music

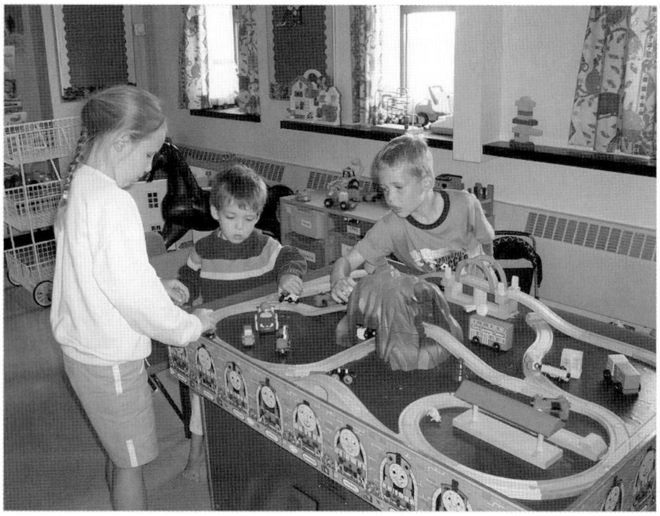

Fig. 3.3 • Children at play in the play room.

by the HPS and children can select their own play activities. When this is not possible it is the responsibility of the HPS or the children's nurse to provide the child with suitable play activities at the bedside (Fig. 3.4).

For suitable toys and activities for ages and stages of development see the website of the National Network for Child Care (2007).

Diversion and distraction

Play can be used to divert or distract a child's attention during painful medical procedures. In distraction the child's attention is diverted from the unpleasant or painful experience through play activities such as blowing bubbles, puppetry or the use of plastic tubes containing brightly coloured oils and foil shapes (Fig. 3.5). Distraction activities should be age-appropriate, for example bubbles and musical story books may be appropriate for younger children while older children may prefer to listen to music of their choice through headsets (Fanurik et al 2000).

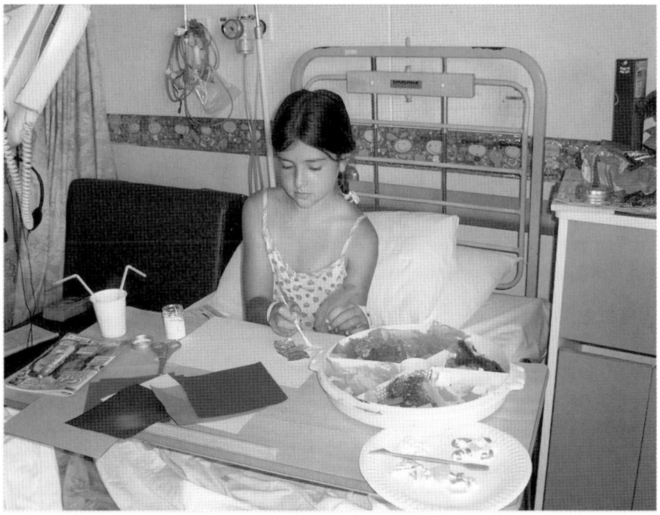

Fig. 3.4 • Child at play in bed.

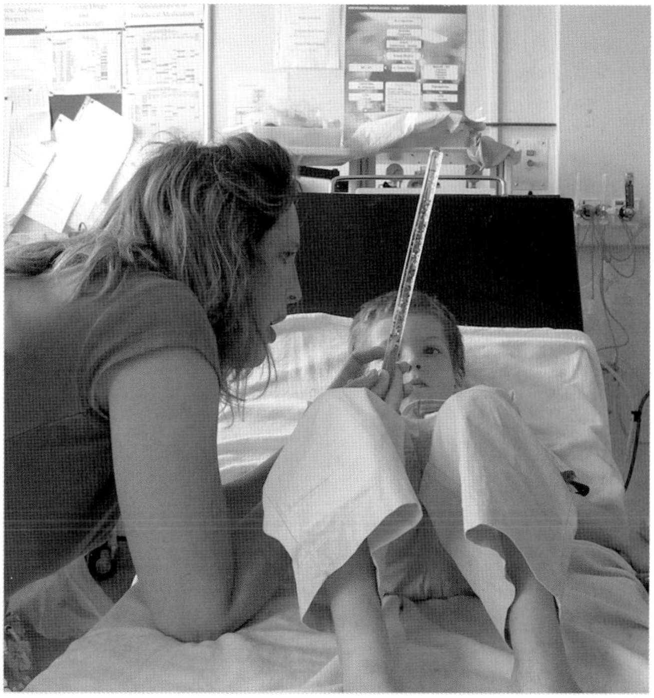

Fig. 3.5 • Use of sparkle wands or bubbles for diversion.

When thinking about distraction techniques it is important to note that children cope with painful or stressful procedures in different ways according to their personality, their experiences and their locus of control – the degree to which outcomes are perceived as inevitable or the result of one's own actions (Rotter 1966). It may be important for some children to retain control by watching the procedure. In this case the use of distraction techniques would be inappropriate.

Medical play modalities

According to Delpo & Frick (1988) there are two types of therapeutic play, which they call directed play and non-directed play. Directed play has very specific outcomes that are decided by the adult who guides the play; examples of this would be preparation for hospital or for medical procedures. Non-directed play refers to play in which the adult provides the setting and the play materials but the child controls all other aspects of the play activity; an example of this is free medical play in which children are given access to real medical equipment and their subsequent play activity is supervised but not controlled by the adult.

Brennan (1994) describes non-directed medical play as a way of allowing children to examine and use medical equipment in a safe environment, while Lutz (1986) suggests that medical play allows adults to observe children's anxieties and misconceptions about medical procedures. They are then able to correct them. When using non-directive techniques it is important that children have access to the types of medical equipment that they have been or will be exposed to during stressful or painful medical and nursing procedures. It is also essential that free medical play is undertaken under the supervision of an adult who can provide feedback to the child and correct any misconceptions arising through the play (Children's Memorial Hospital 2006).

McCue (1988) identifies four distinct conceptual types of medical play (Fig. 3.6):

1. Role rehearsal or role reversal medical play, in which the child takes on the role of medical personnel to rehearse or relive medical events on models such as stuffed toys or commercially produced medical dolls.
2. Medical fantasy play, in which the child engages in medical play but without the equipment, using ordinary play materials to act out medical experiences. In this way the child can avoid contact with objects they are afraid of while still playing out issues of concern.
3. Indirect medical play, in which the child engages in activities that are indirectly related to the hospital theme, such as jigsaw puzzles and hospital games.

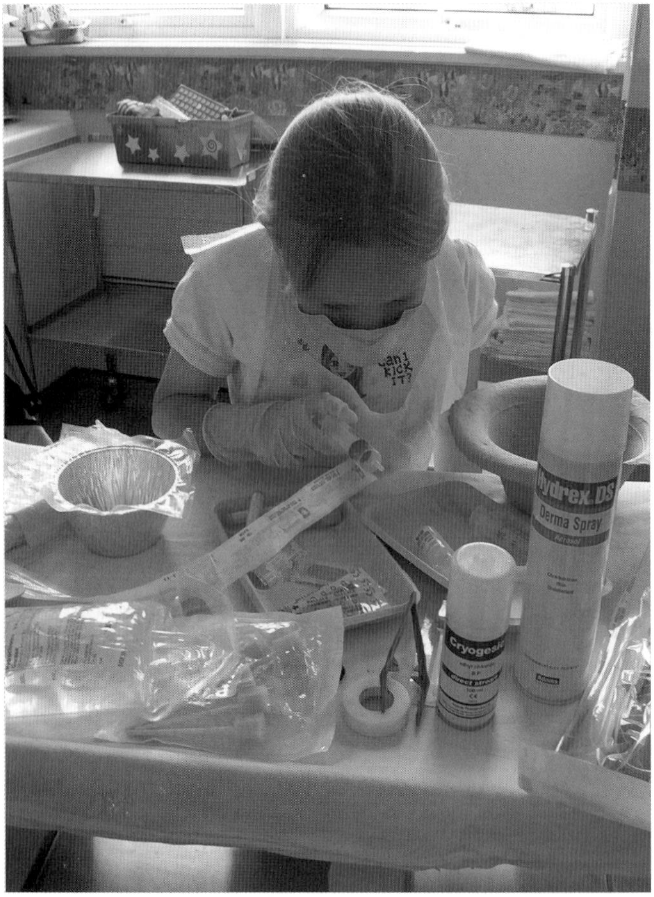

Fig. 3.6 • Medical play table with appropriate medical equipment.

4. Medical art: painting, drawing and collage, sometimes using medical equipment and so on.

For more information about medical play see Children's Memorial Hospital (2006), and for age-appropriate medical play activities see the website of the Children's Hospital, Omaha (2007).

Preparation for hospital and medical procedures

Preparation for hospital

Hospitalisation and in particular surgery have long been recognised as stressful events for children. Fantasies provoked by surgery may include the fear of mutilation or even castration or the concept of hospitalisation as a well-deserved punishment for something they have done wrong. Children's nurses and HPSs can use therapeutic play preparation to help children to develop a more rational understanding of the hospital environment and the purpose of surgery.

Preparation for hospital and surgery has been shown to reduce stress and promote recovery (Demerest et al 1984). Consequently many children's hospitals and children's units in the UK now provide preadmission preparation programmes for children undergoing planned surgery and their families (Box 3.2). Before undertaking play preparation it is important to establish what the child already knows and understands so that play activity can be geared towards meeting the needs of the individual child and family, and the child's fantasies and misconceptions can be addressed during the preparation procedure (Chambers 2007b).

Filmed modelling (Melamed & Siegel 1975) is a preparation method in which children are exposed to a film in which their role is modelled by another child who demonstrates expected behaviour. The rationale for this is that the child will model his or her behaviour on that of the child in the film.

Children who are admitted for surgery in an emergency should receive as much information as their condition permits.

Box 3.2. Content of the prehospital preparation programme

- Before admission, play and other preparation materials can be delivered to the child's home. These may include information books for parents and colouring books showing the process of the day surgery day for the child.
- At the preparation clinic, information for the child and family should be age-appropriate and preferably include filmed modelling (see above), play preparation for the siting of a cannula (see video clip) and whenever possible a visit to the anaesthetic and recovery rooms.
- Timing: whenever possible this should be related to the age and cognitive development of the child, with older children being given more time to develop coping skills and younger children being given a shorter time, as they quickly forget information.
- Sensory information (see bolstering).
- Pain management should be discussed with both the child and the family.

Preparation for medical procedures

Therapeutic play activities are also used to prepare children for medical and nursing procedures such as the insertion of an intravenous cannula. They are usually undertaken in the form of directed medical play modalities (Delpo & Frick 1988), during which the child is exposed to medical equipment and procedures in a non-threatening environment. The procedure to be undertaken is demonstrated for the child using anatomically correct dolls, for example Zaadi dolls (Figs 3.7 and 3.8), stuffed body outline dolls (Fig. 3.9; Gaynard et al 1991) or even the child's own toy.

During preparation the child should be exposed to all the sensory information associated with the procedure, for example the anaesthetic cream of choice. Preferably the child should be able to undertake the procedure on the doll under the supervision of the HPS or the children's nurse.

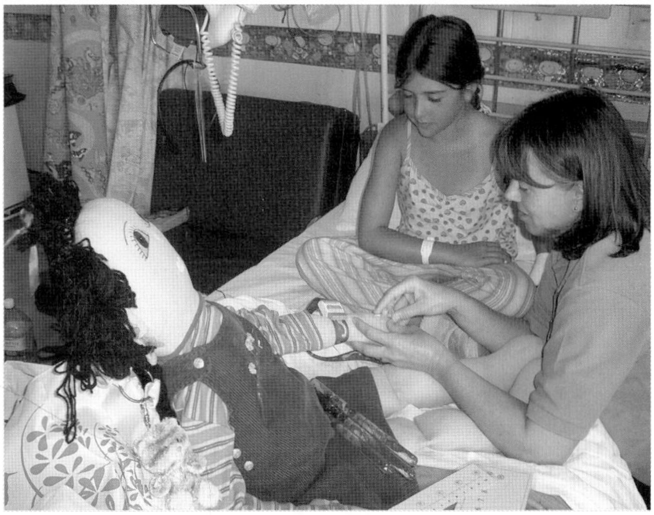

Fig. 3.8 • Child being shown cannulation using a Zaadi doll.

Post-procedural play

Therapeutic play activity following procedures or hospitalisation is less well developed than preprocedural play (Chambers 2007b); however, Heiney (1991) suggested that there are three acute stress points for the child in any medical procedure: before, during and after the event. Further, she proposes that the aftermath may be the most difficult time for the child, who is trying to comes to terms with the experience and may be in discomfort or pain. An examination of children's anxiety levels before and after venepuncture suggests that for most children good play preparation reduces anxiety and is enough to carry them through the aftermath (Chambers 2003). Even so, postprocedural play may be effective in reducing the anxiety of those children who display overt distress behaviour following a procedure, because it allows the child to relive the experience and, through the play, to communicate the fears and anxieties that have been provoked. At the same time postprocedural play allows the

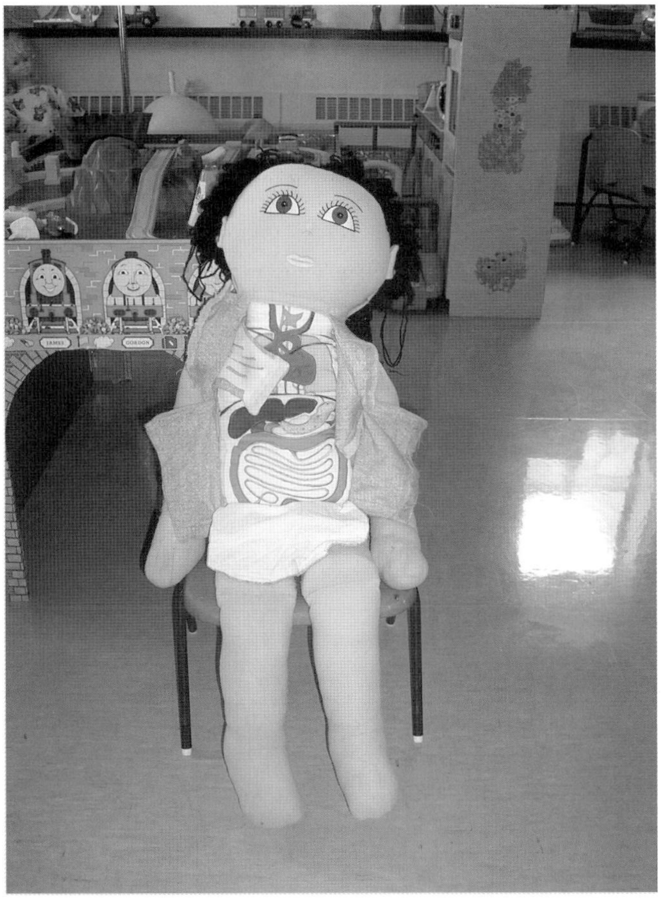

Fig. 3.7 • A Zaadi doll.

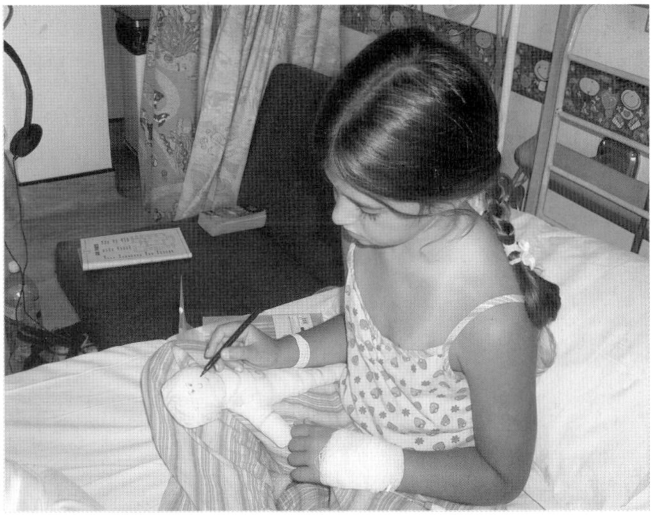

Fig. 3.9 • Girl with a stuffed body outline doll.

child to become the 'aggressor' while the HPS, the children's nurse or toys become the 'victims'. This role reversal permits children to master and come to terms with their experiences, boosting their personal control and developing their coping skills (LaMontagne 1993).

Other play activities to support the sick child

Guided imagery, 'a form of relaxed, focused concentration, is a natural and powerful coping mechanism' (Ott 1996: 34). Guided imagery can be used to help children to relax and cope with pain and procedures. It involves using the child's imagination therapeutically and focusing the concentration, making the child oblivious to the surrounding environment. It is important that the child is able to practise the technique prior to its use during a procedure, and it should be noted that guided imagery is not effective for every child.

Techniques for supporting self-esteem and body image

Children who are sick or hospitalised, especially chronically ill children, may have difficulties in maintaining a high self-esteem or forming a normal body image (Hart et al 1992). Because the way in which children see themselves and their bodies is important for good mental health, it is the role of the HPS or the children's nurse to bolster the child's self-image. Therapeutic play activities can be designed to promote self-esteem and positive body image.

Art, books and music

The use of storytelling, drawing and painting, and music (art and music therapy) all have a role in the care of the sick or hospitalised child. However, these activities are outside the remit of this chapter.

Therapeutic play activities

Two activities are described below. The first is the use of the body outline doll (Fig. 3.10), because this doll can be used for a number of therapeutic play activities. The second is an example of tension relief, expressing anger and putting children in control. This activity also allows children to become familiar with syringes in a non-medical way. For further activities you are referred to Hart et al (1992) and to the PowerPoint presentation and video clip.

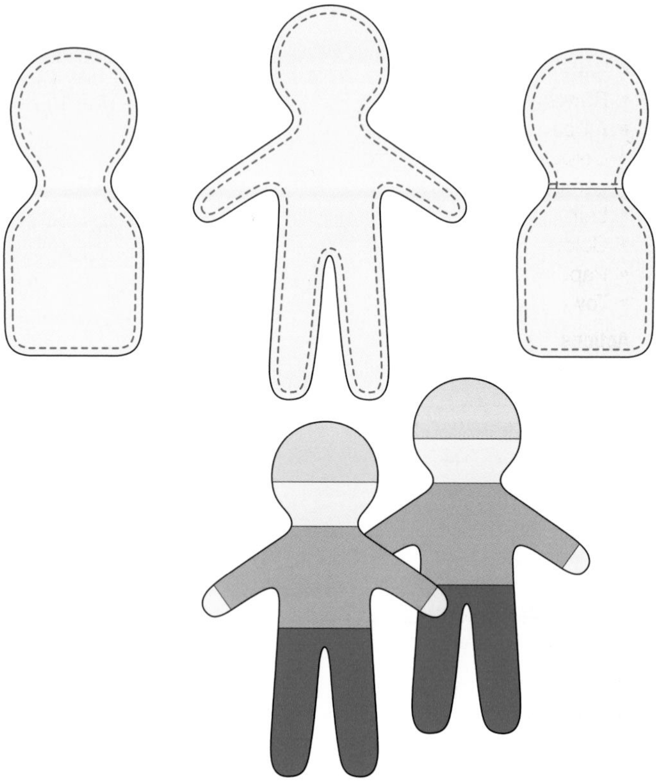

Fig. 3.10 • Pattern for a body outline doll. (From Gaynard et al 1991)

Procedures Box 3.1 The use of body outline dolls

Age range
From 3 years to adolescence

Equipment
- Stuffed body outline doll made of muslin, stuffed with polyester and without clothing or other features
- A set of non-toxic permanent marker pens

Action
Give the doll and markers to the child.
Reason *The child can create his or her own doll.*

Action
Tell the child that the doll and markers are theirs to keep after discharge from the hospital.
Reason *To help develop a therapeutic relationship.*

Action
Tell the child to use the markers to create her or his own doll.
Reason *To distract and divert the child and encourage creative activity.*

Action
Explore with the child the doll he or she has created.
Reason *To provide opportunities for children to process information and express fears.*

Action
Use the doll to demonstrate medical and nursing procedures such as venepuncture, cannulation and lumbar puncture.
Reason *To provide age-appropriate information in a child-friendly way.*

Procedures Box 3.2 Syringe target practice

Age range
From 5 years to adolescence

Reasons
- To become familiar with and to handle syringes.
- To reduce anxiety associated with syringes.
- To permit communication about feelings and fears associated with syringes.
- To reduce anger and tension.
- To put the child in control as the aggressor, not the victim.

Equipment
- 10-mL syringes
- Water
- Bowls for water
- A4 paper
- Coloured pens, pencils or paints
- Laminating material
- Laminator
- Coloured sticky tape
- Paper towels
- Towels or old sheets to protect the floor

Actions
Give the children pieces of A4 paper and pencils, pens or paints.

Ask them to draw something in the hospital that they are anxious about (e.g. doctor, nurse, syringe or intravenous fluids).

Reason *Permits children to express their anxiety about medical equipment and personnel.*

Action
Ask children to give their picture a score from 1 to 10.

Reason *Permits children to grade their level of anxiety associated with medical equipment and personnel.*

Action
Laminate the pictures.

Reason *To make them waterproof.*

Action
Protect the floor with old sheets or towels.

Reason *To prevent accidents.*

Action
Line up the pictures at the child's eye level.

Reason *To accommodate accuracy of shooting.*

Action
Explain to the children how to use the syringes to squirt water at the targets.

Reasons *Children become the aggressors, not the victims. Water squirting allows tension release.*

Action
Add up the scores.

Reasons *Children have a sense of achievement and mastery. Children have an increase in self-esteem.*

Now test your knowledge

- What is play?
- What is therapeutic play?
- What are the functions of play in hospital?
- What is the difference between directed and non-directed medical play?
- What are the advantages of play in preparing children for hospital and medical procedures?
- Plan therapeutic play activities for an 8-year-old boy with cystic fibrosis nursed in isolation. Consider boredom, self-esteem and body image, and lack of companionship.
- Consider how you might use therapeutic play activities in the accident and emergency department for a child who has a fractured radius and ulna.
- As a community nurse how might you use therapeutic play to support a child having sutures removed at home following an appendicectomy?

References

Alcock D, Goodman J, Feldman W, McGrath P, Park M, Cappelli M (1985) Environment and waiting behaviours in emergency waiting areas. Children's Health Care 13:174–180

Bolig R (1984) Play in hospital settings. In Yawkley TD, Pellegrini AD (eds) Child's play: developmental and applied. Lawrence Erlbaum, Hillsdale

Bolig R (1990) Play in health care settings: a challenge for the 1990s. Children's Health Care 19(4):229–233

Brennan A (1994) Caring for children during procedures: a review of the literature. Pediatric Nursing 20(5):451–458

Chambers MA (1993) Play as therapy for the hospitalised child. Journal of Clinical Nursing 2(6):349–353

Chambers MA (2001) Towards a definition of therapeutic play: a concept analysis. MSc paper. Royal College of Nursing Institute, London

Chambers MA (2003) The effects of post-procedural play on the anxiety levels of school aged children following venepuncture. MSc thesis, Royal College of Nursing Institute, London

Chambers MA (2007a) The value of play. In Chambers MA, Jones S (eds) The surgical nursing of children. Elsevier, London (in press)

Chambers MA (2007b) The context of care in surgical nursing. In Chambers MA, Jones S (eds) The surgical nursing of children. Elsevier, London (in press)

Children's Hospital, Omaha (2007) Online. Available: http://www.chsomaha.org/g5-bin/client.cgi?G5button=138

Children's Memorial Hospital (2006) Medical play. Online. Available: http://www.childrensmemorial.org/parents/support/medPlay.asp 4 May 2006

Clatworthy S (1981) Therapeutic play: effects on hospitalized children. Children's Health Care 9(4):108–113

Delpo EG, Frick SB (1988) Directed and non-directed play as therapeutic modalities. Children's Health Care 16(4):261–267

Demerest DS, Hooke JF, Erickson MT (1984) Preoperative intervention for the reduction of anxiety in pediatric surgery patients. Children's Health Care 12(4):179–183

Douglas J (1993) Psychology and nursing children. Macmillan, Basingstoke

Fanurik D, Koh JL, Schmitz ML (2000) Distraction techniques combined with EMLA: effects on I/V insertion pain and distress in children. Children's Health Care 29(2):87–101

Garvey C (1997) Play. Fontana, London

Gaynard L, Goldberger J, Laidley LN (1991) The use of stuffed, body outline dolls with hospitalized children and adolescents. Children's Health Care 20(4):216–224

Gilman CM, Frauman AC (1987) Use of play with the child with chronic illness. ANNA Journal 14(4):259–261

Gunner M (1986) Human development psychoneuroendocrinology: a review of research on neuroendocrine responses to challenge and threat in infancy and childhood. In Lamb M, Brown A, Rogoff B (eds) Advances in developmental psychology, vol. 4. Lawrence Erlbaum Associates, Hillsdale, p 51–101

Hall C, Reet M (2000) Enhancing the state of play in children's nursing. Journal of Child Health Care 4(2):49–54

Hart R, Mather P, Slack JF, Powell MA (1992) Therapeutic play activities for the hospitalized child. Mosby, St Louis

Harvey S, Hales-Tooke A (1972) (eds) Play in hospital. Faber, London

Heiney S (1991) Helping children through painful procedures. American Journal of Nursing 91(11):20–24

Hoffman I, Flutterman E (1971) Coping with waiting: psychiatric intervention and study in the waiting room of a pediatric oncology clinic. Comprehensive Psychiatry 12:67–81

Ispa J, Barrett B, Kim Y (1988) Effects of supervised play in a hospital waiting room. Children's Health Care 16(3):195–200

Jay S, Ozolins M, Elliott C, Caldwell S (1983) Assessment of children's distress during painful medical procedures. Health Psychology 2:133–147

LaMontagne LL (1993) Bolstering personal control in child patients through coping interventions. Pediatric Nursing 19(3):235–237

Landsdown R (1996) Children in hospital: a guide for family and carers. Oxford University Press, Oxford

Lutz W (1986) Helping hospitalized children and their parents cope with painful procedures. Journal of Pediatric Nursing 1:24–32

McCue K (1988) Medical play: an expanded perspective. Children's Health Care 16(30):157–161

McGrath P (1987) An assessment of children's pain: a review of behavioural, physiological and direct scaling techniques. Pain 31:147–176

Melamed BG, Siegel LJ (1975) Reduction of anxiety in children facing hospitalization and surgery by the use of filmed modelling. Journal of Consulting and Clinical Psychology 43:511–521

Miles MS (1981) Play therapy: a review of theories and comparison of some techniques. Issues in Mental Health Nursing 3:63–75

National Network for Child Care (2007) Better kid care: play is the business of kids. Online. Available: http://www.nncc.org/Curriculum/better.play.html

Ott MJ (1996) Imagine the possibilities! Guided imagery with toddlers and pre-schoolers. Pediatric Nursing 22(1):34–38

Pederson C (1995) Effects of imagery on children's pain and anxiety during cardiac catheterisation. Journal of Pediatric Nursing 10(6):365–374

Piaget J (1951) Play, dreams and imitation in childhood. Routledge, London

Rodin J (1983) Will this hurt? Royal College of Nursing, London

Rotter JB (1966) Social learning and clinical psychology. Prentice Hall, New York

Save the Children Fund (1989) Hospital: a deprived environment for children? The case for hospital play schemes. Save the Children Fund, London

Sines JO, Pauker JD, Sines LK (1974) The Missouri Children's Picture Series (MCPS): Iowa City

Spencer H (1898) The principles of psychology. D Appleton, New York

Spielberger C, Edwards C, Lushene R, Monturi J, Platzek S (1973) The State–Trait Anxiety Inventory for Children. Consulting Psychologists Press, Palo Alto

Taylor J, Muller D, Wattley L, Harris P (1999) Nursing children: psychology, research and practice, 3rd edn. Stanley Thornes, Cheltenham

Vessey JA, Mahon MM (1990) Therapeutic play and the hospitalised child. Journal of Pediatric Nursing 5(5):328–333

Williams YB, Powell M (1980) Documenting the value of supervised play in a pediatric ambulatory care clinic. Children's Health Care 9(1):15–20

Wilson K (2000) Play therapy. In Davies M (ed.) Blackwell encyclopaedia of social work. Blackwell, Oxford

Wirt RD et al, (1977) Multidimensional evaluation of child personality Los Angeles: Western Psychological Services

4 Infection prevention and control

Maria Bennallick

It is evident that healthcare-associated infections (HCAIs) cost the National Health Service dear. The estimated cost per year is approximately £1 billion, with approximately 8–10% patients in hospitals in England at any one time with an HCAI (National Audit Office 2000). Five thousand patients have their deaths attributable directly to HCAI, with another 20 000 patients having HCAI as a contributory factor. It has been estimated that 15–30% of these infections are preventable (Plowman et al 1999). So it is clear that lives could be saved if good infection prevention and control was implemented by all staff at all times.

Chain of infection

For infection to spread from person to person certain factors need to be present. These can be described as the chain of infection and are represented in Figure 4.1.

Source of infection

The source or reservoir of infection may be a patient or member of staff with an infection, a piece of equipment, food or water, the environment or an animal. All these reservoirs are where microorganisms such as bacteria and viruses can survive (McCulloch 2000).

Modes of transmission

There are three main modes of transmission, the methods used by microorganisms to leave the source or reservoir of infection:

1. Direct contact: for example impetigo, a staphylococcal skin infection, is spread by direct contact with lesions (Gillespie & Bamford 2003).
2. Indirect contact: for example a blood-borne virus such as hepatitis B could be spread on a contaminated needle (Heyman 2004).
3. Air: for example a respiratory infection such as tuberculosis is transmitted by droplets spread through the air (Heyman 2004).

Person at risk

Although it could be argued that all people are at risk of infection, some groups of individuals are more at risk than others. In particular, the very young, the very old, surgical patients, immunosuppressed individuals and those undergoing invasive procedures as well as the malnourished are particularly susceptible to infection (McCulloch 2000).

Way in

A microorganism can only end its journey by entering the susceptible individual and thereby completing the chain of infection. The ways in include the skin, ingestion, inhalation, mucous membranes, the invasive procedure and sexual contact.

Breaking the chain

As with any chain, it becomes useless if one of the links is broken. Infection prevention and control policies, procedures and practices are designed to break the chain of infection. These include source isolation, use of personal protective clothing and, most important of all, hand washing.

Standard principles for preventing healthcare-associated infections

These precautions should be applied by all healthcare practitioners when caring for all hospital in-patients. They include environmental hygiene, hand hygiene, the use of personal protective equipment and the use and disposal of sharps (Pratt et al 2007).

Hand hygiene

The hands are covered in microorganisms, some of which are part of the resident flora and some of which can be classified as transient. Transient microorganisms are those that are picked up during care activities and can then be transported to another person, eventually resulting in an infection.

Decontamination of the hands is a key aspect of infection prevention and control. It is important that the hands are decontaminated using the correct technique at the appropriate times and using the most suitable decontamination agents (Table 4.1). Hands must be decontaminated before and after each episode of patient contact (Fig. 4.2).

Care of hands

It is important to look after your hands when working in healthcare. Moisturising hands and maintaining skin

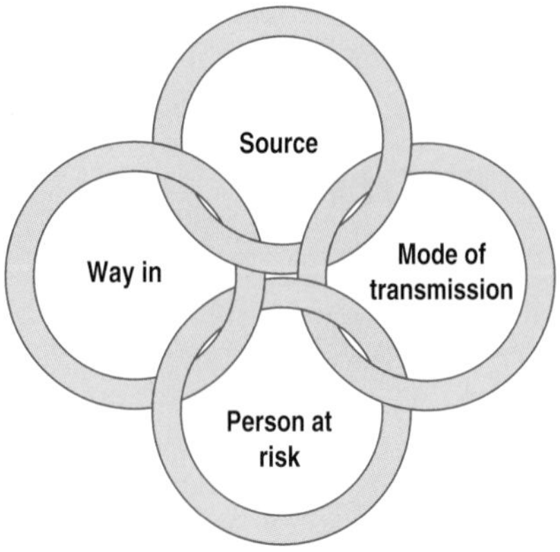

Fig. 4.1 • The chain of infection.

integrity is necessary outside working hours. Nails should be kept short and smooth. Any rough edges around the nails and nail beds can provide an environment for microbial growth.

Hand washing

The equipment required is as follows.

- A hand wash basin with elbow-operated or non-touch mixer taps is preferable.
- Liquid soap or antimicrobial skin disinfectant.
- Paper hand towels.
- A foot-operated waste bin.

Nicol et al (2004) describe the hand-washing procedure.

Procedures Box 4.1 Hand washing

Action
Set the taps to run water at a temperature and speed that are comfortable.

Reason *Setting a comfortable temperature results in more effective hand washing.*

Action
Apply liquid soap or skin disinfectant in sufficient quantity to create a lather.

Reason *Enough solution should be applied to maximise the effectiveness of the product.*

Action
Rub the hands together briskly, ensuring that all areas of the hands and wrists are covered in lather; this should be done for at least 10–15 s.

Reason *Any areas of the hands that are missed may result in microorganism transmission.*

Action
Rinse the soap or disinfectant off the hands, ensuring that all is removed and holding the hands facing downwards.

Reason *Residual soap may result in skin irritation.*

Action
Turn off the taps using your elbows or using a non-touch technique if required.

Reason *Avoids recontamination of the hands.*

Action
Dry the hands thoroughly using disposable paper towels, starting with the fingertips and working down the rest of the hands and wrists.

Reason *Thorough drying will reduce the microbial growth on the hands and also reduce the risk of soreness.*

Action
Dispose of the paper towels in a foot-operated bin using a non-touch technique (Nicol et al 2004).

Reason *Avoids recontamination of the hands by touching the bin lid.*

Hand decontamination: alcohol

This procedure uses alcohol-based hand rub or gel.

Procedures Box 4.2 Hand decontamination: alcohol

Action
Apply alcohol rub or gel in sufficient quantity to cover both hands and wrists.

Reason *Enough solution should be applied to maximise the effectiveness of the product.*

Action
Rub the hands together briskly, ensuring that all areas of the hands and wrists are covered in alcohol; this should be done for at least 10–15 s until the hands feel dry and not sticky.

Reason *Any areas of the hands that are missed may result in microorganism transmission.*

Table 4.1. Hand hygiene

Situations	Type of products
Before and after contact with patients or their environment. After any contact that may result in hands becoming contaminated. Before handling food. No organic matter on the hands.	Alcohol-based hand rub or gel or soap and water
Organic matter present on the hands.	Soap and water. Antimicrobial hand wash.
Before performing an invasive procedure.	Alcohol-based hand rub or gel or antimicrobial hand wash.

Use of personal protective equipment

The use of non-sterile gloves, disposable aprons and eye and mouth protection provides protection for staff and reduces the opportunity for microorganism transmission (Infection Control Nurses Association 1999). The type of personal protective equipment required depends on the level of risk associated with the activity about to be undertaken (Table 4.2).

Use of non-sterile gloves

The equipment required is non-sterile latex, vinyl or nitrile gloves. Gloves must comply with the standard set by the British Standards Institution (2000). Alternatives to latex gloves should be available to be used by staff and/or patients who have latex sensitisation.

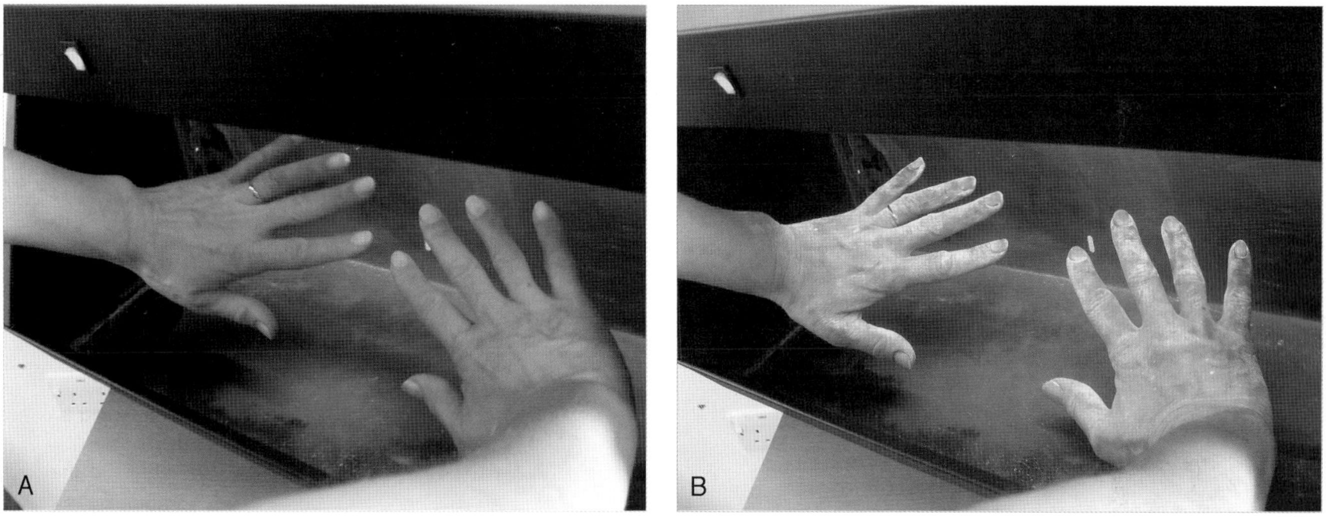

Fig. 4.2 • (**A**) Uncontaminated and (**B**) contaminated hands.

Table 4.2. Personal protective equipment

Activity risk	Protective clothing	Comment
No risk of contact with blood and/or body fluids (e.g. taking a pulse)	None required.	Hand decontamination is required before and after every patient contact.
Contact with blood and/or body fluids expected but *low risk of splashing* (e.g. removing an intravenous cannula)	Non-sterile gloves and disposable apron.	Hands must be decontaminated after apron and glove removal.
Contact with blood and/or body fluids expected and *high risk of splashing* (e.g. surgical procedures)	Non-sterile gloves and disposable apron. Eye and mouth protection.	Hands must be decontaminated after removal of personal protective clothing.
Source isolation	Non-sterile gloves and disposable apron. Face mask may also be required.	Details of specific requirements depend on the organism that is being isolated.

(From Wilson 2006.)

Gloves should be used as single-use items, being put on immediately before carrying out a clinical procedure and being removed immediately after completion of the procedure (Pratt et al 2007).

Use of disposable aprons

Disposable plastic apron are used to protect clothing by reducing the risk of contamination.

Procedures Box 4.3 Use of non-sterile gloves

Action
Decontaminate your hands thoroughly.

Reason *The use of gloves does not negate the need for thorough hand decontamination.*

Action
Choose a pair of gloves that are well fitting.

Reason *Gloves that do not have a good fit may affect the dexterity of the user.*

Action
Following use, remove the gloves without touching the wrists or hands.

Reason *Reduces the risk of hand contamination.*

Action
Dispose of used gloves in a clinical waste bin with foot-operated action.

Reason *Contaminated gloves are classed as clinical waste and should be disposed of accordingly.*

Action
Decontaminate your hands thoroughly.

Reason *Hands may still become contaminated even though gloves are worn.*

Procedures Box 4.4 Use of disposable aprons

Action
Decontaminate your hands thoroughly.

Reason *Hands should always be decontaminated prior to carrying out a clinical procedure.*

Action
Place the apron over the head, avoiding contact with hair and clothing.

Reason *Avoids contamination of the hands.*

Action
Tie loosely around the waist.

Reason *Allows splashes of water to run off the apron and not gather around the waist.*

Action
After use remove the apron by breaking the neckband, folding the apron down, breaking the waist ties and folding the apron, touching only the side of the apron next to the clothing.

Reason *Avoids contamination of clothing during the process of removing the apron.*

Action
Dispose of the used apron in a clinical waste bin with foot-operated action.

Reason *Contaminated aprons are classed as clinical waste and should be disposed of accordingly.*

Action
Decontaminate your hands thoroughly.

Reason *If organic matter is present on the hands then soap and water should be used to wash the hands.*

Use of masks and eye protection

Eye protection and masks should be available for use in clinical settings in which there is a risk of splashing of blood and/or body fluids on to the face. Surgical and obstetric procedures are those most commonly requiring this type of personal protective equipment (Wilson 2006).

Use and disposal of sharps

A sharp is defined as any item that may cause a laceration or puncture the skin, for example needles, scalpel blades, suture removers and glass (Fig. 4.3; Wilson 2006).

A sharps injury is defined as an injury sustained following contact with a sharp. Clearly the risk of a healthcare worker acquiring an infection from a sharps injury is related to the degree of contamination of the sharp, the severity of the injury sustained and the presence of a pathogenic organism on the

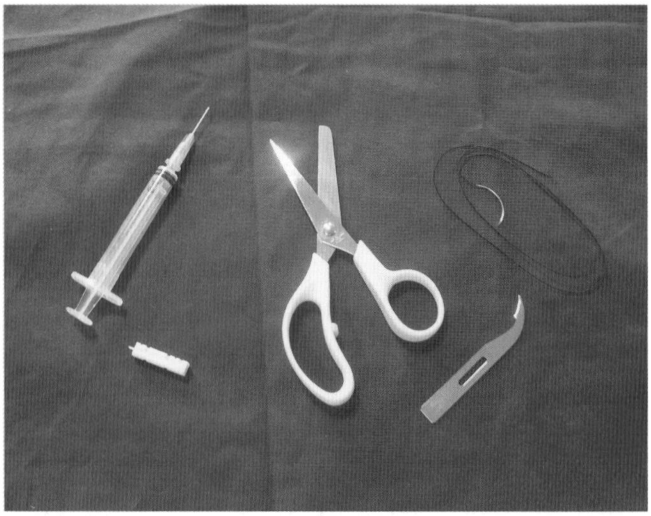

Fig. 4.3 • Sharps.

Procedures Box 4.5 Use and disposal of sharps

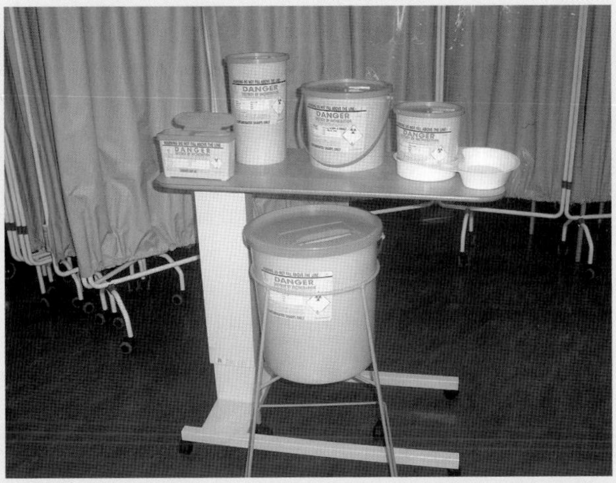

Action
Take a sharps disposal container with you when carrying out a procedure that entails the disposal of a used sharp.

Reason *Disposal of used sharps as near as possible to the point of use reduces the risk of injury.*

Action
Never resheath a used needle.

Reason *Resheathing of a used needle increases the risk of a sharps injury.*

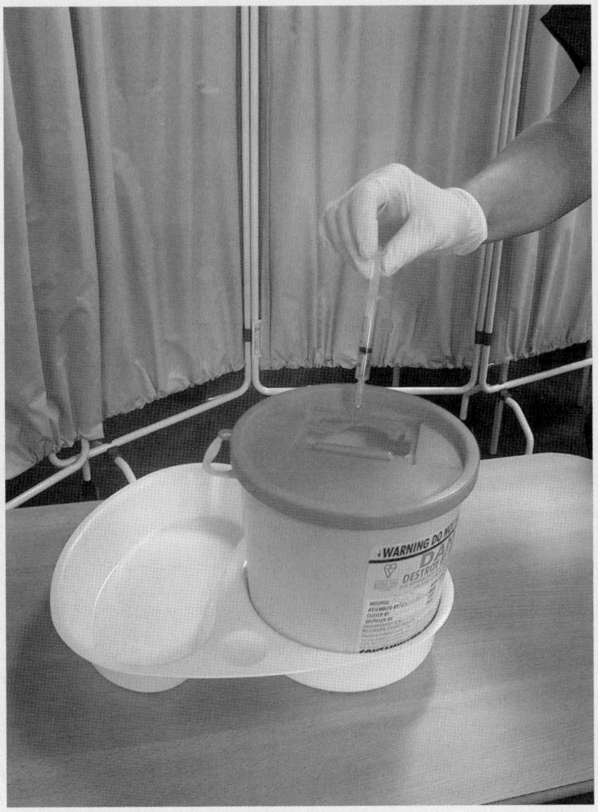

Action
Dispose of the used needle and syringe as a complete item into an approved container.

Reason *Removing the needle from the syringe increases the manipulation of the device and therefore increases the risk of a sharps injury.*

Action
Always dispose of sharps that you have used, and do not pass them to anyone else to dispose of.

Reason *Passing sharps to others increases the risk of sustaining an injury.*

Action
Keep sharps disposal containers out of the reach of children.

Reason *Reduces the risk of a child sustaining a sharps injury; sharps disposal containers are brightly coloured and would attract the attention of children if within their reach.*

Action
Sharps disposal containers should be sealed when two-thirds full and disposed of according to hospital policy; they should *not* be placed inside a yellow bag for disposal.

Reason *Overfilling sharps disposal containers increases the risk of sustaining an injury.*

sharp. There have been a number of cases of healthcare workers who have acquired a blood-borne virus such as human immunodeficiency virus (HIV) or hepatitis B (Wilson 2006).

Disposal of waste

It is important that any waste produced in the clinical setting is segregated appropriately at the point of production. This is to ensure that the waste enters the correct waste management stream and therefore poses the minimum of risk to waste handlers (Wilson 2006). There are also considerable financial and environmental costs involved in waste disposal, which are optimised when the correct procedures are followed (Hilton 2004).

All bags and containers used in the disposal of waste must comply with appropriate legislation (Fig. 4.4 and Table 4.3; Health Services Advisory Committee 1999).

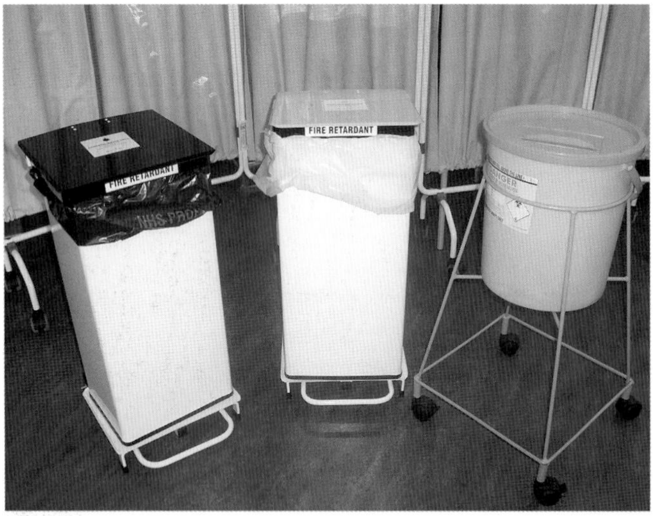

Fig. 4.4 • Containers for the disposal of waste.

Table 4.3. Disposal of waste

Type of waste	Colour of bag	Method of disposal
Household waste (e.g. paper, flowers, hand towels)	Black	Landfill
Clinical waste (e.g. material that is contaminated with blood and body fluid, gloves, aprons)	Yellow	Incineration
Sharps (e.g. needles, syringes, broken glass)	Yellow sharps disposal bin	Incineration

(From Health Services Advisory Committee 1999, with permission of HSE Books.)

Spillages

All spillages of blood and/or body fluids should be dealt with promptly by an appropriate member of staff. The procedure for dealing with such a spillage will vary between organisations, but the same principles will apply.

Patient equipment

Patients have a right to expect that equipment and medical devices that are to be used as part of their care delivery have been decontaminated appropriately and are safe to be used. It is important that manufacturer's recommendations are followed when decontaminating equipment of any sort.

Checking sterile equipment

It is important that equipment that should be sterile is checked before use on a patient. Equipment should be checked for any breaks in the wrapping. If the wrapping has become wet the equipment should not be used, as this would allow for organism

Procedures Box 4.6 Dealing with spillages

Action
Put on a disposable apron and disposable, non-sterile gloves.
Reason *Reduces contamination of the hands and clothing while carrying out the procedure.*

Action
Absorb the liquid using disposable paper towels and dispose of these in a yellow clinical waste bag.
Reason *Helps limit the spread of contaminated fluid.*

Action
Disinfect using 1% sodium hypochlorite solution (1000 ppm) or chlorine-based granules left for 2 min; these should not be used on urine, as this will result in toxic fumes.
Reason *Inactivates any virus that may be present.*

Action
Clean and dry the area using general purpose detergent with reference to local cleaning procedures.
Reason *Removes all contaminated material.*

Action
Remove protective clothing and place it in a yellow clinical waste bag.
Reason *Breaks the chain of infection.*

Action
Wash your hands thoroughly.
Reason *Ensures that the hands are decontaminated before carrying out another procedure.*

Table 4.4. The three levels of decontamination

Decontamination	Definition
Cleaning	The physical removal of organic matter and some microorganisms using detergent and water. Drying following cleaning is very important to reduce microbial growth.
Disinfection	A process by which harmful organisms are removed but spores are not usually destroyed.
Sterilisation	A process that destroys all microorganisms and spores.

Table 4.5. Type of decontamination

Level of risk	Equipment	Decontamination
Low	To be used or has been used on intact skin	Cleaning: wash with detergent and water and dry
Medium	Has been used on mucous membranes or is likely to be contaminated with easily transferable microbes	Disinfection or sterilisation
High	Penetrates the skin and/or mucous membranes or enters a sterile cavity of the body	Sterilisation

transmission through the wrapping and present a risk of microbial contamination

There are three levels of decontamination (Table 4.4).

The type of decontamination required for a piece of equipment that has been used depends on what the equipment is to be used for. This is described in Table 4.5.

Single-use devices

Single-use products are labelled with the words 'single use' or similar and marked with the symbol shown in Figure 4.5. An example is shown in Figure 4.6.

A single-use device is intended to be used once only and then discarded. For example, needles, syringes, cannulae and

Fig. 4.5 • Symbol meaning single use only.

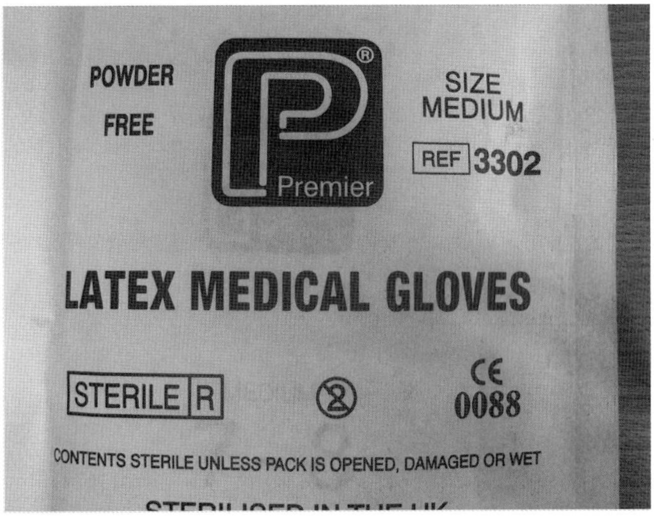

Fig. 4.6 • A single-use product: gloves.

Procedures Box 4.7 Source isolation precautions

Action
Nurse the patient in a single room.

Reason *This is essential for patients with infections spread by the airborne or respiratory droplet route; it is also preferable for patients with infections spread by direct contact.*

Action
Limit patient movement.

Reason *Reduces the risk of transmission of the organism.*

Action
Personal protective equipment should be put on before entering the isolation room.

Reasons *Gloves and aprons should be worn when dealing with infective material (e.g. respiratory secretions, diarrhoea, vomit). Masks should be worn for certain procedures when respiratory secretions are being dealt with.*

Action
Following care delivery the personal protective equipment should be removed and disposed of into a yellow clinical waste bag inside the isolation room.

Reason *Ensures that the infective organism is less likely to spread outside the isolation room.*

Action
Hands should be washed inside the isolation room.

Reason *Removes any contamination of the hands acquired during the care of the patient.*

Action
Hands should be decontaminated using alcohol rub or gel on leaving the room.

Reason *Ensures that any subsequent contamination of the hands is removed on leaving the room.*

urinary catheters are all single-use items. Therefore any piece of equipment designated as single use should not be decontaminated but should be disposed of as clinical waste after use. If a staff member prepares a single-use product for further use, then legal liability for the safe performance of the product is transferred from the manufacturer to the staff member or to the organisation that employs him or her.

Single-patient use

An item that has been identified as single-patient use may be used on more than one occasion but should not be used by more than one patient (e.g. nebulisers and nasal cannulae). The piece of equipment should be decontaminated after each use but should be disposed of when no longer required by the patient or at the duration recommended by the manufacturer.

Equipment sent for repair

All patient equipment (e.g. pressure-relieving mattresses) should be cleaned prior to leaving the ward, department or clinic for loan, service or repair. This is in order to minimise the risk of infection to those who are required to work on such pieces of equipment.

All equipment presented for service or repair must be provided with a decontamination certificate according to local policies (Medical Devices Agency 2003).

Following decontamination all equipment should be correctly reassembled according to the manufacturer's guidance. Staff must be adequately trained to be able to disassemble and reassemble equipment and check that it is operating normally before reuse.

Responsibility for cleaning of patient equipment should be agreed locally.

Source isolation precautions

The purpose of source isolation is to minimise the risk of transmission of pathogenic organisms from the source patient to others at risk (Wilson 2006). Successful source isolation is achieved by ensuring that procedures are followed appropriate to the route of transmission of the organism being isolated.

Standard precautions, as described above, should be followed for all patients at all times. In addition, when patients are known to have or are suspected of having an infectious disease, extra precautions may be required. These include nursing patients in single rooms, and wearing gloves, aprons and masks as appropriate in relation to how the infecting pathogen is spread, e.g. gloves and aprons to be worn when nursing a patient with streptococcal impetigo (Heyman 2004).

Examples of common infections in children that should be isolated in clinical practice are shown in Table 4.6.

Aseptic technique

Many invasive procedures that are carried out in clinical practice require an aseptic technique to be used to minimise the risk of introducing pathogens into a vulnerable part of the body (Hilton 2004). The aim of the technique is to reduce contamination during the process of the invasive procedure. Clinical teams are required to demonstrate high standards of aseptic technique (Department of Health 2003).

How to put on a pair of sterile gloves

Sterile gloves are always packaged with the cuffs folded down so that they can be put on without contamination by the hands. The first glove to be put on should be handled only by the cuff, and the second glove should be touched only by the other gloved hand.

Clinical procedures that require to be carried out using an aseptic technique include:

- redressing acute wounds
- urinary catheterisation
- cannulation
- care of central venous catheters.

Table 4.6. Childhood infections requiring isolation in clinical practice. Reprinted with permission from the American Public Health Association.

Infection or disease	Transmission	Infectivity	Isolation
Bronchiolitis	Droplet and direct contact with secretions	While symptomatic (around 5 days)	Required: single room
Chickenpox (varicella zoster virus)	Direct contact, droplet or airborne spread of secretions	1–2 days before onset of rash and up to 5 days after first appearance of vesicles	Required: single room – only immune individuals should enter the room
Impetigo: staphylococcal or streptococcal	Direct contact with lesion	Duration of the lesions	Required: contact precautions
Measles	Droplet and direct contact with nasal and throat secretions	From just before the rash appearing until 4 days after	Required: single room

Table 4.6. Childhood infections requiring isolation in clinical practice—cont'd

Infection or disease	Transmission	Infectivity	Isolation
Meningococcal meningitis	Direct contact with respiratory droplets, nasal and oral secretions	Until organism no longer present in secretions	Required until 24 h after appropriate treatment
Viral meningitis	Faeco–oral or respiratory spread	Before and during acute illness	Not required
Meticillin-resistant *Staphylococcus aureus*	Direct contact with infected or colonised skin or lesions	Until culture negative	Required: follow local policy
Mumps	Respiratory droplet and direct contact with saliva	7 days before symptoms to 9 days after	Required: single room
Rotavirus	Faeco–oral and/or possibly respiratory spread	Up to 8 days after the onset of symptoms	Required: enteric precautions
Respiratory syncytial virus	Droplet and direct contact with secretions	While symptomatic (around 5 days)	Required: single room
Scabies	Skin-to-skin contact	Until treatment has been applied	Required until 24 h after effective treatment given
Tuberculosis (pulmonary)	Airborne droplet	While there are viable bacilli present in sputum	Required: single room
Whooping cough	Direct contact with respiratory droplets and airborne	Very infectious in early stages, but this is reduced after 3 weeks	Required: single room

(From Heyman 2004.)

Procedures Box 4.8 How to put on a pair of sterile gloves

Action
Open the non-sterile outer packaging.

Reason *This should be done on a large, clean, dry surface to reduce the risk of contamination.*

Action
Decontaminate the hands.

Reason *Hands should always be decontaminated prior to applying sterile gloves.*

Action
Open the inner sterile wrapping, exposing the gloves with the palms facing upwards.

Reason *The gloves are placed in this position to facilitate putting them on without the risk of contamination.*

Action
Pick up the first glove by the cuff, making sure that the only contact made by the hands is with the inside of the glove.

Reason *Avoids the risk of contamination of the glove by the hand.*

Action
Holding the glove in one hand slip the other hand into the glove, making sure that nothing is touched by the gloved hand.

Reason *If this does not feel comfortable at this stage wait until the other glove is put on before adjusting it.*

Action
Slide the fingers of the gloved hand under the folded cuff of the remaining glove and pick it up.

Reason *Ensure that only the outside of the second glove is touched by the gloved hand.*

Action
Put the glove on to the second hand by pulling steadily through the cuff, taking care not to contaminate this glove with the ungloved hand.

Reason *A slow, steady technique is more likely to result in the glove being put on successfully.*

Action
Adjust the fingers of both gloves until they fit comfortably.

Reason *Make sure that only the outside of the gloves are touched by both hands.*

Procedures Box 4.9 Carrying out aseptic technique

Action
Decontaminate the hands and put on a disposable apron.

Reason *Protects clothing from the risk of contamination.*

Action
Ensure that the trolley is clean; it is not always necessary to clean the surface before every use.

Reason *Local policies should be followed.*

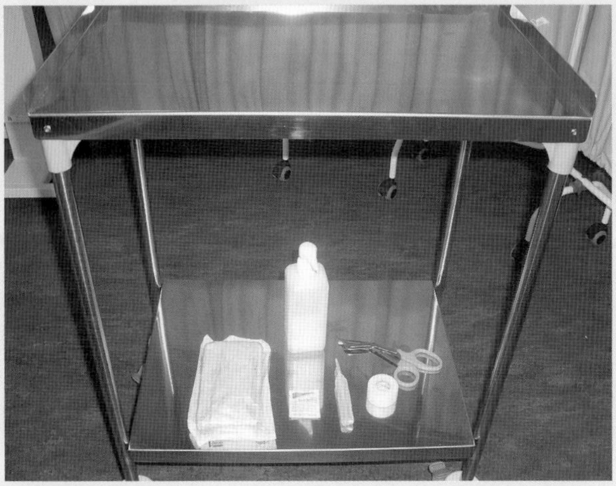

Action
Collect all equipment required for the procedure and place it on the bottom shelf of the trolley, having checked for sterility and expiry date.

Reason *All sterile equipment should be within date and have intact packaging.*

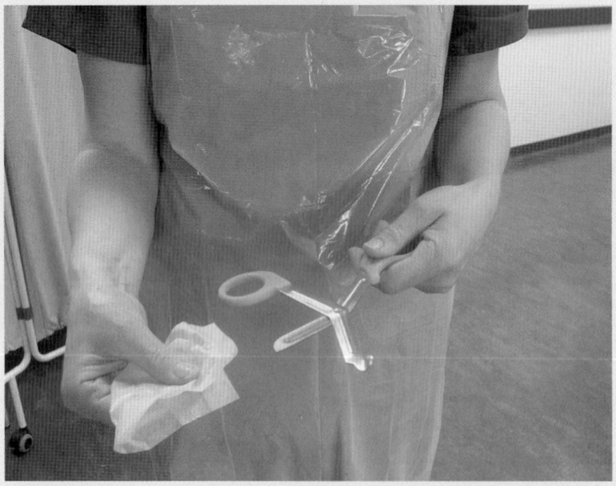

Action
Prepare scissors if cutting non-sterile tape by washing, drying and decontaminating using alcohol wipes.

Reason *Sterile scissors are required only if being used on sterile equipment that is to be in contact with high-risk areas of the body.*

Action
Take the trolley to the patient.

Action
Open the outer packaging of the dressing pack and place on the top of the trolley without allowing the outside packaging to touch the inside wrap.

Reason *The outside wrapping is contaminated and should not come into contact with the sterile equipment inside the packaging.*

Action
Open the dressing pack wrapping by touching only the corners of the wrapping paper; this will create a sterile field.

Reason *Do not touch any other part of the wrapping, as this will result in contamination of the sterile field.*

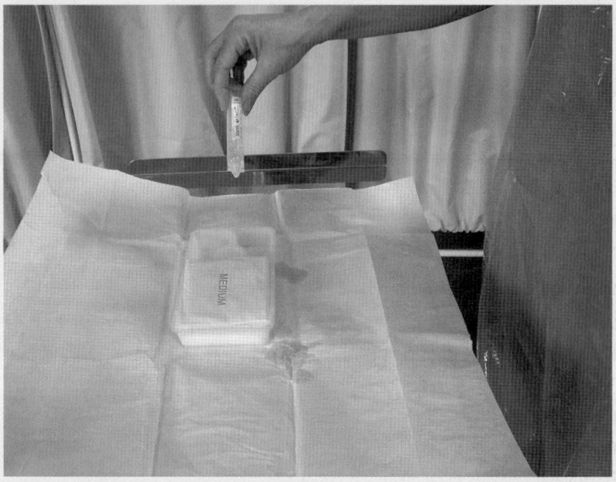

Action
Pour solution for cleansing wounds and open sterile dressing, etc., on to the sterile field without contamination.

Reason *This should be done without making contact between the solution and the sterile field.*

Action
Loosen the patient's dressing.

Action
Decontaminate your hands.

Reason *Hands should always be decontaminated prior to applying sterile gloves or handling sterile equipment.*

Action
Place a hand into the sterile yellow waste bag and use this to organise the contents of the dressing pack on the sterile field.

Reason *The waste bag acts as a glove and allows handling of sterile equipment without the risk of contamination.*

Action
Remove the patient's soiled dressing using the hand inside the waste bag.

Reason *Reduces the risk of contaminating the hands while removing the soiled dressing.*

Action
Turn the waste bag inside out with the used dressing inside and attach the bag to the side of the trolley nearest the patient.

Reason *Placing the bag nearer to the patient reduces the risk of contamination of the sterile field when disposing of soiled swabs and dressings.*

Procedures Box 4.9 Carrying out aseptic technique—cont'd

Action
Put on sterile gloves without contamination of the outside of the gloves.

Reason *See How to put on a pair of sterile gloves procedure box.*

Action
Carry out the invasive procedure or dressing, etc.

Reason *National and local policies and guidance should be followed in all aspects of the procedure.*

Action
Dispose of any sharps in a sharps bin.

Reason *Minimal handling of sharps is recommended to reduce the risk of a needlestick injury.*

Actions
Remove gloves and place them in the waste bag.

Wrap all used disposable equipment in the sterile field and place in the waste bag.

Seal the waste bag and place in a clinical waste bin.

Action
Decontaminate your hands.

Reason *All clinical procedures should be followed with hand decontamination to reduce the risk of cross-infection.*

Key definitions

- Aseptic: free of microorganisms.
- Colonisation: microorganisms present at a body site without any evidence of symptoms of illness or infection.
- Commensal: a microorganism that is part of the normal flora of the body (e.g. *Escherichia coli* in the gut).
- Disinfection: a process that reduces the level of microorganisms to a level that is not harmful. Spores may not be removed.
- Endogenous infection: an infection caused by microorganisms originating from the patient's own body.
- Exogenous infection: an infection caused by a microorganism originating from a source other than the patient's own body.
- Fomites: inanimate objects that may be vehicles of transmission of microorganisms.
- Healthcare-acquired infection: an infection acquired during a period of healthcare.
- Infection: damage of body tissue by microorganisms or toxins released by microorganisms.
- Microorganism: an organism that is not visible to the naked eye.
- Nosocomial infection: healthcare-acquired infection (see above).
- Pathogen: a disease-causing microorganism.
- Sterilisation: a process that destroys all microorganisms and spores.
- Virus: an organism that can only replicate inside another cell.

See Damani (2003) and Wilson (2006).

References

British Standards Institution (2000) Medical gloves for surgical use. BSI, London

Damani NN (2003) Manual of infection control procedures, 2nd edn. Greenwich, London

Department of Health (2003) NICE guidelines – infection control, prevention of healthcare associated infection in primary and community care. Department of Health, London

Gillespie XX, Bamford XX (2003) Medical microbiology and infection at a glance. Blackwell, Oxford

Health Services Advisory Committee (1999) Safe disposal of clinical waste. HSE Books, Sudbury

Heyman DL (ed.) *(2004)* Control of communicable diseases manual, 18th edn. American Public Health Association, Washington, DC

Hilton P (2004) Fundamental nursing skills. Whurr, Chichester

Infection Control Nurses Association (1999) Glove usage guidelines. ICNA and Regent Medical, London

McCulloch J (2000) Infection control: science, management and practice. Whurr, Chichester

Medical Devices Agency (2003) Management of medical devices prior to repair service or investigation (MDA) DB2003(05)

National Audit Office (2000) The challenge of hospital acquired infection. HMSO, London

Nicol M, Bavin C, Bedford-Turner S, Cronin P, Rawlings-Anderson K (2004) Essential nursing skills. Mosby, Edinburgh

Plowman R, Graves N, Taylor L et al (1999) Socio-economic burden of hospital acquired infections. Department of Health, London

Pratt LJ, McDougall C, Wilcox MH (2007) epic 2: National Evidence-based Guidelines for Preventing Healthcare Associated Infections in NHS Hospitals in England. Journal of Hospital Infection 655:S1–S64

Wilson J (2006) Infection control in clinical practice, 3rd edn. Baillière Tindall, London

5 The principles of handling children

Karen Jeffery • Jane Swain

Theoretical approach

The risks associated with the lifting and handling of children are complex. This chapter outlines some of the risks involved and offers guidance on how to minimise these risks. Basic principles to be considered are presented, together with some examples of how these principles can be followed in specific situations. It is stressed, however, that each situation is different, and an assessment of individual circumstances must be made for each situation. Handlers need appropriate manual handling training, provided by their employer, before engaging in handling activities.

ALERT
The principles of handling children are complex. Each situation must be judged separately and a thorough assessment undertaken. The needs of both the child and the handler must be considered. Manual handling must comply with national and local policy and guidelines.

Legislation

Manual handling accounts for 40% of all sickness-related absence in the National Health Service (Department of Health 2004a), at a cost of £400 million a year (Department of Health 2004b). The application of safer techniques when handling children is therefore beneficial for the handler as well as the child being handled.

This chapter looks at the manual handling issues faced by nurses and healthcare workers and also informal carers working with children. There is a common misconception that children, being (mostly) small compared with adults, do not pose a risk to carers in relation to musculoskeletal injury. As will be explained later any lifting can pose a risk, as can the postures and stooping involved in caring for children and managing associated equipment. The reader needs to use this chapter in conjunction with the policies and legislation relating to the work area. The National Health Service learning unit on manual handling (National Health Service 2007) provides an introduction to the risks and the principles of safer handling and is recommended to those with little prior handling experience.

The healthcare team have a legal (Health and Safety at Work Act 1974, Management of Health and Safety at Work Regulations 1999, Manual Handling Operations Regulations 1992) and professional (Nursing and Midwifery Council 2004) responsibility to handle patients safely in a manner that is not undignified or degrading (Human Rights Act 1998). The Health and Safety at Work Act (1974) sets out the employer's duty to ensure the 'health, safety and welfare' of employees (and also informal carers such as parents) within the healthcare setting. It is important to understand, however, that the employer's duty under Health and Safety at Work Act is not absolute, as the duty to protect employees and others is qualified by the phrase 'as far as is reasonably practicable'. This, together with the Human Rights Act (1998), may mean that there are occasions when some risk to the handler may be legally permissible. The needs of the handler should to be balanced with the needs and rights of the child (Mandelstam 2005).

To comply with legislation and promote best practice for both handlers and those being handled, most healthcare and social service providers have developed 'safer' or 'minimal' lifting policies, acknowledging that 'no lifting policies' are unworkable, as some lifting may be essential in certain circumstances (e.g. lifting a small child). The Manual Handling Operations Regulations (1992) set out four steps to guide handlers in the decision-making process, which in turn should promote safer handling. These are as follows:

- Avoid manual handling operations involving risk of injury (so far as is reasonably practicable).
- Assess task, load, environment and capabilities of handlers when hazardous manual handling activities cannot be avoided.
- On the basis of the assessment, plan the handling operation to reduce the risk of injury to the lowest reasonably practicable level, using equipment as necessary.
- Review the assessment each time a manoeuvre is performed and modify the plan if necessary.

Avoid

First consider if the move is necessary and avoid unnecessary manoeuvres. When possible, children should be encouraged to move themselves but may need handler guidance. The handler needs to communicate at a pitch conversant with the child's level of understanding. Pain relief should be given if required, which may aid the child in moving by himself or herself.

Assessment of risk

Having established that it is not appropriate to avoid handling interventions, an assessment should be carried out. Babies may be light in weight but can still pose a handling challenge, such as getting them out of the cot or carrying them to the pushchair. Even a pushchair can pose a problem if not appropriately designed for the needs of the handler. All these activities require an assessment of risk.

Guidance in the Manual Handling Operations Regulations (1992) suggests four aspects of risk that need to be assessed:

1. Task to be performed
2. Individual capability
3. Load
4. Environment.

This is the TILE principle.

Task

The task to be performed must be clearly defined. Preparing children may take longer than the task itself, which can lead handlers to put themselves at risk. Stooping, twisting and bending inappropriately are hazards to be considered and avoided. Can the task be broken down to make it easier for the handler? What assistance can the child give? Does the manoeuvre need to be timed to get the child's full cooperation?

Individual

Some individuals are more at risk than others, for example pregnant women and those with previous back injury. Each individual handler needs to be aware of her or his own limitations.

Load

The child may be unpredictable or uncooperative and heavier than the safe lifting threshold. Children may have complex needs that will affect the manoeuvre.

Environment

The environment in which the manoeuvre is taking place needs consideration. There may be constraints caused by equipment, furniture and toys, so preparation of the environment is essential. The hospital setting is designed with handling in mind; however, this may not be the case for children in their own homes.

Reducing risk

Preparing children for a manoeuvre requires their cooperation. In order to achieve this explanations need to be given that are appropriate and at the child's level of understanding. For some this will be through play and simple verbal explanation, for others it will be through gestures and body language.

Children able and willing to move can be very resourceful. All that is needed is the carer's ability to tap into their level of understanding and encourage them to move themselves. The use of play is a valuable tool to help the handler and child. Thinking what would be a fun way to get a manoeuvre accomplished will assist the handler to choose a manoeuvre that will promote the child's cooperation. Many children, despite their limited ability, still want to be independent, and much can be achieved if the carer is able to motivate the child.

Children can, however, be highly unpredictable and at times uncooperative. Those with complex needs may have poor or increased muscle tone and have abnormal patterns of movement. They may need to be positioned in such a way as to promote good body posture, all of which the handler needs to take into consideration.

Giving children some control and say over what should happen to them is also important (Department of Health 2003). A child who chooses how a manoeuvre is carried out is more likely to comply. However, this choice should not compromise the safety of the handler or child.

Position of the handler

In order for the handler to be in the safest position to handle (Fig. 5.1), the following posture must be adopted:

- To maintain stability, the feet should be placed about shoulder width apart, with one foot slightly in front of the other, pointing in the direction of movement.
- To protect the back and avoid stooping, the normal curvatures at the neck and lumbar region should be maintained and twisting and bending sideways avoided.

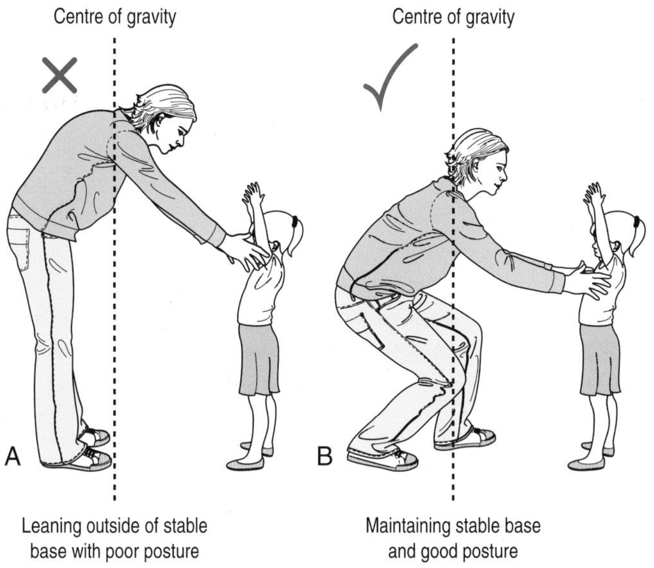

Fig. 5.1 • Stable base and posture of the handler: **(A)** leaning outside a stable base with poor posture; **(B)** maintaining a stable base and good posture.

- The manoeuvre should be powered by the leg and buttock muscles, keeping the knees and hips slightly flexed.
- Ensure that the load is kept close to the body (the optimum position for lifting), with the elbows close to the waist.

Avoiding postural strain

Many childcare activities, although not involving lifting or carrying, can present a postural risk, for example bathing and playing with children on the floor. Both these activities involve prolonged working at a low level. The carer should prepare for these activities, and a risk assessment using TILE will help alert the carer to these risks and the reduction strategies necessary. If the TILE principle is applied, for example, to bathing a child (Table 5.1) a number of questions arise. This will help to identify the risks involved.

Equipment

There is an array of equipment on the market to assist in handling, some specifically designed for use with children.

Low-cost mobility aids such as rope ladders, monkey poles, hand blocks, sliding sheets, handling belts and transfer boards (banana and pat) are useful aids to handling. Research has shown, however, that despite the usefulness of these they are still being under-utilised (Owen 1988, Swain et al 2003). It is recommended that children should have their own moving aids, especially if there is a long-term need, as sharing of equipment carries the additional risk of cross-infection (Barnett et al 1999). When slings are going to be used by more than one child there should be sufficient quantities, enabling washing and prevention of cross-infection.

Equipment should not be improvised, as it will not have been tested as safe. All equipment must be manufactured and

Table 5.1. Application of TILE to bathing a baby

	Risk assessment	Reducing risk
Task	Stooping, static posture, twisting, pushing or pulling, risk of sudden movement, carrying over a distance, lifting or lowering into the bath	Prepare for the task, as it may not be possible to leave a child without additional assistance. Use a crib or pushchair to transport the baby to the bathroom rather than carry. Use a changing tallboy to undress and dress the baby, as it is of a suitable height. The use of a baby or hydraulic bath or sink may be more appropriate than a conventional bath (Fig. 5.2). When this is not available handlers should position themselves to reduce undue stretching or bending.
Individual	A handler who has health problems, is pregnant or is in need of training	The handler should be appropriately trained, utilising the help of more than one handler if necessary. The handler may be better equipped to handle a load early in the day rather than at the end of a long shift, requiring a change in the child's normal routine.
Load	A child who is bulky, difficult to grasp, unstable, unpredictable or uncooperative	Utilise appropriate equipment to help in the procedure (e.g. bath net or seat, Fig. 5.3). Time the manoeuvre to get the child's full cooperation.
Environment	A bathroom that may have space constraints, slippery or unstable floors, extremes of temperature, poor lighting and ventilation and toys for the child to play with	Toys are a great hazard in any environment that children frequent. Ensure that these assist with the bathing and do not pose a hazard. Some children get cold quickly requiring the use of heaters. These should be used with caution and should comply with safety standards and local policy. Ensure that the floor does not become wet and slippery, particularly hazardous when the child is splashing about.
Other factors	Handler inappropriately dressed and a child with additional considerations, such as having an intravenous infusion or wound dressing	Handlers should wear clothing that will not hinder movement. However, parents are usually unaware of the risk that high-heeled shoes or tight clothing pose. The handler needs to consider this when engaging the help of others. Intravenous infusions and other such equipment may require the help of additional handlers to reduce the risk these pose.

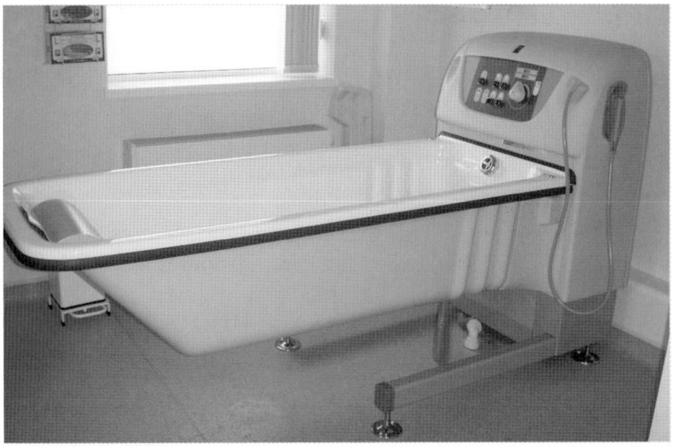

Fig. 5.2 • A hydraulic bath.

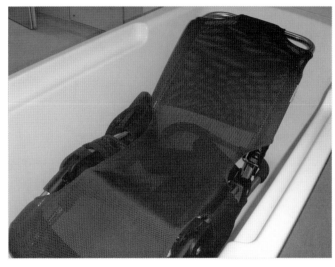

Fig. 5.3 • A bath net.

tested as suitable for the purpose intended and well maintained. This complies with the Provision and Use of Work Equipment Regulations (Health and Safety Executive 1992) and Lifting Operations and Lifting Equipment Regulations 1998 (Health and Safety Executive 2005a,b). Some additions to equipment as in relation to aids for children (Swain & Jeffery 2005) can make them more 'user'-friendly. This, however, must not compromise the safety of the product or the child (Fig. 5.4).

Mechanical aids such as hoists and stand aids will be required by some children. For equipment requiring slings a variety of sizes and patterns should be available to suit children (Fig. 5.5) of different ages. Slings should be of the correct size and type and clearly identified in the child's handling plan.

Parent handler

Many parents lift their children without thought of the implications to themselves (Griffin & Price 2000), which is particularly hazardous for those with children with long-term handling needs. The healthcare provider has a duty to prevent risks to the health and safety of not only employees but also informal carers such as parents (Health and Safety at Work Act 1974). Under the Nursing and Midwifery Council's code of professional conduct (2004), nurses have a duty to act in the best interest of patients, and it may often be in children's best interest for them to be handled by their parent or usual carer. It is necessary therefore to ensure that carers are also conversant with the principles of safer handling. This is particularly important for those families in which the child is likely to need assistance over a period of time, for example when caring for a child with a disability (Fig. 5.6). The nurse has a duty to both child and carer to ensure that they are using appropriate techniques (Nursing and Midwifery Council 2004). Involving the carer in the assessment and planning stage is vital to ensure that this happens.

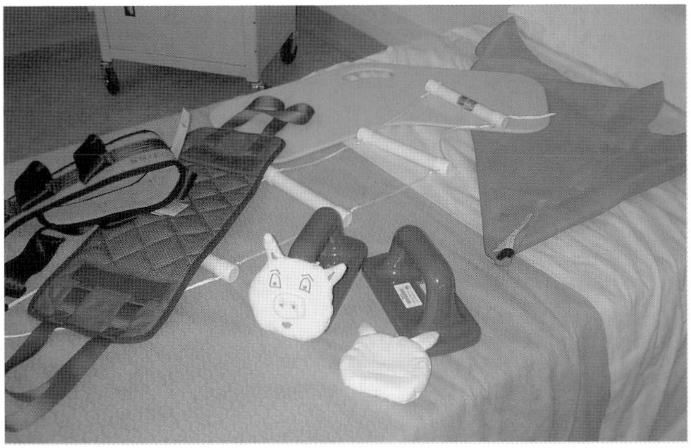

Fig. 5.4 • Handling equipment with pig motifs attached to handling blocks.

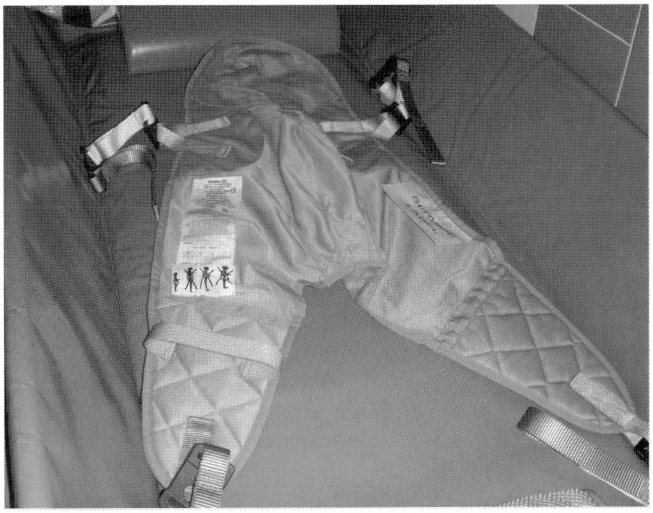

Fig. 5.5 • Child size sling for hoist.

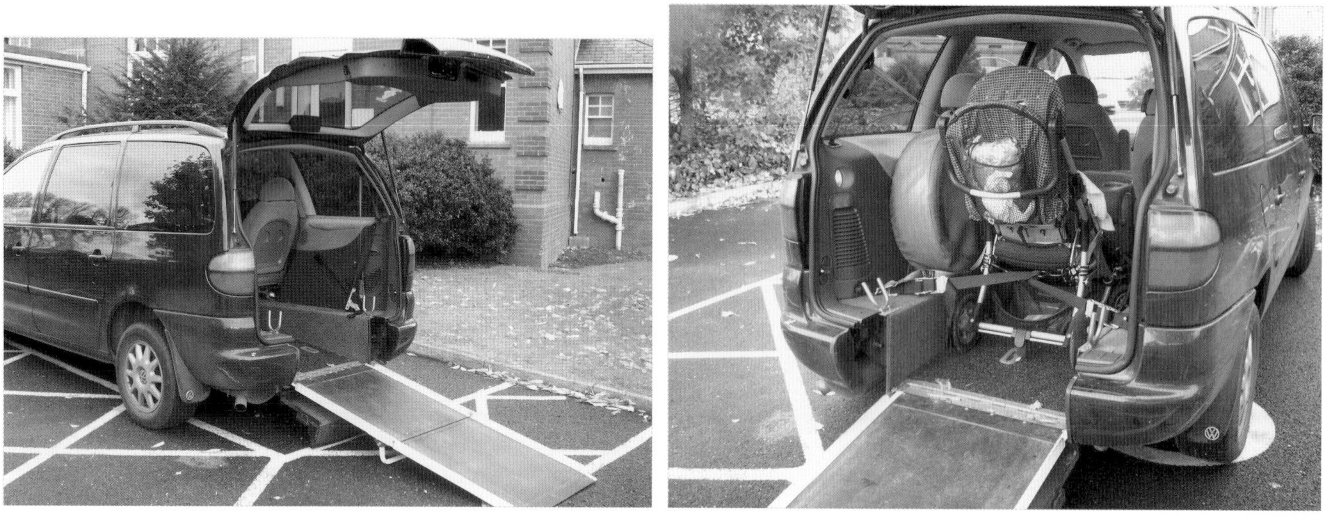

Fig. 5.6 • Rear access mobility car for buggy with ramp.

Review

A child's conditions can change over a short period of time for the better or worse; it is therefore important to review the handling assessment prior to all manoeuvres to ensure that the handling instructions do not compromise the safety of the child or handler and to modify the handling plan if necessary.

Practical approach

When assessing the risk of handling children it is important to consider the following factors together with those already identified:

- Size
- Weight
- Ability
- Need.

The SWAN analysis is a useful way of building on the task, individual, load and environment elements of the TILE risk assessment.

Size and weight

Size and weight of children vary greatly. Children of identical ages can be markedly different in weight and height, with one 5-year-old being on the 5th and another on the 95th centile; however, both children demonstrate normal growth patterns. It is therefore important not to assume that children of the same age will be the same size.

The lifting of a young baby may seem to be low risk to most carers, as the weight of the child may fall within recognised limits (Table 5.2). These weight limits indicate a reasonably safe load for about 95% of handlers. It should be noted that a handler can carry the greatest load when it is close to them and between waist and upper thigh height in relation to the body. A lesser load can be tolerated if the arms are outstretched or held higher or lower than indicated above. However, these weights must be viewed in context, as there are many other factors that need to be considered, such as the ability and position of the handler, the child and the environment in which the manoeuvre is taking place.

Ability

The ability of the child will vary according to her or his developmental age, level of understanding and disability, and whether she or he is ill or technologically dependent (attached to equipment needed to sustain life or optimise health). The handler will need to understand how this will affect the child's ability in order to consider the best way to prepare a child and carry out a manoeuvre.

Need

Differences in size, weight and ability mean that children will have different needs. These should be considered in any handling assessment. However, handlers will need to think not only how a manoeuvre should be performed but also how this information is to be conveyed to the child and who it is to be conveyed by. Many children rely on their parents for guidance. Involving parents therefore in imparting such information may help get the child's cooperation when a stranger may not.

Tables 5.3–5.11 look at some of the specific problems posed when handling children in different situations, identifying risks and giving suggestions on how these risks may be reduced. There may be other solutions appropriate to the context in which the manoeuvre takes place.

Table 5.2. Lifting thresholds for women and men related to child's age

	Close to body		Away from body	
	Boy	*Girl*	*Boy*	*Girl*
Women holding load at				
Shoulder height	7 kg (5.5 months)	7 kg (6 months)	3 kg (newborn)	3 kg (newborn)
Elbow height	13 kg (2 years)	13 kg (2.25 years)	7 kg (5.5 months)	7 kg (6 months)
Knuckle height (with arms down by side)	16 kg (3.5 years)	16 kg (3.75 years)	10 kg (11 months)	10 kg (1 year)
Top third of thigh to mid calf height	13 kg (2 years)	13 kg (2.25 years)	7 kg (5.5 months)	7 kg (6 months)
Mid lower leg height	7 kg (5.5 months)	7 kg (6 months)	3 kg (newborn)	3 kg (newborn)
Men holding load at				
Shoulder height	10 kg (11 months)	10 kg (1 year)	5 kg (2 months)	5 kg (2.5 months)
Elbow height	20 kg (5.75 years)	20 kg (6 years)	10 kg (11 months)	10 kg (1 year)
Knuckle height (with arms down by side)	25 kg (7.75 years)	25 kg (8 years)	15 kg (3 years)	15 kg (3.5 years)
Top third of thigh to mid calf height	20 kg (5.75 years)	20 kg (6 years)	10 kg (11 months)	10 kg (1 year)
Mid lower leg height	10 kg (11 months)	10 kg (1 year)	5 kg (2 months)	5 kg (2.5 months)

(After Health and Safety Executive 2004.)

Table 5.3. Lifting a baby out of a cot with one handler

	Reducing risk
Size	The handler should lift from the side closest to the baby to avoid stretching, being aware of restrictions posed by the cot sides, which can sometimes hinder bending of knees (Figs 5.7 and 5.8). Height-adjustable cots should be used (Kitson 2000).
Weight	The maximum weight a handler can lift will vary with where the child is being lifted from and the handler's position and ability. Care should be taken that this does not exceed those recommended.
Ability	A baby up to the age of 6 months will be totally dependent on the carer, with little ability to assist in the manoeuvre. Knowledge of child development will assist the handler when assessing and planning the manoeuvre.
Need	The baby needs to be lifted safely and be well supported. Wrapping a small baby in a light blanket may make the child easier to grasp. A baby who is hypo- or hypertonic will have specific handling needs, and advice should be sought from the appropriate therapist.

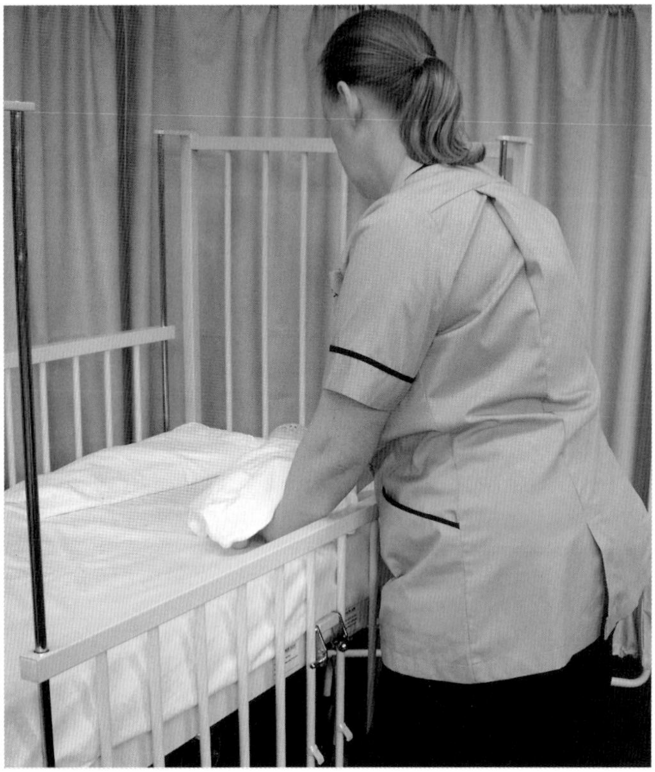

Fig. 5.7 • Lifting a baby out of a cot.

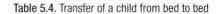

Table 5.4. Transfer of a child from bed to bed

	Reducing risk
Size	A hard transfer board or inflatable transfer mattress may be used (Fig. 5.9). The use of extension straps to prevent the carer over-reaching ensures that a stable base is maintained.
Weight	The weight of the child will dictate the number of handlers required and may require many depending on the child.
Ability	Children requiring this manoeuvre are usually in a passive or an unconscious state or physically disabled and so unable to assist, needing additional consideration (e.g. correct positioning of limbs).
Need	Lots of encouragement in addition to physical support is needed for the conscious child, who may be afraid of falling between beds. Getting the child to focus on an object such as a toy on the receiving bed may assist in the manoeuvre.

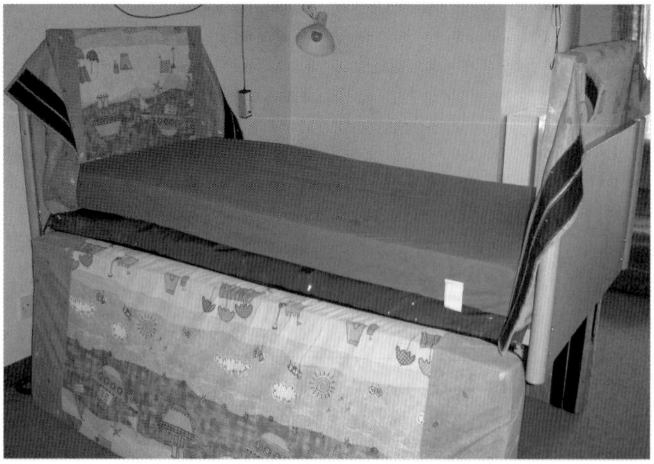

Fig. 5.8 • A bed with adjustable sides.

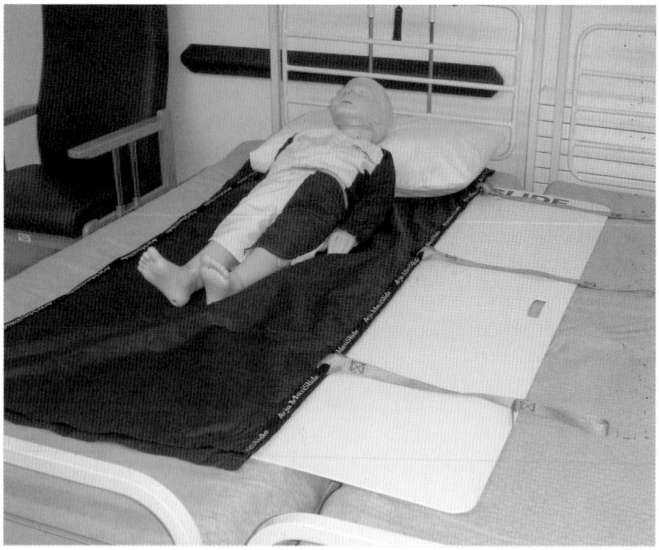

Fig. 5.9 • A transfer board.

Table 5.5. Picking a child up from the floor

	Reducing risk
Size	A small child can be lifted from the floor by one handler. The handler needs to kneel to one side of the child and lift him or her on to the knee then towards the chest prior to standing (Fig. 5.10).
Weight	Use of mechanical handling aids, such as the hoist, may be needed for the bigger child.
Ability	An inflatable cushion (which requires the child to have good sitting balance), a hoist or a transfer scoop (Betts & Mowbray 2004) may be required for the less able child.
Need	Children need space to play in order to develop. The child who presents a challenge when getting up from the floor could have an alternative play area such as a raised playpen.

Table 5.6. Assisting a child to stand from sitting

	Reducing risk
Size	It is important that children sit in appropriately sized chairs so that they can place their feet on the floor, facilitating them to stand. Assisting the child sitting in the middle of a large chair may cause the handler postural strain, as it is difficult to get close to the child.
Weight	The weight of the child is less significant than her or his ability to assist in the manoeuvre.
Ability	The child must be able to weight bear and be able to assist the handler, which requires his or her full cooperation. The handler needs to time the manoeuvre to achieve this, and it should not be performed when the child is tired or in pain.
Need	The child needs know what is expected of her or him and requires an age-appropriate explanation.

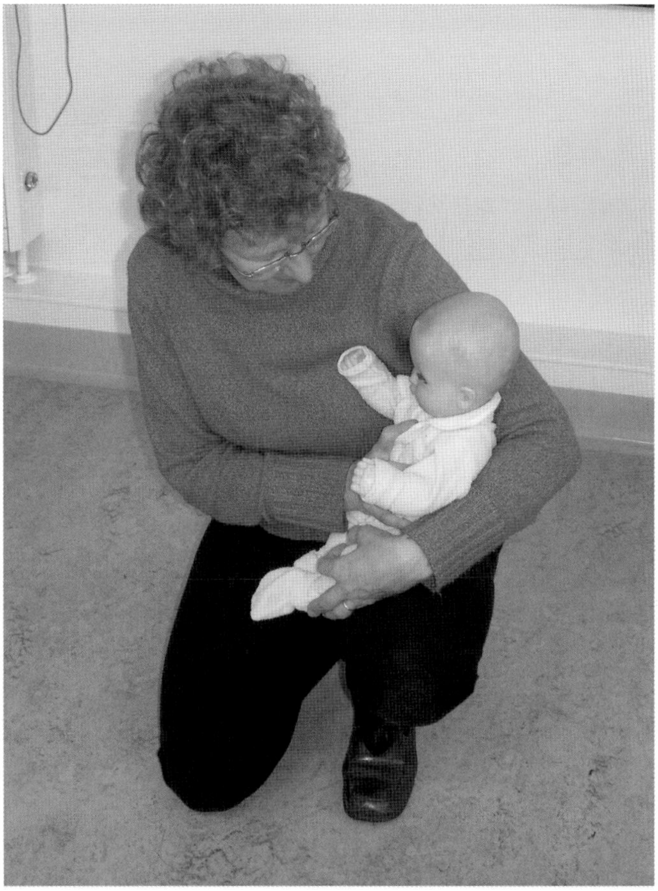

Fig. 5.10 • Picking a child from the floor.

Table 5.7. Sitting a child up in bed

	Reducing risk
Size	Small children in adult size beds may necessitate the handler placing the knee on the bed to get close to the load. A back raiser with straps (Fig. 5.11) can help the handler remain in a good position when sitting the child.
Weight	Profiling beds are the ideal but may not be safe for smaller children; however, they are useful in high-dependency areas where the child remains supervised at all times.
Ability	A rope ladder attached to the bottom of the bed can assist the child to sit independently. Numbering or colour coding the rungs can help the child to use this with minimal instruction.
Need	Cooperation of the child can be achieved through play. Attaching small toys to the rope ladder can encourage the child to use this to full effect without compromising safety.

Table 5.8. Hoisting a child

	Reducing risk
Size	Each hoist (Fig. 5.12) should have a number of slings to suit children of various sizes. Using too large a sling may cause the child to feel insecure or slip, causing a potential hazard. Always refer to the manufacturer's instructions.
Weight	Most children will fall well below the maximum weight for most hoists. However, with obesity levels rising in children consideration should be given to the maximum weight each hoist can take.
Ability	The cooperation of the child is required, and care must be taken that limbs and head are supported and do not get trapped.
Need	Most children approached correctly will see this manoeuvre as a great adventure, but careful explanation or demonstration may be required. Dignity, privacy and comfort must be maintained if the child's ongoing cooperation is to be maintained.

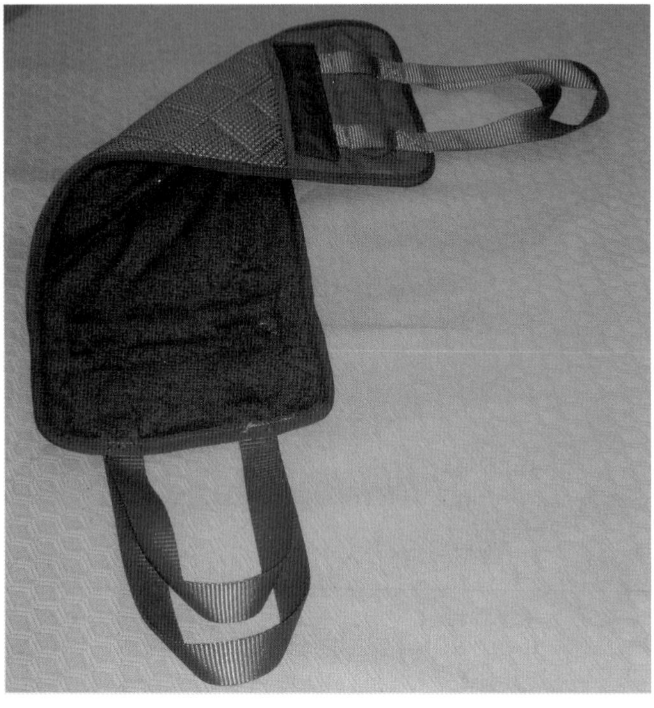

Fig. 5.11 • A back raiser with straps.

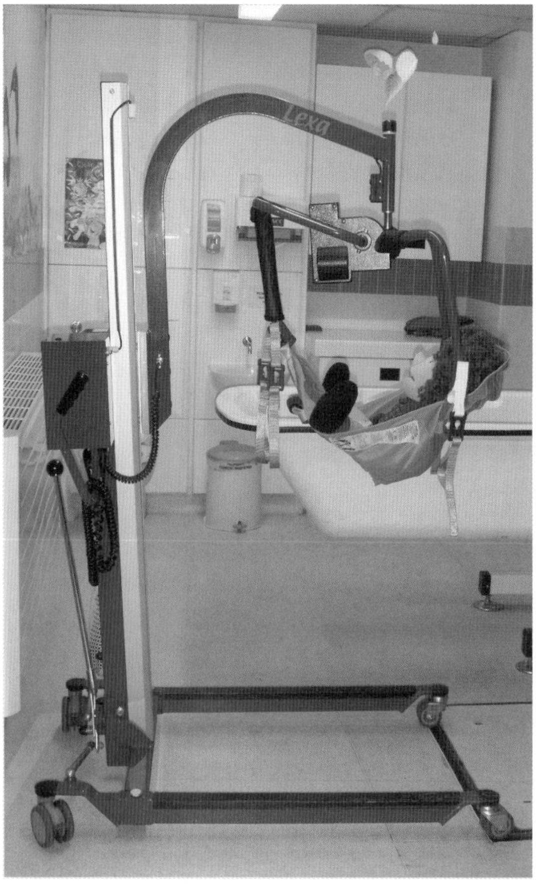

Fig. 5.12 • A hoist.

Table 5.9. Bathing a larger child

	Reducing risk
Size	The bigger child will normally be able to bathe with minimal assistance unless ill or physically compromised. An appropriately sized bath will assist greatly in this manoeuvre.
Weight	Equipment such as hydraulic baths (Fig. 5.2), a hoist and a bath net that cradles the less able child in the bath (Fig. 5.3) may be required.
Ability	This will vary from child to child. The use of steps and non-slip mats may assist the independent child and reduce handler intervention.
Need	Safety is paramount, not only for the child but also for the handler. Remember, children like to splash about in the bath, making the floor hazardous. Ensuring that the floor is dry before embarking on any manoeuvre is vital.

Table 5.10. Administering intravenous medication

	Reducing risk
Size	A small child in a large bed could mean that the nurse has to stoop or stretch to access the intravenous site (Fig. 5.13). Ensuring that the bed is at an appropriate height with the nurse sitting in a chair close to the bed will reduce postural strain and over-stretching.
Weight	Even a small limb can become heavy if held. Ideally the limb should be placed flat onto a pillow or bed to ensure the comfort of the child and nurse during the procedure.
Ability	Some children may require persuasion and distraction to allow the nurse time to deliver the medication.
Need	It may be appropriate for the child to sit on the parent's lap for emotional security and comfort during the procedure.

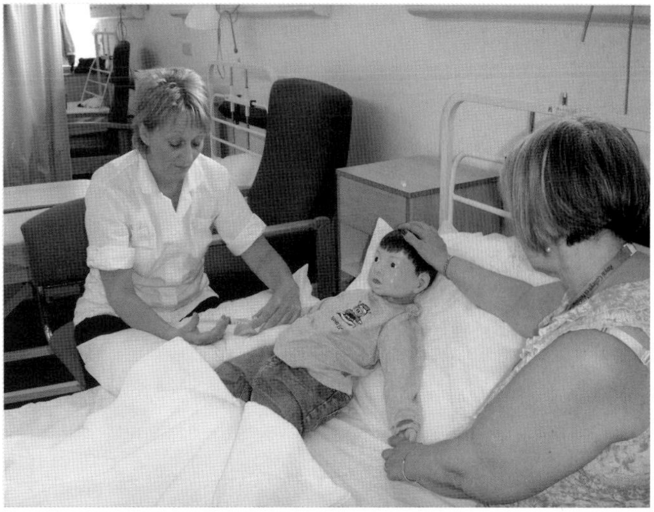

Fig. 5.13 • Administering intravenous medication.

Table 5.11. Putting a child into a car seat

	Reducing risk
Size	The size of the child, seat and car will vary. Some children will have their seat in the front and others in the back of the car, which restricts access for the handler. The handler must avoid twisting and stooping when securing the child and seat.
Weight	The weight of the child and sometimes that of the seat will need to be considered.
Ability	Some children will be able to climb into their car seat, and when possible this should be encouraged.
Need	The law requires children in cars to be appropriately secured (Department for Transport 2005). For the severely disabled a specially designed vehicle in which the child can be wheeled via ramps into a secure holding may be available (see Fig. 12.4). For others the seat can be mounted on to a frame over the existing seat, which rotates through 90° to face outwards, enabling the handler easier access (National Back Pain Association & Royal College of Nursing 1997).

Occasionally handlers may come across a manual handling problem for which no appropriate options can be found. In this instance a manual handling adviser should be consulted.

Conclusion

The principles of safer manual handling must be applied to all situations when caring for children. Care must be taken not to think that children do not pose a handling risk if young or small. A thorough assessment should be carried out on all children who need handling, no matter what their ability. It is, however, the principles that are important and should be applied to all manoeuvres the handler is likely to encounter. Each manoeuvre should be addressed considering the size, weight, ability and need (SWAN) of the child together with the task, individual, load and environment (TILE). The child should be encouraged to cooperate with the manoeuvre and be adequately prepared. Consideration should be given to the timing of or alternatives to the manoeuvre for the child who is uncooperative, and when possible the parents should be involved. Parents should, however, be alerted to poor handling practices and if necessary be taught about safer manual handling techniques as part of the holistic package of care.

Now test your knowledge

Jenny is a 7-year-old who has cerebral palsy. She requires regular therapy at the local child development centre. During a visit you notice mum struggling to lift Jenny in and out of her buggy. When asking mum how she is getting on with Jenny's care it becomes clear that she is now finding it extremely difficult to lift her:

- What risks can you identify in this particular manoeuvre – to mum and to Jenny?
- What advice can you give to reduce these to the lowest level?

References

Barnett J, Thomlinson C, Perry R, Marshall R, Macgowan AP (1999) An audit of the use of manual handling equipment and their microbiological flora: implications for infection control. Journal Hospital Infection 43(4):309–313

Betts M, Mowbray C (2004) The falling and fallen person and emergency handling. In Smith J (ed.) The guide to the handling of people, 5th edn. RCN and NBPA, London

Department for Transport (2005) Consultation, compulsory seat belt/child restraint wearing. Online. Available: http://www.dft.gov.uk/groups/dft_rdsafety/documents/page/dft_rdsafety_038198. hcsp 10 Jan 2006

Department of Health (2003) Getting the right start: National Service Framework for Children; Standard for Hospital Services. TSO, London

Department of Health (2004a) Back in work. TSO, London

Department of Health (2004b) Back in work: key messages. Online. Available: http://www.nhs.uk/backinwork/whatsup.htm 22 Nov 2006

Griffin SD, Price VJ (2000) Living with lifting: mothers' perception of lifting and back strain in childcare. Occupational Therapy International 7(1):1–20

Health and Safety at Work Act (1974) HMSO, London

Health and Safety Executive (1992) Provision and Use of Work Equipment Regulations. HMSO, London

Health and Safety Executive (2004) Getting to grips with manual handling: a short guide. HSE, Suffolk

Health and Safety Executive (2005a) Lifting Operations and Lifting Equipment Regulations 1998. HMSO, London

Health and Safety Executive (2005b) Simple guide to Lifting Operations and Lifting Equipment Regulation 1998. Online. Available: http://www.hse.gov.uk 17 Dec 2006

Human Rights Act (1998) TSO, London

Kitson J (2000) Mind your back: variable height cots. Paediatric Nursing 12(4):26–27

Management of Health and Safety at Work Regulations (1999) HMSO, London

Mandelstam M (2005) Manual handling in social care: law, practice and balanced decision making. In Smith J (ed.) The guide to the handling of people, 5th edn. Backcare, Middlesex

Manual Handling Operations Regulations (1992) UK Government Statutory Instrument no. 2793. HMSO, London

National Back Pain Association, Royal College of Nursing (1997) The guide to the handling of patients, 4th edn. RCN and NBPA, Middlesex

National Health Service (2007) Learning for the NHS by the NHS. Online. Available: http://www.clu.nhs.uk

Nursing and Midwifery Council (2004) Code of professional conduct: standards for conduct performance and ethics. NMC, London

Owen BD (1988) Patient handling devices: an ergonomic approach to lifting patients. In Aghazadeh E (ed.) Trends in ergonomic/human factors. Elsevier Science, London, p 721–728

Swain J, Jeffery K (2005) Advantages of low cost mobility aids in healthcare settings. International Journal of Therapy and Rehabilitation 2(7):316–319

Swain J, Pufhal E, Williamson G (2003) Do they practice what we teach: a survey of manual handling practice amongst student nurses. Journal Clinical Nursing 12:296–306

6 Supportive holding of children during therapeutic interventions

Karen Jeffery

Introduction

This chapter discusses principles that can be applied when holding or immobilising children during clinical procedures. It is not a definitive guide to all forms of supportive holding but provides a repertoire of skills, enabling practitioners to adapt to changing circumstances and procedures.

Holding or immobilising children is a practice used to ensure success in carrying out therapeutic and diagnostic interventions. This is particularly common for younger children, who may find it difficult to sit still during procedures such as venepuncture or medical examination. It requires practitioners to hold the child, enabling a procedure to be carried out safely and quickly, thus reducing the child's stress. Nurses would justify their practice by working under the premise that they are acting in the best interest of the child in accordance with their code of professional conduct (Nursing and Midwifery Council 2004).

Holding or immobilising children can be justified only if practitioners have a good working knowledge of legislation, policy and child development (Jeffery 2002). Used routinely restraining or holding could be viewed as abusive (Folkes 2005) or inhumane (Pearch 2005). There are those, however, who would argue that the acceptability of the practice is dependent on place and time (Meadows 1993). Therefore what is acceptable today may not be tomorrow.

Holding, if inappropriate, could be subject to scrutiny under the 1998 Human Rights Act, article 3: 'a right not to be tortured or subject to treatment or punishment which is inhumane or degrading' (Power 2002). Holding therefore should be used only as a last resort because, as Robinson & Collier (1997) found, being held appears to cause more distress to the child than the procedure itself.

ALERT
Supportive holding should be used only as a last resort and in line with national and local policy.

Definition

In order to understand what is meant by *holding*, it is important to examine the language currently used in the literature and identify the most appropriate definition.

Many terms have been identified to describe the holding of children for clinical procedures, from therapeutic restraint (Jeffery 2002) to clinical holding (Lambrenos & McArthur 2003) and therapeutic holding (American Academy of Pediatrics 1997). For ease of understanding, reference will be made to the Royal College of Nursing guidelines (2003), which refer to 'immobilising' or 'holding the child still' to prevent further discomfort or pain. This does not imply restraint, which requires additional force (Royal College of Nursing 2003) and is used in situations in which children may be a danger to themselves or others. Immobilising or holding should leave the reader in no doubt of the intention.

Consent

Before embarking on any therapeutic intervention, consent must be obtained. For those caring for children this is not a simple process. Not only is consent necessary for the procedure but also for the way this may be executed, including the need to hold. The Royal College of Nursing (2003) states that immobilising or holding should be with the child's and parent's permission, something that could be argued may not always be possible. There may be situations in which the child is unable to give consent. In an emergency, for example, holding a young child to replace a misplaced tracheostomy tube may be the only means of ensuring the child's survival. The practitioner may be required to act immediately with little or no time to gain the child's consent, acting under the premise of best interest.

A 15-month-old may not understand the need to be held for an immunisation, which a parent wishes the child to have. Would nurses in this situation be in breach of their code of professional conduct and be acting in the best interest of the child by refusing to enable immunisation? Is it acceptable to hold the child against her or his will, with their parent's consent, momentarily, to provide immunity to a perhaps life-threatening disease? To answer yes or no is looking at the issue simplistically. Obtaining valid consent from a child will largely depend on the situation, the law and the child's level of understanding.

Minors (a person under 18 years old) can consent to treatment providing they have sufficient understanding as to the consequences of their actions (Children Act 1989). However, the legal position regarding competence is different for children aged over and under 16 (Department of Health 2001a). In law (Family Law Reform Act 1969), 16- or 17-year-olds can consent to treatment providing they:

- understand the information that has been presented
- believe this information
- retain it long enough to make a decision (Medical Protection Society 2005).

Unlike for adults, refusal to treatment by 16- or 17-year-olds appears less clear and may be overridden by either a person with parental responsibility or the court (Department of Health 2001b). It could be argued that if children are competent to consent they should also be competent to refuse treatment. Some practitioners could view a child's refusal to treatment as meaning they do not understand the consequence of their actions, when they would have been deemed competent if they had consented.

Dealing with an older child who refuses treatment is complex; it would be impossible to hold the child without his or her consent. To do this would be viewed as restraint, putting those involved at risk of being charged with assault, battery or false imprisonment. In order to prevent this, care must be taken to ensure that all avenues of support and preparation have been explored and, if necessary, alternative methods of care considered that may be more acceptable to the child. Often it is the child's misconception of what is about to happen to him or her that causes the refusal. Careful preparation is not a quick alternative and requires time and patience, something that may not be available, as discussed earlier. Practitioners must be very clear that whatever action they take (and that may be to do nothing) is in the best interest of all concerned and if necessary be able to stand up in a court of law and justify this.

Nurses' responsibility

Once consent has been obtained (according to local policy) it is the nurse's responsibility to help the child through the procedure to reduce adverse effects and distress (Willock et al 2004). This may include deciding whether to hold or not. Some nurses may feel uncomfortable about holding a child, and some (27%) may ask a parent to do this for them (Robinson & Collier 1997), exonerating them from the task. Ethically this should be questioned. Some parents, however, may want to hold their child while others may see this as the role of the nurse. Whoever is responsible for holding should always consider the child's best interest. Remember, nursing care of children is open to scrutiny for many years, with some 18-year-olds taking legal advice for something that happened to them in the past, putting nurses in a vulnerable position.

There are measures nurses can take to safeguard themselves when considering to hold, and that is to adopt principles of good practice (Royal College of Nursing 2003). These are that there is:

- an ethos of caring
- a consideration of legal implications
- an openness about who decides what is in the child's best interest
- a clear mechanism for staff to be heard if they disagree with a decision to hold the child
- a holding policy that is relevant to the child and setting
- appropriately trained staff to carry out holding techniques.

Nurses need to adopt these principles to safeguard themselves against possible litigation in the future.

Training

The code of professional conduct states that all nurses should work within their own capabilities (Nursing and Midwifery Council 2004) and would be negligent if they embarked on procedures for which they have not had training, yet very few nurses are routinely taught about holding techniques (Pearch 2005). It could be argued, however, that although holding techniques are not taught per se, nurse education provides a philosophy that encourages the application of safe practice through knowledge of consent, ethics, child development, legislation and policy. Is this enough? There are limited applications of this issue within an educational context (Valler-Jones & Shinnick 2005), and with little evidence on the subject this question is difficult to answer.

Clinical holding policy

Problems arise when (a) there is no specific policy in place to cover the practice of supportive holding or (b) it is implied through other polices, such as restraint. Guidelines need to be clear, transparent and easy to follow. They must 'hold up' in a court of law and withstand scrutiny by those able to pass judgement on their suitability.

As part of a clinical holding policy, Lambrenos & McArthur (2003) devised an algorithm to assist staff when faced with the issue of supportive holding. The aim of the algorithm was to help practitioners in the decision-making process. In devising their policy Lambrenos & McArthur recognised the importance of staff knowing about their legal, moral and ethical obligations and the use of alternative techniques such as pain relief, distraction therapy and relaxation. This suggests that practitioners need a wealth of knowledge when faced with the decision to hold or not.

Algorithms, although useful, cannot be used in isolation but need to be supported by a written policy expanding on the issues identified. This in turn needs to be understood by knowledgeable practitioners with the necessary skills to interpret the policy and algorithm correctly.

The child health holding algorithm shown in Figure 6.1 was devised by a modern matron (Jayne Deaves) and university lecturer (Karen Jeffery) after scrutinising Lambrenos & McArthur's (2003) work. The policy, although devised primarily for use within a general children's ward, was also designed to be used in other areas in which children may be nursed.

The algorithm was split into three sections: preprocedure action, action during procedure and postprocedure action. This three-stage approach was meant to assist practitioners in their understanding of the holding process.

Preprocedure action

In the preprocedure stage of the algorithm an appropriate person should be identified to lead the intervention. His or her

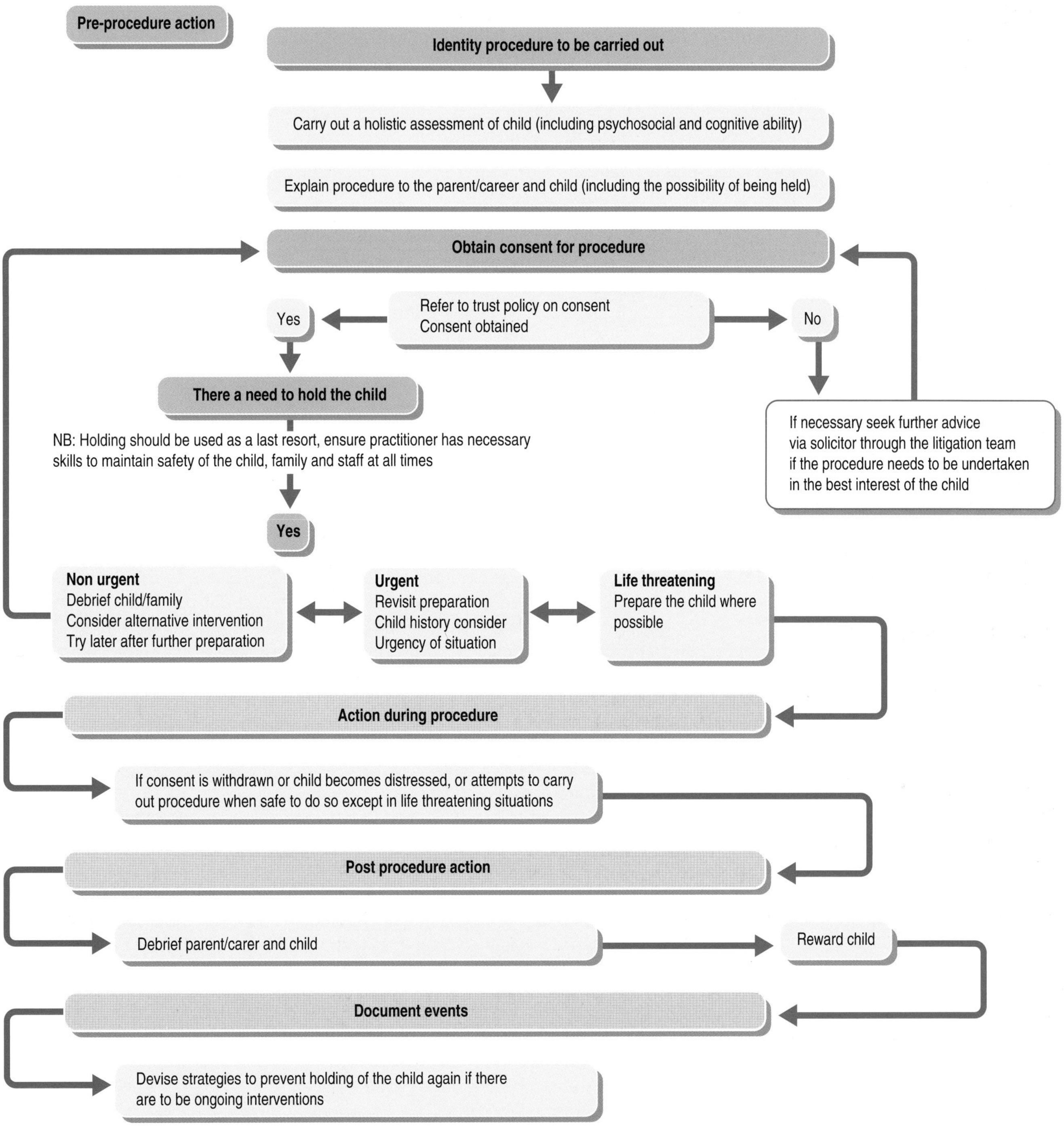

Fig. 6.1 • Child-holding algorithm. This algorithm must be supported with a written policy.

role is to ensure that the child and parent (or guardian) have been adequately prepared and that consent has been given. He or she then decides if it is in the best interest of the child to be held. This person must:

- have the expertise to follow the algorithm
- have the underpinning knowledge to interpret this to the best effect
- lead other members of the care team through the intervention
- be responsible for documenting events.

Holding should be used only to promote the child's safety, and practitioners should use mechanisms to avoid the need to hold whenever possible. Given the right preparation and encouragement even very young children can cooperate, with children adequately prepared displaying significantly less distress than those who are not (Kolk et al 2000).

Preparation

Preparing a child for an intervention can be achieved in many ways. This can be through the use of dolls, puppets, play equipment and age-appropriate descriptions. One such age-related description could be through reading a story. An example would be a story about a cat curled up in a basket, which can then be used as an analogy to explain the position the child needs to be in when undergoing, for example, a lumbar puncture. It may be necessary to enrol the use of the play specialist to assist in the child's preparation. Careful planning and sensitive preparation for an intervention is important in minimising undue stress, anxiety and trauma (Willock et al 2004) and in all but emergency situations should not be rushed.

The time needed to prepare for an intervention is dependent on the child's condition, whether the intervention is non-urgent or urgent, and whether failure to carry this out would be life threatening. For the child in a life-threatening condition very little preparation time may be available. Care must be taken that preparation is not at the expense of the child's overall condition, which could change rapidly.

Communication

It is important to communicate effectively with the child. Explanations need to be appropriate for the child's level of understanding, avoiding the use of jargon. Care should be taken not to be too graphic; however, honesty is important. If a procedure is going to be unpleasant, denying this will cause the child to lose trust in those performing the intervention; the child will then be reluctant to assist in the future, which will have a knock-on effect for those caring for them thereafter. Words should be chosen that will somehow soften what is meant, such as 'sore' rather than 'painful'. Clear explanations should be given prior to and during the procedure on why holding is necessary, what will happen and what the child may feel, hear or smell (Willock et al 2004). This is particularly important for children who are not in a position to see what is going on. Appropriate use of body language and tone of voice should also be demonstrated.

Choice

Children can be cooperative if they understand what is required of them and are allowed to make choices. Real choices over aspects of treatment should be offered wherever possible (Department of Health 2003). This can be as simple as who loosens the tape on a dressing, or choosing where the procedure should be carried out. This will empower the child, give them more control over the procedure and provide some distraction (Willock et al 2004).

Parental or carer involvement

Parental or guardian involvement in care is important and has been debated at some length over the past few decades. Playing some part in their child's hospitalisation is regarded as helpful for both child and family (Department of Health 1996). Parents are able to provide emotional support during technical procedures, providing they have access to information that is understandable and developmentally, ethically and culturally appropriate (Department of Health 2003). They and the child need to know if a procedure is unpleasant or painful before consenting to an intervention. Parental consent will not always mean parental involvement. The wishes of parents must always be respected, with their role clearly defined.

Parents can also play a major role in preparing their child for an intervention, providing they are not anxious or have had unpleasant experiences themselves (Smalley 1999). Time may be needed to help parents overcome their own anxiety before being able to assist in preparing their child.

Action during procedure

Supporting a child through an intervention requires the practitioner to be competent in holding techniques. Care must be taken during the hold not to injure the child or compromise her or him in any way. Body, head and limbs should be held in a natural position, avoiding pressure to face, neck, chest, abdomen, genitalia and other parts of the body and ensuring that breathing and circulation are not compromised (Orr & Richards 2004). Not only must practitioners be able to support the child safely, they must also be able to assist with distraction techniques and continually assess the child and the situation. They need to be able to reassure the child throughout and act as the child's advocate. This may mean stopping the procedure to give more pain relief or stop the procedure (at an appropriate point) if consent is withdrawn (Department of Health 2003).

Holding the child is not a licence to complete an intervention at all cost. If any members of the team feel uncomfortable or if the child becomes distressed they must voice their concerns and act accordingly, with the underlying philosophy being the child's best interest.

Risks for the child

Deciding to hold a child is not without risk. Reflecting on these prior to, during and after the procedure and reducing these to the lowest level possible is vital, being proactive rather than reactive.

The boxes below highlight examples from practice in which supportive holding techniques are used by practitioners. Some of the risks associated with these particular manoeuvres are also identified and suggestions made to help the practitioner to reduce these risks and promote best practice.

Time limit

Holding should be performed in accordance with existing (local) policies such as the maximum number of attempts or time it takes before the procedure is stopped and either handed over to someone more senior or postponed. The length of time the child

Procedures Box 6.1 Risks of supportive hold during venepuncture

1

Risk
Undue movement of child during hold

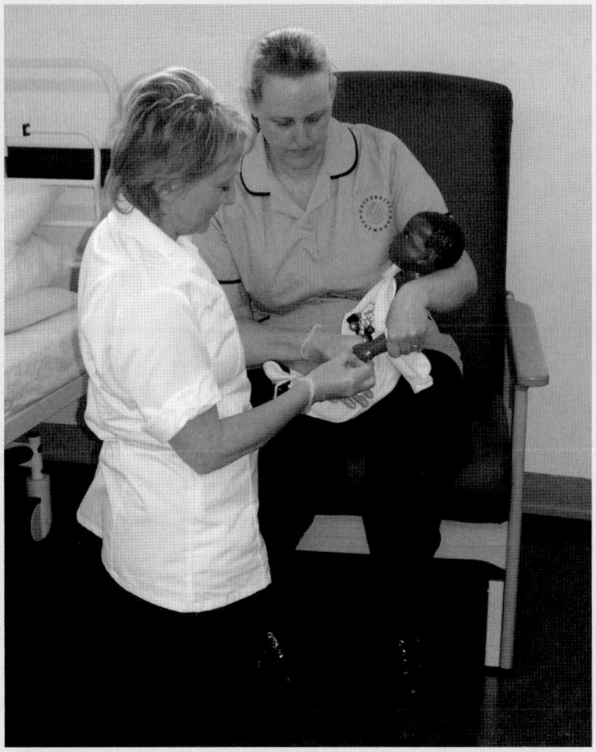

Action
Support the child on the lap of the parent or nurse or according to local policy.

Reason *Prevents undue movement during the procedure.*

Action
The child's nearest arm can rest behind the handler's back.

Reasons *Can allow the doctor to work from behind the carer, out of the child's sight, or in front.*
Position allows for holder or bystander to distract child.

Action
Encourage distraction through play.

Reason *Reduces undue stress.*

2

Risk
Stress of child being held

Action
Provide clear explanation throughout.

Reasons *Reduces stress to child and parent.*
Promotes cooperation and concordance.

Action
Apply local analgesic as prescribed.

Reasons *Relieves pain of procedure.*
Promotes cooperation.

Action
Be prepared to stop if the child becomes too distressed and consent is withdrawn.

Reason *To comply with local and national policy on consent.*

3

Risk
Skin-to-skin trauma when holding the limb

Actions
Check that the hold is not too tight and fingertips are not digging into the child's arm.

Provide a cushion between the practitioner's hand and the child's arm through the use of, for example, a gauze swab.

Reason *For comfort and prevention of skin-to-skin trauma.*

Procedures Box 6.2 Risks of supportive hold during lumbar puncture

1

Risk
Maintaining the correct position during hold

Action
Prepare the child, giving developmentally appropriate explanations and preparation for correct position (e.g. 'nose to knees', 'curl like a hedgehog').

Reasons *Reduces stress to child and parent.*
Promotes cooperation and concordance.
Encourages correct position for procedure.

2

Risk
Restraining rather than supporting the child in the position

Action
Support the child; care must be taken not to restrain the child in this position.

Reason *Provides continuing support and correct positioning of the child.*

Procedures Box 6.2 Risks of supportive hold during lumbar puncture—cont'd

2 **Continued**

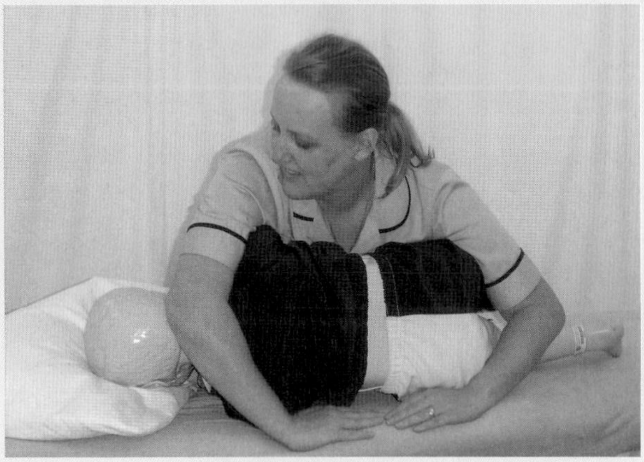

Action
The practitioner's arms should rest gently in the position shown to support the child.

Reason *Prevents undue movement, which may be dangerous during lumbar puncture.*

Action
Continually explain the holding technique to the child.

Reason *Reduces stress and promotes concordance.*

3

Risk
Distress of child and family due to hold

Action
Give clear explanations throughout the procedure.

Reason *Reduces stress.*

Action
Be prepared to stop if the child becomes distressed and consent is withdrawn.

Reason *To comply with local and national policy on consent.*

Procedures Box 6.3 Risks of supportive hold during throat and ear examination

1

Risk
Undue movement during hold

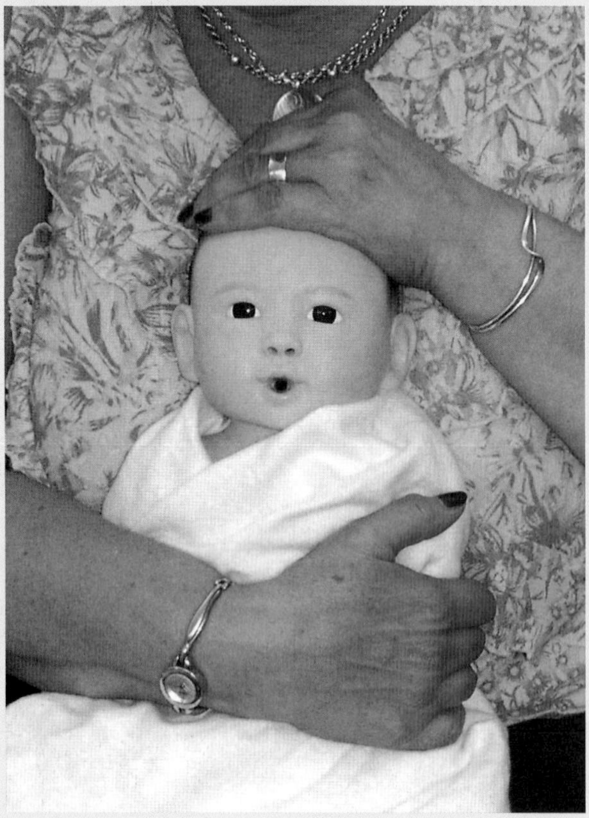

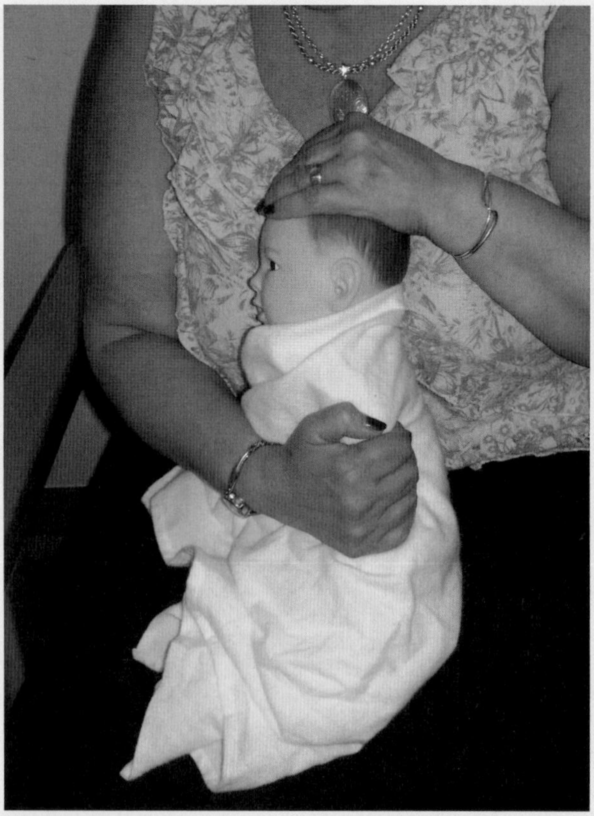

Actions
Sit the child on the lap of the parent or nurse.
Support the child's head and body.

Procedures Box 6.3 Risks of supportive hold during throat and ear examination—cont'd

1 Continued

Reason *Prevents undue movement during procedure and ease of examination.*

Action
Give clear instruction to the parent on holding technique.

Reason *Promotes parental participation.*

2

Risk
Non-concordance necessitating the need to hold

Actions
Consider which examination should be undertaken first.

If the child is likely to gag during the throat examination, consider leaving this till last or give the child a choice on which examination should be undertaken first.

Reasons *Promotes self-esteem and mastery.*
Reduces the need to hold.

3

Risk
Holding the child too tightly

Actions
Observe for signs of stress and release the hold if safe to do so.

Continue to give clear instruction to the parent.

Reason *Promotes safety of the child, prevents harm and reduces stress.*

4

Risk
Distress of child and family due to hold

Action
Give clear explanations throughout the procedure.

Reason *Reduces stress.*

Action
Be prepared to stop if the child becomes distressed and consent is withdrawn.

Reason *To comply with local and national policy on consent.*

Procedures Box 6.4 Risks of supportive hold when administering oral medication

1

Risk
Non-concordance necessitating the need to hold

Action
Give the child a choice if there is one (e.g. cup or spoon).

Reason *Promotes cooperation and mastery.*

Action
Allow child to choose who gives the medication (e.g. nurse or parent).

Reason *May prevent the need to hold or reduce the time the child is held.*

2

Risk
Difficulty in holding a baby

Action
Lightly swaddle during procedure.

Reasons *For ease of holding.*
Light swaddling prevents overheating and allows some body movement.
Provides support during hold.

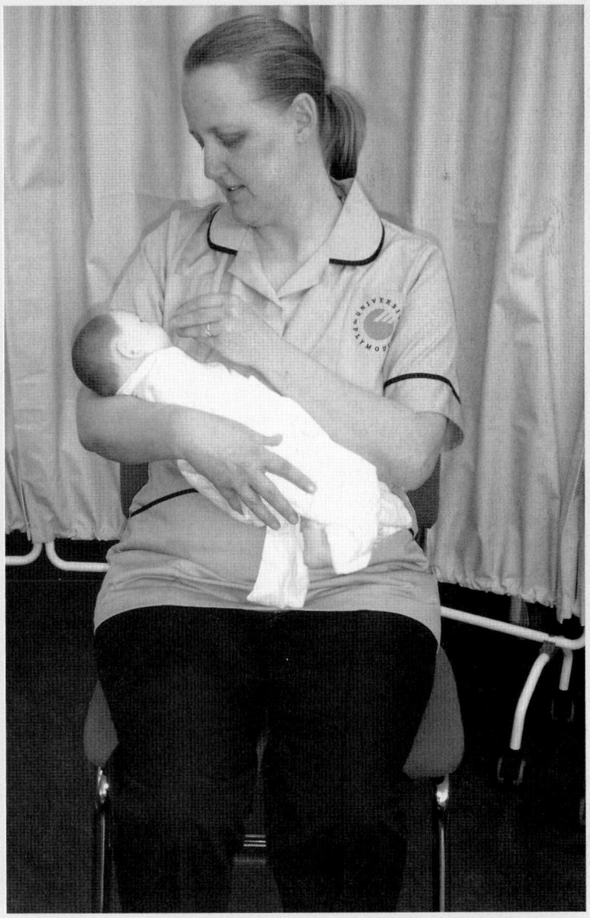

Procedures Box 6.4 Risks of supportive hold when administering oral medication—cont'd

3

Risk
Difficulty in holding a toddler

Action
Sit the child on the parent's or nurse's lap; the child's nearest arm to the handler should be behind the handler's back – the handler can then hold the child's other hand.

Reason *This is the ideal position for giving encouragement and support throughout.*

4

Risk
Choking during holding procedure

Action
Use an oral syringe, medicine cup or spoon.

Reason *Enables delivery of medicine at an appropriate rate to prevent choking.*

Action
Deliver medicine at a rate the child can swallow.

Reason *Reduces stress during the hold and prevents choking.*

5

Risk
Distress of child and family due to hold

Action
Give clear explanations throughout the procedure.

Reason *Reduces stress.*

Action
Be prepared to stop if the child becomes too distressed and consent is withdrawn.

Reason *To comply with local and national policy on consent.*

Procedures Box 6.5 Risks of supportive hold when administering an intramuscular injection

1

Risk
Undue stress during preparation of injection, necessitating the need to hold

Actions
Prepare the injection out of sight of the child.

Explain the procedure to parent and child.

Do not let the child dwell on the procedure for too long.

Reasons *Reduces stress.*
Promotes cooperation.
Reduces the need for supportive hold.

2

Risk
Non-concordance during hold

Action
When possible give the child a role (e.g. holding a swab or plaster); this should be held in the hand closest to the nurse delivering the injection.

Reasons *Provides distraction.*
Provides choice.
Prevents the child putting her or his hand in the way of the needle.

Action
Provide some form of distraction through the use of a toy.

Reasons *Provides distraction.*
Reduces stress of procedure.

3

Risk
Undue movement during the hold

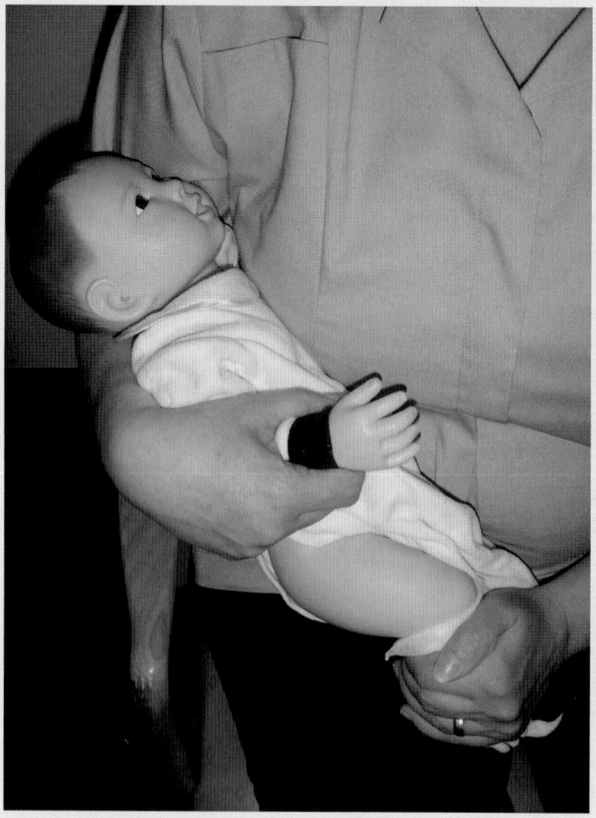

Procedures Box 6.5 Risks of supportive hold when administering an intramuscular injection—cont'd

3 Continued

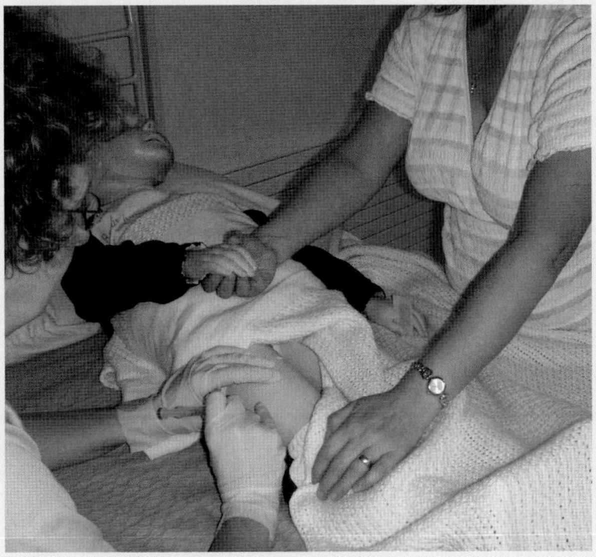

Actions
This usually requires the assistance of a nurse and another according to local policy.

The younger child should be sat on the parent's or nurse's lap, with an older child lying on the bed.

One person should place his or her hand on the child's leg or knee and gently hold the child's hand while the nurse administers the injection.

Reasons *Safe delivery of injection.*

4

To comply with local policies and procedures.

Risk
Distress of child and family due to hold

Action
Give clear explanations throughout the procedure.

Reason *Reduces stress.*

Action
Be prepared to stop if the child becomes distressed or consent is withdrawn.

Reason *To comply with local and national policy on consent.*

is subject to a stressful intervention should also be judged and the procedure stopped if this exceeds unacceptable levels. This is difficult to measure even for the most experienced practitioner. The use of a pain score may be one way of ascertaining this, but it must be introduced prior to the intervention, with the child having a good understanding of how this should be used.

Postprocedure action

Postprocedure action is about making the child feel comfortable. Children should have some place where they can retreat to after the intervention. This shows the child that the procedure is over and helps him or her to feel secure (Orr & Richards 2004). The child's bed and bed space may be an appropriate area for the child to retreat to, ensuring a safe haven. This can be particularly difficult in high-dependency units where the child may be too sick to be moved. In such instances the practitioner should look at other ways to promote a sense of safety for the child.

Reward

Whatever the outcome of the intervention or how the child behaved, she or he should be praised. At no time should children feel that they are being punished for the way they behaved during a procedure but rewarded for the things that went well. Stickers and certificates are readily available and will often aid in the child's compliance, particularly if chosen beforehand.

Documenting events

Documenting events in detail is vital, as practitioners could be called to account (in the case of children) many years after an event. This should include:

- why the child needed to be held in the first instance
- who held the child
- where the hold took place (e.g. the treatment room)
- the method used to immobilise or hold the child (particularly important in cases of child abuse, in which the holder could easily be accused of causing bruises)
- the length of time the child was held
- techniques needed to reduce the need to be held in the future (particularly important for those children who require ongoing treatment).

Debrief

Last, debrief the child, patent or guardian and members of the care team, reflecting on what went well and what did not. As Wilkinson (1999) implies, reflection is useful in contributing to the practitioner's knowledge and informs nursing practice, which is important.

Children coming into the hospital should not have to deal with negative events as well as their condition because, as Bijttebier & Vertommen (1998) found, children with a history of negative experiences show greater levels of anxiety and are less positive than those with positive or neutral experiences. It is therefore important to reflect on the negative or unpleasant nature of hospitalisation, such as holding a child against his or her will, and ensure whenever possible that this is avoided.

Conclusion

If there is a need to hold, remember to consider the three stages identified in the algorithm. Do not move into the second stage of the algorithm unless all options have been explored. Holding a child should not be used as a means to get the procedure 'over and done with' for the sake of those carrying out the intervention. Remember, the child's welfare is paramount.

If it is necessary to hold a child this must be done having obtained consent from those in a position to give it and with the child's best interests in mind. All involved in the process must be clear about what is meant by holding a child and be able to differentiate this from restraint. There should be a clear line of responsibility, with each practitioner knowing her or his role and what to do if she or he has a problem.

Remember, children of today will be adults of tomorrow able to question practice from the past (Jeffery & Deaves 2007). If practitioners can justify their action under the premise of acting in the best interest of the child and in accordance with current policy and legislation, this will be deemed as best practice. However, best practice today may not be so in the future, with practitioners needing to ensure that they remain up to date in the practice of supportive holding.

Now test your knowledge

Joshua is 14 years old and suffers from cystic fibrosis. He has refused, despite his mother consenting, to have his blood taken at his yearly update in the outpatient department. This is a fairly routine examination and in the past his drug regimen has been altered as a result of changes. Clearly he is too big to be held against his will.

- Discuss the options open to Joshua and the medical and nursing team.
- What would be the implication for you and the medical team if you were to try to force Joshua to have his blood taken?

References

American Academy of Pediatrics (1997) The use of physical restraint interventions for children and adolescents in the acute care setting. Pediatrics 99(3):497–498

Bijttebier P, Vertommen H (1998) The impact of previous experience on children's reactions to venepuncture. Journal of Health Psychology 3(1):39–46

Children Act (1989) HMSO, London

Department of Health (1996) Welfare of children and young people in hospital. Department of Health, London

Department of Health (2001a) Seeking consent working with children. Department of Health, London

Department of Health (2001b) Reference guide to consent for examination or treatment. Department of Health, London

Department of Health (2003) Getting the right start: the National Service Framework for Children, Young People and Maternity Services – Standard for Hospital Services. Department of Health, London

Family Law Reform Act (1969) HMSO, London

Folkes K (2005) Is restraint a form of abuse? Paediatric Nursing 17(6):41–44

Human Rights Act (1998) HMSO, London

Jeffery K, Deaves J (2007) Translating policy and guidelines into practice: an education practice synergy. Journal of Children's & Young People's Nursing 1(2):93–97

Jeffery K (2002) Therapeutic restraint of children: it must always be justified. Paediatric Nursing 14(9):20–22

Kolk AM, Van Hoof R, Fiedeldij Dop MJC (2000) Preparing children for venepuncture. The effects of an integrated intervention on distress before and during venepuncture. Child: Care, Health and Development 26(3):251–260

Lambrenos K, McArthur E (2003) Introducing a clinical holding policy. Paediatric Nursing 15(4):30–33

Meadows R (1993) ABC of child neglect. BMJ Publishing, London

Medical Protection Society (2005) GP registrar: consent children and young people, MPS survey results, elderly patients, Mental Capacity Act, summer 9. Online. Available: http://www.mps.org.uk/gpregistrar 1 Nov 2005

Nursing and Midwifery Council (2004) The NMC code of professional conduct, performance and ethics. NMC, London

Orr J, Richards M (2004) Guidelines for supportive holding: child health. MP60. Royal Cornwall Hospitals NHS Trust, Truro

Pearch J (2005) Restraining children for clinical procedures. Paediatric Nursing 17(9):36–38

Power K (2002) Implications of the Human Rights Act 1998. Paediatric Nursing 14(4):14–19.

Robinson S, Collier J (1997) Holding children still for procedures. Paediatric Nursing 9(4):12–14

Royal College of Nursing (2003) Restraining, holding still and containing children and young people. RCN, London

Smalley A (1999) Needle phobia. Paediatric Nursing 11(2):17–20

Valler-Jones T, Shinnick A (2005) Holding children for invasive procedures: preparing student nurses. Paediatric Nursing 17(5):20–22

Wilkinson J (1999) Implementing reflective practice. Nursing Standard 13(21):36–40

Willock J, Richardson J, Brazier A, Powell C, Mitchell E (2004) Peripheral venepuncture in infants and children. Nursing Standard 17(18):43–50

Section Two
Assessment of the child

7

Interpretation of observations

Sue Syers

In a typical year a preschool child will visit his or her general practitioner an estimated six times, and a school-aged child two to four times. Up to a half of under 1-year-olds and one-quarter of older children will attend the local emergency department. One in eleven children will be referred to the hospital for outpatient care, and one in ten for admission for an acute illness (Department of Health 2004). With the development of children's assessment units, most of these children will be sent home again after a period of observation. It is therefore vital that accurate, ongoing assessments of the child are undertaken. Often the first person to meet the child on arrival on a ward or unit is a nurse, therefore it is essential that nurses develop good assessment skills to ensure that the child is treated appropriately.

The physical assessment of a sick child is a multifactorial process that can initially appear complex but very quickly becomes second nature. This process covers areas such as the recording of basic physical readings (e.g. temperature, pulse, respirations and blood pressure) and full system assessments (e.g. neurological and respiratory assessments). It is important to remember that a good assessment is much more than just the recording of numbers; the best information is gained from well-developed observational and listening skills. The physical assessment is more to do with the analysis and interpretation of findings rather than the act of obtaining the information. Some of the practical procedures related to taking a temperature, pulse and respiratory rate are described in other parts of this book; this chapter will concentrate more on the interpretation of the information.

General assessment

General assessment encompasses all aspects and acts as an overview of the whole child. The majority of this assessment can be carried out from a distance or while obtaining a nursing history and weighing the child. The colour of the child should be noted, looking to see if she or he is pale, cyanosed, mottled, flushed or jaundiced. Are there any obvious birthmarks, bruises or rashes? What is the general appearance of the child? Is she or he clean and are there any dysmorphic features?

Next it is important to look at the interaction of the child with the parents, surroundings and strangers. Is the child alert, lethargic, agitated or drowsy? How much stimulation is required to obtain a reaction, and is the reaction appropriate for the age of the child? Is the child interested in playing or looking at pictures, or is he or she disinterested and sleepy? Is the child holding himself or herself in a normal position or is he or she unusually floppy (hypotonic) or stiff (hypertonic)?

Temperature

This is the aspect of assessment that often raises the most amount of anxiety in both parents and children (Kelly & Morin 1996, Kramer et al 1985). Many people perceive an increase in temperature to be dangerous to the child and an indication of the severity of illness (Campbell & McIntosh 1998, Kelly & Morin 1996, Kramer et al 1985). In reality the height of a fever does not necessarily bear any relation to the severity of the underlying condition, nor is it in itself dangerous to the child. Many common viral infections will give rise to very high fevers, when in contrast a child with meningitis may have only a slight rise in temperature. It is true that 3–5% of children will suffer from a convulsion in response to a high fever (Ashwill & Droske 1997, Campbell & McIntosh 1998); however, it has also been shown that this is most likely due to the rapid rise in temperature rather than the fever itself (Ashwill & Droske 1997, Campbell & McIntosh 1998).

Despite this the temperature reading is a valuable asset within the assessment and can have an effect on other readings such as pulse and respirations, which can be raised in the presence of a fever. It is therefore not only essential that an accurate measurement is taken using an appropriate method for the individual child but also that the method used is documented clearly (see Ch. 8). It is also important to note the environmental temperature and conditions, as these can have an effect on the child's temperature: an infant can rapidly develop a 'fever' when over-wrapped in blankets in a warm room. Conversely infants' large surface area also causes them to lose heat rapidly if left uncovered, thus masking a fever.

Infants utilise oxygen to maintain their temperature (Robertson 1993), and therefore it is important to remember that a sick infant whose oxygen levels may be low may actually record a low temperature. Therefore assessing the temperature of a child is not a case of 'Has the child got a fever?' but more an issue of 'What is the temperature?', 'Does this fit with the other findings?' or 'Is there too much of a variance?'

Respiratory

The most common reason for parents to seek medical assistance for their child is an acute respiratory infection (Gill & O'Brien 2003). The assessment of the respiratory system involves assessing the rate of breathing, the type of respirations, any noise on breathing, cough, chest movement, the colour of the child, the ability to feed or talk, the oxygen saturation level, nasal flaring and the position of the child. A large amount of the assessment of breathing can and should be done from a distance without even touching the child.

Position and appearance of the child

Children who are in severe respiratory distress will hold themselves in particular ways, for example children with a severe asthma attack will often adopt a Buddha-type posture in which they are supporting the upper body by placing their hands on their knees. An infant with an upper airway narrowing may lie with his or her head slightly extended in an attempt to open the airway. You should note the position that the child has adopted and the degree of distress that is apparent. Is the child cradled in mum's arms, sleeping quietly and comfortably? Or is she or he restless and sleepy, with eyes rolled back and neck extended over a parent's arm and with an outstretched body? Both children may well look asleep, but one is exhausted and very ill while the other is obviously coping well with the illness. It is important to know what the child was like on arrival, as this can often be very different to the child that the doctor sees a few minutes later after oxygen therapy has been commenced. Is the child pink, pale, mottled or cyanosed? Is the cyanosis restricted to the peripheries, central or both?

Chest movement

As the severity of the respiratory illness increases so does the effort required by the child to maintain adequate respirations. You should note whether the chest is moving symmetrically or whether it appears that one side of the chest is expanding more than the other. Look for any evidence of an increase in the effort of breathing, as this will indicate an increase in the severity of the condition (Mackway-Jones et al 2005):

- Flaring of the alae nasi (nasal flaring) occurs in children and infants in an attempt to increase the airflow into the lungs.
- The use of accessory muscles, especially the sternomastoid muscle, is common in all children with severe disease. Evidence of the use of these accessory muscles is seen in the infant whose head appears to be bobbing up and down with each breath. In the older child the shoulders will rise up and down with each breath.
- The intercostal muscles aid the expansion of the chest cavity. In infants and young children the chest wall is very compliant and flexible. This means that in times of respiratory difficulty and increase in effort of the intercostal muscles the child's or infant's chest will recess in between and/or under the ribs. This is known as recession and is usually differentiated as intercostal recession (in between the ribs), subcostal recession (under the ribs) or sternal recession, which is the pulling in at the base of the sternum. The presence of recession above the age of 6 years is an indication of severe disease.

You should be wary of children who look unwell and in whom all other aspects of the respiratory assessment indicate a severe respiratory condition even though they are not demonstrating an increase in the work of breathing. This could be an indication of a child who is fatigued, has a degree of cerebral depression and/or has an underlying neuromuscular disease (e.g. Werdnig–Hoffmann or spinal muscular atrophy). Infants are the most likely to fatigue, as they rely heavily on diaphragmatic breathing (Mackway-Jones et al 2005).

Type and rate of respirations

Normal respiratory rates vary with the age of the child (Table 7.1).

The rate can be affected by various other factors, such as fever, pain, circulatory failure and fear, and therefore needs to be assessed along with the type of respirations to give a clearer picture. Are the respirations gentle and quiet, jerky or laboured? Is the child struggling to breathe and distressed? Is the pattern of respirations regular, irregular, periodic, deep or shallow? Tachypnoea is classified as rapid, shallow breathing and is an indication of an increase in ventilation requirements. Rapid deep breathing (sigh) is an indication of metabolic acidosis, as seen in children with diabetes (Gill & O'Brien 2003, Mackway-Jones et al 2005).

Table 7.1. Respiration rate, heart rate and systolic blood pressure in children of different ages

Age (years)	Respiration rate (breaths/min)	Heart rate (beats/min)	Systolic blood pressure
<1	30–40	110–160	70–90
1–2	25–35	110–150	80–95
2–5	25–30	95–140	80–100
5–12	20–25	80–120	90–110
>12	15–20	60–100	100–120

(From Mackway-Jones et al 2005, with permission of BMJ Books and Blackwell Publishers.)

Respiratory noises

There are three main noises that may be heard when the child breathes: stridor, wheeze and grunting. Each has a very different cause:

1. Stridor. This is a harsh, vibrating; shrill sound (Weller 2004) usually heard on inspiration in the presence of a laryngeal or tracheal obstruction (e.g. croup). If the obstruction is severe it may also be heard on expiration.
2. Wheeze. This is a rasping or whistling sound (Weller 2004) heard on expiration when there is a narrowing or an obstruction of the airway. Wheeze is most commonly seen with asthma and is associated with a prolonged expiratory phase.
3. Grunting. This occurs mainly in infants and is an indication of severe respiratory distress. It is generated by the infant exhaling against a partially closed glottis in an attempt to maintain a degree of continuous positive airway pressure (Robertson 1993).

Repeat observations are required to truly assess respiratory function.

It is important to note any environmental factors that may affect these, such as a cool room, which can reduce the child's ability to respond appropriately to hypoxia. Additionally any other factors, such as a fever or an underlying medical condition, may alter the respiratory rate without any underlying respiratory problem and can give the appearance of recession (e.g. abdominal distension or a very thin infant).

Heart rate

The heart rate is affected by various external and internal factors, such as hypoxia and/or shock, in which it will initially increase but then decrease. It is therefore very important to remember that on its own the heart rate will tell you very little about the condition of the child. Other factors that will initiate a normal rise in heart rate are fever, excitement, crying and fear. In fact the heart rate can increase by 10 beats/min for each 1° rise in temperature (Gill & O'Brien 2003). When assessing the heart rate it is important to think about not just the rate and whether it is within normal limits for the child (Table 7.1) but also whether it is regular or irregular in pattern. Are there any extra beats or particularly strong beats as compared with the main beat? The pulse volume is also important to note, especially in a sick child who may be displaying other signs such as those of dehydration, sepsis or shock. The method for taking a pulse is described in Chapter 8.

Capillary refill time

This is the time taken for the capillary bed to refill with blood after being exposed to pressure to empty the bed. Cutaneous pressure is applied to a digit or centre of the sternum for 5 s. The pressure is then released and the number of seconds that it takes for the capillaries to refill and the skin colour to return to normal is counted (Fig. 7.1). This should be less than 2 s. A slower time indicates poor perfusion, which can be a sign of shock. However, a low ambient temperature can reduce the specificity of this test. Additionally if the child has a fever that is in the rising stage the peripheral circulation may well be shut down and the refill time will be delayed. In this instance it is advisable to use the centre of the sternum. This test should be undertaken alongside other assessment tools and the results interpreted accordingly, for example a prolonged capillary refill time and raised heart rate could indicate a fever, anxiety, hypoxia or hypovolaemia.

Blood pressure

The blood pressure is a reading that is often overlooked in children, as it is considered difficult and usually normal. It is unusual to find abnormal blood pressure readings in children, as their bodies compensate for the disease processes very well. Although hypertension may be found following a severe head injury and in children with severe renal disease, hypotension in children is a preterminal sign and would therefore be found only in an extremely sick child. It is therefore important to remember to check the blood pressure in any child, as this provides a

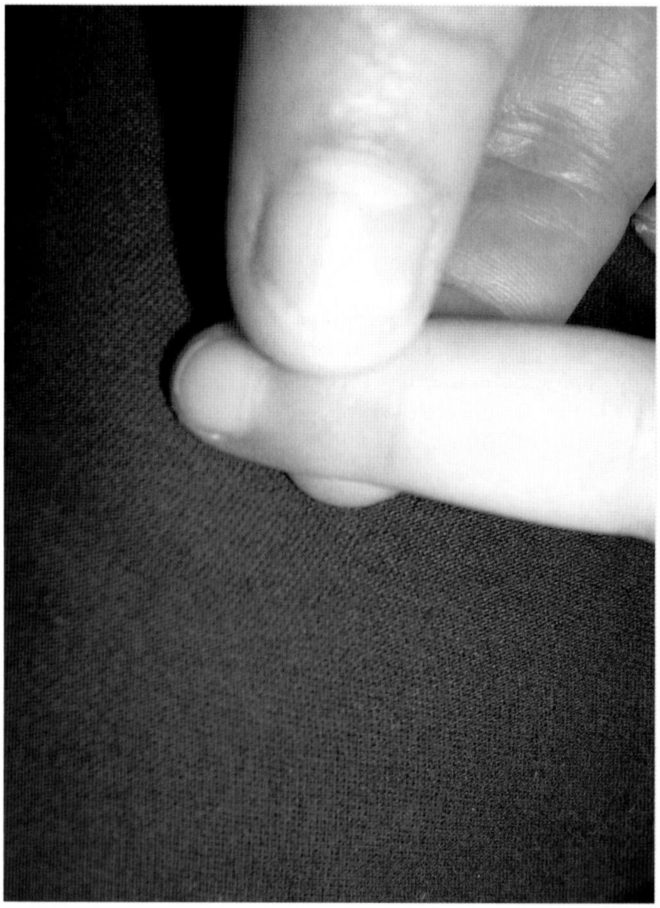

Fig. 7.1 • Assessing capillary refill time.

baseline when normal and indicates a potentially serious condition when abnormal. The normal values for blood pressure vary with the age of the child and can be found in Table 7.1, although the systolic pressure can be estimated by using the child's age as 80 + (age in years × 2). The method for obtaining a blood pressure reading is discussed in Chapter 9.

Level of hydration

The normal circulating blood volume in children varies with age and is approximately 100 mL/kg at birth and 80 mL/kg at 1 year. The total amount of water in the body also decreases with age, with a level of 800 mL/kg in the neonate and 600 mL/kg at 1 year, two-thirds of which is intracellular and one-third extracellular (Mackway-Jones et al 2005). Under normal circumstances the child's kidneys can maintain normal hydration even in the presence of a poor fluid intake. The recommended normal fluid requirements are set out in Table 7.2.

Table 7.2. Recommended normal fluid requirements in children

Body weight	Daily fluid requirement (mL/kg)	Hourly fluid requirement (mL/kg)
First 10 kg	100	4
Second 10 kg	50	2
Subsequent kg	20	1

Dehydration occurs when the fluid loss is at a greater rate than the kidneys can cope with, such as in children with gastroenteritis, diabetic ketoacidosis or urinary tract infection; chronic renal failure may also present like this. Very young children and infants are also more at risk of developing dehydration due to their greater surface area, mass ratio and therefore higher insensible losses (Gill & O'Brien 2003). Their high basal metabolic rate and increased febrile response to infection also increase the amount of fluid loss (Gill & O'Brien 2003).

There are three forms of dehydration:

1. Isotonic dehydration, in which there is an equal loss of sodium and water
2. Hypotonic or hypernatraemic dehydration, in which the loss of water is greater than the loss of sodium
3. Hypertonic or hyponatraemic dehydration, in which the loss of sodium is greater than the loss of water.

Most children in the UK are admitted with mild to moderate hypotonic dehydration and are lethargic and 'flat'. Hypertonic dehydration is more likely to make the child irritable and cranky and give a doughy feel to the skin.

There are many signs and symptoms that enable the detection and assessment of the severity of dehydration; these are shown in Table 7.3. The most obvious ones, which reflect a loss of interstitial fluid and can be detected with a 3% loss of fluid upwards, are:

- sunken anterior fontanelle (3%)
- dull, sunken eyes (3%)
- dry tongue and mouth (3%)
- decreased skin turgor (8%)
- lethargic and weak cry (8%).

Table 7.3. Dehydration assessment

Clinical sign	Mild (3%)	Moderate (8%)	Severe (> 8%)
Mucous membranes	Dry	Dry	Dry
Eyes	Sunken	Sunken	Sunken
Skin turgor[a]	Instant recoil	Recoil in 1–2 s	Recoil in > 2 s
Peripheral circulation	Normal peripheries	Normal peripheries	Decreased perfusion
	Capillary refill in 1–2 s	Capillary refill in 1–2 s	Capillary refill in > 2 s
Neurological status	Normal	Drowsy and irritable	Increasingly drowsy and irritable
Respirations	Normal	Deep acidotic breathing	Increasingly deep, rapid and acidotic

[a]Pinch skin of abdomen and note time taken for skin to recoil.
(From Armon et al 2001, with permission.)

As the dehydration progresses fluid is lost from the intravascular volume and is reflected in:

- diminished pulse volume
- diminished urinary output
- reduced capillary refill time
- reduced blood pressure, which would be a very late sign and is classified as a preterminal sign.

Oxygen saturation

This is the non-invasive peripheral monitoring of the oxygen saturation of haemoglobin in arterial blood (S_aO_2) and has been widely used since 1988 (Robertson 1993). Unless the child is receiving oxygen therapy the S_aO_2 reading is a good indication of the efficacy of breathing (Mackway-Jones et al 2005); however, it is possible to have an S_aO_2 reading of nearly 100% and still be close to death if receiving high-flow oxygen (Stroobant & Field 2002). These monitors work on the principle of Beer's law, which states that the concentration of a substance can be determined by the absorption of light passing through it (Jevon & Ewens 2002). The reading that they give is an indication of the percentage of haemoglobin saturated with oxygen at the time (Schutz 2001).

There are a number of different sensor probes available depending on the make of the monitor. In general there tends to be an adult finger probe, a paediatric finger probe and a multisite or infant probe (Fig. 7.2). It is essential that the correct sensor probe is used, as the wrong size could allow ambient light to distort the readings.

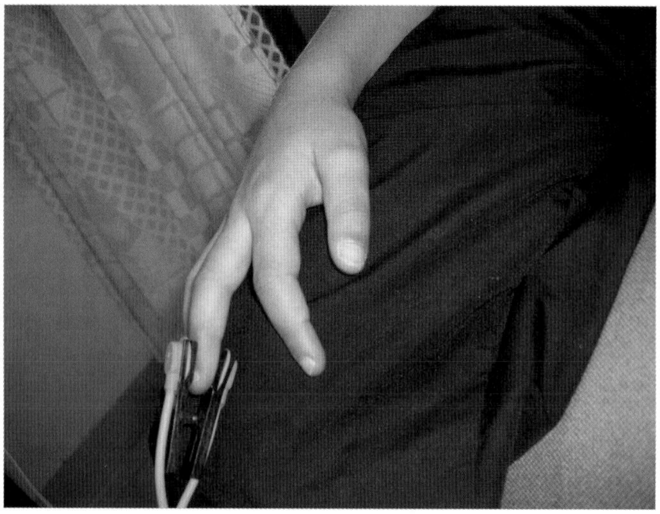

Fig. 7.2 • Finger probe measuring oxygen saturation.

Procedures Box 7.1 Measuring oxygen saturation

Action
Decontaminate hands.

Reason *Prevents cross-infection.*

Action
Switch on the monitor and sensor probe and ensure that the infrared light source is working.

Reason *Checks that the monitor is functioning.*

Action
Check the alarm limits and ensure that they are suitable for the age of the child.

Reason *Enables safe monitoring of the child.*

Action
Select the desired sensor site, which should be warm and well perfused with a good capillary refill time.

Reason *The accuracy of the reading can be affected by the ambient temperature of the limb or digit it is taken from.*

Action
Select an appropriately sized sensor probe and attach it to the desired site; there are red infrared diodes on one side of the probe and a detector on the other, and these should be directly opposite each other on either side of the sensor site.

Reasons *It is important to ensure that the sensor is protected from the ambient light.*
The processor within the monitor then analyses the changes in light absorption in the pulsatile blood flow through the capillary bed (Schutz 2001).

Action
If no reading is acquired then resite and/or shield the probe.

Reasons *If the monitor is unable to provide a reading from a site that is clean and well perfused then it could be that too much light is getting on to the sensor.*
If the sensor is too large for the site or positioned incorrectly then shielding the probe will not work (Schutz 2001, Stroobant & Field 2002).

Action
Verify the accuracy of the reading by checking that the waveform is regular and has a good volume to it and compare the recorded heart rate and the child's apical rate or pulse.

Reason *If they do not correlate then the reading in unreliable; in these cases the probe should be resited.*

Action
If the monitor is to be left on the patient for continuous monitoring then it is essential that the probe site is checked hourly and changed every 4–6 h.

Reason *Prevents skin damage under the probe sensor (Medical Devices Agency 2001).*

Action
All readings should be documented, along with the probe site and time that the probe site was last checked and changed.

Reason *Maintains accurate patient records.*

Oxygen saturation monitors have a level of error of ± 2% in the 70–100% range (Robertson 1993) but are less accurate at readings of < 70% in the presence of carbon monoxide and in a shocked child with poor perfusion (Mackway-Jones et al 2005). The accuracy of the reading can also be affected by various factors including the haemoglobin level in the blood, the temperature of the digit or limb used, the arterial flow to area, the percentage of inspired oxygen, the amount of ambient light seen by the sensor, the venous return at the probe site and the patient's oxygenation ability (Mackway-Jones et al 2005, Schutz 2001). Movement of the sensor probe, nail varnish and/or dirt under the sensor will also adversely affect the accuracy of any reading obtained. In cases of carbon monoxide poisoning in which the carbon monoxide binds heavily to haemoglobin the oxygen saturation reading is falsely high and cannot be relied on (Hampson 1998).

Height, weight and head circumference

The most rapid changes in weight occur during the first year of life. An average birth weight of 3.5 kg would have increased to 10.3 kg by the age of 1 year. After that time, weight increases more slowly until the pubertal growth spurt (Campbell & McIntosh 1998). As most drugs and fluids are given as the dose per kilogram of body weight it is important to determine a child's weight as soon as possible. The most accurate method for achieving this is to weigh the child on scales; however, in an emergency this may be impracticable. In this situation the child's weight may be estimated by one of a number of methods:

- The Broselow tape uses the height (or length) of the child to estimate weight. The tape is laid alongside the child and the estimated weight read from the calibration on the tape. This is a quick, easy and relatively accurate method.
- If a child's age is known and it is between 1 and 10 years, the following formula may be useful:

weight (kg) = 2(age in years + 4).

The formula method has the added advantage of allowing an estimation of the weight to be made before the child arrives in hospital so that the appropriate equipment and drugs may be arranged. Whatever the method, it is essential that the carer is sufficiently familiar with it to be able to use it quickly and accurately under pressure.

Growth within expected limits is probably the best indicator of health during infancy and childhood (Bickley 2000). Any opportunity to measure the height and weight of a child should be taken so that any failure to thrive or over-nutrition can be identified early. Look for measurements above the 97th and below the 3rd centiles or any indication that a child's weight or height has crossed the centiles. Any large variation between height and weight should also be examined.

Ensure that the scales used are suitable for the age of the child (e.g. basin scales for infants and children who are unable to sit unsupported) and that they have been calibrated regularly. Children younger than 3 years should be weighed naked (Royal College of Nursing 2006), and the reading should be taken when the child is still. Check the weight against expected weights for a child of that age (Table 7.4) and with previous weights recorded for the child. All weights and heights should be plotted in kilograms on a centile chart and any spurious readings reported.

Head circumference should be measured at every examination within the first 2 years of life and plotted on a centile chart (Bickley 2000, Royal College of Nursing 2006). It is an indicator of brain growth (Gill & O'Brien 2003) and as such any crossing of the centiles is abnormal. It is good practice to take parental measurements if concerned with head circumference,

Table 7.4. Expected weights for children of different ages

Age (years)	Guideline for average weight from formula (kg)	Average weight from growth charts (kg)	
		Girls	***Boys***
1	10	7.25–12.5	7.75–13.5
2	12	9–16.25	9.5–16.8
3	14	10.5–19.75	11–20
4	16	12–23.25	12.25–23
5	18	13.25–27.25	14–26.5
6	20	15–32	16.5–30.5
7	22	16.5–37.5	17–35
8	24	18–44	18.5–42
9	26	20–51	20–49
10	28	22–59	22–56
11	–	23.5–66	24–63
12	–	26–71	25.5–69
13	–	29–75	28–76
14	–	33.5–79	31–84
15	–	37–84	35–92

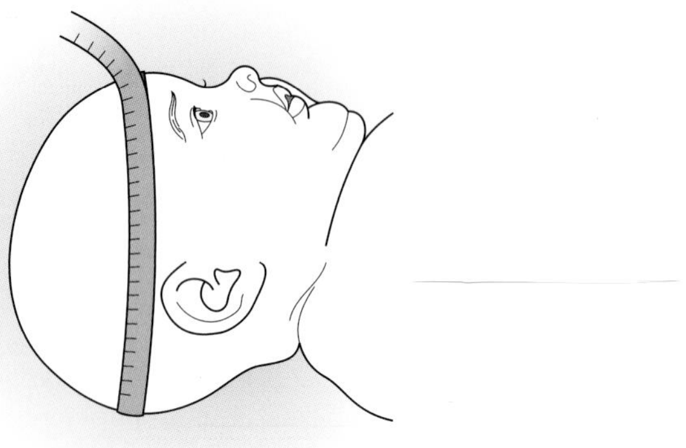

Fig. 7.3 • Using a tape to measure the head circumference of an infant.

as this will give an indication of the expected head circumference of the child.

The infant should be laid supine and then, using a non-stretchable cloth or soft plastic or paper tape, stretch the tape over the occipital, parietal and frontal prominences (Fig. 7.3); note the reading at the greatest measurement.

For further information and guidance on the use of centile charts see the website of the Royal College of Paediatrics and Child Health (2007).

Summary

All the above aspects of your assessment are useful only when looked at as a whole and not individually. A child who is pale, finding it difficult to talk and raising her or his shoulders using the whole body to take each breath is clearly quite sick regardless of the respiratory rate. The most important factors are the general colour and condition of the child. Is the child pale, grey, flushed, mottled or blue? Is he or she relaxed or distressed, and how much effort does it take him or her to breathe? How is the child sitting or positioning himself or herself, and is he or she able to talk or feed?

The oxygen saturation reading is a good back-up indicator of the child's condition; it should not be used in isolation. Be wary of the child who is receiving oxygen, as the oxygen saturation reading may be giving falsely comforting readings; use blood gases and visual assessment to confirm your assessment.

Any attendance of a child for assessment is an opportunity to undertake a general health check. Take the opportunity to obtain a height, weight and head circumference (if appropriate), as any static measurements may be an indication of disease (Gill & O'Brien 2003). Additionally you may not be aware of any problems that the health visitor may be having in monitoring the child; do not assume that somebody else will be aware of a problem. Document everything that you do, see and hear; even seemingly unimportant facts may turn out to be vital when added to further information gained by others or at a later date.

The best tools for undertaking a good paediatric assessment are your eyes closely followed by your ears. The use of machines is increasing within paediatrics, but readings must always be checked against the information that is provided by your eyes and ears. This skill of assessment is the most important skill that you have and one that should continually develop throughout your career.

Now test your knowledge

- What factors influence the heart rate of children?
- What effect does a rise in temperature have on heart rate?
- What effect may a cold room have on a hypoxic child?
- What signs would indicate increased effort in breathing in children?
- What are the three forms of dehydration?
- How is a progressive loss of fluid reflected in:
  - pulse volume
  - urinary output
  - capillary refill time
  - blood pressure?
- In which situations are oxygen saturation monitors less effective?
- How often should an oxygen saturation probe site be changed in continuous monitoring?
- What formula can used to calculate a child's weight between the ages of 1 and 10 years?

References

Armon K, Lakhanpaul M, Stephenson T (2001) An evidence and consensus based guideline for acute diarrhoea management. Archives of Disease in Children 85:132–142

Ashwill JW, Droske SC (1997) Nursing care of children. Principles and practice. Saunders, Edinburgh

Bickley L (2000) Bates' pocket guide to physical examination and history taking, 3rd edn. Lippincott, Philadelphia

Campbell AGM, McIntosh N (1998) Campbell and McIntosh and Arneil's textbook of paediatrics, 5th edn. Churchill Livingstone, Edinburgh

Department of Health (2004) National Service Framework for Children, Young People and Maternity Services: children and young people who are ill. Department of Health, London

Gill D, O'Brien N (2003) Paediatric clinical examination made easy, 4th edn. Churchill Livingstone, London

Hampson N (1998) Pulse oximetry in severe carbon monoxide poisoning. Chest 114:1036–1041

Jevon P, Ewens B (2002) Monitoring the critically ill patient. Blackwell Science, Oxford

Kelly L, Morin K. (1996) Improving caretakers' knowledge of fever management in preschool children: is it possible? Journal of Pediatric Health Care 10(4):167–173

Kramer M, Naimark L, Leduc D (1985) Parental fever phobia and its correlates. Pediatrics 75(6):1110–1113

Mackway-Jones K, Molyneux E, Phillips B, Wieteska S (eds) (2005) Advanced paediatric life support – the practical approach, 4th edn. BMJ Books, Blackwell Publishers, Oxford

Medical Devices Agency (2001) Tissue necrosis caused by pulse oximeter probes. Medicines and Healthcare Products Regulatory Agency, London

Robertson NRC (1993) A manual of neonatal intensive care, 3rd edn. Edward Arnold, London

Royal College of Nursing (2006) Malnutrition. What nurses working with children and young people need to know and do. RCN, London

Royal College of Paediatrics and Child Health (2007) Growth reference charts for use in the United Kingdom. Online. Available: http://www.rcpch.ac.uk/doc.aspx?id_Resource=1746

Schutz S (2001) Oxygen saturation monitoring by pulse oximetry. AACN procedure manual for critical care, 4th edn. Saunders, Edinburgh

Stroobant J, Field D (2002) Handbook of paediatric investigations. Churchill Livingstone, Edinburgh

Weller B (2004) Nurses' dictionary, 23rd edn. RCN, Baillière Tindall, London

8 Assessment of temperature, pulse and respiration

Marion Aylott

The cornerstone of nursing assessment is the measurement of temperature, pulse and respirations (TPR). Together with blood pressure measurement (see Ch. 9) these are popularly known as vital signs. Oxygen saturation may be included based on hospital or unit policy. The measurement and assessment of vital signs, as the name suggests, refers to the measurement of vital or critical physiologic functions. The measurement and monitoring of vital signs provides one of the most important keys to the child's health status and is an efficient method for monitoring a client's condition, identifying problem areas or assessing a client's response to medical and/or nursing treatment. Indeed, the measurement of body temperature in the seriously sick child is important, as hypothermia and hyperthermia have profound effects on the cardiovascular, pulmonary, neurological and haemostatic systems (Smith et al 2005). The assessment of TPR is probably the most important aspect of your work, because without a good assessment there is almost no other reliable way to determine serious illness in a child before collapse.

Definitions

- Temperature is defined as an objective measurement of the relative warmth or coolness of a substance.
- Pulse rate is a measurement of the heart rate or the number of times the heart beats per min.
- Respiratory rate is the number of breaths a person takes per min.

Body temperature

Humans are homeothermic, that is, they have the ability of the body to regulate heat (Candy et al 2006). The internal temperature is kept relatively constant, with only minor deviations from the normal range of core body temperature, which is 36.6–37.8 °C. Good health is associated with a range of normal temperature. Possible reasons for deviation include:

- prolonged, heavy exercise
- illness
- accident, for example near drowning
- poisoning, for example alcohol or drug overdose
- inadvertent postoperatively due to anaesthetic agents
- deliberate harm
- extreme conditions of hot and cold
- therapeutic (Smith et al 2005).

Physiologic body processes actively generate, conserve, dissociate or redistribute heat. These processes are coordinated by a region of the hypothalamus that acts as a thermostat for the body (Lissauer & Clayden 2001). Thermosensory impulses from the skin and central receptors are integrated and compared with a thermostatic set point range. This set point range is from approximately 36.4 to 37.3 °C (Holtzclaw 1993). Any deviation above or below this range causes the body to initiate physiological responses that lead to heat loss or gain as required.

The body consists of three thermal compartments: the core, the shell and the skeletal muscle (McChance & Huether 2006). The core includes all the body's inner organs. Each of these inner organs has its own metabolic rate, blood flow and preferred working temperature range. The shell, which consists of skin and subcutaneous fat, serves as an insulator for the core. The skeletal muscle acts as an insulator during low activity states or as a heat producer during increased muscle activity such as shivering or exercising. Under normal circumstances the body controls its temperature within a very tight tolerance, with the core being 2–4 °C warmer than the periphery. Heat moves along a temperature gradient from warmer to cooler areas. Therefore in hypothermia, heat will be transferred from the warm core to the cooler peripheral compartment, resulting in a greater degree of core hypothermia. It is important to remember that neonates, infants and young children have a much larger core compartment as compared with the adult, which also extends closer to the body surface due to general body morphology and less muscle and adipose tissue, which act as a thermal insulator (Chamley et al 2005).

The temperature gradient between the core and the periphery is regulated mainly by a thermoregulatory vasoconstriction mechanism (McChance & Huether 2006). This is of particular importance when considering the site of body temperature measurement, particularly in the child, as stated above. Vasoconstriction and vasodilation influence the amount of heat lost to the environment by controlling the distribution of blood near the body surface. Heat transfer occurs through radiation, evaporation, conduction and convection (Potter et al 2003). The anterior hypothalamus senses an elevated body temperature and triggers heat loss mechanisms such as sweating, vasodilation of blood vessels and inhibition of heat production. In contrast the posterior hypothalamus senses a low temperature and triggers heat conservation mechanisms, which include vasoconstriction and compensatory heat production by shivering. Vasomotor activity also influences blood flow to a region and can significantly raise or lower temperature to specific organs (Chamley et al 2005). Body temperature is also influenced by hormonal changes, some related to age, and diurnal variations (Neill & Knowles 2004).

Heat is produced in the body by metabolism, which is the chemical reaction in all body cells. Food is the primary source of fuel of this chemical reaction. The amount of energy used for metabolism is the metabolic rate. Heat is produced as a by-product of metabolism. Activities that increase chemical reactions increase the metabolic rate. The basal metabolic rate (BMR) is the amount of heat produced by the body at absolute rest. The average BMR depends on body surface area, which is proportionally greater in infants and children as compared with adults (Chamley et al 2005). Thyroid hormones have a significant effect on BMR. Increased production of thyroid hormones increases the rate of chemical reactions and increases BMR. Conversely, decreased thyroid levels decreases BMR. Voluntary muscle movements, for example shivering, also increase BMR.

Table 8.1 provides a glossary of terms associated with the measurement of body temperature.

Measuring body temperature

We measure temperature because good health is associated with a range of normal temperature. Temperature measurement is arguably one of the most common assessments within

Table 8.1. Glossary of terms associated with body temperature measurement

Term	Definition
Afebrile	Absence of fever
Ambient temperature	Temp erature of the immediate surrounding environment
Axilla	Armpit
Core temperature	Deep tissue temperature within the central part of the body (brain, heart, lungs) not influenced by environmental temperature
Febrile	State of elevated temperature (fever)
Hyperpyrexia	Heat loss is unable to keep pace with excess heat production (> 41°C)
Hyperthermia	Elevated body temperature
Hypothermia	Decreased body temperature (< 35°C)
Malignant hyperthermia	Hereditary condition of uncontrolled heat production that occurs in susceptible persons who receive certain anaesthetic drugs
Pyrexia	Elevation of body temperature up to 41°C
Pyrogens	Bacteria and viruses that cause a rise in body temperature
Rectum	Back passage
Thermometer	Temperature-sensing instrument
Tympanic	Ear canal

nursing practice and provides a critical tool in detecting fever in children. Interventions are frequently based on temperature assessment, as fever may indicate inflammatory or infectious processes. Instruments used to measure temperature must be thoroughly evaluated for accuracy.

Vigilant and accurate assessment of thermal balance is an important factor in the recognition of the seriously sick child and young person (Department of Health 2004). Disease, injury or pharmacological therapy can impair thermoregulation, leaving children vulnerable to uncontrolled gain or loss of heat. We also measure body temperature to track the thermal effect of environmental exposure, hypothermia and hyperthermia, and to monitor and control deliberate warming or cooling of the body for therapeutic purposes. Body temperature is therefore commonly measured to confirm the presence or absence of fever or hypothermia. The presence of fever or hypothermia and its severity are vital indicators that its causes need careful investigation and prompt treatment (El-Radhi & Barry 2006). However, there remains considerable controversy in the research literature regarding the most appropriate method, such as infrared ear-based thermometer (tympanic), chemical dot thermometer (e.g. Tempa.dot) and glass or electric thermometer.

The current gold standard for measuring core body temperature is a thermistor placed in the pulmonary artery, coronary artery or brain (Box 8.1; McKenzie & Osgood 2004). This deep tissue measurement sites are clinically inaccessible, and the risk associated with their invasive nature far outweighs their clinical benefit in most situations (Chaturverdi et al 2004). Therefore a variety of practical alternative body sites, such as the rectum, the axilla (armpit), sublingual (under the tongue), the skin and the tympanic membrane (ear canal), have been used clinically to measure body temperature (Box 8.1). However, there is also controversy with regard to which of these constitutes the best indirect core anatomical site. Ideally, valid and reliable temperature measurement should reflect the child's current thermal status. The gold standard, the ideal thermometer:

- is accurate and reliable
- is safe
- is comfortable
- is child-friendly
- is linear
- is rapid
- is non-invasive
- has minimal risk of cross-infection
- can be readily disinfected
- is easy to use.

Box 8.1. Temperature-monitoring sites

Core (deep)

- Pulmonary artery
- Distal oesophagus
- Tympanic membrane
- Nasopharynx

Shell (surface)

- Mouth
- Axilla
- Bladder
- Rectum
- Skin surface (forehead, abdomen)

However, irrespective of best instrument and most appropriate site, individual practitioner variation or an error in temperature measurement technique might seriously influence the validity and reliability of the measurement and evaluation of a child's health condition (Sund-Levander et al 2004). It is also important to be mindful that the supposedly simple task of measuring a child's temperature can be made difficult and hence inaccurate and unreliable if the child is restless, combative or uncooperative. The nurse must not only be knowledgeable in selecting the best instrument and the most appropriate site and be skilful in using the instrument in that site efficiently but also be skilful in preparing and engaging the child. These factors are vital if the measurement is to be taken effectively.

In recent years there has been a proliferation of research studies that have investigated the accuracy of different thermometers and measurement sites in an effort to determine evidence-based best practice. The results on initial review are somewhat contradictory. However, close scrutiny of the research by a panel of experts has led to the development of an evidence-based guideline by the National Institute for Health and Clinical Excellence (2006) that is currently under public review.

Obtaining an accurate temperature in the actual or potentially sick child is vital. As discussed, temperatures vary throughout the body. Therefore the optimal site must be selected. The core thermal compartment is composed of highly perfused tissue and yields a uniform temperature that is high compared with the rest of the body. The temperature of blood returning to the right side of the heart is thought to be the most accurate clinical measurement of core body temperature (Chamley et al 2005). However, a pulmonary artery catheter is necessary to measure this temperature. Nasopharyngeal and oesophageal sites are thought to correlate well with pulmonary artery catheter temperature, but again these are unsuitable for general use as they are invasive and uncomfortable.

Urinary catheters with a thermistor port tend to read slightly behind pulmonary artery catheter temperatures, and again this method is unnecessarily invasive in most instances. Contrary to traditional (recent) opinion the rectum is an area of low blood flow and therefore does not accurately reflect core body temperature (Robinson et al 1998), particularly when there is evidence of poor peripheral circulation. Oral temperature measurement is dependent on technique and affected by many environmental factors, for example recent hot or cold drinks and child cooperation. It is also important to be aware of the advantages and disadvantages of a thermometry device in order that the most appropriate device is selected (see Table 8.2).

Table 8.2. Advantages and disadvantages of temperature measurement instruments

Instrument	Advantages	Disadvantages
Glass mercury	• Accurate • Easy access and convenient • Minimally invasive	• Dwell time: 6–7 min • Unsafe: glass breakage, mercury poisoning, cross-infection • Glass is porous and mercury can evaporate within 6 months of manufacture, which affects accuracy
Electronic or digital	• Convenient • Non-invasive • Reduced risk of cross-infection • Quick: takes 40–80 s • Provides choice of route: oral or axilla • Readings approximately 0.4°C below pulmonary artery temperature	–
Tempa.dot	• Fast temperature reading (oral, 1 min; axilla, 3 min) • Stabilisation period: 10 s • Comfortable for all ages • Easy to use • Provides choice of route: oral or axilla • Readings approximately 0.4°C below pulmonary artery temperature	• Ambient temperatures affect results • Readings start at 35.5°C • Influenced by vasomotor activity
Infrared tympanic membrane	• Fast and easy to use • Wide temperature range: 20–42.2°C • Reduced risk of cross-infection • Not influenced by environmental temperature • Good correlation with pulmonary artery temperature (within 0.1–0.6°C) due to close proximity to internal carotid artery and hypothalamus • Preferred by children	• Ear tug required to direct towards tympanic membrane (important for accuracy) • Inaccuracies in small babies in neonatal period (under 4 weeks of age), as difficult to ensure that probe is inserted properly (currently under review with neonatal instruments) • Ear infections reduce temperature reading by 0.1°C • Presence of cerumen causes under-reading by 1°C

For example, in the care of a hypothermic child it is important to be aware of the temperature range of the monitoring device chosen, as many digital electronic thermometers will record temperatures only as low as 34.6°C even though the child's true temperature may be lower (Molton et al 2001).

ALERT
Environmental and accidental ingestion concerns regarding mercury mean that mercury-in-glass thermometers are no longer recommended (Medicines and Healthcare products Regulatory Agency 2006).

Research suggests that as the tympanic membrane shares the same blood supply as the hypothalamus, the tympanic thermometer will reflect a core temperature (Akinyinka 2002). There is some conflicting research regarding its accuracy, which is thought to be due to user technique and failure to apply ear tug appropriately (Betta et al 1997, Childs et al 1999, Craig et al 2000). It must be remembered that chemical dot (Macqueen 2001) and electronic thermometers (Craig et al 2002) rely on conductive heat transfer, whereas tympanic infrared thermometers measure naturally occurring electromagnetic radiation and require a direct view of the tympanic membrane (eardrum), hence the need for an ear tug to straighten the ear canal (El-Radhi & Patel 2006). A number of researchers were highly critical of the accuracy of infrared ear thermometry (Androkites et al 1998, Banitalebi & Bangstead 2002, Craig et al 2002, Jean-Mary et al 2002, Lanham et al 1999). However, these studies were fundamentally methodologically flawed, as their gold standard comparison was rectal temperature. Table 8.3 demonstrates the comparative advantages and disadvantages of indirect core temperature measurement sites.

Table 8.3. Advantages and disadvantages of indirect measurement sites

Site	Advantages	Disadvantages
Axilla	• Safe • Easily accessible • Reasonably comfortable • Accurate when ambient temperature stable	• Accurate in afebrile infants and children only • Requires constant supervision because of risk of displacement • Inaccurate when peripheral vasoconstriction present • Inaccurate when evaporation of sweat present • Sensitivity in detecting fever reported as only 28–33% • Affected by fluctuating ambient temperature • Detection of fever poor
Skin	• Safe • Easy to use • Comfortable	• Inaccurate when peripheral vasoconstriction present • Insensitive: frequently records normal temperature despite elevated body temperature • Poor correlation between skin and core temperature • Affected by ambient temperature
Oral	• Safe in children over 5 years old • Not affected by ambient temperature • Easily accessible • Runs approximately 0.5°C lower than pulmonary artery temperature • More accurate than axillary site • Oxygen, mouth breathing and tachypnoea do not influence results	• Correct placement is important for accuracy – readings can vary by 1°C from right and left posterior sublingual pocket to beneath the frenulum • Requires cooperation of child • Not suitable for children with cognitive development equivalent to under 5 years • Hot and cold drinks influence results
Rectum	• Not influenced by ambient temperature	• Correct depth of placement and dwell time are important for accuracy • Time-consuming • Psychologically frightening, embarrassing • Requires privacy • Rectal temperature lags significantly during thermal change – up to 1 h • Accuracy affected by depth of insertion, presence of stool and local blood flow • Inaccurate compared with pulmonary artery, especially when there is thermal imbalance that is hypo- and hyperthermia • Inaccuracy due to insulating effect of faecal material in rectum and coliform bacterial action • Infectious hazard • Rectal perforation risk
Tympanic	• Fast and easy to use • Reduced risk of cross-infection • Not influenced by environmental temperature • Good correlation with pulmonary artery temperature (within 0.1–0.6°C) due to close proximity to internal carotid artery and hypothalamus • Preferred by children	• Ear tug required to direct towards tympanic membrane (important for accuracy) • Inaccuracies in children under 3 years; however, compared with oral and rectal not pulmonary artery • Ear infections reduce temperature reading by 0.1°C • Presence of cerumen causes under-reading by 1°C

Because the aim of temperature measurement is usually to detect or exclude the presence of fever, use of the rectum and skin site is not recommended as the detection rate is poor due to vasomotor response in illness, as discussed earlier. Furthermore the rectal route is not recommended as there are concerns regarding its safety (Rush & Wetherall 2003) and acceptability (Pickersgill et al 2003). Recommendations made by the National Institute for Health and Clinical Excellence (2006) are summarised in Table 8.4.

Table 8.4. Recommendations made by the National Institute for Health and Clinical Excellence (2007)

Age group	Recommended method	Contraindications
Baby in the neonatal period (first 4 weeks of life)	Electronic thermometer in axilla	• Tympanic, as difficult to ensure that probe is positioned properly in ear canal • Oral route is unsafe
Infant of 4 weeks of age to child of 5 years of age	One of the following: • electronic thermometer in axilla • chemical dot thermometer (e.g. Tempa.dot) in axilla • infrared tympanic thermometer	• Oral route is unsafe • Oral route may provide inaccurate measurement, as child must be able to understand the need to hold a thermometer under his or her tongue while a measurement is taken
Child over 5 years of age	One of the following: • electronic thermometer in axilla or oral • chemical dot thermometer (e.g. Tempa.dot) in axilla or oral • infrared tympanic thermometer	–

Procedures Box 8.1 Preparation for temperature measurement

Actions

1. Determine the appropriate method and site for temperature measurement, taking into consideration age, level of understanding and level of alertness:
   - Consider the National Institute for Health and Clinical Excellence guidance (2006), as in the *Temperature measurement using a Tempa.dot* procedure box.
2. Explain the procedure to the child and the parent(s) using developmentally appropriate language. You may need to:
   - use play through the use of dolls to prepare the child
   - give the child time to familiarise herself or himself with the equipment that you might use, for example a stethoscope
   - use distraction therapy such as bubble blowing
   - work in collaboration with parents and/or a play specialist (this can be helpful)
   - give the child a choice of preferred method.
3. Gather the equipment required and check for cleanliness and working order.
4. ALWAYS wash your hands and check the identity of the child.
5. CAUTION: do not use any thermometer unless you have been properly trained and have practised under supervision with the particular type of device to be used.
6. Intense physical activity can raise the temperature, so be sure to give the child time to cool down before taking the temperature.

   Consumption of hot or cold drinks or food immediately beforehand may affect the outcome. If taking the child's temperature via the oral route, wait 20 min before taking the temperature.

Procedures Box 8.2 Temperature measurement using a Tempa.dot

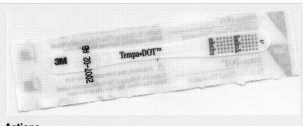

Actions

1. Check the expiry date of the thermometer and that it has been stored correctly.

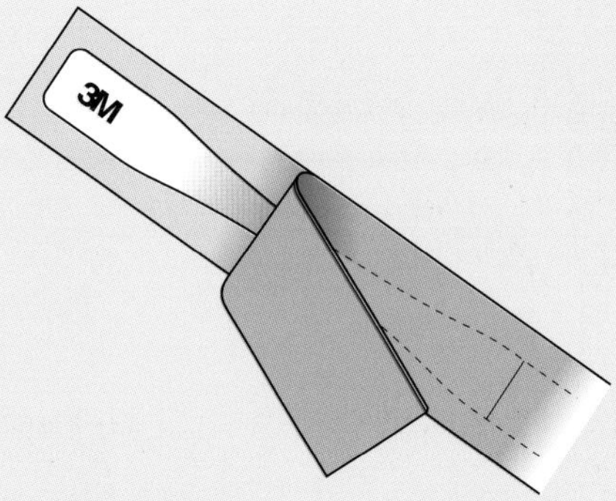

2. Tear off paper cover, being careful not to touch the chemical strip.

Procedures Box 8.2 Temperature measurement using a Tempa.dot—cont'd

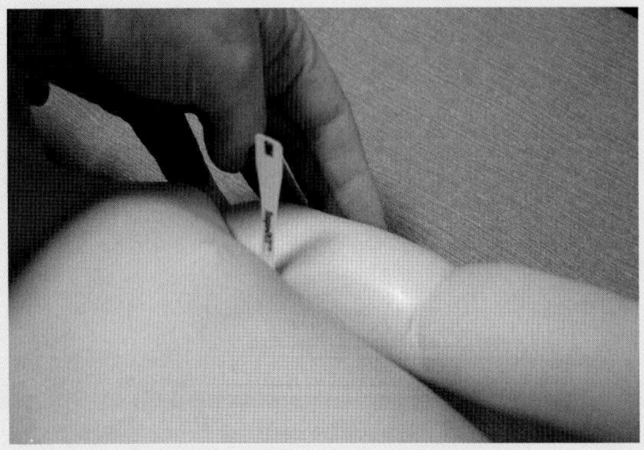

3. The plastic strips can be placed in the axilla of children under 5 years and in the oral cavity or in the axilla of the child over 5.

   Note: regarding oral route, the child must be awake and alert and able to hold the thermometer in his or her mouth under the tongue while the measurement is taken.

Placing in the axilla

Actions

3a. Place the temperature strip (dots facing towards the trunk) high and snugly in the apex of the child's axilla, making sure that it is in contact with tissue not clothing.

3b. Encourage children to hold their arm down by their side – you might need to assist them in this; good tissue contact is essential.

Placing under the tongue

Actions

3a. Ask the child to open her or his mouth.

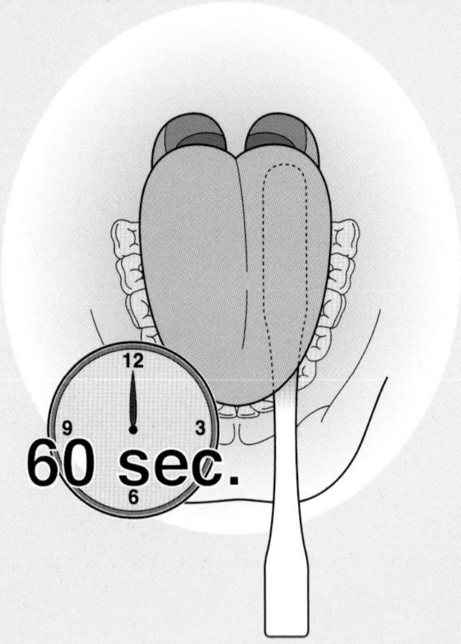

3b. Gently place the thermometer under the tongue in the left or right posterior sublingual pocket.

3c. Ask the child to close her or his lips to hold the thermometer in place.

Actions

4. Leave the thermometer in place for the desired time: oral, 1 min; axilla, 3 min.
5. On removal, taking care not to touch the dot area, allow a stabilisation period of at least 10 s to allow chemical colour development (like a Polaroid photograph); this will make the strip easier to read and interpret.

   (The temperature reading will remain constant once removed from the temperature-taking site.)

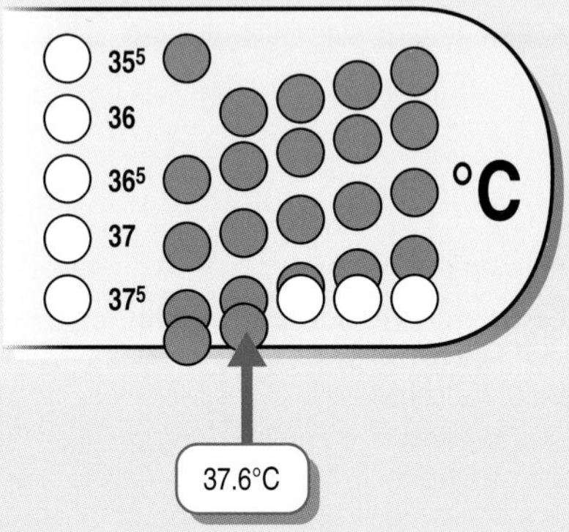

6. Read the temperature measurement using the blue dots as above.
7. Dispose of the temperature strip appropriately and wash your hands.

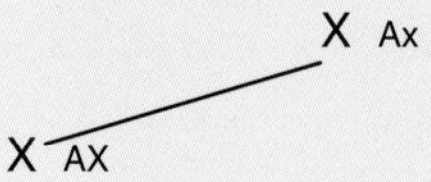

8. Clearly and accurately document the measurement, method and site.
9. Notify the doctor of abnormal readings or as directed by the doctor or senior nurse.

(Some images courtesy of 3M.)

Procedures Box 8.3 Temperature measurement using an electronic thermometer

Actions

1. Check that the thermometer is in good working order.

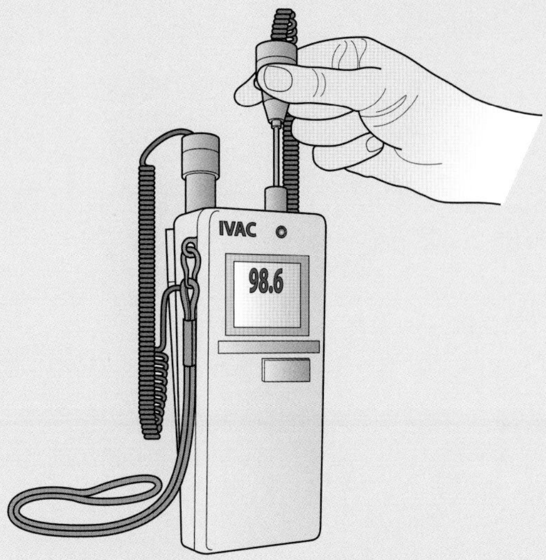

2. With your thumb and forefinger, grasp the base of the probe and withdraw it from the storage well; this action automatically turns on the instrument.
3. Always use a new probe cover and apply it until it snaps into position.
4. The probe can be placed:
   - in the axilla of children under 5 years
   - in the oral cavity or in the axilla of the child over 5.

   Note: regarding the oral route the child must be awake and alert and able to hold the thermometer in her or his mouth under the tongue while the measurement is taken.

   Hold the probe during the entire temperature measurement process and keep the probe tip in contact with sublingual pocket tissues (the richest blood supply is located here) at all times.

   Do not allow the child to reposition the probe.

Placing in the axilla

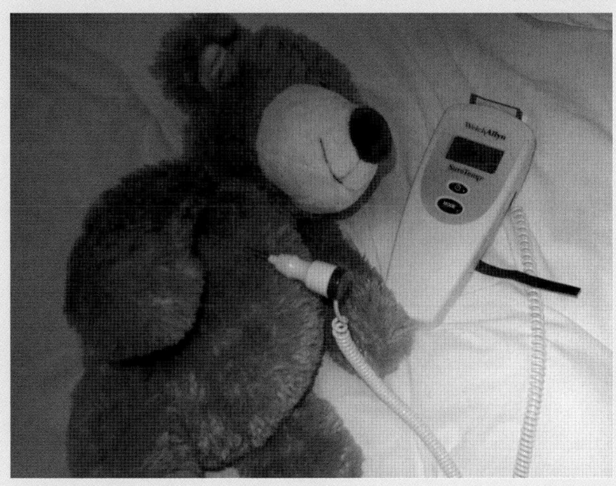

Actions

4a. Check to make sure that the thermometer is set in the 'direct' or 'monitor' mode and plan to spend at least 8 min with the thermometer in place.

4b. Place the probe high and snugly in the apex of the child's axilla, making sure that it is in contact with tissue not clothing.

Encourage children to hold their arm down by their side – you might need to assist them in this.

4c. When the temperature stops changing, after about 8–10 min, read the LED before removing the probe from the axilla.

Placing under the tongue

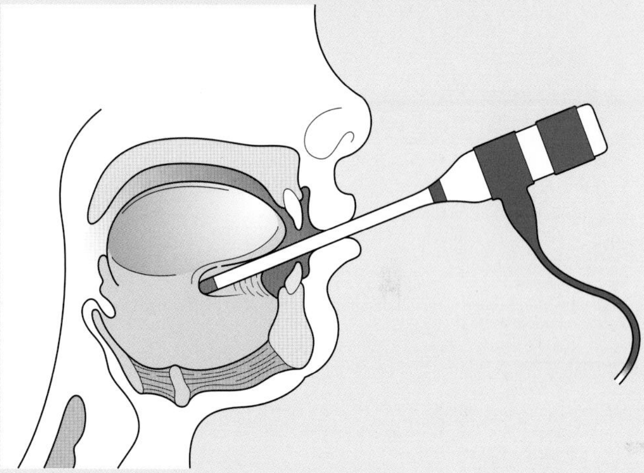

Actions

4a. Check to make sure that the thermometer is set in the 'predictive' mode.

4b. Ask the child to open his or her mouth.

Gently place the thermometer under the tongue in the left or right posterior sublingual pocket.

Ask the child to close his or her lips to hold the thermometer in place.

Encourage the child to relax the tongue over the probe, not hold the tongue away from the probe.

4c. When the audible signal occurs, the beep, read the temperature display.

Actions

5. Hold the probe as you would a syringe and press the probe ejection button at the base of the probe to eject the used probe cover directly into an appropriate waste container.
6. Return the probe to its storage well. This will automatically turn off and reset the thermometer for the next use.
7. Wash your hands.
8. Clearly and accurately document the measurement, method and site.
9. Notify the doctor of abnormal readings or as directed by the doctor or senior nurse.

(Some images courtesy of the Starship Children's Hospital, Auckland.)

Procedures Box 8.4 Temperature measurement using an infrared tympanic membrane thermometer

Actions

1. Check that the thermometer is in good working order.

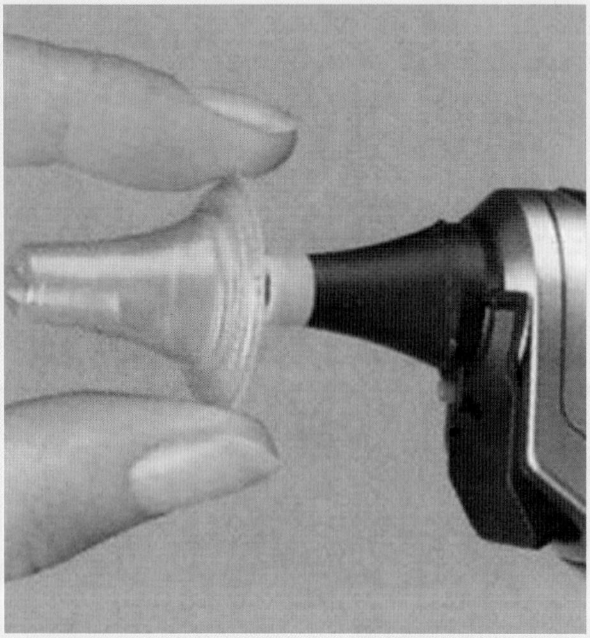

2. Always use a new probe cover and apply it until it snaps into position.

3a. Perform an ear tug to straighten the ear canal to give the thermometer a clear view of the eardrum.

This is NOT suitable for use in babies less than 4 weeks of age.

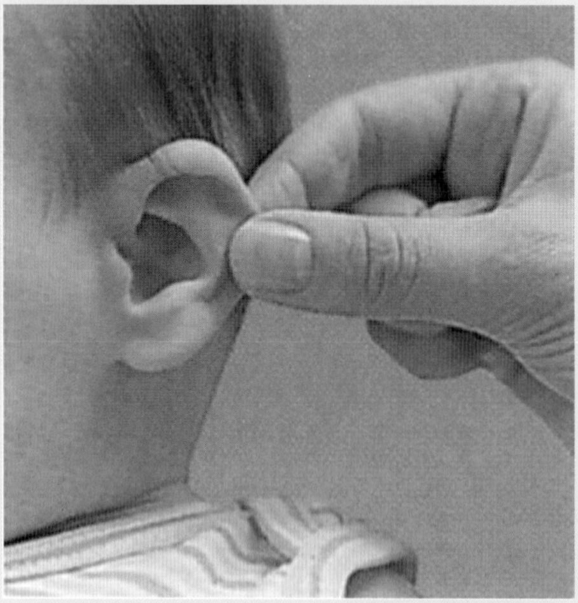

- In children under 1 year, gently pull the ear straight back.

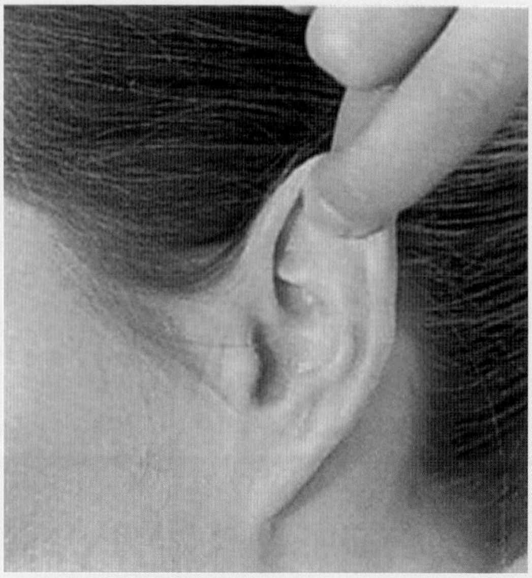

- In children aged over 1 year or an adult, gently pull the ear up and back.

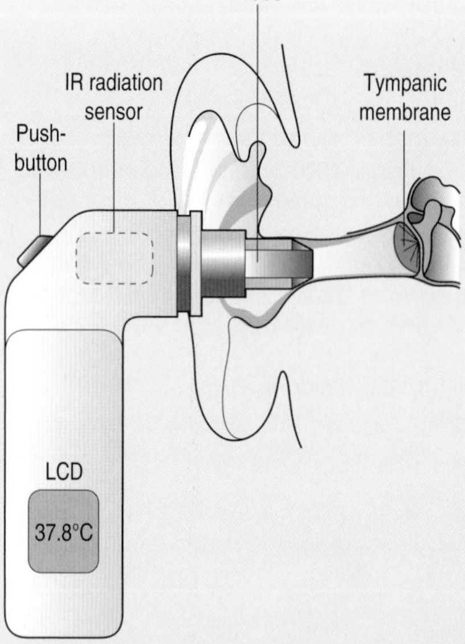

3b. While tugging the ear, fit the probe gently in the ear canal as far as possible and press the activation button.

Release the button when you hear the bleep.

4. Remove the thermometer from the ear canal; the temperature will then be displayed along with the probe cover symbol.
5. Press the ejector button and dispose of the probe cover appropriately and wash your hands.
6. Clearly and accurately document the measurement, method and site.
7. Notify the doctor of abnormal readings or as directed by the doctor or senior nurse.

(Images courtesy of IOP Publishing and Welch Allyn.)

Pulse rate

The pulse rate is a measurement of the heart rate, or the number of times the heart beats per minute (Rudolf & Levene 2006). The pulse is caused by pressure exerted on the arterial wall, causing expansion of the vessel for the brief moment that the wave of pressure passes (Blows 2001). The pulse represents the beating of the heart, specifically the pressure wave caused by the ejection of blood from the left ventricle to the general circulation of the body (Tortora 2005). The ventricles (right and left) have two phases: diastole, or the time when the ventricles 'rest' so they can fill with blood, and systole, the time when the ventricles contract to send blood either to the lungs (from the right side of the heart) or to the rest of the body (from the left side of the heart). Blood from the left side of the heart first enters the aorta, the largest artery in the body. The aorta branches into smaller arteries that carry blood to all parts of the body. The pulse represents the variation in blood pressure from diastole to systole. During diastole blood pressure falls, but it increases after systole as the heart pumps more blood into the arteries. You feel this difference when taking your pulse. As the heart pushes blood through the arteries, the arteries expand and contract with the flow of the blood, and this can be felt in various points in the body as a pulse. Taking a pulse not only measures the heart rate but also can indicate the following:

- Heart rhythm (abnormal rhythm may indicate a heart disorder)
- Strength of the pulse (a weak pulse may indicate a fast heartbeat in which some beats are too weak to feel, for example in heart failure, or a low volume of blood in the circulatory system).

Thus the pulse rate is an indicator of the health of the heart and the arterial circulation (Tortora & Derrickson 2007). Pulse assessment is performed to:

- establish a baseline measurement on a patient's admission or prior to commencement of therapy
- detect any abnormalities from the healthy state or response to therapy.

Table 8.5 provides a glossary of terms associated with pulse and heart rate assessment.

Measuring the child's pulse

Feeling the pulse is much more than counting the heart rate and evaluating the rhythm. It requires a great deal of

Table 8.5. Glossary of terms associated with pulse and heart rate assessment

Term	Definition
Arrhythmia	Irregular pulse/heart rhythm
Bounding pulse	Strong pronounced pulsation that does not disappear easily with pressure
Bradycardia	Slow heart rate
Normal pulse	Easily felt pulsation which withstands moderate pressure
Pulsus alternans	Amplitude of pulse is strong and weak pulse alternatively
Pulse rhythm	The pattern of the pulsations and pauses between them.
Pulse volume	Quality of the pulsations that are felt
Sinus rhythm	Regular pattern of the pulsations and pauses between them
Tachycardia	Fast heart rate
Thready pulse	Pulse not easy to feel. Applying slight pressure will cause it to disappear
Weak pulse	Stronger than a thready pulse. Requires light pressure to disappear

patience and experience to learn to evaluate heart rate, strength and rhythm disturbances. The rate, rhythm and strength of a pulse are assessed by palpation using usually the index, middle and ring fingers. Avoid using the thumb otherwise you might end up counting your own pulse! The pulse is felt at points where a surface artery runs over a bone (see Fig. 8.1). The most common option used, under normal circumstances, is the radial artery (in the forearm) in the child. The radial pulse is found on the inner aspect of the wrist, thumb side against the ridge due to a tendon. However, radial pulses are not easy to palpate in the infant less than 1 year of age. The brachial artery pulse that occurs along the inner aspect of the upper arm, beneath the brachial muscle and against the humerus, is easier in infants (see *Temperature measurement using an infrared tympanic membrane thermometer* procedure box). Moreover, in young children under 2 years of age counting the peripheral pulse is technically difficult and auscultation of the apical beat is recommended (Margolius et al 1991, Tanner et al 2000). Incidentally, auscultation of the apical beat is recommended for accuracy of measurement in any age group, particularly in children in whom tachycardia is present (Lockwood et al 2004). For the advantages and disadvantages of routine pulse assessment locations see Table 8.6.

An appreciation of the variability of pulse (heart) rate in relationship to age and clinical state in children is important as part of the overall assessment of the presenting child. The heart rate is initially rapid at birth and gradually decreases as the child approaches adolescence (Wallis et al 2005). The heart rate show greatest variability in neonates and infants up to 1 year of age (Sarti et al 2006). Nurses should have a thorough knowledge about the normal and abnormal pulse in order to identify irregularities. You may have no prior knowledge of the patient's 'healthy' pulse rate for comparison, therefore it is important to know the range of normal values that apply to patients of different ages (see Table 8.7). The heart rate of the child varies according to age. The newborn baby born at term (neonate) for the first 4 weeks of life has a typical heart rate of approximately 130–160 beats/min. During puberty the heart rate falls to adult levels of 66–80 beats/min (Department of Health 2004).

Table 8.6. Advantages and disadvantages of routine pulse assessment locations

Pulse site	Advantages	Disadvantages
Radial	• Non-invasive • Easily accessible • Usually easily palpable in children over 1 year of age	• Not easy to palpate in infants • Not easily palpable in obese children • Loses accuracy when cardiac output is low
Brachial	• Easily accessible • Usually easily palpable in infants	• Not easily palpable in obese children • Loses accuracy when cardiac output is low
Apical	• Greater accuracy in children under 2 years of age and those with poor peripheral perfusion	• Invasive • Embarrassment in teenagers

Table 8.7. Normal heart rate ranges

Age (years)	Heart rate (beats/min)
Neonate	130–160
<1	110–160
1–5	95–140
5–12	80–120
<12	60–80

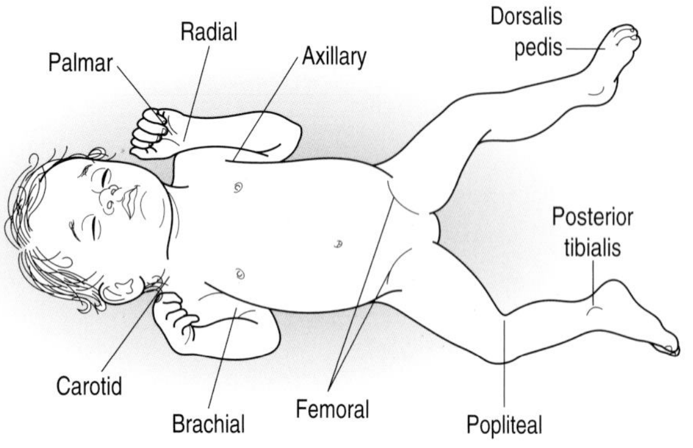

Fig. 8.1 • Pulse assessment locations.

The quality of the pulse should be evaluated first, even when the nurse intends to measure the heart rate by auscultation. It is always important to palpate the quality of the pulse, as this is an important indicator of poor cardiac output and circulatory insufficiency (Marieb 2004). Experience alone will allow the nurse to develop the skill to distinguish the variations in pulses that can exist. Pulses are normal when they are easily palpated with a smooth upstroke and down slope. Weak and thready pulses are not easily felt in the periphery and may be caused by a number of factors including shock or extreme tachycardia (>200 beats/min). A 'bounding' high-pressure pulse may be caused by fever, for example. These types of pulses are graded in order to describe them qualitatively (see Table 8.8). An alternating strong and weak pulse pressure (during sinus rhythm) is termed *pulsus alternans*, which is a cardiovascular phenomenon associated with heart failure although the exact mechanism is not understood (Weber 2003).

After determining the quality of the pulse, the child's resting pulse and heart rate should be evaluated. A pulse count through palpation or auscultation of heart rate and rhythm is best accomplished during quiet alert or sleep states of infants and children, as it is virtually impossible to auscultate heart rate in a crying child and the resultant measurement is likely to be wholly inaccurate. Abnormalities of heart rate commonly encountered in children include sinus bradycardia and sinus tachycardia. Sinus means 'normal rhythm'. Sinus bradycardia is defined as a heart rate less than is normal for the child's age and is generally due to predominance of the parasympathetic nervous system regulation (Tortora 2005). Any trigger that results in vagal stimulation will cause a transient decrease in heart rate and subsequent bradycardia. Sinus tachycardia is defined as a heart rate greater than is normal for the age of the child (Tortora 2005). It is triggered by a variety of intrinsic and extrinsic stimuli that place greater demands on the heart, for example stress and exercise. Under normal circumstances removal of the triggering stimuli will allow a gradual return of the heart rate to baseline.

Before placing a stethoscope on the chest, the nurse must first understand the nature and origin of audible heart sounds. The heart produces two sounds, often referred to as 'lub' and 'dub'. The first 'lub' is the sound produced by closure of the atrioventricular valves. The second, 'dub', sound is produced by the aortic and pulmonic valves closing behind the ejected blood. These sounds should correspond to the palpated peripheral pulse if felt simultaneously (Marieb 2004). It is important to listen to the left ventricle at the outermost and lowest point of the heart, known as the apex of the heart; this is known as the apex beat (Sneed & Hollerbach 1992). When assessing the heart rate auscultation, use the bell of the stethoscope to auscultate over the fourth intercostal space (in the under 8 years) and fifth intercostal space in the mid-clavicular line (in the over 8 years). You can practise locating these landmarks on yourself. Begin by locating the suprasternal notch. Feel for the hollow U-shaped depression just above the sternum, in between the clavicles (shoulder bones). Locate the sternum (breastbone), immediately below the notch. The sternum has three parts: the manubrium, the body and the xiphoid process. Walk your fingers down the manubrium a few centimetres until you feel a distinct bony ridge, the manubriosternal angle. This ridge is continuous with the second rib and a useful place to start counting ribs (Bates 1995). Palpate lightly to the second rib on the left side of the chest and slide your finger down to the second intercostal space. (Intercostal spaces are always numbered by the rib above.) Using the intercostal spaces count down to the fourth intercostal space (under the fourth rib). When auscultating the heart rate of the infant and young child, place the bell of the stethoscope in this space in what is called mid-clavicular line. This is an imaginary line drawn straight down the left side of the chest halfway along the clavicle. When auscultating the heart rate of the older child (over 8 years) and adult, locate the fifth intercostal space and again place the bell of your stethoscope in the mid-clavicular line (Fig. 8.2). This is where it is easiest to auscultate the apical heart beat clearly (James & Smith 2005).

Despite the availability of electrical monitoring equipment to measure pulse rate through pulse oximetry, research evidence suggests that in order to obtain an accurate pulse rate counting the pulse over a full minute by palpation or auscultation remains the best method. Inaccuracies through over-reliance on pulse oximeters have been reported in the literature (Mower et al 1996, Lockwood et al 2004).

Errors in measurement have been reported in the literature due to the period over which the pulse and heart rate are counted. Studies have compared pulse and heart rate counted using 15-, 30- and 60-s count periods (Hollerbach & Sneed 1990). Pulse and heart rate measurement in children under 12 years of age counted over a 60-s period resulted in least variability. A study by Margolius et al (1991) found that rapid respiratory rates in infants counted on auscultation using a stethoscope were more accurate than those counted using pulse palpation. Tachycardia is often associated with weak and irregular heart rhythms, which can make palpation difficult and the resultant rate measured unreliable.

There is no research evidence base to determine how frequently a pulse should be assessed in a given situation

Table 8.8. Assessing pulse force: grading system

Grade	Pulse
3 +	Full, bounding
2 +	Normal
1 +	Weak, thready
0	Absent

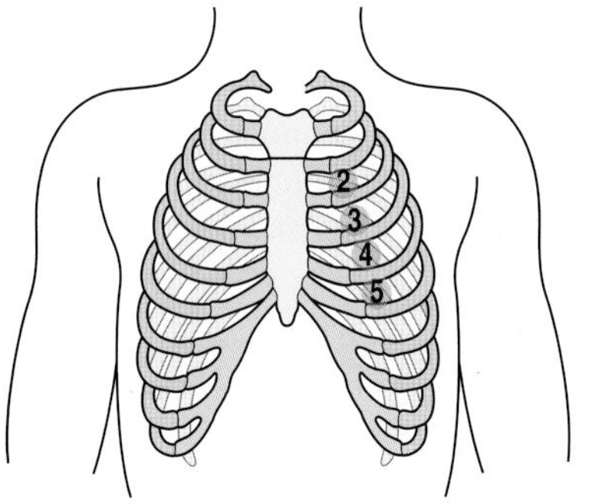

Fig. 8.2 • Locating the apical heartbeat.

Procedures Box 8.5 Pulse measurement

Actions

1. Determine the appropriate method and site for pulse and heart rate measurement, taking into consideration age and likely tachycardia.
2. Explain the procedure to the child and the parent(s) using developmentally appropriate language. You may need to:
   - use play through the use of dolls to prepare the child
   - give the child time to familiarise himself or herself with the equipment that you might use, for example a stethoscope
   - use distraction therapy such as bubble blowing
   - work collaboratively with parents and/or a play specialist (this can be helpful).
3. Ensure that the child is sitting or lying comfortably; in particular ensure that the child's forearm is in a comfortable position not raised to a level above the heart.
4. You will require a watch with sweep second hand or digital read-out.
5. ALWAYS wash your hands and check the identity of the child.

Palpating the radial pulse (>1 year)

Actions

6a. Place the index, middle and sometimes ring finger as well over the artery, which is located on the anterior surface of the thumb side of the wrist.
Apply gentle pressure.
Avoid obstructing the child's blood flow.
Using the watch, count the pulsations that are felt where the artery rests against the bone.

6b. Note the rate, rhythm and strength of the pulse over a 60-s period.

Palpating the brachial pulse (<1 year)

Actions

6a. Place the index, middle and sometimes ring finger as well over the artery, which is located on the anterior surface of the thumb side in the antecubital fossa.
Apply gentle pressure.
Avoid obstructing the child's blood flow.
Using the watch, count the pulsations that are felt where the artery rests against the bone.

6b. Note the rate, rhythm and strength of the pulse over a 60-s period.

Auscultating the apical heart beat (<2 years with or without tachycardia)

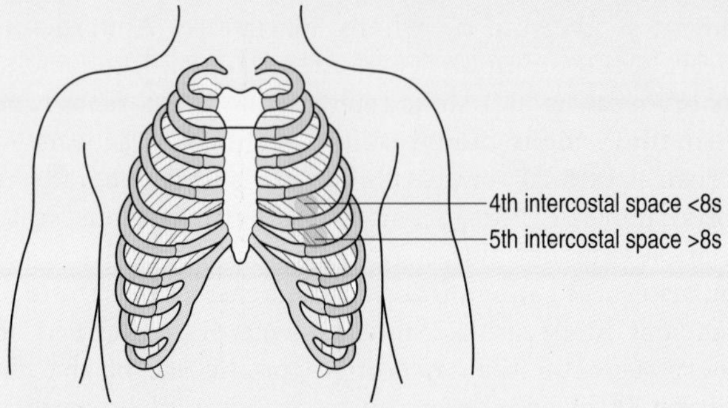

Actions

6a. Place the bell of the stethoscope gently on the left side of the anterior chest in the mid-clavicular line in the:
   - fourth intercostal space (<8 years of age)
   - fifth intercostal space (>8 years of age).

6b. Note the rate and rhythm of the apical heartbeat over a 60-s period.

Actions

7. Make the child comfortable.
8. Clearly and accurately document the measurement, method and site.
9. Notify the doctor of abnormal readings or as directed by the doctor or senior nurse.

(Evans et al 1999, Lockwood et al 2004). The pulse is generally taken at a frequency determined by a child's condition, for example immediately following surgery a child will require a pulse assessment every 15 min, compared with a child undergoing long-term rehabilitation, who might require a pulse assessment once a day unless otherwise indicated.

Respiration

Respiratory illness is the commonest cause of morbidity in young children (Advanced Life Support Group 2005), as children are predisposed to upper and lower airway obstruction by their anatomy and physiology. The main predisposing factors are as follows (Bew 2006):

- The smallest diameter of the upper airway at the cricoid is only 4 mm in an infant. Even 1 mm of oedema reduces the diameter of the airway by 75% and will increase the work of breathing by 16 times.
- The upper and lower airway mucosa is loosely adherent to the submucosa and prone to swelling.
- The tongue base is large relative to the jaw and the oropharyngeal space is smaller, so for the first 3–6 months of life infants are obligate nasal breathers.
- Cartilaginous structures are compliant, and increased respiratory effort causes subcostal, intercostal and sternal recession with decreased efficiency of the chest wall.
- Metabolic rate and oxygen consumption are high compared with in the child over 12 years and the adult.
- Functional residual capacity is smaller and the diaphragm is a less efficient muscle due to fewer fatigue-resistant fibres as compared with the child over 12 years and the adult.

Overall respiratory reserve is, therefore, small and fatigue occurs sooner. Early recognition of impending respiratory failure is vital. Respiratory failure due to oxygenation failure is caused by insufficient oxygen (P_aO_2 <8.0 kPa) being transferred into pulmonary capillaries to maintain normal levels, but normal carbon dioxide (CO_2 <6.0 kPa) levels can be maintained (British Thoracic Society 2002). CO_2 is far more soluble than O_2 and so can perfuse across the alveolar–capillary border when O_2 cannot, for example when there is an increased fluid barrier in pulmonary oedema. Respiratory failure due to ventilation failure occurs when insufficient volumes of gas ventilate the alveoli due to a low respiratory rate and/or low tidal volumes, reflected by the observation of shallow breathing. As well as hypoxaemia (P_aO_2 <8.0 kPa; British Thoracic Society 2002) there is insufficient clearance of CO_2 and therefore hypercapnia develops (CO_2 >6.0 kPa). If this is allowed to continue, the child will also become acidotic (pH <7.33). Anticipation and early detection of each type of respiratory failure depends on astute clinical assessment. Assessment is the cornerstone of safe and effective practice and goes hand in hand with the process of prioritising a sick child's needs. However, respiratory assessment is particularly challenging in the infant and preschool child due to the inability and/or unwillingness to cooperate. Successful respiratory assessment of the child with difficulty breathing demands that the nurse remain acutely aware of the fragility of the dyspnoeic child. Although it is important to work out what assessment data reveal, it is equally important to be clear about what it does not say (Aylott 2006a).

Table 8.9 provides a glossary of terms associated with the assessment of respiration.

Measuring respirations

It is useful to evaluate children for important signs of respiratory problems in a logical physiological and anatomical order, and assessment of respiratory rate is a key parameter that is often under-assessed. There is very little research relating to the measurement of respiratory rate, and these studies focus on the accuracy of respiratory rate measurement and respiratory rate as a marker for respiratory dysfunction. The value of respiratory rate as an indicator of potential respiratory dysfunction has been investigated, and results of studies are conflicting across the age span. One study found that only 33% of children presenting to an emergency department with an oxygen saturation level below 90% (normally 97–98%), indicating respiratory dysfunction and a need for oxygen therapy, had an increased respiratory rate (Hooker et al 1992). However, the authors speculate that this might be secondary to the apparent lack of cooperation in a toddler who may be anxious because of any number of causes, in a distressed child with an abnormal pattern and rate of breathing, or in an adolescent in whom the clinician may fail to appreciate tachypnoea by applying the 'normals' for a younger child. This was certainly the case in the later findings of Rusconi et al (1994). Later researchers (Aldous 2000, Brookes et al 2003, Rajesh et al 2000) found that if respiratory rate was 'carefully' measured by appropriately trained practitioners, then respiratory rate is a sensitive and reasonably reliable marker of respiratory dysfunction in children, especially infants less than 1 year of age. The pattern of breathing of children provides a useful tool for assessing the respiratory system and can provide important clues of cardiorespiratory distress (Monaghan 2005).

Assessing respiration, like the pulse, is much more than counting the rate. Respirations are evaluated by rate, rhythm, depth and character (quality). Again it requires a great deal of patience and experience to learn to evaluate heart rate, strength and rhythm disturbances. An appreciation of the variability of respiratory rate in relationship to age and clinical state in children is important as part of the overall assessment of the presenting child (Kelsey & McEwing 2006). The respiratory rate is initially rapid at birth and gradually decreases as the child approaches adolescence (Rusconi et al 1994, Wallis et al 2005). Respiratory rate shows greatest variability in neonates and infants up to 1 year of age (Department of Health 2004). Nurses should have a thorough knowledge about the normal and abnormal respiratory rate in order to identify abnormalities. You may have no prior knowledge of the infant's or child's 'healthy' respiratory rate for comparison, therefore it is important to know the range of normal values that apply to patients of different ages (see Table 8.10).

The respiratory rate is the number of breaths a person takes per minute. One respiration is counted by one up-and-down movement of the child's chest. The rate is best measured when a person is at rest. The pattern of breathing includes the respiratory rate, rhythm and effort required by the child to breathe. One-off recordings are of little clinical use other than to provide a baseline (Simoes et al 1991). Serial assessments of respiratory rate, rhythm and effort, known as 'work of breathing', should be measured and recorded at a frequency appropriately determined by the child's overall presenting condition; this provides the best data for the early detection of the child with a deteriorating serious illness (Monaghan 2005).

Table 8.9. Glossary of terms associated with respiration assessment

Term	Definition
Apnoea	A pause in breathing of more than 20 s or a pause of shorter duration associated with bradycardia or cyanosis
Bradypnoea	Slow breathing rate
Dyspnoea	Difficulty breathing
Eupnoea	Normal rate and depth of ventilation
Periodic breathing	Cycles of short respiratory pause up to 20 s followed by an increase in respiratory rate
Tachypnoea	Fast breathing rate
Ventilation	Movement of gases in and out of lungs

Table 8.10. Normal respiratory rate relating to age

Age (years)	Respiratory rate (breaths/min)
Neonate	30–60
<1	35–45
1–5	25–35
5–12	15–25
>12	12–16

Normal respiratory rate in the child is between 12 and 60 breaths/min. Respiratory rhythm should be regular. Respiratory depth (as seen in the amplitude or excursion of chest wall movement) should also be the same between breaths. Regular respiratory rate, rhythm and depth are interrupted occasionally by a large breath (called a 'sigh') in healthy children (Gill & O'Brien 2002). Periodic breathing is defined as a pause in breathing of more than 20s or a pause of shorter duration associated with bradycardia or cyanosis (American Academy of Pediatrics 2003). Periodic breathing is a normal pattern of respiration in premature infants during active or rapid eye movement (REM) and quiet or non-REM sleep. It persists in young infants but decreases in percentage as the youngster matures. In term infants, periodic breathing is most often confined to active (REM) sleep. Persistence of periodic breathing that occurs during long portions of sleep may be abnormal and reflect immaturity or an abnormality of brainstem respiratory control. Unfortunately, clear norms regarding appropriate percentages of periodic breathing across age groups are not yet available.

Assessing respiratory function in small children can be challenging. The nurse should consider the child's age and developmental level to plan an assessment approach. An important first step in assessing the chest of an infant or a toddler is to help the small child feel comfortable. Some nurses carry an extra stethoscope for use by the child. It may be helpful to start with playing a game, using either a favourite doll or a stuffed animal, or by involving the parent. The nurse can listen to the animal's or parent's chest first and then apply the stethoscope to the child's chest. A small child may feel more secure and cooperate more if he or she sits on a parent's lap during the examination. When examining a school-age child, the nurse might help the child draw and label a picture of the lungs. The first method and most commonly used method of assessing respiratory rate involves simply counting the number of breaths for 1 min by counting through direct visualisation how many times the chest rises. In doing the assessment keep in mind that abdominal breathing is common and normal in infants. Respiratory rates may increase (tachypnoea) with fever, with illness and with other medical conditions (see Box 8.2).

Box 8.2. Causes of tachypnoea and bradypnoea

Causes of tachypnoea

- Exertion
- Fever
- Pain
- Acute respiratory distress
- Heart failure
- Anaemia

Causes of bradypnoea

- Raised intracranial pressure
- Excessive sedation
- Alcohol
- Benzodiazepines
- Illicit drug use
- Morphine

Despite the availability of electrical monitoring equipment to measure respiratory rate (Brookes et al 2003), research evidence suggests that in order to obtain an accurate respiratory rate, counting respirations for a full minute by either visualisation or auscultation remains the best method (Lovett et al 2005). Inaccuracies in respiratory measurement have been reported in the literature. One study compared respiratory rate counted using 15-, 30- and 60-s count periods (Simoes et al 1991). Respiratory rate measurement in children under 12 years of age counted over a 60-s period resulted in least variability. Hooker et al (1992) found that rapid respiratory rates in infants counted on auscultation using a stethoscope were 50% more accurate than those counted using chest visualisation. Increased respiratory rates are often associated with shallow breathing, which can make direct visualisation difficult and the resultant rate measured unreliable. The movement of air in and out of the respiratory system produces breath sounds that can be auscultated. Breath sounds are transmitted through the chest wall and may be heard through the diaphragm (flat piece) of a stethoscope placed firmly against the chest wall. Auscultation of the lungs is the recommended technique for measuring respiratory rate and assessing airflow through the tracheobronchial tree when there is tachypnoea and/or shallow breathing (Lockwood et al 2004). When auscultating breath sound in young children use the bell of the stethoscope. The bell is a more sensitive indicator of sounds and detects softer, lower pitched sounds than the stethoscope diaphragm. Assess the child for signs of laboured breathing, such as retractions, and look for colour changes in the lips and nail beds. If retractions are noted look for the location of the retractions:

- Suprasternal retractions are seen above the clavicle and sternum
- Intercostal retractions occur between the ribs
- Subcostal retractions may be seen below the lower costal margin of the ribcage
- Substernal retractions may be seen below the xiphoid process.

Procedures Box 8.6 Respiratory rate assessment

Actions

1. Determine the most appropriate method for respiratory rate measurement, taking into consideration age and likely tachypnoea.
2. Wash hands and check the identity of the child.
3. Gather the stethoscope if using auscultation.
4. Children may alter their respiratory pattern if they are made aware that you are counting their respirations, so pretend to be taking a pulse or listening to the heartbeat while counting the respiratory rate over 60 s.
5. While counting respiratory rate observe respiratory depth and note symmetry or asymmetry.
6. Assess the presence and equality of chest rise and fall incorporating the abdomen in children younger than 8 years.
7. If using auscultation to measure respiratory rate, place the diaphragm of the stethoscope just underneath the clavicles in the mid-clavicular line anteriorly or just below the inferior edge of the scapulae posteriorly.
8. While counting respirations also note signs of increased work of breathing.
9. Document your observations and repeat as indicated by the intervention and child's condition.
10. Report to a doctor any abnormality immediately.

If the child has retractions look for compensatory respiratory mechanisms such as nasal flaring during inspiration, grunting during expiration, or the use of accessory muscles in the neck and shoulders. The majority of a resting inspiration is due to diaphragmatic contraction; there should be very little apparent chest movement (Aylott 2006a). During normal inspiration diaphragmatic contraction displaces abdominal viscera towards the spine and the abdominal wall moves in passively, that is, the chest and abdomen move out together. It should therefore be intuitive that contraction of the abdominal muscles (abdominal effort) can only assist with expiration. However, it is important to be aware that paradoxical abdominal movement is a manifestation of severe respiratory distress. Paradoxical (asynchronous) abdominal movement occurs when increased intercostal contraction draws the diaphragm and abdominal viscera outwards on inspiration and the abdominal wall moves in, that is, the chest and abdomen move in opposite directions (Aylott 2006b). This can occur due to decreased lung compliance and upper airway obstruction. Much information can be gleaned from simply observing the breathing pattern of the child. One should look for the postural manifestations of dyspnoea, such as an extended neck, abducted elbows, open mouth breathing, an anxious facial expression, increased abdominal movement and paradoxical abdominal movement. Straightening of the neck and open mouth breathing occur in children over 1 year of age (Aylott 2006a).

Conclusion: putting it all together

An assessment of vital signs, TPR gives an overview of the child's general health. These measures, which indicate the effectiveness of circulatory, respiratory and neural body functions, offer a quick and efficient way to monitor a child's condition, identify problems and evaluate her or his response to interventions. Early recognition of subtle alterations that signal the need for medical or nursing intervention promotes better health outcomes (Department of Health 2004). Therefore, it is imperative that the children's nurse accurately assess these values. However, vital signs are not infallible indicators. These data need to be interpreted so that the significance of the reading or of serial readings in relation to the child's condition is assessed. This requires the nurse to be familiar with evidence-based measurement techniques and equipment in order to determine if accurate data were obtained, as well as knowledge regarding what is being measured and the potential physiological impact of the results obtained. TPR data measurements are integrated with other physiological, psychological and behavioural assessment to determine the child's condition or stability. Common to all methods of data measurement are the requirements that the nurse is accurate, appropriately trained and consistent in technique, in the use of the specific instrument and in documenting the result. Records should reveal patterns of variation over time.

Now test your knowledge

- What would be the most effective method of assessing the temperature of a 1-year-old infant?
- What is the normal range of TPR for a child this age?
- You are asked to recommend a temperature-measuring device to the accident and emergency department. What would you choose and why?
- What trend do you see in infants' and children's respirations as they grow older?
- How you would explain to a student what the pulse actually represents?

References

Advanced Life Support Group (2005) Advanced paediatric life support: the practical approach, 4th edn. BMJ Publishing Group, London

Akinyinka OO (2002) Infrared ear thermometry versus rectal thermometry in children. Lancet 360(9333):584–585

Aldous MB (2000) A respiratory rate of ≥ 60 breaths per minute had high sensitivity for detecting hypoxia in infants. Evidence Based Medicine 5(5):152–153

American Academy of Pediatrics (2003) Health in child care manual, 4th edn. AAP, Elk Grove Village

Androkites A, Werger AM, Young ML (1998) Comparison of axillary and infrared tympanic membrane thermometry in a pediatric oncology outpatient setting. Journal of Pediatric Oncology Nursing 15(4):215–222

Aylott M (2006a) Developing rigour in observation of the sick child: part 1. Paediatric Nursing 18(8):38–44

Aylott M (2006b) Observing the sick child: part 2a. Respiratory assessment. Paediatric Nursing 18(9):38–44

Banitalebi H, Bangstead HJ (2002) Measurement of fever in children – is infrared thermometry reliable? Tidsskrift for den Norske laegeforening 122(28):2700–2701

Bates B (1995) A guide to physical examination and history taking, 6th edn. Lippincott, Edinburgh

Betta V, Cascetta F, Sepe D (1997) An assessment of infrared tympanic thermometers for body temperature measurement. Physiological Measurement 18:215–225

Bew S (2006) Acute and chronic airway obstruction. Anaesthesia and Intensive Care 7(5):164–168

Blows WT (2001) The biological basis of nursing: clinical observations. Routledge, London

British Thoracic Society (2002) Non-invasive ventilation in acute respiratory failure. Thorax 57:92–211

Brookes CN, Whittaker JD, Moulton C, Dodds D (2003) The PEP respiratory monitor: a validation study. Emergency Medical Journal 20:326–328

Candy D, Davies G, Ross E (2006) Clinical paediatrics and child health. Saunders, Edinburgh

Chamley CA, Carson P, Randall D, Sandwell M (2005) Developmental anatomy and physiology of children: a practical approach. Churchill Livingstone, Edinburgh

Chaturverdi D, Vilhekar KY, Chaturvedi P, Bharmbe MS (2004) Comparison of axillary temperature with rectal or oral temperature and determination of optimum placement time in children. Indian Pediatrics 41:600–603

Childs C, Harrison R, Hodkinson C (1999) Tympanic membrane temperature as a measure of core temperature. Archives of Disease in Childhood 80(3):262–267

Craig JV, Lancaster GA, Taylor S, Williamson PR, Smyth RL (2000) Temperature measured at the axilla compared with rectum in children and young people: systematic review. British Medical Journal 320(7243):1174–1178

Craig JV, Lancaster GA, Taylor S, Williamson PR, Smyth RL (2002) Infrared ear thermometry compared with rectal thermometry in children: a systematic review. Lancet 360(9334):603–609

Department of Health (2004) Spotting the sick child. Department of Health, London

El-Radhi AS, Barry W (2006) Thermometry in paediatric practice. Archives of Disease in Childhood 91(4):351–356

El-Radhi AS, Patel S (2006) An evaluation of tympanic thermometry in a paediatric emergency department. Emergency Medical Journal 23:40–41

Evans D, Hodgkinson B, Berry J (1999) Vital signs: a systematic review no. 4. Joanna Briggs Institute. Online. Available: http://joannabriggs.edu.au

Gill D, O'Brien N (2002) Paediatric clinical examination made easy, 4th edn. Churchill Livingstone, London

Hollerbach AD, Sneed NV (1990) Accuracy of radial pulse assessment by length of counting interval. Heart and Lung 19:258–264

Holtzclaw BJ (1993) Monitoring body temperature. AACN Clinical Issues 4(1):44–55

Hooker EA, Danzl DF, Brueggmeyer M, Harper E (1992) Respiratory rates in pediatric emergency patients. Journal of Emergency Medicine 10:407–410

James N, Smith N (2005) Treatment of heart failure in children. Current Paediatrics 15:539–548

Jean-Mary MB, Dicanzio J, Shaw J, Berstein HH (2002) Limited accuracy and reliability of infrared and axillary and aural thermometers in a pediatric outpatient population. Journal of Pediatrics 14(5):671–676

Kelsey J, McEwing G (2006) Respiratory illness in children. In Glasper EA, Richardson J (eds) A textbook of children's and young people's nursing. Churchill Livingstone, Edinburgh

Lanham DM, Walker B, Klocke E, Jennings M (1999) Accuracy of tympanic readings in children under 6 years of age. Pediatric Nursing 25(1):39–43

Lissauer T, Clayden G (2001) Illustrated textbook of paediatrics, 2nd edn. Elsevier, London

Lockwood C, Conroy-Hiller T, Page T (2004) Systematic review: vital signs. Centre for Evidence-Based Nursing, Adelaide

Lovett PB, Buchwald JM, Sturmann K, Bijur P (2005) The vexatious vital: neither clinical measurements by nurses nor an electronic monitor provides accurate measurements of respiratory rate in triage. Annals of Emergency Medicine 45(1):68–76

McChance KL, Huether SE (2006) Pathophysiology: the biologic basis for disease in adults and children, 5th edn. Mosby, St Louis

McKenzie JE, Osgood DW (2004) Validation of a new telemetric core temperature monitor. Journal of Thermal Biology 29:605–611

Macqueen S (2001) Clinical benefits of 3M Tempa.DOT thermometer in paediatric settings. British Journal of Nursing 10(1):55–58

Margolius FR, Sneed NV, Hollerbach AD (1991) Accuracy of apical pulse rate measurements in young children. Nurse Research 40:378–380

Marieb EN (2004) Human anatomy and physiology, 6th edn. Addison-Wesley, San Francisco

Medicines and Healthcare products Regulatory Agency (2006) Device bulletin no. 42. Department of Health, London

Molton AH, Blacktop J, Hall CM (2001) Temperature taking in children. Journal of Child Healthcare 5(1):5–10

Monaghan A (2005) Detecting and managing deterioration in children. Paediatric Nursing 17(1):32–35

Mower WR, Sachs C, Nicklin EL, Safa P, Baraff LJ (1996) A comparison of pulse oximetry and respiratory rate in patient screening. Respiratory Medicine 90:593–599

National Institute for Health and Clinical Excellence (2006) Feverish illness: assessment initial management in children younger than 5 years of age: first draft for consultation. NICE, London

Neill S, Knowles H (2004) The biology of child health: a reader in development and assessment. Palgrave Macmillan, Basingstoke

Pickersgill J, Fowler H, Bootham J, Thompson K, Wilcock S, Tanner J (2003) Temperature taking: children's preferences. Paediatric Nursing 15(2):22–25

Potter P, Schallom M, Davis S, Sona C, McSweeney M (2003) Evaluation of chemical dot thermometers for measuring body temperature of orally intubated patients. American Journal of Critical Medicine 12(5):403–407

Rajesh VT, Singh S, Kataria S (2000) Tachypnoea is a good indicator of hypoxia in acutely ill infants under 2 months. Archives of Disease in Childhood 82:46–49

Robinson JL, Seal RF, Spady DW, Joffres MR (1998) Comparison of oesophageal, rectal, axillary, bladder, tympanic and pulmonary artery temperatures in children. Journal of Pediatrics 133:553–556

Rudolf M, Levene M (2006) Paediatrics and child health, 2nd edn. Blackwell Publishing, Oxford

Rusconi F, Castagneto M, Porta N et al (1994) Reference values for respiratory rate in the first 3 years of life. Pediatrics 94(3):350–355

Rush M, Wetherall A (2003) Temperature measurement: practice guidelines. Paediatric Nursing 15(9):25–31

Sarti A, Savron F, Ronfani L, Pelizzo G, Barbi E (2006) Comparison of three sites to check the pulse and count heart rate in hypotensive infants. Pediatric Anesthesia 16:394–398

Simoes EA, Roark R, Berman S, Esler LL, Murphy J (1991) Respiratory rate: measurement of variability over time and accuracy of different counting periods. Archives of Disease in Childhood 66(10):1199–1203

Smith JJ, Bland SA, Mullett S (2005) Temperature – the forgotten vital sign. Accident and Emergency Nursing 13:247–250

Sneed NV, Hollerbach AD (1992) Accuracy of heart rate assessment in atrial fibrillation. Heart and Lung 21:125–128

Sund-Levander M, Grodzinsky E, Loyd D, Wahren LK (2004) Errors in body temperature assessment related to individual variation, measuring technique and equipment. International Journal of Nursing Practice 10:216–223

Tanner M, Nagy S, Peat JK (2000) Detection of infant's heart beat/pulse by caregivers: a comparison of 4 methods. Journal of Pediatrics 137:429–430

Tortora GJ (2005) Principles of human anatomy, 10th edn. Wiley, Danvers

Tortora GJ, Derrickson B (2007) Introduction to the human body: the essentials of anatomy and physiology, 7th edn. Wiley, Danvers

Wallis LA, Healy M, Undy MB, Maconochie I (2005) Age related reference ranges for respiration rate and heart rate from 4 to 16 years. Archives of Disease in Childhood 90(11):1117–1121

Weber M (2003) Pulsus alternans a case study: pediatric care. Critical Care Nurse 23:51–54

9 Assessment of blood pressure

Eileen P. Brennan

Measuring blood pressure (BP) in children requires practice, specialist skills and knowledge. It is particularly challenging, especially in the younger age group. Many babies and small children dislike being held still and are often frightened of the procedure. The technical difficulty of measuring BP in children is well documented (Beevers et al 2001, Dillon 1988, Portman et al 2004). Inaccurate measurement can result in children being exposed to unnecessary investigations and treatments or at worse high readings can be dismissed as inaccurate, exposing children and adolescents to many of the high-risk complications associated with uncontrolled hypertension. The long-term health risks in children can be considerable, therefore it is essential that clinical guidelines for measuring BP be used in order to ensure best practice and optimise health outcomes for this vulnerable group.

Definition

Blood pressure is defined as 'the force exerted by blood against the walls of blood vessels due to contraction of the heart and influenced by the elasticity of the vessel walls' (Tortora 2006). Maintenance of normal BP is dependent on the balance between the cardiac output and the peripheral vascular resistance (Beevers et al 2001).

Phases

There are two main phases of a BP: the systolic phase and the diastolic phase. The systolic represents the pressure when the heart is beating and the diastolic represents the pressure when the heart is at rest (Edwards 1997).

A BP is made up of five Korotkoff sounds, which are defined as follows:

- Phase 1: the first appearance of faint, repetitive, clear tapping sounds that gradually increase in intensity for at least two consecutive beats – this is the systolic BP.
- Phase 2: a brief period may follow during which the sounds soften and acquire a swishing quality. An auscultatory gap may occur here in some patients (usually children and infants with severe hypertension); this is when sounds may disappear altogether for a short time.
- Phase 3: the return of sharper sounds, which become crisper to regain, or even exceed, the intensity of phase 1 sounds. The clinical significance, if any, of phases 2 and 3 has not been established.
- Phase 4: the distinct, abrupt muffling sounds, which become soft and blowing in quality.
- Phase 5: the point at which all sounds finally disappear completely; this is the diastolic pressure, although this is under debate, and current recommendations suggest that both phase 4 and phase 5 should be recorded, especially in children (Beevers et al 2001).

Systolic versus diastolic readings

In children, measuring the systolic BP is a preference because it is easier to measure and has greater accuracy and reproducibility (National High Blood Pressure Education Program Working Group on Hypertension Control in Children and Adolescents 1996). A diastolic BP is not always present in children and can often be zero (O'Sullivan et al 2001). There is increasing evidence that the height of the systolic BP is a better predictor of morbidity and mortality than the diastolic (Beevers et al 2001); furthermore the long-term benefits of lowering the systolic BP strongly correlate with a decrease in morbidity and mortality (Sorof et al 2002).

A normal BP is age-, height- and gender-related, and there is a range of acceptable limits for each age and group. BP levels for the 50th to the 99th percentile are defined by the National High Blood Pressure Education Program Working Group on Hypertension Control in Children and Adolescents (1996).

Conditions with high and medium risk of blood pressure anomalies

Blood pressure is not routinely measured in well children in the UK. However, there are children who fall into risk categories of having or developing BP problems; special attention needs to be focused in the areas listed in Box 9.1. A BP should be measured regularly and then monitored if the initial reading is shown to be outside normal ranges. The National Heart, Lung, and Blood Institute and the American Academy of Paediatrics recommend routine BP monitoring of all children from the age of 3 years in an attempt to reduce the growing numbers of strokes and cardiovascular problems in adulthood. However,

Box 9.1. Conditions with high and medium risk of blood pressure anomalies

High risk

- Premature babies
- Babies nursed in special care following a acute illness
- All children with urological problems
- All renal abnormalities
- Cardiac children
- Children with neurological problems
- Any children with vasculitis problems
- During a critical illness
- Children receiving intravenous infusion, especially plasma expanders (i.e. colloids, albumin or blood transfusion)

Medium risk

- Oncology
- Obese children
- Children with eating disorders
- Family history of hypertension
- Children with a persistent history of headaches
- Children who are failing to thrive
- Children presenting in accident and emergency departments with symptoms of any of the above
- Children on medications that can cause hypertension (steroids, nephrotoxic drugs, erythropoietin, to mention a few)

the concern among paediatricians in the UK is the growth in unnecessary investigations caused by incorrect measurement, especially in the younger age group. Unfortunately in the UK there are very few resources available where young children can have their BP measured accurately; in some cases high measurements on automated monitors have been misdiagnosed as artificially high readings or misinterpreted as machine error. No follow-up for BP monitoring places these seemingly well children at high risk of strokes or organ failure. The detection of abnormal BP in children is important because hypertension often relates to an identifiable and potentially treatable disease process; untreated hypertension is associated with significant morbidity and mortality (Falkner 2004, Morgenstern & Butani 2004, Pappadid & Somers 2003).

If a small child is suspected of having a high BP, she or he should have a four-limbed BP measurement performed (Perloff et al 1993). In older children BP should be measured on both arms. In general the limb with the highest reading should then be used (McAlister & Straus 2001). It is recommended that three successive readings at 2-min intervals should be measured at the first assessment (Flynn 2004).

Variability in BP can be common in children. Causes include:

- time of day
- meals
- anxiety
- drugs
- temperature
- sleeping (Beevers et al 2001) (sleeping BP on average is 10% less than waking BP).

Measuring children's blood pressure

There are two main methods of BP monitoring: direct and indirect. A direct BP can be performed only when the child has an arterial line in situ; this is regarded as the gold standard or 'true' BP (Derrico 1993). This is obviously not always practical to perform and is rarely performed outside critical care areas. The indirect methods are more commonly performed but there are several different ways to achieve a measurement of indirect BP:

- Sphygmomanometer with stethoscope (auscultation)
- Sphygmomanometer with Doppler (ultrasound)
- Sphygmomanometer with palpation
- Dinamap or various automated monitors (usually oscillometric).

Auscultation using a sphygmomanometer and stethoscope or Doppler is the method of choice for most healthcare professionals treating children with BP problems. This method of measurement requires more time, knowledge and skills; however, it remains the only non-invasive consistent and accurate method of measuring infants' and children's BP under the age of 5 (Beevers et al 2001).

Oscillometric devices (automated monitors: Dinamap) have widely replaced manual manometers in most paediatric settings, resulting in an excess of devices flooding the market, most of which do not fulfil the accuracy criteria protocol recommended by the Taskforce on Blood Pressure Control in Children (Morgenstern & Butani 2004). There are advantages of using oscillometric devices; however, only a limited number have been reported to be accurate. Many of the studies validating the oscillometric monitors have been carried out with adults or in critical care areas, where children are often immobile, which significantly reduces one of the major inaccuracies: that of movement artefact. In practice, movement artefact and cuff error are responsible for the majority of inconsistent and high measurements obtained in small children, making the readings impossible to interpret. Additional factors that contribute to errors of measurement are:

- heart arrhythmias
- heart block
- a poor pulse volume
- variable BP measurements
- distress experienced from discomfort caused by the procedure
- very high BP
- medical conditions such as cerebral palsy, autism, fitting and hyperactivity.

ALERT
When measuring BP with an automated monitor, if a reading is not within normal limits on repeated measurement it is recommended that the BP is measured manually.

Comparisons of BP readings using manual and oscillometric devices demonstrate that the two methods are not comparable, and the oscillometric device demonstrated differences ranging from −4 to +24 mmHg, significantly higher in the under 8 age group (Park et al 2001). It is always advisable to check if devices have been validated for use in the under 5 years age group.

Cuff size

Correct measurement of BP in children requires use of a cuff that is appropriate to the size of the child's upper right arm. For such a cuff to be optimal the cuff bladder length should cover 90–100% of the circumference of the arm (Morgenstern & Butani 2004). The bladder width to length ratio must be at least 1:2. It should be noted that not all commercially available cuffs are manufactured with this ratio and different brands vary considerably, as there is no standardisation in any of the products seen in clinical environments. The most common cause of error in BP measurement for both manual and automated methods is the selection of the correct cuffs size (Beevers et al 2001). It is well recognised that 'under-cuffing', i.e. the use of a cuff that is too small, leads to erroneously high BP readings, whereas overly large cuffs do not seem to generate significant errors (Morgenstern & Butani 2004). However, the most probable explanation for inappropriate cuff selection is the labelling of the cuffs (infant, small child, adult and outsized adults): cuff selection is often chosen by label as opposed to measuring the cuff to fit the child. The wide disparity in cuff size further complicates the situation, leaving some normotensive children labelled with having hypertension.

Monitors used to measure blood pressure

The types of manometer most frequently used were the aneroid and mercury. Mercury is felt to be more accurate; however, for health and safety reasons areas are replacing them with other models. The aneroid manometer requires recalibration frequently and will often have to be sent back to its manufacturer (Markandu et al 2000). In reality, clinical settings require monitors that require less maintenance, such as the Accoson green light, which seems to fulfil many of the criteria set out by the British Hypertension Society. This, together with a Doppler (ultrasound), is considered to be the most accurate method of measuring the systolic BP in the under fives.

Table 9.1 lists monitors used to measure BP.

Table 9.1. Monitors used to measure blood pressure

Method	Advantages	Problems
Sphygmomanometry (auscultatory)	• Paediatric BP normative data based on it • Portable • Inexpensive • Widely available	• Inaccuracies in measurement if skills for taking manual BP are not maintained • Observer biases • Incorrect cuff size used • Poor results if equipment is not well maintained
Mercury	• Still regarded as the gold standard • Minimal maintenance required	• Concerns about environmental contamination
Aneroid	• Measures the same parameters as mercury	• Easily lost calibration • Cannot be recalibrated easily
Accoson Green light 300	• Validated as comparable with the mercury manometer • Reduces digital bias • Speed deflation rate light display • Self-calibrating each time the apparatus is switched on • Reduces inappropriately rapid deflation rate	• Additional training would be required

Table 9.1. Monitors used to measure blood pressure—cont'd

Method	Advantages	Problems
Oscillometry (automated)	• Easy to use • Convenient • Requires less training • Eliminates observer biases	• Very few of the many devices on the market have been validated for use in children • Limited numbers of cuff sizes available • First reading effect (3–5 mmHg higher than subsequent readings) • High initial inflation pressures cause discomfort • Inaccuracy in the under fives • Motion artefacts • Limited normative data available for small children • Oscillometric devices measure mean arterial BP and then calculate systolic and diastolic values • Equipment is heavy and bulky • Reported to become more inaccurate in measurement in the range of severe hypertension

BP, blood pressure.

Procedures Box 9.1 Blood pressure measurement

1

Preparation for blood pressure measurement

Actions
The equipment required should be gathered and checked for leaks and damage.

The sphygmomanometer meniscus should be at zero and not obscured.

The cuff, bladder, tubing, connections, inflation bulb and valves should be clean and in a good condition.

Reasons *Ensures accuracy of reading.*
It is recommended that sphygmomanometers should be recalibrated every 6 months.

Action
Nylon cuffs should be wiped with disinfectant wipes between patients, and fabric cuffs should be washed regularly.

Reason *Reduces the risk of cross-infection.*

Actions
Select the appropriate size cuff.

Ideally the length of the bladder (rubber tubing inside the cuff) should completely encircle the child's arm (the range markings on many cuffs vary depending on the brand and are not useful ranges in children).

Reason *The higher the blood pressure (BP), the more inaccurate the reading will be if an incorrect cuff size is used.*

2

Measuring the blood pressure

Action
Wash your hands.

Reason *Reduces the risk of cross-infection.*

Action
The child should be in a warm environment.

Reason *Allows for an accurate assessment of BP.*

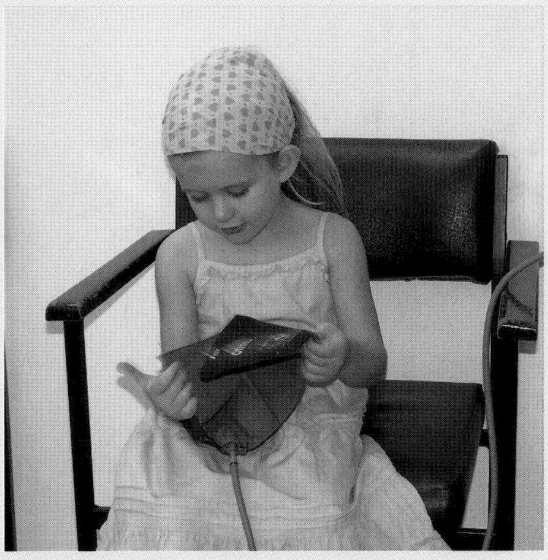

Actions
Explain the procedure using toys and dolls to prepare young children.

If necessary give the child and parents time to familiarise themselves with the equipment; a play specialist can be very useful during the preparation stage if the child is nervous.

Reason *Reduces the child's anxiety.*

Action
It is recommended that BP should be taken 1.5 h after the last feed.

Reason *Allows for an accurate assessment of BP.*

Procedures Box 9.1 Blood pressure measurement—cont'd

2 Continued

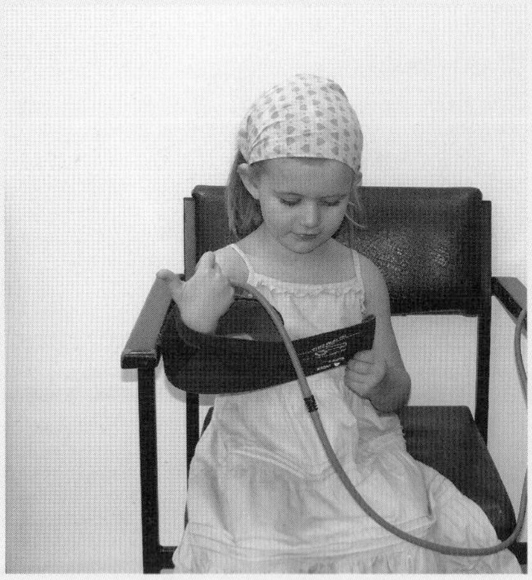

Action
The child should be advised to sit and relax in a quiet environment for 3-5 min before the BP is taken.

Reason *Allows for an accurate assessment of BP.*

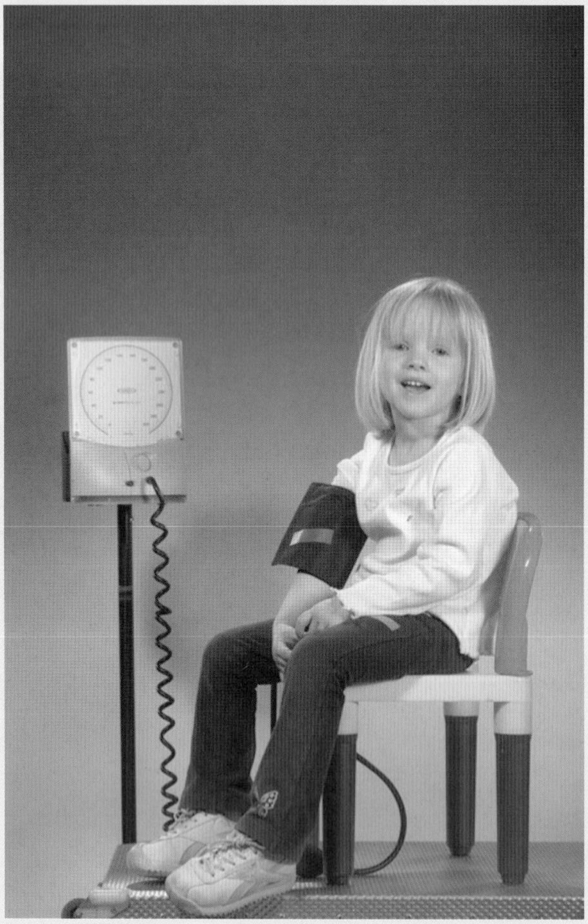

Actions
The child should be in a seated position with her or his legs uncrossed and feet on the ground.

If the child is in bed and the BP has to be measured on the leg, the lying position is recommended.

Action
Tight or restrictive clothing should be removed.

Reason *Allows for an accurate assessment of BP.*

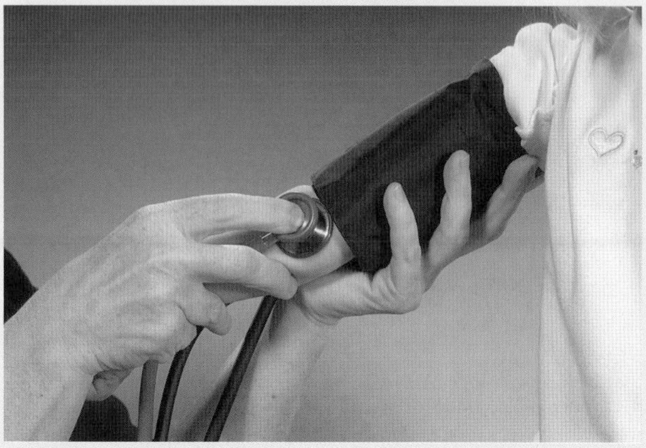

Action
Position the child's arm horizontal at the level of the mid-sternum, well supported.

Reason *If the child's arm is below heart level, BP can be overestimated by up to 10 mmHg, and if above the level of the mid-sternum it can be underestimated by the same amount.*

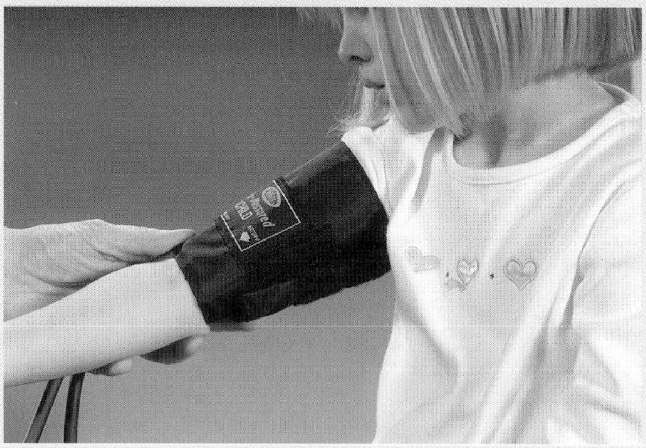

Actions
Apply the correct sized cuff over the area of maximal pulsation of the superficial artery, radial for the intecubital fossa arm and dorsalis pedis on the leg, centre of the bladder over the artery.

The width of the bladder should be at least two-thirds of the length of the arm from olecranon to acromion (or the largest cuff that can be fitted on the arm and still allow auscultation; Dillon 1988).

The cuff should fit firmly and be well secured.

The lower edge of the bladder should be 1 cm above the pulse.

Procedures Box 9.1 Blood pressure measurement—cont'd

2 Continued

The tubing from the BP cuff should not cross the auscultatory area.

Reason *Provides an accurate reading of the BP.*

Action

The manometer should be positioned vertical at eye level, not more than 3 feet from the observer.

Reason *Allows the practitioner to read the manometer accurately.*

Action

The practitioner should be comfortably positioned.

Reason *Allows the practitioner to be able to inflate and deflate the cuff gradually with ease.*

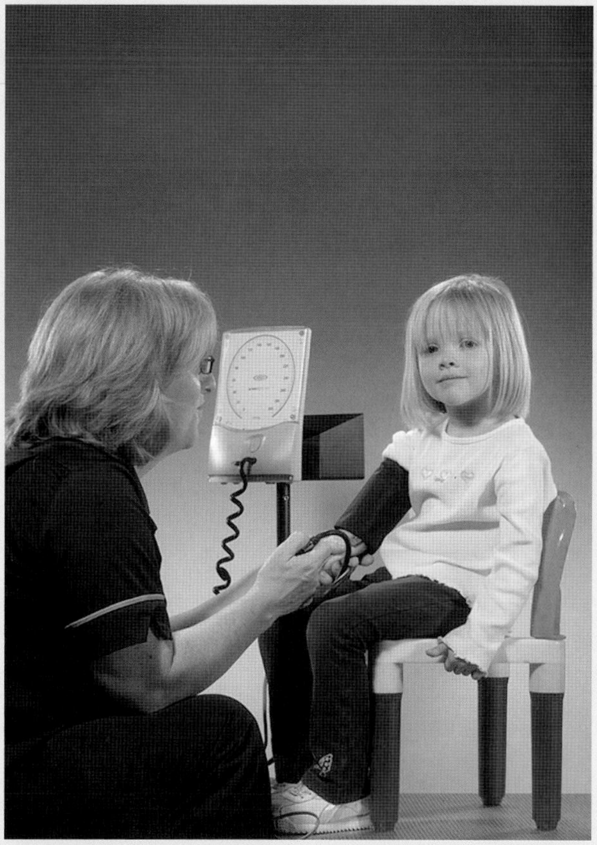

Actions

First an estimation of the systolic BP should be measured by palpation.

Inflate the cuff over 3–5 s, noting when pulsation disappears, then deflate the cuff (this gives the estimated systolic pressure; Beevers et al 2001).

Reason *Prevents underestimation of systolic pressure by misreading Korotkoff phase 3 after the auscultatory gap as Korotkoff phase 1 (Beevers et al 2001, Perloff et al 1993).*

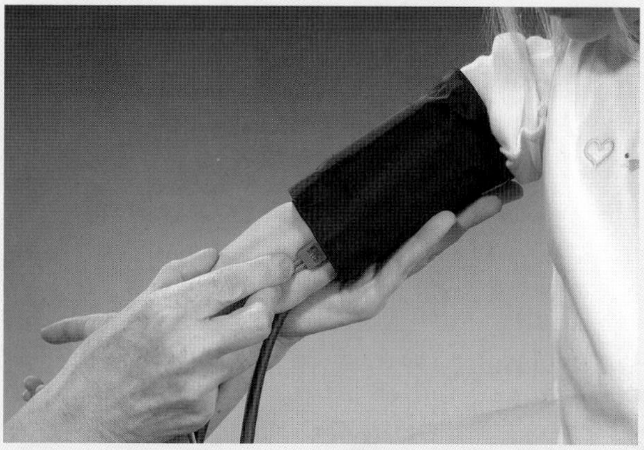

Actions

Place the stethoscope (or Doppler or fingers to palpate) gently over the artery.

Try not to press too firmly or touch the cuff (see above).

Inflate the bladder rapidly and steadily to a pressure of 30 mmHg above the previously estimated systolic BP.

Reduce the pressure at 2–3 mmHg.

The point at which repetitive, clear tapping sounds (phase 1) first appear for at least two consecutive beats gives the *systolic BP* (McAlister & Straus 2001)

The point at which repetitive sounds disappear (phase 5) gives the *diastolic BP* (auscultation only).

Then continue to completely deflate the cuff rapidly (McAlister & Straus 2001).

Both measurements should be taken to the nearest 2 mmHg (Beevers et al 2001).

A diastolic BP may not be present in some groups of patients and can sometimes be zero.

The diastolic pressure should be recorded at the point at which muffling of the repetitive sounds is taken (phase 4).

There may be a 'silent' or 'auscultatory' gap at which sounds disappear shortly after the systolic phase is heard; this should be documented if it is noted and care must be taken to ensure that the systolic phase is heard and the return of the sounds after the gap is not thought to be the systolic BP.

If the reading is difficult to ascertain, which is common in small children, it may be easier to find a second person to assist with the measurement.

Action

If it is necessary to repeat the BP the cuff should be allowed to fully deflate, then a minute should elapse before the next measurement is taken.

The same limb and cuff size should be used for repeated measurements to ensure consistency. The right arm would usually be the limb of choice. (Normative distribution data for BP are calculated on readings from the right arm.)

Reason *Minimises venous congestion and reduces the possibility of inaccurate readings.*

Procedures Box 9.1 Blood pressure measurement—cont'd

2 Continued

Actions
The BP should be written down as soon as it is recorded.

The limb in which the pressure is being recorded and the position of the subject and the equipment used (stethoscope, Doppler, palpation) should be noted.

Record the limb and the cuff size used each day.

If the patient is anxious, restless, distressed or in pain a note should be made on the BP chart.

Action
Wash your hands and clean the equipment after use.

Reason *Reduces the risk of cross-infection.*

Now test your knowledge

Question 1

The most accurate non-invasive method to obtain a BP in children is:

a direct BP (arterial)
b sphygmomanometer (manual)
c oscillometry (Dinamap)
d automated BP (24-h monitor)

Question 2

The most preferable method to obtain a systolic BP using a sphygmomanometer in the under fives is:

a auscultation (stethoscope)
b Doppler
c palpation
d visible motion of mercury

Question 3

How do you choose the most accurate cuff size to use in measuring BP in any age group?

a Use the cuff size label (infant, young child, child)
b Measure the size using the cuff that covers 90–100% of the arm circumference
c Use the cuff that looks like it best fits the arm or leg
d Use the largest cuff possible

Question 4

Using a cuff that incorporates a bladder that is too small (too short, too narrow or both) is likely to result in:

a an underestimation of BP
b an overestimation of BP
c no diastolic reading
d no systolic reading

Question 5

What would you expect to be the difference in sleeping and waking BP?

a No difference
b 2% difference
c 5% difference
d 10% difference

Question 6

If the BP measurement needs to be retaken, how long should elapse before the second measurement?

a 10 s
b 30 s
c 1 min
d 10 min

Question 7

When using any form of BP-measuring equipment, list the five most important principles for measuring BP accurately.

References

Beevers G, Lip G, O'Brien E (2001) ABC of hypertension, 4th edn. BMJ Books, London, p 17–48

Derrico D (1993) Comparison of blood pressure measurement methods in critically ill children. Dimensions of Critical Care Nursing 12(1):31–39

Dillon MJ (1988) Blood pressure. Archives of Disease in Childhood 63:347–349

Edwards S (1997) Recording blood pressure. Professional Nurse Study Supplement 13(2):S8–S11

Falkner B (2004) Development of blood pressure norms in children. In Portman R, Sorof J, Ingelfinger J (eds) Paediatric hypertension. Humana Press, Totowa, p 97–106

Flynn J (2004) Neonatal hypertension. In Portman M, Sorof J, Ingelfinger J (eds) Paediatric hypertension. Humana Press, Totowa, p 351–370

McAlister F, Straus S (2001) Evidence based treatment of hypertension. Measurement of blood pressure: an evidence based review. British Medical Journal 322:908–911

Markandu N, Whitcher F, Arnold A, Carney C (2000) The mercury sphygmomanometer should be abandoned before it is proscribed. Journal of Human Hypertension 14:31–36

Morgenstern B, Butani L (2004) Casual blood pressure measurement methodology. In Portman R (ed.) Pediatric hypertension. Humana Press, Totowa, p 77–96

National High Blood Pressure Education Program Working Group on Hypertension Control in Children and Adolescents (1996) Update on the. 1987 Task Force Report on High Blood Pressure in Children and Adolescents: a Working Group Report from the National High Blood Pressure Education Program. Pediatrics 98(4):649–658

O'Sullivan J, Allen J, Murray A (2001) A clinical study of the Korotkoff phases of blood pressure in children. Journal of Human Hypertension 15:197–201.

Pappadid S, Somers M (2003) Hypertension in adolescents: a review of diagnosis and management. Lippincott Williams & Wilkins, Philadelphia, p 370–378

Park MK, Menard SW, Yuan C (2001) Comparisons of auscultatory and oscillometric blood pressure. Archives of Pediatric and Adolescent Medicine 155(1):50–53

Perloff D, Grim C, Flack J (1993) AHA medical/scientific statement: special report. Human blood pressure determination by sphygmomanometry. Circulation 88(5):2460–2467

Portman R, Sorof J, Ingelfinger J (2004) Paediatric hypertension. Humana Press, Totowa

Sorof J, Cardwell G, Franco K (2002) Ambulatory blood pressure and left ventricular mass index in hypertensive children. Hypertension 39:903–908

Tortora (2006) Anatomy and Physiology. John Wiley and Sons, Indianapolis

10 Neurological assessment

Ruth Trengove

A thorough and structured neurological assessment provides the nurse with a baseline of the neurological status of the child. The need for accurate neurological assessment in paediatric practice is particularly relevant due to the increased incidence of head injury in young children, although neurological status may also be impaired by illness or intoxication (Advanced Life Support Group 2005, Ferguson-Clark & Williams 1998).

Knowledge of children's normal physiological and psychological growth and development is essential in the early detection of deteriorating neurological status. In addition, knowledge of the developmental history specific to the individual child is also necessary. Parents and carers are therefore absolutely vital to the effectiveness of the neurological assessment process (Ferguson-Clark & Williams 1998).

Rapidly deteriorating levels of consciousness can occur in children, with devastating consequences. Children's nurses therefore require additional skills to promptly interpret and act on a deteriorating neurological status. Such prompt action not only saves lives but will also reduce the risk of residual neurological damage resulting from hypoxia, hypotension or raised intracranial pressure (Ferguson-Clark & Williams 1998).

Raised intracranial pressure

A child with a deteriorating conscious level and/or who complains of headache or nausea, or begins vomiting may be developing raised intracranial pressure.

The skull is a rigid, unyielding structure containing the brain, blood, and interstitial and cerebrospinal fluid. There is no space to accommodate expanding lesions such as oedema, haematoma or tumours, which can cause pressure within the skull known as raised intracranial pressure. The cerebral blood vessels are compressed, compromising perfusion of the cerebral tissues. If the cause is not treated the increased pressure will lead to brain death.

Causes of raised intracranial pressure are listed in Box 10.1 (Davies & Hassell 2001, Waterhouse 2005).

Coma scales

A coma scale is a tool on which to record repeated neurological observations to provide an initial baseline and then a trend of the child's neurological status.

Coma scales were developed to standardise and minimise variability in the nursing and medical assessment of patients with impaired levels of consciousness, to monitor progress and to provide a guide to prognosis (Ferguson-Clark & Williams 1998).

Primary assessment of neurological disability

An extremely rapid assessment of conscious level during the initial, critical stage of assessing the child's illness or injury can be achieved using the AVPU scale, although assessment and management of the child's airway, breathing and circulation must always take priority. The AVPU scale assigns the child to one of four categories:

A: *Alert*

V: responds to *Voice*

P: responds only to *Pain*

U: *Unresponsive* to all stimuli

A child who responds only to pain or who is unresponsive has a significant and extremely concerning altered level of consciousness. Senior, experienced assistance should be summoned immediately, as intubation to secure the child's airway may be necessary (Advanced Life Support Group 2005).

Secondary and ongoing assessment of neurological disability

The National Institute for Clinical Excellence (2007) stipulates the use of the Glasgow Coma Scale (GCS) for the assessment of all head injury patients. However, it is also considered to be effective in assessing cerebral function in patients at risk of neurological deterioration regardless of the underlying pathology (Jevon 2004). Originally developed by Jennell & Teasdale in 1974, the GCS has since been modified and is currently well recognised and widely used.

The GCS evaluates the patient's ability to perform three key activities:

1. Eye opening
2. Verbal response
3. Motor response.

Box 10.1. Causes of raised intracranial pressure

- Extradural, subdural or intracerebral haematoma
- Cerebral oedema (due to injury, infection, hypoxia, sodium imbalance, renal problems)
- Encephalitis, meningitis
- Tumours
- Thrombus or embolism
- Hypercapnia (raised carbon dioxide in the blood)
- Hydrocephalus (increased volume of cerebrospinal fluid)
- Metabolic: renal or hepatic disease, electrolyte imbalance

Numbers are assigned to each separate observation then totalled together to give a coma score between 3 and 15. The lower the score, the poorer the neurological status. The maximum score of 15 indicates that the patient is awake, alert and completely responsive. The lowest score of 3 indicates a totally unresponsive patient (Waterhouse 2005). A GCS score of 8 or less is equivalent to a P or U on the AVPU scale (Advanced Life Support Group 2005).

The GCS should not be used in isolation, and other neurological assessment indicators including pupil reaction, limb movements and physiological signs should always be used in conjunction with it (Addison & Crawford 1999).

The original GCS was considered unsuitable for use in children. However, it has since been modified for use in paediatric practice, making the assessment and desired responses correlate to differing stages of child development (Campbell & Glasper 1995).

There are various adaptations of both the adult and the paediatric GCS, and the appearance and layout of neurological observation charts vary between differing hospital trusts. The Advanced Life Support Group (2005) recommends the GCS shown in Table 10.1 for those under and over 4 years old. However, the National Institute for Clinical Excellence (2007) guidelines also recommend using a grimace score to replace verbal response in preverbal or intubated children (Table 10.2).

Eye opening

Eye opening assesses the level of arousal or wakefulness, which is controlled by the reticular activating system in the brainstem (Shah 1999). If the child's eyes do not open spontaneously on your approach assess his or her response to speech. Ask the parent or carer to call the child's name gently initially, and if there is no response increasingly loudly, then ask the child to open his or her eyes.

Verbal response

Verbal response assesses the child's orientation, articulation and memory. It is important to pose questions using words and phrases familiar to the child and appropriate to developmental understanding (Ferguson-Clark & Williams 1998). The Paediatric GCS (Table 10.1; Advanced Life Support Group 2005) accommodates the assessment needs of preverbal children, although the National Institute for Clinical Excellence (2007) guidelines recommend a grimace score in this age group (Table 10.2).

Irritability and a high-pitched cry may be suggestive of meningeal irritation (Ferguson-Clark & Williams 1998). If

Table 10.1. Glasgow coma scales

Glasgow coma score *Response in child aged 4–15 years*	*Score*	**Paediatric Glasgow coma score** *Response in child aged < 4 years*
Eye opening		
Spontaneously	4	Spontaneously
To verbal stimuli	3	To verbal stimuli
To pain	2	To pain
No response to pain	1	No response to pain
Best motor response		
Obeys verbal commands	6	Spontaneous or obeys verbal commands
Localises to pain	5	Localises to pain or withdraws from touch
Withdraws from pain	4	Withdraws from pain
Abnormal flexion to pain (decorticate)	3	Abnormal flexion to pain (decorticate)
Abnormal extension to pain (decerebrate)	2	Abnormal extension to pain (decerebrate)
No response to pain	1	No response to pain
Best verbal response		
Oriented and converses	5	Alert, babbles, coos, words to usual ability
Disoriented and converses	4	Fewer than usual words, spontaneous irritable cry
Inappropriate words	3	Cries only to pain
Incomprehensible sounds	2	Moans to pain
No response to pain	1	No response to pain

Table 10.2. Best grimace response

Response	Score
Spontaneous normal facial or oromotor activity	5
Less than usual spontaneous ability or only response to touch stimuli	4
Vigorous grimace to pain	3
Mild grimace to pain	2
No response to pain	1

the child cannot verbally respond due to a tracheostomy or an endotracheal tube this is usually recorded on the observation chart with the letter T (Waterhouse 2005).

Motor response

Motor response assesses the brain's ability to translate sensory input into an appropriate motor response by effectively and consistently obeying simple verbal commands (Waterhouse 2005). The Paediatric GCS (Table 10.1; Advanced Life Support Group 2005) accommodates those too young to understand and comply with a verbal command. Best practice guidelines recommend asking the child to obey two different commands (Lower 2002). Avoid asking the child to squeeze the assessor's fingers, as an involuntary grasp reflex may occur that may not accurately reflect the child's condition (Shah 1999).

In infants under 6 months of age the best motor response will be flexion to pain, whereas children above this age can effectively localise pain (Davies & Hassell 2001). Fine motor control is not achieved until early childhood, therefore motor assessment should be based on the child's developmental ability (Ferguson-Clark & Williams 1998).

ALERT

If the child does not open her or his eyes, verbalise or elicit a motor response to verbal stimuli, progress to assessing these activities in response to a painful stimulus. A child who responds only to pain has a significant and extremely concerning altered level of consciousness. Senior, experienced medical assistance should be summoned immediately (Advanced Life Support Group 2005).

Painful stimulus

Painful stimulus assesses the brain's ability to recognise something is hurting and the patient's ability to attempt to remove the pain source (Waterhouse 2005). The methods for painful stimulus in children are controversial. However, there is a general consensus that painful stimulus is necessary in children with a significantly decreased conscious level (Ferguson-Clark & Williams 1998).

To avoid unnecessary distress, initially touch or gently shake the child to determine a deeper level of consciousness. If there is no response a painful stimulus will need to be applied (Waterhouse 2005).

Central painful stimulus can be delivered using the following methods (Advanced Life Support Group 2005, Ferguson-Clark & Williams 1998):

- Pulling the frontal hair
- Sternal pressure: rub the sternum with the knuckles of your clenched fist
- Trapezius squeeze: pinch the trapezius muscle, where the head meets the shoulder, between your thumb and first two fingers of one hand (ineffective in children under 5 years old because of the under-developed trapezius muscle)
- Supraorbital ridge pressure: apply pressure to the notch or groove in the bony ridge along the top of the eye.

Supraorbital ridge pressure should be applied only by practitioners trained to apply it correctly and only in a child in an extremely deep level of unconsciousness (Huband & Trigg 2000, Waterhouse 2005).

Apply the chosen stimulus and gradually increase the intensity for approximately 30 s. Rotate sites to prevent bruising (Ferguson-Clark & Williams 1998).

Best arm response should be assessed when applying painful stimuli, as it is the brain and not the spinal response that is being assessed. Spinal reflexes can cause limb flexion even in confirmed brainstem death (Waterhouse 2005).

Pupil reaction

Pupil reactions, controlled by the third cranial nerve, are integral to effective neurological assessment (Hazinski 1992). Pupil dilation, inequality and unreactivity may be indicative of serious brain disorders (Advanced Life Support Group 2005). Pupillary changes will occur on the same side of the body as the lesion. The use of a pupil measurement scale promotes accurate recording of pupil sizes (Fig. 10.1; Davies & Hassell 2001).

Pupil sizes should be assessed before shining a light into the eye to ensure they are of an equal size and a regular shape (Shah 1999). Some people have irregular or unequal pupil sizes normally (Waterhouse 2005). A unilateral dilated pupil indicates raised intracranial pressure. Bilaterally dilated pupils may be due to hypoxia or drugs (e.g. atropine), whereas opiates (e.g. morphine) constrict the pupils (Davies & Hassell 2001).

Both pupils should constrict briskly and equally to light. Reactions are recorded as follows:

- Brisk reaction: +
- No reaction: –
- Sluggish reaction: S

A sluggish reaction or dilated unequal pupil indicates a deteriorating neurological condition requiring immediate

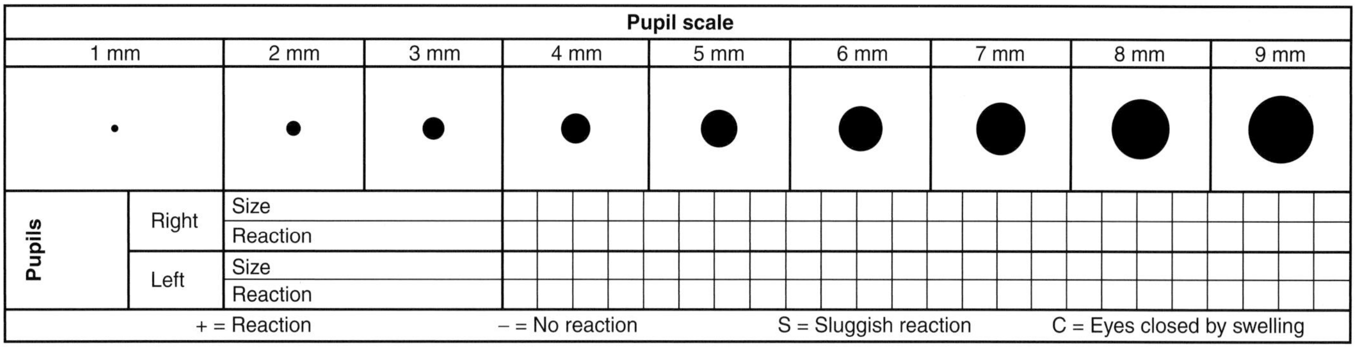
Pupil scale
1 mm
2 mm
3 mm
4 mm
5 mm
6 mm
7 mm
8 mm
9 mm
Pupils
Right
Size
Reaction
Left
Size
Reaction
+ = Reaction
– = No reaction
S = Sluggish reaction
C = Eyes closed by swelling

Fig. 10.1 • Pupil reaction.

medical intervention (Shah 1999). A hippus response occurs when the pupil initially constricts then immediately redilates to light. Meningitis may evoke a bilateral hippus response, although unilateral hippus is concerning (Davies & Hassell 2001).

When eyes are closed by orbital swelling this should be recorded on the observation chart with the letter C (Waterhouse 2005).

Limb movement

Limb movement is assessed to detect a developing hemiparesis resulting from raised intracranial pressure. Limb weakening will occur on the opposite side of the body to the brain lesion (Shah 1999).

Assess each of the four limbs separately. Ask the child to lift their arm or hold their hand and ask them to push or pull away. Similarly, ask them to raise their leg off the bed or push or pull their feet towards your hand (Shah 1999, Waterhouse 2005).

Posturing

Posturing is an abnormal and severely concerning motor function. Opisthotonus, when the neck and back arch backwards towards the buttocks, may suggest meningeal irritation. Decorticate (flexion of the arms with the legs extended) and decerebrate (extended arms and legs) are abnormal postures suggesting serious signs of cerebral dysfunction (Advanced Life Support Group 2005, Davies & Hassell 2001).

Physiological assessment

Temperature, pulse, respirations, blood pressure and oxygen saturations should be recorded (National Institute for Clinical Excellence 2007). Altered temperatures may indicate damage to the thermoregulatory hypothalamus in the brain. The brainstem controls blood pressure, heart rate and respiration (Shah 1999). Raised intracranial pressure causes dramatic changes in vital signs as the brain becomes increasingly hypoxic and ischaemic. Arterial blood pressure is increased in the body's attempt to perfuse the brain. As a result heart and respiratory rates are decreased and the breathing pattern is impaired, often varying from hyperventilation to Cheyne–Stokes respiration to apnoea. This is a very late and preterminal sign of cerebral damage known as Cushing's triad (Advanced Life Support Group 2005, Hickey 1997).

Rapid brain growth is accommodated in children under 3 years of age by unfused skull sutures. The anterior fontanelle remains open until approximately 18 months of age. Bulging or tenseness of this area in the infant at rest may suggest raised intracranial pressure (Ferguson-Clark & Williams 1998). An initial capillary blood glucose test must also be performed in any patient with decreased level of consciousness (Advanced Life Support Group 2005).

Frequency of assessment

The National Institute for Clinical Excellence guidelines (2007) recommend that head-injured patients with a GCS score below 15 should be reassessed half-hourly until the maximum score of 15 is achieved. Patients with a GCS score of 15 should be assessed half-hourly for 2 h, hourly for 4 h, then 2-hourly thereafter. Any deterioration in the score indicates a need to revert to half-hourly observations and an immediate medical review.

Discontinuation of neurological observations is based on clinical judgement once the patient is consistently stable and the underlying cause has been rectified (Waterhouse 2005). Observations must never be omitted because the child is sleeping. The child may be unconscious rather than asleep (Ferguson-Clark & Williams 1998).

Continuity of assessment

The same practitioner should complete assessments on the same patient throughout her or his shift. At handover both nurses should assess the child's neurological status together and reach an agreement on their findings (Ferguson-Clark & Williams 1998). Teaching should be given to all new nursing staff on the neurological assessment tool specific to the employing hospital trust (Huband & Trigg 2000).

Procedures Box 10.1 Conducting the neurological assessment

Action
Collect the required equipment:

- neurological observation chart
- blood pressure monitor
- oxygen saturation monitor
- thermometer
- pen torch.

Reason *Avoids unnecessary delay or prolonged assessment.*

Action
In the initial, critical assessment phase of child's injury or illness (following assessment and management of the child's airway, breathing and circulation), assess the child's conscious level on the AVPU scale.

Reason *Gives an extremely rapid and effective assessment of neurological status.*

ALERT
If the child is responsive only to pain, immediately summon senior medical assistance.

Reason *The child has a significant decreased level of consciousness, and intubation and ventilation to secure the airway may be necessary.*

Action
Once the child's condition is stable, commence the full neurological assessment.

Reason *Emergency measures to stabilise the child must always take priority over any neurological assessment.*

Action
Initially establish a baseline in relation to the child's individual developmental history from the parent or carer.

Reason *Allows the assessor to formulate an idea of the child's normal abilities.*

Action
Find out who the child interacts with on a regular basis, and her or his siblings, pets, favourite toys, comforters and daily activities, through a thorough assessment.

Reason *Allows the assessor to pose appropriate questions to the child.*

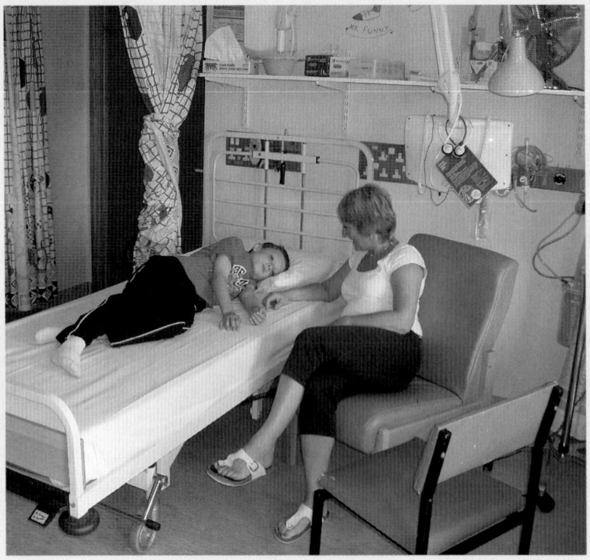

Action
While observing from a distance, note the child's eye opening, vocalisation, motor activity, posture and evidence of seizures.

Reason *The child may react differently if she or he is aware of being watched.*

Actions
In particular, note the following:

- Is the child awake or asleep?
- Is the child playing or resting?
- Is he or she settled and happy or irritable and unhappy?
- Does the child appear to be in pain?
- Has the child been vomiting?
- If crying, is it a normal or high-pitched cry?
- Is the child's colour normal?
- Is the breathing regular and at a normal rate for his or her age?
- If vocalising, is it normal for the child's age and developmental stage?
- Is the child fixing and following with his or her eyes appropriately?
- Is the child using all four limbs appropriately or is he or she reluctant to move one or all of the limbs?
- Does the child's posture appear normal?
- Is there evidence of any seizure activity?

Reason *Allows for an initial assessment without causing any distress to the child.*

Action
Involve the parent or carer in determining whether the behaviour observed is normal for the child.

Reason *The parent or carer will know what is normal and abnormal for the child.*

Actions
Interpret the findings from your covert assessment – is there any cause for concern?

If there is cause for concern seek senior assistance immediately.

Reason *Allows early medical intervention if the neurological condition is concerning.*

Action
If the child has not demonstrated eye opening and verbal and motor responses through observation alone these should be assessed further now.

Reason *Ensures that a thorough assessment is undertaken.*

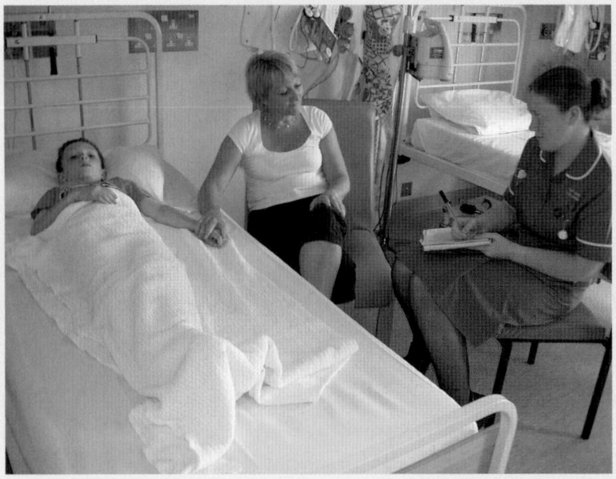

Procedures Box 10.1 Conducting the neurological assessment—cont'd

Action
Explain to the parent or carer what you are going to do next and enlist her or his help in asking the child to obey specific commands.

Reason *The child is more likely to respond to a parent or carer than an unknown healthcare professional.*

Action
Explain to the child what you are going to do in language and terminology appropriate to her or his age and level of understanding.

Reason *Psychologically prepares the child for the procedure, and compliance is more likely to be gained.*

1

Eye opening

Actions
If the child's eyes do not open spontaneously on your approach assess his or her response to speech.

Ask the parent or carer to call the child's name gently initially, and if there is no response increasingly loudly, then ask the child to open his or her eyes.

Reason *Assesses the child's level of arousal and wakefulness.*

2

Verbal response

Action
Initially ask the child approximately three questions appropriate to her or his age and developmental level.

Reason *Allows the assessor to score the response as oriented, disoriented, inappropriate words or incomprehensible sounds.*

Action
In the preverbal child, score against her or his normal vocal ability (Table 10.1) or grimace response (Table 10.2).

Reason *Allows the assessor to score the response as alert and vocalising to usual ability, less than usual words, or spontaneous or less than usual spontaneous grimace response.*

3

Motor response

Action
Ask the child to perform two differing activities, for example 'Hold up your thumb', 'Stick out your tongue' or 'Touch your nose'.

Reason *Assesses the child's ability to translate a verbal command into an appropriate motor response.*

Action
In children too young to comply with verbal commands, observe their spontaneous movements or establish their response to touch.

Reason *Allows for motor response to be assessed in this age group.*

ALERT
A child who has not responded to verbal stimuli, responds only to pain or who is unresponsive has a significant and extremely concerning altered level of consciousness – senior, experienced medical assistance should be summoned immediately.

4

Painful stimulus

Action
If the child does not open his or her eyes, verbalise or elicit a motor response to verbal stimuli, progress to assessing these activities in response to pain.

Reason *The assessor needs to evaluate the child's response to painful stimuli.*

Action
Gently shake the child prior to applying the chosen painful stimulus.

Reason *Confirms a deeper level of consciousness and avoids unnecessary distress to the child.*

Action
Explain to the parent or carer and child what you are going to do.

Reason *Gains the parent's or carer's consent and prepares the child even if he or she appears deeply unconscious.*

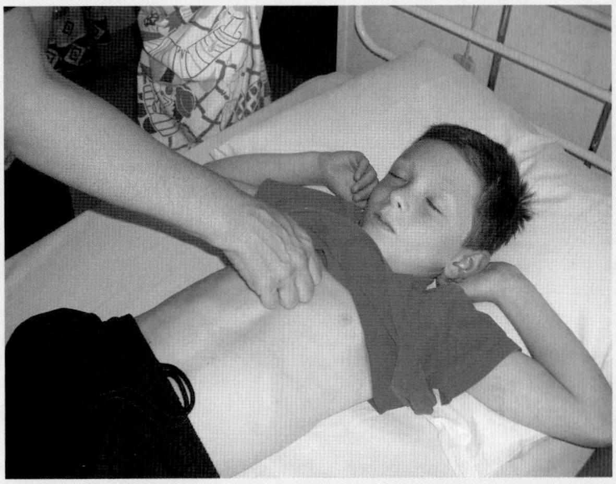

Action
Apply the chosen painful stimulus.

Reason *To observe the child's response to pain.*
Reason *Allows early medical assessment and intervention if neurological status is concerning or deteriorating.*

5

Pupil reaction

Action
Reduce the overhead lighting.

Reason *Enables a better view of the eye and reaction to light stimulus.*

Action
Look into the eyes – are the pupils of equal size and a regular shape?

Reason *Assesses appearance of pupils to detect abnormalities.*

Procedures Box 10.1 Conducting the neurological assessment—cont'd

5 Continued

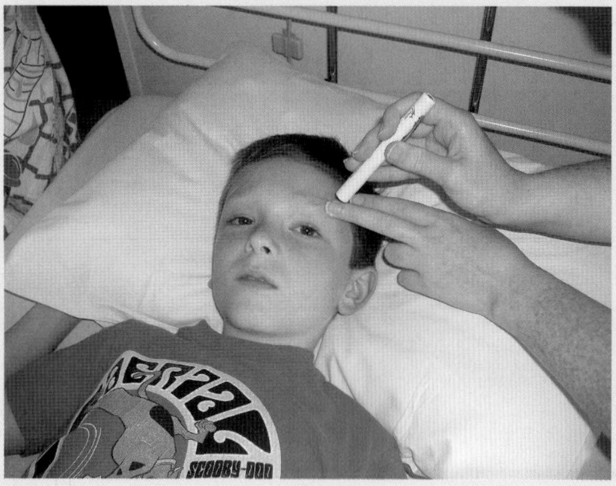

Action
Shine a bright, thin beam from the outer aspect towards the centre of the eye.

Reason *Assesses pupil reaction to light, which should be a brisk constriction.*

Action
Repeat on the other eye after a few seconds.

Reason *Allows the pupil to return to its normal size prior to repeating the procedure.*

Action
It may be necessary to gently hold the eye open, in which case ensure that you wash your hands in advance and inform the child of what you are going to do.

Reason *Prevents cross-infection and promotes psychological support and compliance.*

ALERT
If there is cause for concern, seek senior experienced assistance immediately.

Reason *Allows early medical assessment and intervention if neurological status is concerning or deteriorating.*

6

Limb movement

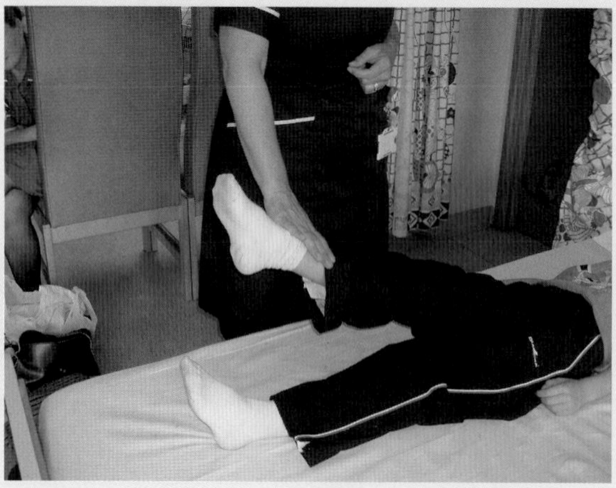

Action
Assess each of the four limbs separately.

Ask the child to lift his or her arm or hold his or her hand and ask him or her to push or pull away.

Then ask the child to raise each leg off the bed or push or pull the feet towards your hand.

Reason *Identifies a weakness on one side of the body, indicating raised intracranial pressure.*

7

Physiological signs

Action
Monitor and record temperature, pulse, respirations, blood pressure and oxygen saturation.

Reason *Detects physiological changes that may indicate raised intracranial pressure.*

Action
Perform an initial capillary glucose blood test.

Reason *To detect and initiate early treatment of hypo- or hyperglycaemia.*

Action
In the restful infant palpate the anterior fontanelle.

Reason *A bulging or tense fontanelle may indicate raised intracranial pressure.*

8

Documentation and interpretation

Action
Document your observations on the neurological assessment chart.

Reason *Keeps a record of findings and trends for analysis.*

Action
Interpret your findings – is there an improvement or deterioration from your previous assessment?

Reason *Promptly interpreting and acting on a deteriorating level of consciousness reduces the risk of morbidity and mortality.*

Actions
Is there any cause for concern?

If there is, immediately report to a senior medical colleague.

Reason *Allows early medical assessment and intervention if neurological status is concerning or deteriorating.*

Action
Assess when the next set of neurological observations should be performed.

Reason *Allows the assessor to plan his or her workload and ensures that the patient is reviewed in a timely manner.*

Action
At handover perform a neurological assessment with the nurse who is taking over responsibility for the patient.

Reason *Ensures continuity of assessment and an agreement on findings.*

Now test your knowledge

Question 1

In addition to head injury consider other situations in which you may undertake a period of neurological assessment.

Question 2

Name and describe the scale that precedes the GCS and provides a rapid assessment of neurological function.

Question 3

Which three responses does the GCS assess and what score is assigned to each category?

Question 4

What may lead you to suspect that a child or young person is developing signs of raised intracranial pressure?

Question 5

Consider which type of painful stimulus you would apply, if necessary, to an extremely drowsy 9-month-old child and how you would achieve it.

Question 6

If a child or young person has left-sided weakness and a sluggish and dilated right pupil, which side of the brain is affected?

Question 7

What score can be used to assess verbal response in a preverbal or intubated child or young person?

Question 8

A 6-year-old child is admitted for a period of observation following a head injury. His GCS score has been 15 since admission and his observations are currently being undertaken every 2 h. He is about to be discharged home when he complains of a headache and feeling sick. What will you do?

Question 9

You are unsure if a 10-year-old girl has a sluggish pupil reaction. Her eyes are dark brown and it is difficult to see a reaction. What could you do?

References

Addison C, Crawford B (1999) Not bad just misunderstood. Nursing Times 95(43):52–53

Advanced Life Support Group (2005) Advanced paediatric life support: the practical approach, 4th edn. Blackwell Publishing, London

Campbell S, Glasper EA (eds) (1995) Whaley and Wong's children's nursing, UK edition. Mosby/Times Mirror International, London

Davies JH, Hassell LL (2001) Children in intensive care. A nurse's survival guide. Churchill Livingstone, London

Ferguson-Clark L, Williams C (1998) Neurological assessment in children. Paediatric Nursing 10(4):29–35

Hazinski MF (1992) Nursing care of the critically ill child, 2nd edn. Mosby-Year Book, St Louis

Hickey JV (1997) The clinical practice of neurological and neurosurgical nursing, 4th edn. Lippincott, New York

Huband S, Trigg E (2000) Practices in children's nursing: guidelines for hospital and community. Churchill Livingstone, London

Jennell B, Teasdale G (1974) Assessment of coma and impaired consciousness: a practical scale. Lancet 2:81–84

Jevon P (2004) Paediatric advanced life support: a practical guide. Butterworth Heinemann, London

Lower J (2002) Facing neuro assessment fearlessly. Nursing 32(2): 58–64

National Institute for Clinical Excellence (2007) Head injury: triage, assessment, investigation and early management of head injury in infants, children and adults. Clinical guideline 56. NICE, London

Shah S (1999) Neurological assessment. Nursing Standard 13(22): 49–56

Waterhouse C (2005) The Glasgow Coma Scale and other neurological observations. Nursing Standard 19(33):56–64

Section Three
Therapeutic interventions

11 Personal hygiene

Laura Gilbert • Gillian McEwing

The skin is the largest organ of the body, and when intact provides a dry surface that is resistant to penetration by microorganisms (Harrison 2006). It is water-resistant and formed from two layers: the epidermis and the dermis. The epidermis is the most superficial layer of the skin, and it is made up of stratified squamous epithelium. It varies in thickness, with a very thin layer being present on the eyelids and more thickness on the palms of the hands and the soles of the feet (Waugh & Grant 2006). The dermis is formed from connective tissue, collagen fibres and elastic fibres. It contains blood vessels, lymph vessels, sensory nerve endings, sweat glands and their ducts, hairs arising from hair follicles and sebaceous glands that secrete sebum, which provides a water-resistant coating to the skin and maintains the softness and pliability of the hair (Waugh & Grant 2006). The skin provides a protective barrier for the entire body, which protects the vital organs of the body from injury and, in addition, forms part of the thermoregulatory mechanism for the body (Madder 2000).

Bathing infants, children and young people

Children's nurses need to be able to assess and meet the hygiene needs of children from birth to adulthood when they are unable to perform these skills themselves. Personal hygiene is an important part of the daily routine for any child whether she or he is at home or in hospital, as it enhances comfort, promotes self-esteem and helps prevent infection by removing microorganisms that could be potentially harmful (Major 2005, Trigg & Mohammed 2006). Feeling clean can be an important social, cultural or religious requirement (Firth 2006, Major 2005). Many children will have their parents, extended family or carers willing to assist in this care, but if the child is attached to monitoring equipment the family may not feel able to bathe or wash their child, or they may not be able to visit at the times when washing or bathing the child may be necessary, and therefore in these circumstances carers must have the knowledge and skills to meet the hygiene needs of children competently and safely.

In infants and young children the skin covers a large surface area in proportion to their body volume (Chamley et al 2005); this large ratio, plus the limited amount of subcutaneous fat present in young children (Tortora 2005) and the fact that the hypothalamus is immature (Leone & Finer 2006), means they can lose heat very rapidly and become hypothermic (Rudolf & Levene 2006). Therefore extra care needs to be taken when bathing infants and young children to ensure that they do not become too cold due to the temperature of the room being too low, the water temperature being too cold or the procedure taking an unnecessary length of time. It is important for nurses to be organised, and all equipment required for bathing and redressing the infant or child must be prepared before the child's clothing is removed (Campbell & Glasper 1995, Trigg & Mohammed 2006).

Bathing should be a relaxing and pleasurable experience that is part of the daily routine for each individual (O'Regan & Fawcett 2006). This procedure also allows time to be in close contact with the child to encourage communication and allow for a thorough observation and assessment of the child's physical condition (Duncan 2004). If possible, meeting the personal hygiene needs of the child should take place in the bathroom, as this is a more familiar environment for the child and provides some privacy (Department of Health 2001, Major 2005).

LINK CHAPTER **1**

The use of bath toys, bubble bath or skin wash suitable for the delicate skin of infants and children can add to the enjoyment for both the child and the adult supervising the bathing.

If a child is confined to her or his bed due to illness or the equipment required to monitor her or his condition, a blanket bath may be undertaken, which will ensure that the integrity of the skin on the whole body is monitored and maintained and should still be a pleasurable activity that the child can take part in by assisting with washing her or his face, hands, abdomen or legs as able.

All nurses must practise care that is evidence-based and ensure that the safety of the child is paramount during any procedure undertaken, including bathing (*Code of Professional Conduct* 1.3 and 1.4; Nursing and Midwifery Council 2004). It must always be remembered that infants and young children must never, under any circumstances, be left alone in a bath even momentarily, as young children can drown in just a few millimetres of water within a very short space of time.

LINK CHAPTER **1**

The assessment of skin integrity in both infants and children is an important part of the nurse's role. The *Essence of Care* framework (Department of Health 2001) requires all nurses to assess, evaluate and enhance the care that is delivered to all patients. This assessment must include the visual assessment of the child's ears, eyes, umbilicus (for infants) and nappy area. All areas of the child's body should be assessed, and the information obtained must be documented in the nursing records. The following aspects of skin integrity should be assessed:

- The colour (pale for that child, which may indicate a low haemoglobin concentration or decrease in the peripheral circulation due to sepsis, dehydration or shock; the presence of Mongolian blue spot; normal skin tone for the individual child)
- The texture of the skin (dry, smooth, moist)
- Skin temperature (warm, cold, sweaty, clammy)
- The presence of rashes or skin conditions (eczema, psoriasis); scabs from chickenpox, measles, etc.; surgical wounds; bruising.

This assessment should be undertaken as quickly as possible, ensuring that the child's privacy and dignity are maintained and that the child does not become cold due to lack of clothing or blankets. The room in which the assessment is undertaken must be warm.

For children with a specific skin condition such as eczema, dermatitis, impetigo, scabies or psoriasis among many others, a specific regimen of skin care will be prescribed and may include the application of bandages or dressings.

Daily bathing may be an important part of the treatment for these and can help to soften hardened scaly skin and previously applied skin creams and lotions (Moules & Ramsay 1998).

LINK CHAPTER **34**

Umbilical cord care

Following birth the umbilical cord is clamped tightly and then cut a few centimetres from the abdominal skin. This forms a stump that becomes dry and stiff, turns brown–black and separates, leaving healthy skin (Fig. 11.1). The blood vessels of the umbilical cord remain patent for a few days after birth and therefore present a dangerous route for infection (Furdon & Clark 2002). It is important that the stump is kept clean and dry to prevent infection (McConnell et al 2004). The use of antiseptics has been shown to delay the cord falling off because the normal skin flora are destroyed that would have attracted leucocytes to the cord and encouraged separation (Zupan et al 2004). The use of alcohol has also been shown to be detrimental, as it is not effective against bacteria and delays cord separation (Oishi et al 2004). Exposure to the air encourages the cord to dry out and separate. If there are any signs of infection, such as raised temperature, inflammation, swelling or redness, then a swab should be taken for microbiological culture (Trigg & Mohammed 2006). The stump usually separates from the healthy abdominal skin after about a week and drops off, leaving the area known as the umbilicus or belly button (Fig. 11.2).

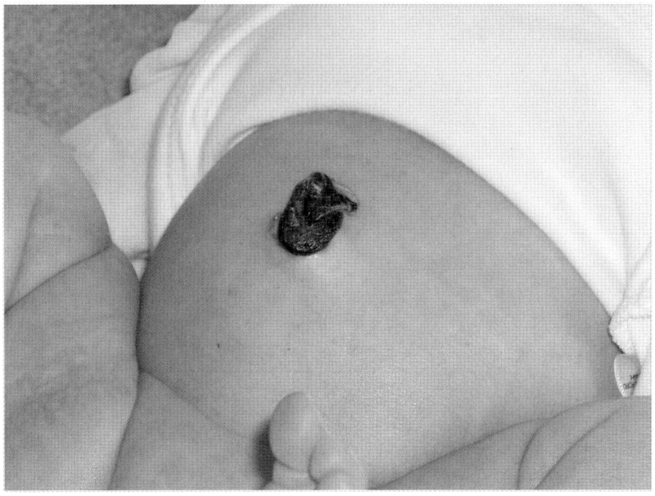

Fig. 11.1 • The umbilical cord.

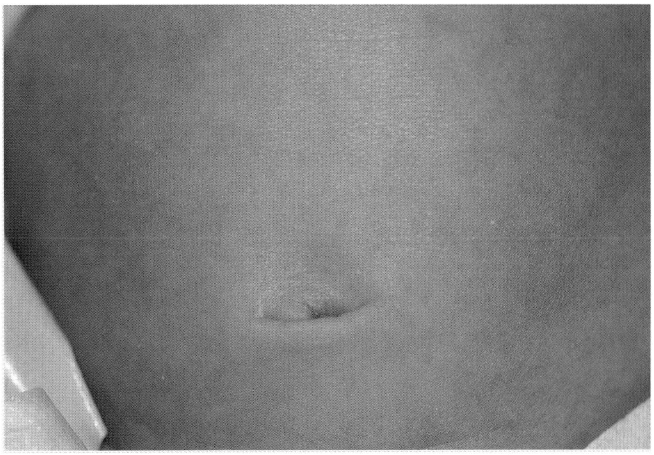

Fig. 11.2 • The umbilicus (belly button).

To encourage the cord to dry out it is recommended that the baby is not bathed for approximately 7–10 days following cord separation (Department of Health 2006).

Contact with urine should be avoided by folding the nappy down below the stump; this will also increase exposure to the air (Zupan et al 2004). Leaving the abdomen exposed or only dressing in loose-fitting clothes will also encourage air to circulate around the stump. The cord should be cleaned only when clinically indicated by the presence of debris (Zupan et al 2004). Cleaning should be performed using cool boiled water and sterile gauze. The stump should be wiped gently using a clean piece of gauze for each sweep. When the debris has been removed the area should be fully dried using dry sterile gauze.

Procedures Box 11.1 Cleaning the umbilical cord

Equipment
- Non-sterile gloves
- Disposable apron
- Sterile bowl
- Sterile water (or boiled water in home environment)
- Sterile gauze swabs
- Waste disposal bag
- Clean changing mat on safe firm surface

Actions
Prepare the room and equipment.

Prepare the gauze and pour the water into the bowl.

Reasons *Avoids delays in the procedure and causing unnecessary distress to the baby.*
Avoids putting the baby at risk.

Action
The room should be warm and draught-free (Boxwell 2001).

Reason *Helps maintain the baby's body temperature.*

Actions
Wash your hands (Department of Health 2003).

Put on gloves.

Reason *Helps prevent cross-infection.*

Action
Place the baby in a supine position on the changing mat and remove only the clothing necessary to expose the cord area (Chamley et al 2005).

Reason *Provides a safe position and ensures that the baby remains warm.*

Actions
Dip the gauze into the water and gently wipe in a sweeping motion around the cord, using a clean piece of gauze each time.

Do not put undue pressure on or pull at the stump (Zupan et al 2004).

Remove all debris, but some black stump residue may remain attached.

Reason *Removes debris and avoids infecting the area.*

Action
Thoroughly dry the area using clean gauze.

Reason *Encourages healing and separation.*

Action
Report and record any signs of inflammation or infection.

Reason *It is important that any possible infection of the cord stump is recognised and is treated immediately if necessary (World Health Organization 1998).*

Baby: minimal hygiene care

Young babies do not get dirty and therefore do not require a full bath each day; however, if the baby has vomited or has had a very dirty nappy this may be required at any time. A minimal cleansing can be given, which involves cleaning the face, neck and nappy area; this is sometimes called a top-and-tail wash (Trigg & Mohammed 2006). When a baby is ill, with cardiac or respiratory problems, a bath can be stressful and exhausting. It may also be unsuitable for a baby with neurological problems. Avoid bathing immediately following a feed, as this may cause the baby to vomit (Lee & Thompson 2007).

Procedures Box 11.2 Minimal hygiene care for a baby

Action
Ensure that the room is warm and free from draughts (Department of Health 2006).

Reason *Ensures that the infant does not become cold while the procedure is taking place; infants have a reduced ability to regulate their body temperature and can lose heat rapidly.*

Actions
Ensure that you have all the equipment close to hand: two clean towels, a clean nappy, clean clothes, perfume-free soap, a sponge or cloth if desired and cotton wool balls.

Be sure that these are ready before you start to bathe the baby or child.

Reason *Ensures that the child is not left unattended at ANY time while the bath is undertaken (Lee & Thompson 2007).*

Action
Use products made for infants, such as soaps with a neutral pH and without preservatives (Gfatter et al 1997).

Action
Remember to talk to the infant while you are providing this care, and respond to any smiles or noises that the infant makes to you.

Reason *Promotes the development of speech and language skills.*

Actions
Ensure that cold water is placed in the bowls to be used before gradually adding hot water.

Use a water thermometer to check the temperature of the water before the infant is lowered into the water.

Reason *Ensures that the water is not too hot, as this could cause damage to the baby's skin (Young 2004).*

Action
Undress the baby and wrap him or her in a towel with the nappy still in place (Boxwell 2001).

Reasons *Protects the nurse from faeces or urine.*
Helps to maintain body temperature.

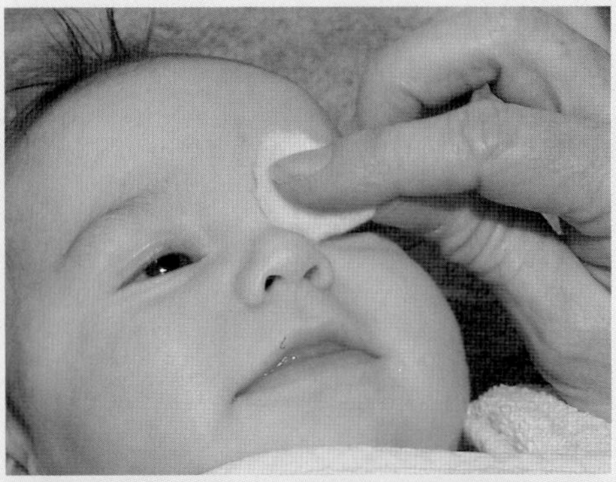

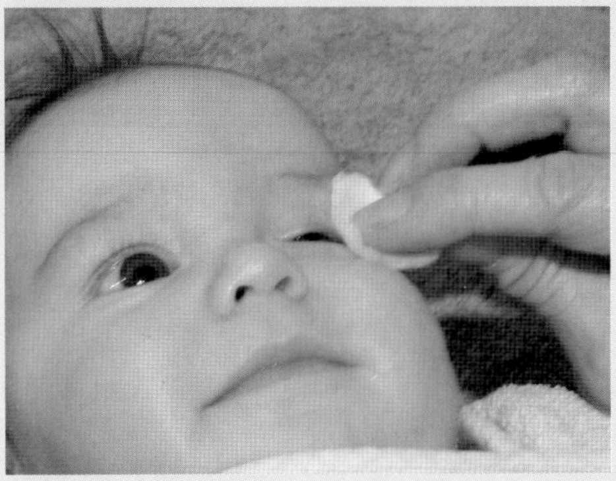

Actions

Using a fresh non-sterile swab for each eye, dip the gauze into the sterile water and clean each eye from the inner area by the nose the other edge at the side of the face.

Discard each swab after use.

Reasons *Avoids cross-contamination from one eye to another.*
Using each swab only once prevents any discharge from one side of the eye being reintroduced into the eye that has been cleaned.

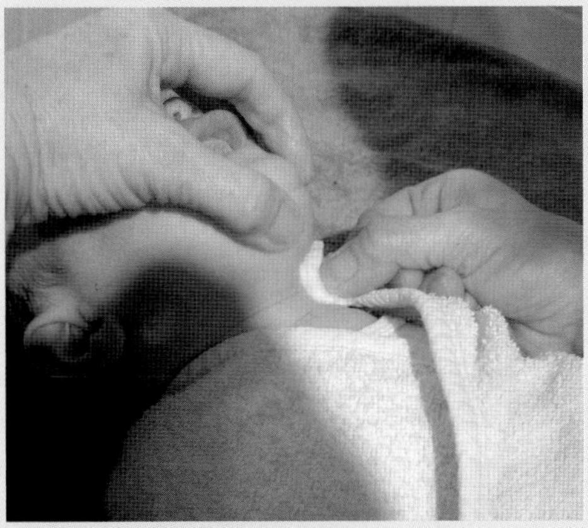

Action

Gently wash the rest of the baby's face and behind the ears as well as under the chin and around the neck folds carefully and pat dry with a clean towel.

Reason *Ensures that any milk, vomit or saliva that may collect in the neck folds and behind the ears is removed to prevent the skin from becoming sore or infected.*

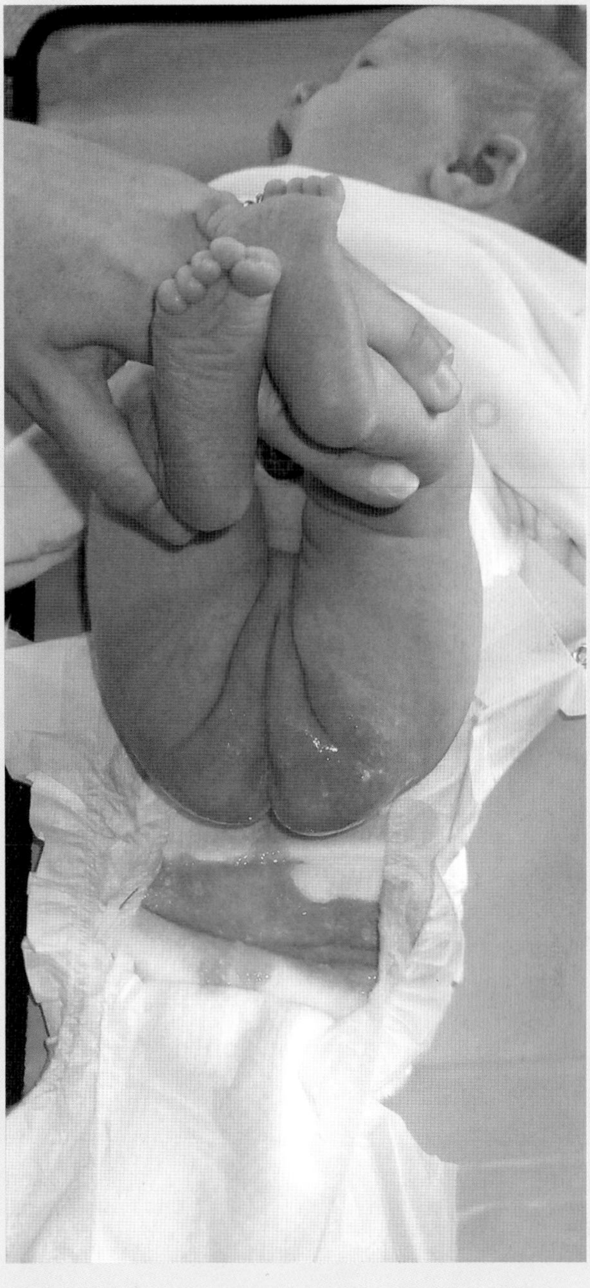

Actions

Put on non-sterile gloves.

Open the towel and remove the soiled nappy.

(Note that gloves are not worn in this photograph, which shows a mother and her baby at home.)

Reason *This is in accordance with hospital universal precautions policies.*

Actions

Gently clean the genital area with a disposable cloth, wiping from front to back, therefore from the vagina to the rectum in girls.

Gently pat dry with a towel.

Procedures Box 11.2 Minimal hygiene care for a baby—cont'd

Reason *Avoids introducing faecal matter and bacteria into the vagina.*

Action
For boys, ensure that the skin underneath the scrotum is clean, and dry it carefully with a towel.

Reason *Ensures that faeces is not left in contact with the skin, as this may cause soreness.*

Action
Observe the skin integrity carefully, documenting accurately and reporting any rashes or soreness observed in the nursing notes.

Action
Apply any creams that may have been prescribed for the treatment of thrush or nappy rash.

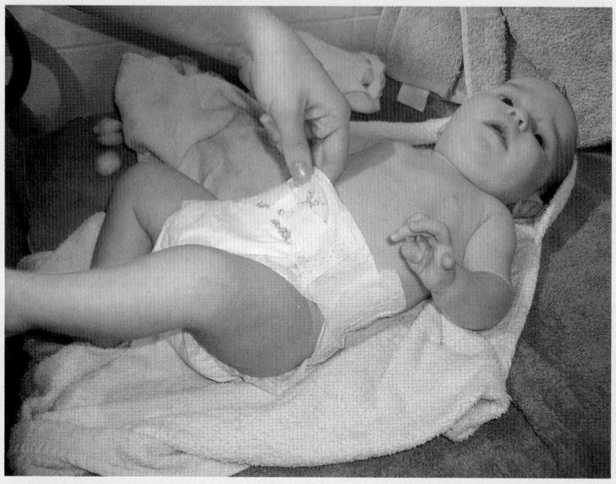

Action
Replace a clean nappy on the baby, ensuring that it is properly fitted.

Reason *Nappies that are too tight will cause friction to the skin, and nappies that are too loose will enable leakage of urine or faeces to occur.*

Action
Re-dress the infant with appropriate clothing for the time of year.

Reason *Ensures that the infant is neither too hot nor too cold.*

Action
Place the baby back in the cot or pram and ensure that the cot sides are in place and that the infant is safe and secure.

Reason *Prevents the infant from rolling over and falling to the ground and becoming injured.*

Action
Document the care given in the nursing notes.

Reason *This is in accordance with the Nursing and Midwifery Council's guidelines for record keeping (Nursing and Midwifery Council 2005).*

Bathing an infant or young child

Infants' and young children's skin is delicate, and bathing helps to maintain its health and texture. They do not need to be bathed daily, and too frequent bathing can lead to drying of the skin. An infant or a young child can be bathed at any time during the day; however, it is not recommended to bath immediately after a feed or meal. Many parents incorporate bathing into the child's prebedtime ritual, as it can relax the child ready for bed.

Procedures Box 11.3 Bathing an infant or young child

Action
Ensure that the room is warm and free from draughts (Department of Health 2006).

Reason *Ensures that the infant or child does not become cold while the procedure is taking place; infants have a reduced ability to regulate their body temperature and can lose heat rapidly.*

Actions
Ensure that you have all the equipment close to hand: two clean towels, a clean nappy, clean clothes, baby shampoo, perfume-free soap, a sponge or cloth if desired and cotton wool balls.

Be sure that these are ready before you start to bathe the baby or child.

Reason *To ensure that the child is not left unattended at ANY time while the bath is undertaken (Lee & Thompson 2007).*

Action
Use products made for infants, such as soaps with a neutral pH and without preservatives (Gfatter et al 1997).

Procedures Box 11.3 Bathing an infant or young child—cont'd

Action
Position the bath at an appropriate height if possible and ensure that it is safe and secure (Smith 2005).

Reason *Maintains good posture and a safe position.*

LINK CHAPTER **1**

Action
Wash your hands and put on a disposable apron.

Reason *Prevents cross-infection and protects clothing (Department of Health 2003).*

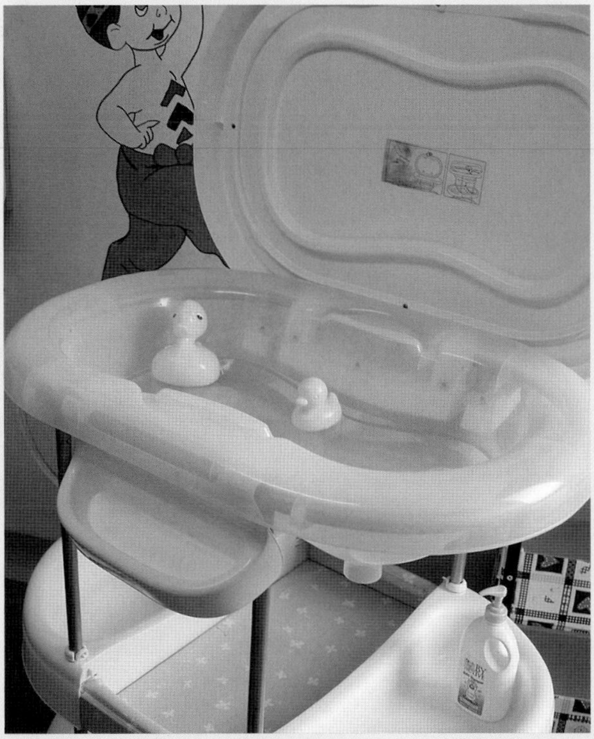

Actions
Run cold water into the baby bath or bathtub and then gradually add hot water until the desired temperature of the water is reached (32–35 °C).

Check the temperature of the water with a bath thermometer before undressing the baby or child.

In a main bath always finish by running cold water in case the tap drips and scalds the child.

Reason *Ensures that the baby or child is not scalded from the water being too hot.*

Action
Add baby bubble bath to the water, if permitted.

Reason *If medical condition allows: excessive use can cause the baby's skin to become dry and may lead to irritation (Cowan & Frost 2006).*

Action
Add clean bath toys to the water.

Reason *To prevent cross-infection all bath toys must be disinfected after each use.*

Action
Undress the baby or child while talking to him or her and explaining what you are about to do.

Reason *Make it fun! It should be a relaxed and pleasurable experience for the child.*

Action
Undress the baby and wrap him or her in a towel with the nappy still in place (Boxwell 2001).

Reasons *Protects the nurse from faeces or urine.*
Helps maintain body temperature.

Action
Place the baby either supine on a clean changing mat or, when seated, across your lap.

Actions
Using a fresh non-sterile swab for each eye, dip the gauze into the sterile water and clean each eye from the inner area by the nose the other edge at the side of the face.

Discard each swab after use.

Reasons *Avoids cross-contamination from one eye to another.*
Using each swab only once prevents any discharge from one side of the eye being reintroduced into the eye that has been cleaned.

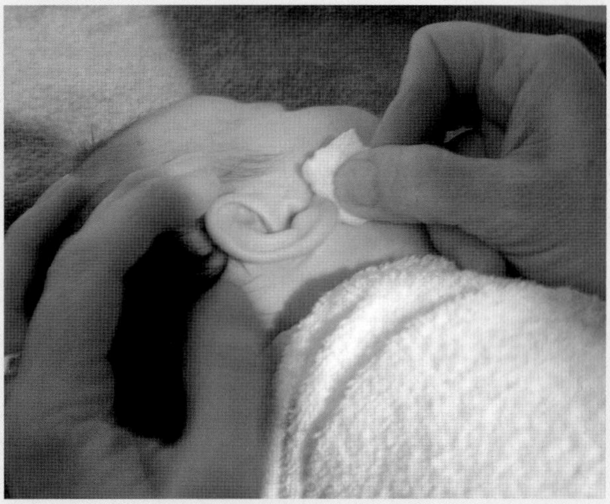

Action
Gently wash the rest of the baby's face and behind the ears as well as under the chin and around the neck folds carefully and pat dry with a clean towel.

Reason *Ensures that any milk, vomit or saliva that may collect in the neck folds and behind the ears is removed to prevent the skin from becoming sore or infected.*

Actions
Put on non-sterile gloves, undo the nappy and clean away any faecal matter with a disposable wipe.

Dispose of the nappy and wipe in a clinical waste bin.

Remove the gloves.

Reasons *This is in accordance with hospital universal precautions policies.*
Prevents the bathwater becoming contaminated with faecal matter.

Procedures Box 11.3 Bathing an infant or young child—cont'd

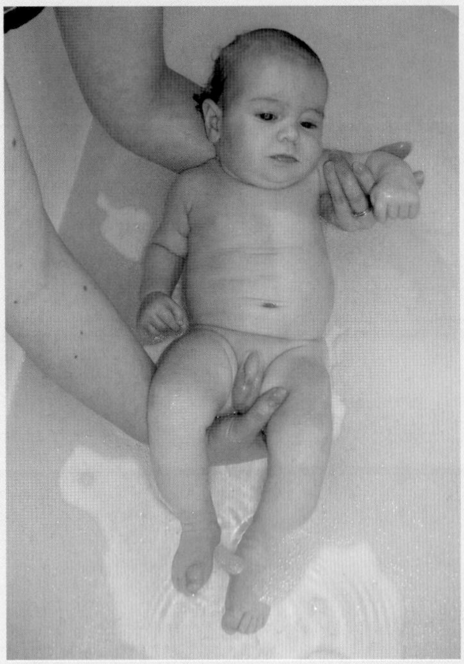

Actions
Hold the baby securely by placing your forearm around the baby's shoulders and holding the top of the upper arm gently to ensure that she or he does not slip beneath the water.

With your other hand supporting the infant's buttocks and upper thighs gently lower the infant into the water.

Reason *Ensures the safety of the baby.*

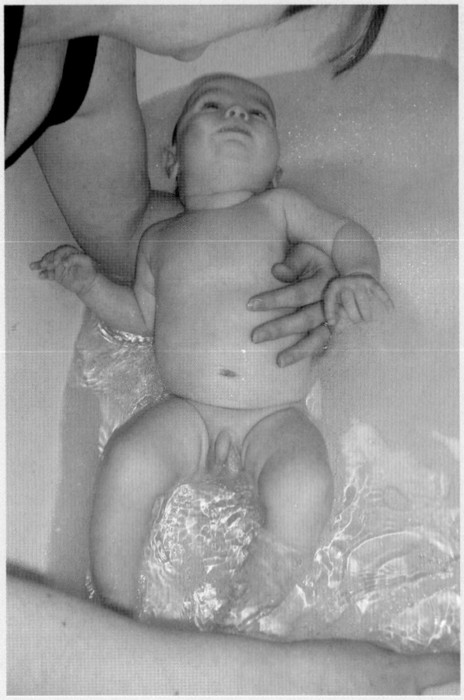

Action
While continuing to hold the baby securely around his or her shoulders, use your other hand to wash the baby with your hand or a clean flannel or sponge.

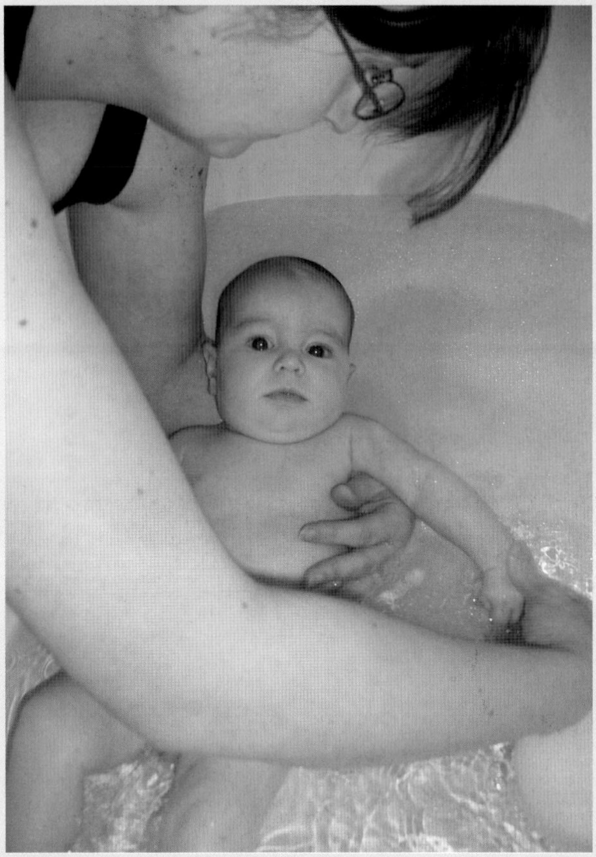

Reason *Maintains the safety of the baby and makes the infant feel safe.*

Action
Pay special attention to cleaning the creases under the arms, the spaces between the fingers and the genital area.

Action
For toddlers and young children, lift them into the bath and make sure that they are sitting on a non-slip bathmat to ensure that they do not slip under the water.

Reason *Maintains the safety of the child and prevents her or him from slipping under the water.*

Action
Stay with the child at ALL times.

Reason *Prevents accidental drowning, which can occur within a few moments.*

Action
Encourage the child to splash and play with bath toys.

Reason *It is good exercise for the child and should be a relaxing and fun experience.*

Actions
Do not allow the water to get cold.

Procedures Box 11.3 Bathing an infant or young child—cont'd

If the hair has been washed, ensure that the hair is towel-dried to prevent excess heat loss from the head.

Reason *Prevents the child from becoming cold.*

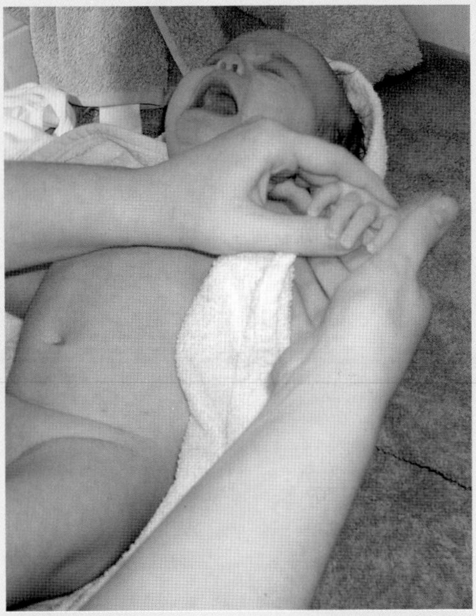

Actions

Lift the child out of the water following the same procedure as when lowering the baby into the water, taking great care, as the baby will be wet and slippery.

Immediately wrap the baby in a clean, warm towel.

Action

Dry the skin carefully, observing the skin integrity for any rashes, bruises or injury; report and record any concerns accurately in the child's notes.

Reason *To document any improvement or deterioration of the skin condition.*

Action

Avoid the use of talcum powder (Department of Health 2006).

Reason *There is a risk of aspiration into the lungs.*

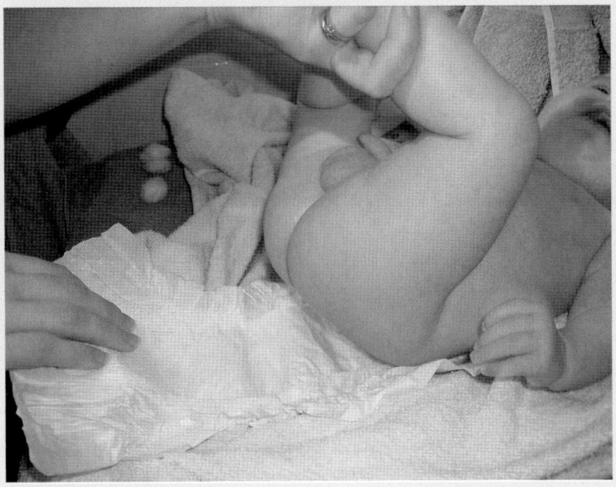

Action

Place a clean nappy on the child and re-dress him or her in the clean clothes.

Reason *Prevents soiling of the clothing with urine or faeces.*

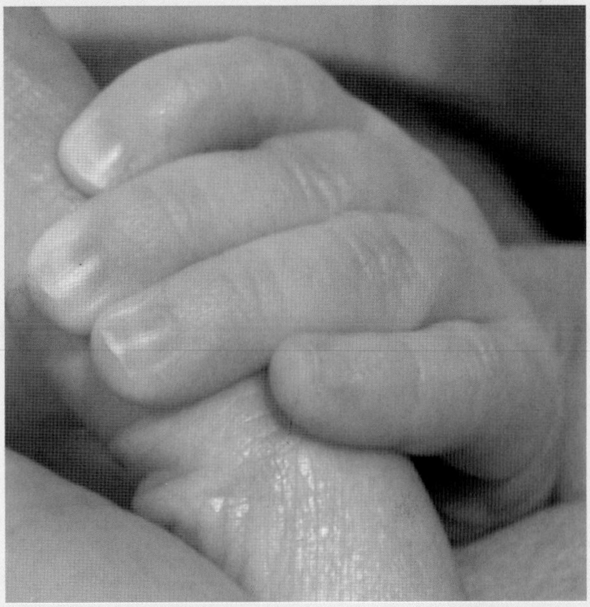

Action

The baby's nails grow rapidly and are very soft and flexible; keep them trimmed using baby nail scissors, which are small with rounded tips.

Reason *If nails grow long or become ragged they can scratch the baby's face or eyes.*

Action

Remember to praise the child.

Reason *Encourages the child to enjoy baths in the future.*

Actions

Brush the child's hair.

Make note of the condition of the scalp and observe carefully for head lice; document findings if necessary.

Return the baby or child to the cot or bed.

Actions

Clean the bath using warm water and detergent and dry it thoroughly to avoid the growth of bacteria (Jamieson et al 2002).

Dispose of clinical waste appropriately.

Reason *Prevents cross-infection.*

Bathing the older child or young person in bed

As children grow they become more independent in meeting their own hygiene needs. However, when they are seriously ill, unconscious or in traction they will need assistance to meet these needs and may require a bed bath. The involvement of the parents should be discussed with the parents and if possible the child or young person; some children prefer the nurse to perform this task (Department of Health 2001, 2003). Some children and young people may prefer a carer of the same gender as themselves; it may be to protect their dignity or for religious or cultural reasons (Trigg & Mohammed 2006).

Procedures Box 11.4 Bathing an older child or young person in bed

Equipment

Ensure that you have all the equipment close to hand:

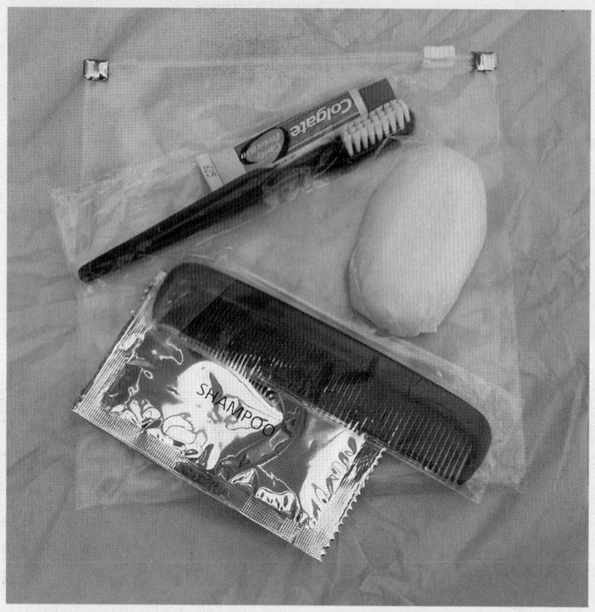

- Two clean towels
- Clean clothes
- Soap
- Two sponges or cloths
- Washbowl with warm water
- Hairbrush
- Toothbrush and toothpaste
- Deodorants and perfumes, if desired
- Clean bed linen and linen skip.

Action
Check that it is a suitable time for the child to have the bath.

Reason *Take into consideration mealtimes, school times and medical rounds and try to avoid the child's favourite television programme.*

Action
Ensure that the room is warm and free from draughts and ensure privacy (Department of Health 2006).

Reason *Ensures that the child does not become cold while the procedure is taking place and maintains dignity and respect.*

Action
Replace the water as necessary to ensure that it remains clean and warm.

Action
Remember to talk to the child or young person while you are providing this care.

Reason *Gives the child or young person the opportunity to discuss any concerns he or she may have and build a relationship with the nurse.*

Action
Raise the bed to a comfortable working height.

Reason *Ensuring that you are comfortable and safe, use manual handling aids as required.*

Action
Loosen and fold back the bedclothes.

Reason *Allows the child to move more freely, and to give you access to assist the child with washing.*

Actions
Assist the child or young person to undress; leave him or her covered with either the sheet or the towel.

Allow the child or young person as much independence as possible.

Reason *Protects dignity and autonomy.*

Action
Assist the child to clean his or her teeth.

Reason *Ensure that toothpaste residue is removed from around the mouth.*

Actions
Assist the child cleanse her or his eyes using a clean corner of the washcloth for each eye.

Rinse the cloth and assist the child to wash the remainder of her or his face, neck and behind the ears.

Wash the hair, if required.

Wash each part of the body in the following sequence:

- Arms: one at a time, carefully cleanse between the fingers and under the arms; check the nails and trim and clean them as required
- Chest and abdomen
- Front of upper legs, lower legs and feet
- Genitalia: use a second washcloth
- Turn the child on to her or his side with assistance and wash the back of the upper legs and buttocks; continue to use the second washcloth.

Older children and young people may prefer to do this themselves.

For boys, when washing the genitalia do not push back the foreskin – simply wash the glans (Firth 2006).

Action
Before washing each area of the body, position a towel either under or around the area.

Procedures Box 11.4 Bathing an older child or young person in bed—cont'd

Reason *Prevents unnecessary wetting of bed clothes.*

Action
Cover the child with a sheet or towel, exposing only the part of the body being cleansed.

Reason *Protects the child's dignity and avoids unnecessary heat loss.*

Action
Ensure that the skin is thoroughly rinsed and dried after washing.

Reason *Avoids soap residue being left on the skin, which may cause irritation.*

Action
Observe the skin throughout the procedure, checking for pressure sores in high-risk areas such as the elbows, heels, occiput and buttocks, as well as for rashes, swellings, etc.

Reason *To identify skin deterioration and respond by using pressure-relieving devices.*

LINK CHAPTER **12**

Actions
Change the bed linen as required.
Help the child dress into clean clothes.
Help the child into a comfortable position.
Assist the child to brush the hair and style it as required.

Action
Document the care given in the nursing notes.

Reason *In accordance with the Nursing and Midwifery Council's guidelines for record keeping (Nursing and Midwifery Council 2005), make note of and report any signs of skin deterioration or inflammation, any physical abnormalities and any signs of poor nutrition or oedema.*

Now test your knowledge

Think about the last time that you were involved with bathing a child on your ward:

- How did you prepare yourself and the child for the bath?
- Was it a blanket bath for a child who was confined to bed, or was the child able to go to the bathroom on the ward?
- What went well about the experience?
- What might you do differently in the future?
- Read the policies and procedures for your hospital trust relating to meeting the hygiene needs of patients.

Hair care

Most children do not require their hair to be washed each day unless they have a scalp condition such as psoriasis. However, weekly or twice-weekly hair washes are an important part of meeting the hygiene needs of infants, children and young people.

The hair should be gently brushed each day, even if a hair wash is not required, and the condition of the scalp and the hair must be noted and documented.

Particular attention must be given to the presence of head lice, as early detection and prompt appropriate treatment are required for the child's comfort and to reduce the risk of the head lice being passed on to other children or adults (Firth 2006).

There are several different preparations that are available for the treatment of head lice, with current advice being the use of aqueous solutions rather than alcohol-based preparations to reduce the incidence of skin irritation and wheeze (Sladden & Johnston 2005). Other treatments, such as daily applications of hair conditioner and careful combing of each section of the hair with a fine-toothed head lice comb to remove the eggs and the lice, are favoured by some parents; however, this is time-consuming and needs to be done for several days to ensure complete removal of all eggs (known as 'nits'). Pharmacists are extremely useful sources of accurate and updated knowledge as to the best treatments for head lice.

A baby's hair can be washed while in the bath or before having a minimal wash or bath:

1. After cleansing the baby's face, keeping the baby wrapped in the towel, hold the baby securely with his or her body extending the length of your lower arm (left arm if you are right-handed), with your hand supporting the head and the legs tucked close to your body.
2. Hold the baby's head over the bowl of water and dampen the baby's hair using a small jug or by cupping water in your free hand (Fig. 11.3). Try not to wet the baby's face or eyes.
3. Apply a small amount (2–3 mL) of baby shampoo to the baby's head and gently massage the scalp. Avoid undue pressure on the fontanelles.
4. Rinse thoroughly and repeat.
5. Dry the head immediately to reduce heat loss.

In the bath, using a cupped hand dampen the scalp, apply shampoo, rinse thoroughly and repeat the wash. Dry the baby carefully when out of the bath.

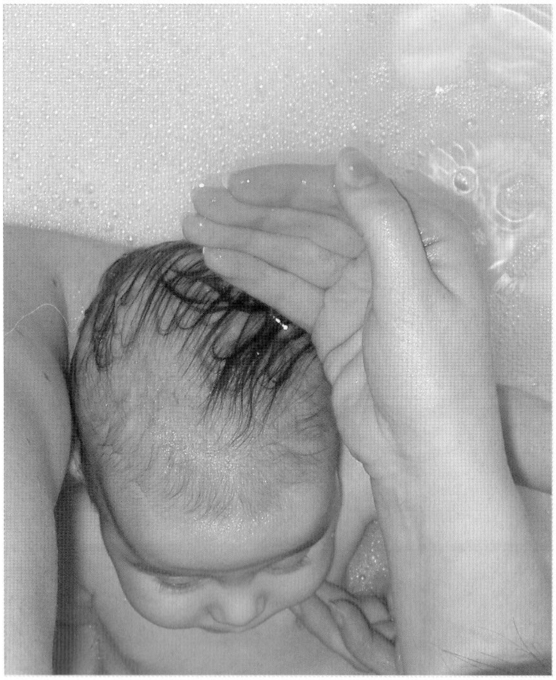

Fig. 11.3 • Washing a baby's hair.

When washing an older child's hair in bed, use the following steps:

1. Pull the head of the bed away from the wall and remove the back of the bed and the pillows. Have bowl of warm water, jug, shampoo, conditioner and towels ready.
2. Position the bowl of water on a low table at the head of the bed.
3. Position the child supine on the bed with his or her head extending beyond the head of the bed over the bowl, with the neck supported by towels and the head supported by the nurse.
4. Using the jug and water dampen the hair (Fig. 11.4).

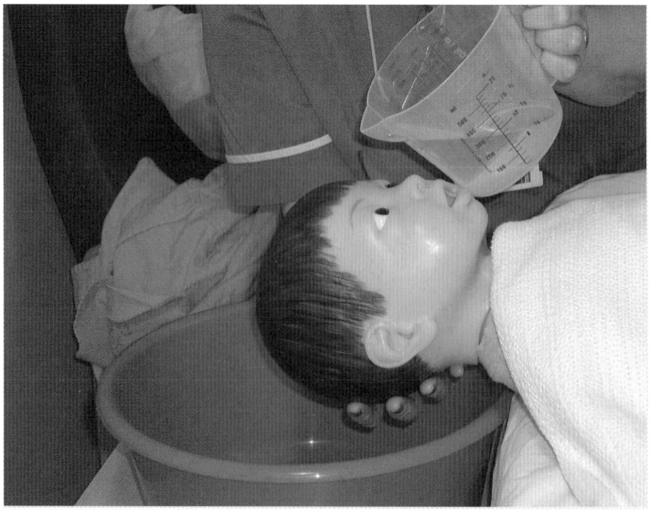

Fig. 11.4 • Washing an older child's hair in bed.

5. Shampoo the hair, rinse, repeat, apply conditioner and rinse thoroughly.
6. Wrap the head and hair in a towel.
7. Move the child down the bed into a more comfortable position.
8. Dry the hair thoroughly, brush and comb, and style.

Now test your knowledge

A 6-year-old girl is admitted to your ward for a routine surgical procedure. The recovery room nurse notifies the ward that the child has been noted to have an infestation of head lice:

- What would you do?
- Whom would you inform?
- How should the child be treated to deal with the head lice?
- What information and advice would you give to the child's parents?

Dental and oral hygiene

The oral cavity is lined by a layer of rapidly dividing mucosal cells; these are replaced every 7–14 days. Beneath the surface of the epithelium there are minor salivary and sebaceous glands, which are important for lubrication (Madeya 1996). Saliva contains several antibacterial factors that suppress bacterial and fungal colonisation; the mechanical action of mastication promotes the washing action of saliva and helps prevent the attachment of microorganisms to the surfaces (Somerville 1999). The condition of the mouth gives an indication of the general health and the quality of life of the individual (World Health Organization 2006). When the mouth is in poor condition it will interfere with the person's ability to communicate verbally and eat or drink and will be uncomfortable (Holman et al 2005). The implementation of oral hygiene helps ensure that the mouth remains healthy.

Dental hygiene should begin when the primary teeth erupt (Trigg & Mohammed 2006). Babies will need assistance to clean their teeth; in the early stages of tooth eruption a foam sponge can be used, and as more teeth erupt a baby toothbrush is more effective (British Dental Health Foundation 2007, Kite & Pearson 1995). Young children will need some encouragement and assistance to clean their teeth effectively; gradually they will become more independent in accomplishing this task. Teeth cleaning should be part of the child's daily hygiene routine. When assisting a child to clean her or his teeth it may be easier to stand or sit behind the child, cradling her or his chin in your hand so you can reach the top and bottom teeth more easily. Children should be supervised when cleaning their teeth until they are at least 7 years old (British Dental Health Foundation 2007).

The aims of oral hygiene are to:

- keep the mucosa and lips clean, soft, moist and intact
- remove food debris and dental plaque
- prevent infection

- maintain the development of healthy teeth and gums
- prevent halitosis
- maintain oral function and adequate oral intake
- alleviate pain and discomfort
- promote dignity, comfort and well-being (Xavier 2000).

Table 11.1 lists some potential oral disorders. Some of the factors contributing to poor oral health are:

- lack of knowledge or motivation to maintain oral hygiene
- impaired or altered physical dexterity
- children with special needs
- inability to take oral fluids (Thurgood 1994)
- poor nutritional status
- insufficient saliva production
- major interventions affecting oral status (e.g. surgery, radiotherapy, chemotherapy)
- immunodeficiency
- childhood illnesses and habits
- foreign body in nose
- oxygen therapy (unhumidified oxygen administered by mask can dry the mouth)
- xerostomia, which has the prime effect of severe and rapid dental decay (Gelbart 1998) and can often lead to oral fungal infection (Sweeney 1998).

Oral care

Before beginning oral care there should be an assessment of the oral cavity (Department of Health 2001, Turner 1996, White 2000). An appropriate assessment tool should be used to determine the care required (Eilers et al 1988, Royal Free Hampstead NHS Trust 2006). The frequency of oral hygiene is more important than the cleaning agents used (Table 11.2; Buglass 1995, Kite & Pearson 1995, Thurgood 1994, Turner 1996). There is no consensus regarding how frequently care should be given or the tools and agents that should be used (Buglass 1995). Tooth brushing is considered the most effective method of plaque control (Kite & Pearson 1995, Ransier et al 1995); the brush should have relatively soft bristles and a small head.

Table 11.1. Some potential oral disorders

Disorder	Description
Xerostomia	A dry mouth.
Stomatitis	Inflammation and infection of the oral mucosa.
Candidiasis (oral thrush)	Caused by a yeast-like fungus, *Candida albicans*, which normally inhabits the vagina and digestive system. It commonly manifests as soft white plaques on the mucosa and tongue.
Gingivitis	Inflammation of the gums, leading to swelling and bleeding. Caused by poor hygiene and the consequent build-up of plaque attacking the damaged tissue (Gelbart 1998). It is the first stage of periodontitis. The highly vascular nature of the mucosal tissue in the gums and subsequent tissue destruction can lead to the formation of a communication channel between the bacteria in the plaque and the bloodstream (Somerville 1999). Gingivitis can lead to tissue and bone destruction and then to tooth loss (Kite & Pearson 1995).
Ulceration	Aphthous ulcers are white, small, punched-out lesions of epithelial surfaces of the mouth, probably of viral origin.

(From Thurgood 1994, with permission.)

Table 11.2. Oral cleaning agents

Agent	Description
Water	Non-irritant, pleasant and moistening but ineffective at plaque removal on its own (Anaissie et al 2002).
Toothpaste	Loosens debris and plaque, has a pleasant taste and is refreshing. Fluoride content prevents dental caries. Dries mucosa if not rinsed adequately.
Hydrogen peroxide	Antiplaque effect but can be painful, uncomfortable and unpleasant. May burn mucosa (British National Formulary for Children 2007).
Sodium bicarbonate	Loosens mucus but has an unpleasant salty taste and may burn or irritate mucosa.
Lemon and glycerine	Stimulates saliva production but can cause reflex exhaustion of saliva process and is hypertonic and acidic. Lemon causes decalcification of tooth enamel.
Chlorhexidine solution	Effective against plaque and has local anaesthetic properties but has an unpleasant taste and discolours tooth enamel (Berry & Davidson 2006).

Foam swabs on sticks or large cotton buds can be used (Fig. 11.5), but these are often ineffective at removing plaque from teeth and gums (Pearson 1996). They can be useful at reaching the recesses of the gums and under the tongue, which can be difficult using a toothbrush. Extreme caution needs to be exercised when using swabs (Fig. 11.6) with young children or those with learning disabilities, as biting the end of the swab may cause the foam to break away from the stick and be swallowed or choke the child. Wrapping a gauze swab around forceps or a gloved finger is no longer recommended practice.

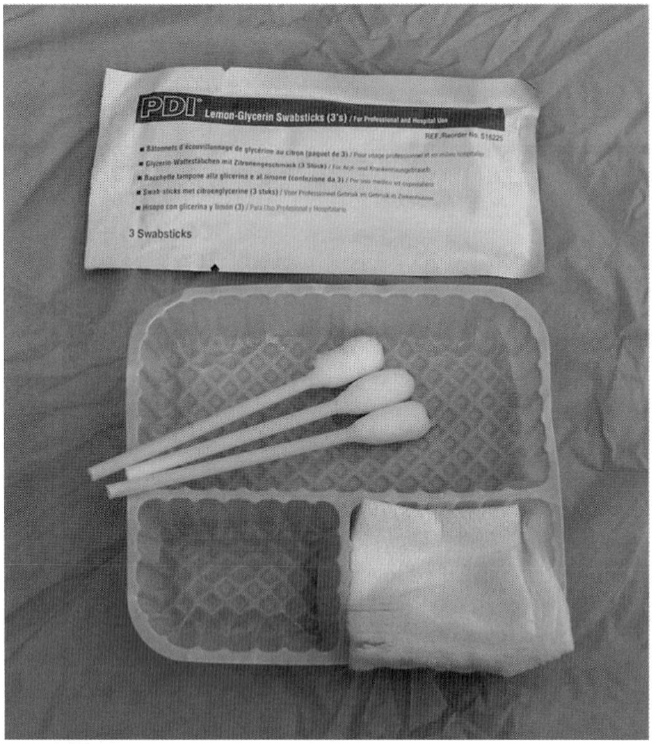

Fig. 11.5 • Cotton buds can be used for oral care.

Tests have proved that certain electric toothbrushes are better at removing plaque. Electric toothbrushes can also be better for children, who may be more inclined to brush regularly because of the novelty of using an electric toothbrush. Children's toothpastes have about half the level of fluoride that adult toothpastes have. They still provide extra protection for the teeth, but as children have a tendency to 'eat' their toothpaste there is less risk of them taking in too much fluoride (British Dental Health Foundation 2007).

This procedure is more difficult if the child is unconscious. Mouth care remains an essential element of patient hygiene. The main danger of the procedure is aspiration of fluids into the lungs. Therefore to avoid this children must be positioned on to their side. The head should be lower than the body, which can be achieved by removing the pillows and lowering the head of the bed. Once this is accomplished, gravity will enable the secretions to drain out of the mouth and avoid aspiration into the lungs. Oral suction should be available during the procedure to be used if necessary. Fluid may pool in the side of the mouth, from where it can be easily suctioned (Kozier et al 2004).

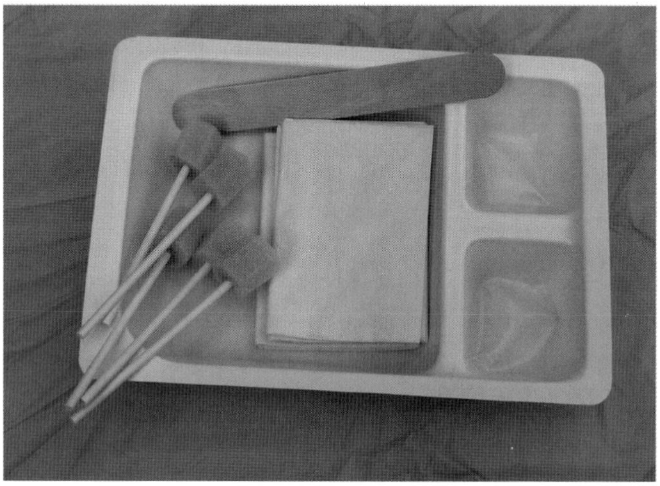

Fig. 11.6 • Foam sticks for use in oral care.

Procedures Box 11.5 Brushing a child's teeth

Equipment

- Torch
- Toothbrush and paste
- Tongue depressor
- Soft paraffin
- Kidney dish, if required
- Suction equipment, if appropriate
- Clean procedure gloves
- Tissues or wipes
- Mouth care pack
- Mouthwashes and medication, if prescribed

Action
Explain and discuss the procedure with the child and family.
Reason *Gains their assent and cooperation.*

Action
Wash your hands thoroughly with soap and water and dry.
Reason *Prevents cross-infection.*

Actions
Prepare equipment.

Solutions, if required, should be prepared immediately before use.

Equipment should be clean and dry.
Reason *Minimises bacterial contamination.*

Action
Inspect the child's mouth, using a torch and spatula if appropriate.
Reason *To assess and monitor the condition of the mouth.*

Procedures Box 11.5 Brushing a child's teeth—cont'd

Actions
Using toothbrush and toothpaste, brush the teeth and gums.

If more comfortable for the child, use foam sticks and appropriate solution.

Reasons *Removes debris and plaque from the teeth, which could provide a growth medium for pathogenic organisms. Stimulates gingival tissue to maintain tone and prevents circulatory stasis (Kite & Pearson 1995, Ransier et al 1995, Thurgood 1994).*

Actions
Tilt the bristle tips to a 45° angle against the gum line.

Move the brush in small circular movements, several times, on all the surfaces of every tooth.

Brush with firm strokes away from the gum margins.

Work methodically around the mouth.

Reason *Ensures that plaque and debris are removed and not forced into gum margins.*

Actions
Encourage the child to spit into a disposable bowl, rinse the mouth with clean water and spit it out again; repeat as necessary.

Provide tissues to dry lips and face as necessary.

Reasons *Removes loosened debris from the mouth. Rinsing reduces the drying effect of fluoride residue from toothpaste on the lips (Hampton & Collins 2003).*

Action
Apply soft yellow paraffin or lip balm to the lips.

Reason *It acts as an occlusive barrier that retains moisture and prevents drying and cracking of the lips (Gibson & Stone 2004, Turner 1996).*

Action
Clean and dry all equipment and return it to the child's bedside cupboard.

Reason *Removes organisms from the equipment and avoids cross-infection.*

Action
Wash and dry your hands.

Reason *Avoids cross-infection.*

Now test your knowledge

Question 1
How often should you clean a child's teeth?

Question 2
How often should you change your toothbrush?

Question 3
Name three indications of a healthy mouth.

Question 4
Name three predisposing factors contributing to an unhealthy mouth.

Question 5
What is the importance of regular flossing?

Question 6
What would you use to moisten dry lips?

References

Anaissie E, Prenzak SR, Dignani M (2002) The hospital water supply as a source of nosocomial infections: a plea for action. Archives of Internal Medicine 162(13):1483–1492

Berry AM, Davidson PM (2006) Beyond comfort: oral hygiene as a critical nursing activity in the intensive care unit. Intensive and Critical Care Nursing 22:318–328

Boxwell G (2001) Neonatal intensive care nursing. Routledge, London

British Dental Health Foundation (2007) Online. Available: http://www.dentalhealth.org.uk

British National Formulary for Children (2007) British National Formulary for Children. BMJ Publishing, London

Buglass EA (1995) Oral hygiene. British Journal of Nursing 4(9):516–519

Campbell S, Glasper EA (eds.) (1995) Whaley and Wong's children's nursing. Mosby, London

Chamley CA, Carson P, Randall D, Sandwell M (2005) Developmental anatomy and physiology of children: a practical approach. Churchill Livingstone, Edinburgh

Cowan ME, Frost MR (2006) A comparison between a detergent baby bath additive and baby soap on the skin flora of neonates. Journal of Hospital Infection 7:91–95

Department of Health (2001) Essence of care. Department of Health, London

Department of Health (2003) Winning ways: working together to reduce healthcare associated infection in England. Department of Health, London

Department of Health (2006) Birth to five. Department of Health, London

Duncan A (2004) Personal hygiene: skin care. In Dougherty L, Lister S (eds) Royal Marsden manual of clinical nursing procedures, 6th edn. Blackwell, Oxford, p 580–586

Eilers J, Berger AM, Petersen MC (1988) Development, testing, and application of the oral assessment guide. Oncology Nursing Forum 15(3):325–330

Firth M (2006) Head lice. Cited in Glasper E, McEwing G, Richardson J (eds) Oxford handbook of children's and young people's nursing. Oxford University Press, Oxford

Furdon SA, Clark DA (2002) Assessment of the umbilical cord outside the delivery room. Advances in Neonatal Care 2(4):187–197

Gelbart M (1998) All mouth. Nursing Times 94(46):26–28

Gfatter R, Hackl P, Braun F (1997) Effects of soap and detergents on skin surface pH, stratum corneum hydration and fat content in infants. Dermatology 195(3):258–262

Gibson F, Stone J (2004) Mouthcare clinical procedure guideline. Great Ormond Street Hospital for Children NHS Trust, London

Hampton S, Collins F (2003) Tissue viability: a comprehensive guide. Whurr Publishing, London

Harrison M (2006) Caring for children: the role of the immune system in protecting against disease. In Glasper A, Richardson J (eds) A textbook of children's and young people's nursing. Elsevier, Edinburgh

Holman C, Roberts S, Nicol M (2005) Promoting oral health. Nursing Older People 16(10):37–38

Jamieson EM, McCall JM, Whyte LA (2002) Clinical nursing practice, 4th edn. Churchill Livingstone, Edinburgh

Kite K, Pearson L (1995) A rationale for mouth care: the integration of theory with practice. Intensive and Critical Care Nursing 11:71–76

Kozier B, Erb G, Berman A, Snyder S (2004) Fundamentals of nursing: concepts, processes and practice, 7th edn. Pearson Prentice Hill, Upper Saddle River

Lee LK, Thompson KM (2007) Parental survey of beliefs and practices about bathing and water safety and their children: guidance for drowning prevention. Accident Analysis and Prevention 39:58–62

Leone TA, Finer NN (2006) Fetal adaptation at birth. Current Paediatrics 16:269–274

McConnell TP, Lee CW, Couillard M, Sherrill WW (2004) Trends in umbilical cord care: scientific evidence for practice. Newborn and Infant Nursing Reviews 4(4):211–222

Madder SS (2000) Human biology, 6th edn. McGraw-Hill, Boston

Madeya M (1996) Oral complications from cancer therapy: part 1 – pathophysiology and secondary complications. Oncology Nursing Forum 23(5):801–807

Major C (2005) Meeting hygiene needs. In Baille L (ed.) Developing practical nursing skills, 2nd edn. Hodder Arnold, London

Moules T, Ramsay J (1998) The textbook of children's nursing. Stanley Thornes, Cheltenham

Nursing and Midwifery Council (2004) Code of professional conduct. NMC, London

Nursing and Midwifery Council (2005) Guidelines for records and record keeping. NMC, London

Oishi T, Iwata S, Nonoyama M, Tsuji A, Sunakawa K (2004) Double-blind comparative study on the care of the neonatal umbilical cord using 80% ethanol with or without chlorhexidine. Journal of Hospital Infection 58:34–37

O'Regan H, Fawcett T (2006) Learning to nurse: reflections on bathing a patient. Nursing Standard 20(46):60–64

Pearson LS (1996) A comparison of the ability of foam swabs and toothbrushes to remove dental plaque: implications for nursing practice. Journal of Advanced Nursing 213:62–69

Ransier A, Epstein JB, Lunn R, Spinelli J (1995) A combined analysis of a toothbrush, foam brush, and a chlorhexidine-soaked foam brush in maintaining oral hygiene. Cancer Nursing 18(5):393–396

Royal Free Hampstead NHS Trust (2006) Online. Available: http://www.bahnon.org.uk/Professional%20Guidelines/OralCare.doc

Rudolf M, Levene M (2006) Pediatrics and child health. Blackwell Publishing, Oxford

Sladden MJ, Johnston GA (2005) More common skin infections in children. British Medical Journal 330:1194–1198

Smith J (2005) The guide to the manual handling of people, 5th edn. Backcare, Middlesex

Somerville R (1999) Oral care in intensive care setting: a case study. Nursing in Critical Care 4(1):7–13

Sweeney P (1998) Mouth care in nursing – part 1. Common oral conditions. Journal of Nursing Care spring:4–7

Thurgood G (1994) Nurse maintenance of oral hygiene. British Journal of Nursing 3(7):332–353

Tortora GJ (2005) Principles of human anatomy, 10th edn. Wiley, Danvers

Trigg E, Mohammed T (2006) Practices in children's nursing guidelines for hospital and community. Elsevier, London

Turner G (1996) Oral care. Nursing Standard 10(28):51–56

Waugh A, Grant A (2006) Ross and Wilson anatomy and physiology in health and illness, 10th edn. Churchill Livingstone, Edinburgh

White R (2000) Nurse assessment of oral health: a review of practice and education. British Journal of Nursing 9(5):260–266

World Health Organization (1998) Care of the umbilical cord: a review of the evidence. Online. Available: http://www.who.int/rht/documents/MSM98-4/MSM-98-4.htm

World Health Organization (2006) Oral health in aging societies: integration of oral health and general health. WHO, Geneva

Xavier G (2000) The importance of mouth care in preventing infection. Nursing Standard 14(18):47–51

Young AE (2004) The management of severe burns in children. Current Paediatrics 14:202–207

Zupan J, Garner P, Omari AAA (2004) Topical umbilical cord care at birth. Cochrane Database of Systematic Reviews, issue 3, article no. CD001057. DOI: 10.1002/14651858. CD001057.pub2

12 Pressure ulcer care in children

Rosemary Smith • Donald Todd

Pressure ulcers are painful. They can cause disfigurement including alopecia, increase the risk of infection and ultimately may be life-threatening (Samaniego 2004). Ninety-five per cent of all pressure ulcers are thought to be preventable (Thomas & James 2002); it is therefore vitally important in the interests of the child and his or her family, as well as good nursing practice, to be able to recognise pressure ulcer risks quickly and thereby prevent their subsequent development (Willock & Maylor 2004).

Previously, pressure ulcers have been known as decubitus ulcers or pressure sores. They are defined as 'an area of localised damage to the skin and underlying tissue caused by pressure or shear or a combination of these' (Baldwin 2002).

It is important to bear in mind that other forms of skin lesion can appear similar to pressure ulcers, but their cause, outcome and treatment may well be different (Defloor et al 2005). For example, incontinence of urine or faeces can cause excoriation and skin breakdown around the perineal area. This is especially true for babies and children still in nappies or for children with continence problems. Bed rest combined with poor toileting routines can also compound this problem. The use of adhesive tapes and dressings to hold cannulae in place, secure nasogastric tubes to the face, secure urinary catheters to the leg, or secure wound dressings, and so on, may well be common practice. However, their subsequent removal can cause shearing on the skin and consequently lead to skin breakdown and breaches to skin integrity. This is especially problematic on fragile skin such as that of neonates, babies and infants, or of children with skin conditions such as eczema. It is therefore important to differentiate between a pressure ulcer and other forms of skin lesion.

Pressure ulcers differ from other skin lesions in that they result from shear and/or pressure forces. They tend to be over bony prominences (although they can develop over any dependent skin surface), be of circular or regular shape and occur in one spot only with defined edges. They range from non-blanching erythema to full-thickness tissue damage and necrosis (Gunningberg 2005). Other skin lesions, however, depending on the causative factor, are rarely necrotic and tend to be superficial without the involvement of a bony prominence. They are usually dispersed, with no regular shape or defined edge. The healthy surrounding skin may also become macerated, especially if there is excessive moisture present (Nursing and Midwifery Practice Development Unit 2002).

There are four classes of pressure ulcer (Willock et al 2005):

- A *stage 1* ulcer is described as a non-blanching erythema of intact skin.
- A *stage 2* ulcer is described as blistered skin that is partial thickness involving the epidermis and/or dermis.
- A *stage 3* ulcer is a superficial ulcer described as tissue damage involving full-thickness skin loss with damage and/or necrosis of subcutaneous tissue; it extends down to fascia but not through.
- A *stage 4* ulcer involves extensive destruction, necrosis and possible damage to muscle, bone and supporting structures, with or without full-thickness skin loss (Curley et al 2003).

Incidence

There is a general consensus that there is little robust evidence regarding the prevalence and incidence of pressure ulcers in children (Silverwood 2004). This is partly due to the lack of research, often impeded by ethical constraints, into the topic, combined with the lack of a paediatric risk assessment tool. However, the 2003 National Pediatric Pressure Ulcer Survey in the USA showed a 4% prevalence rate (Curley et al 2003), while two surveys conducted in Great Britain using multiple in-patient units showed a 2.2% prevalence and a 5.6% incidence (Waterlow 1997, Willock & Maylor 2004). Incidence is significantly lower in children than in adults (Baldwin 2002). A lower incidence rate in children may be attributed to a number of factors (Defloor et al 2005). Unless there is an underlying medical condition children's skin is better perfused than that of adults. Children's skin also has good amounts of collagen and elastin and is still growing and therefore should be healthier than adult skin. The child's skin should therefore be stronger and able to withstand greater pressure and shearing forces. However, this does not mean that children are not susceptible to pressure ulcers, with those who are at greatest risk being the critically ill (Willock & Maylor 2004). It also cannot be assumed that the risk of formation of ulcers in children is the same as that in adults (Murdoch 2002).

Areas of pressure ulcer risk

As already discussed, children's skin is different from that of adults. So too are many aspects of the rest of the child's anatomy. As previously mentioned, pressure ulcers often develop over bony prominences. In comparison with adults, neonates and infants have larger heads relative to the rest of their body, therefore the most common site for pressure area development in children is the occiput (Fig. 12.1). This is followed by the sacrum then the scapula, while the most common area for an adult is the sacrum. Other areas of the body susceptible to pressure ulcers are the heels, knees, elbows, buttocks, nose and ears, and if nursed prone then the sternum, iliac crests, auricle of the ear, upper lip and corner of the mouth become more susceptible (Fig. 12.2; Willock & Maylor 2004).

Patients at risk from pressure ulcers

Children with additional underlying conditions are increasingly susceptible to pressure ulcer formation. For example:

- Children with neurological conditions may have areas of sensory impairment and/or have limited motor function, resulting in them not being able to move off pressure areas or feel the pressure or friction building up over pressure areas.
- Children with musculoskeletal conditions, with abnormal anatomy or who are obese may have limited mobility as a result, again reducing their ability to move off pressure areas or, because of their abnormal anatomy, pressure areas may have increased friction, shearing or pressure.
- Children who are malnourished or who have medical problems such as diabetes, cardiac conditions or respiratory conditions that require medications that could cause altered tissue perfusion will be more susceptible to pressure ulcers.
- Children in pain with inadequate analgesia will be unwilling to move or change position, thus increasing their risk for pressure ulcer formation.

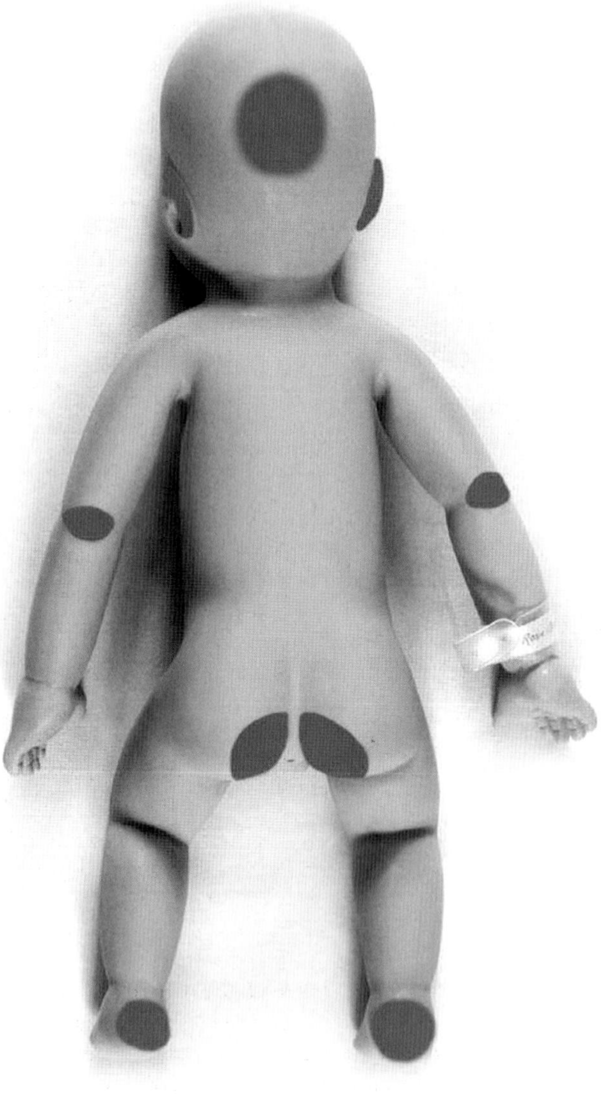

Fig. 12.1 • Areas of pressure ulcer risk in the neonate and infant.

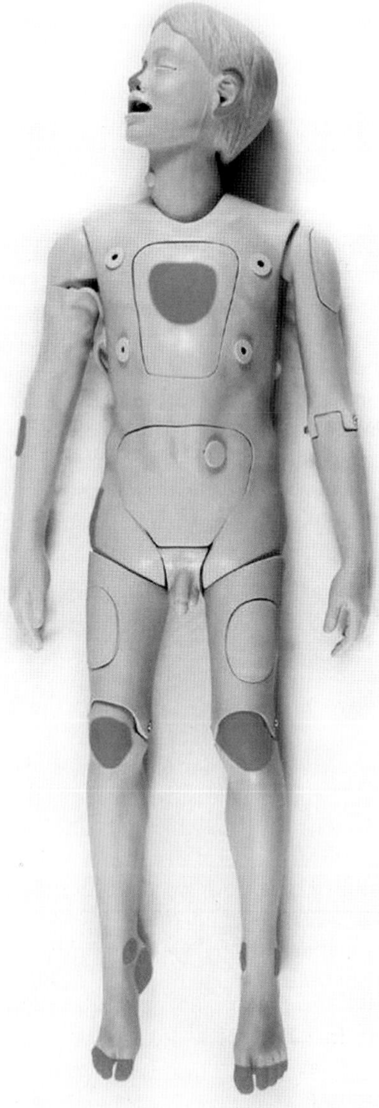

Fig. 12.2 • Areas of pressure ulcer risk in the older child.

- Very young children and neonates have fragile immature skin, which as a result will have increased susceptibility to friction and pressure.
- Incontinence can increase the likelihood of pressure ulcer problems, as the skin becomes wet and macerated and subsequently has reduced integrity.
- The acutely critically ill child is also susceptible for a variety of reasons, such as immobility, poor tissue perfusion, poor dietary intake, medication, pain, incontinence and the use of monitoring and medical equipment. For this reason more pressure ulceration is observed in the multidisciplinary paediatric intensive care unit and neonatal unit (Willock & Maylor 2004).

There is some suggestion that all children should be considered at risk (Murdoch 2002). Home-acquired pressure ulcers should also not be ignored (Samaniego 2004), particularly as there is greater emphasis on community care these days, with children being cared for on a lifelong basis at home wearing splints or braces or in wheelchairs.

Causes of pressure ulcers

Nursing and medical interventions carried out to care for these children can themselves cause pressure ulceration. Equipment commonly used to care for children can increase pressure or friction over the skin, particularly over the areas already mentioned that are susceptible to ulceration (Willock & Maylor 2004). Pressure ulcers have been found to be caused by catheters, electrocardiogram leads, oxygen saturation probes, nasogastric tubes, endotracheal tubes (Zollo et al 1996), orthopaedic casts and splints (Muller & Nordwall 1994, Okamoto et al 1983), wheelchairs, earrings (Phelan 1980) and presumably other cosmetic jewellery that is becoming popular these days. Up to 50% of pressure ulcers are caused by equipment (Willock & Maylor 2004).

Prevention

In 2000 the Royal College of Nursing recommended that 'one of the first activities in preventing pressure ulcers is the early identification of individuals who are susceptible to developing them'. This should preferably be done within the first 6 h of admission, or if the admission is an acute emergency then it should be done immediately on admission. Pressure ulcer and skin integrity assessment should then be carried out at regular intervals, the frequency of which will depend on the care setting or when the patient's care or condition changes. Skin and pressure ulcer assessment should be done by a practitioner suitably trained and competent in doing so. The Department of Health 1993 suggested that this need not be a trained member of staff; however, accountability for skin assessment and pressure ulcer prevention would still be with the registered practitioner.

Adjuncts to assist with relieving pressure can also be used, particularly for patients known to be at risk, the choice of adjunct used being dependent on the pressure ulcer assessment and scoring. Equipment choice can be as simple as using soft linen or using cushions, towels, padding or gel pads over areas at risk from ulceration, or in more difficult cases pressure-relieving mattresses can be used, of which there are a number of types available (Willock & Maylor 2004).

To date there is no reliable evaluation or research evidence on the clinical and cost effectiveness of most of the pressure-relieving equipment that is available (Thomas & James 2002). The choice of pressure-relieving adjunct will also be determined by local hospital policy. The use of pressure-relieving adjuncts, however, is only effective if they are implemented and used as soon as the patient is identified as being at risk (Thomas & James 2002).

Please note that the use of water-filled gloves as an adjunct is not advised, as the fluid pressure in the gloves is no less than the ordinary mattress and will therefore not be adequate enough to alleviate pressure (Silverwood 2004).

Assessment

Given the complexity of pressure ulcers in children there is as yet no consensus on an assessment tool; the tools available at present are adaptations of adult tools. However, an assessment tool alone is not sufficient. Assessment tools must be used in conjunction with vigilance (Willock et al 2005) and early recognition of pressure ulcer signs through regular skin checks and, when appropriate, the use of pressure-relieving adjuncts (Nursing and Midwifery Practice Development Unit 2002).

Pressure risk assessment should take place within 6 h of admission to the healthcare setting and additionally if the condition deteriorates (National Institute for Clinical Excellence 2003, Nursing and Midwifery Practice Development Unit 2002). Risk assessment should involve both formal and informal procedures, and any tools used must not replace clinical judgement (National Institute for Clinical Excellence 2003).

There are several non-validated tools, such as Pattold (Olding & Paterson 1998), Bedi (Bedi 1993), Pickersgill (Pickersgill 1997), Waterlow (Waterlow 1997) and Barnes (Barnes 2004) available, based primarily on experience with critically ill children. The Waterlow paediatric tool assesses and advises on nursing actions (Willock et al 2004), while the Starkid Skin Scale (Suddaby et al 2005) and the Neonatal Skin Risk Assessment Scale (Huffines & Lodgson 1997) have limited evidence of validity within paediatric settings. The Braden Q Scale, however, is an adaptation of the adult Braden Scale (Quigley & Curley 1996), which has since been validated for identifying those in paediatric intensive care units at risk of stage 2 ulceration (Curley et al 2003). Criticism has been levelled over its applicability to all children in any setting, because it does not take into account developmental differences in children, the presence of enteral feeding, or any non-invasive technological support that may be in use while caring for a critically ill child in a paediatric intensive care unit.

The Braden Q tool is a summated scale with seven subscales (mobility, activity, sensory perception, moisture, friction and shearing, nutrition and tissue perfusion). Each subscale is ranked on a four-point system, with four being the maximum. The scoring range is 7–28; the lower the score, the greater the risk of stage 2 ulcers, a score of 16 being the predictability value (Curley et al 2003). This scale has since been modified, because in a predictability study it was recognised that there were difficulties in scoring all categories on admission (Curley et al 2003). The Modified Braden Q Scale uses only three subgroups (mobility, sensory perception and tissue perfusion), the predictability score this time being 7. However, it should be reiterated that neither tool has been validated for all settings, nor are they applicable for children who have any underlying conditions, for example normally poor tissue perfusion (Curley et al 2003).

Two other scales with limited validity, both derived from the Braden Q Scale, are the Starkid Skin Scale, which assesses the hospitalised child requiring intensive prevention measures (Suddaby et al 2005), and the Neonatal Skin Risk Assessment Scale used for neonates. In one study it had a reported sensitivity of 83% and a specificity of 81%. The tool scores the general physical condition, activity and nutrition of the neonate. Unlike the other tools it is a high score instead of a low score that predicts a high-risk profile (Huffines & Lodgson 1997).

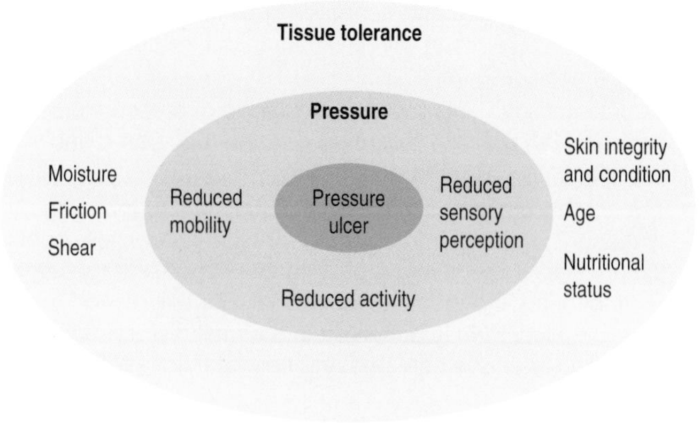

Fig. 12.3 • A framework for evaluating pressure ulcer risk.

While there is a lack of a robust valid formal assessment tool, most tools have a similar basis but consideration has to be given to their use alongside clinical judgement. A conceptual framework that encompasses the commonalities within the various tools and not only considers factors such as reduced activity, sensory perception and mobility but also includes the extrinsic and intrinsic factors that affect tissue tolerance could be a useful adjunct for consideration when evaluating pressure ulcer risk (Bergstrom et al 1987). Figure 12.3 shows an example of such a framework.

Procedures Box 12.1 Pressure ulcer care in children

Action
Using the locally agreed policy tool, assess the child's skin integrity as soon as possible after admission at a convenient time, such as when bathing or changing a nappy.

Reason *To assess the skin condition as soon after admission as possible:*

- *a pressure ulcer risk score is obtained as soon as possible*
- *the procedure is completed at a time that is least distressing to the child*
- *direct decision making regarding the need for pressure-relieving devices is possible.*

Action
Record the assessment of the skin in the notes.

Reason *Provides documented evidence of the condition of the child's skin at time of admission.*

Action
If skin breakdown is detected ensure that local wound policy is implemented and adapt the child's care plan to reflect this as necessary.

Reason *Provides documented evidence for the condition and care of any wounds.*

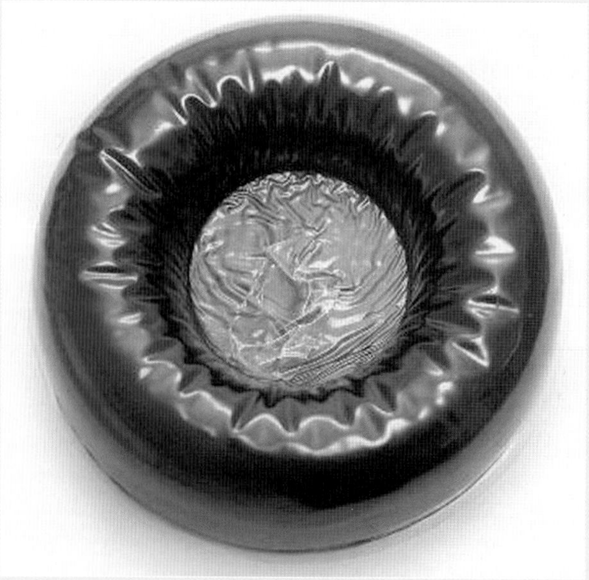

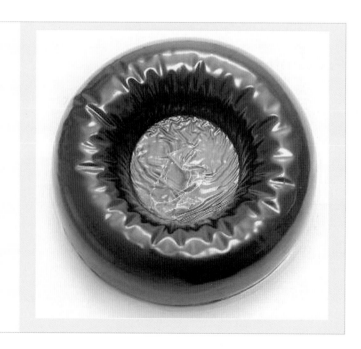

Procedures Box 12.1 Pressure ulcer care in children—cont'd

Action
Using locally agreed policy provide pressure-relieving adjuncts such as mattresses, if necessary, and document this in the notes.

Reasons *Provision of pressure-relieving equipment will assist in prevention of pressure ulcer formation.*
Documentation in the notes provides evidence and informs other staff if equipment is used and what is used.

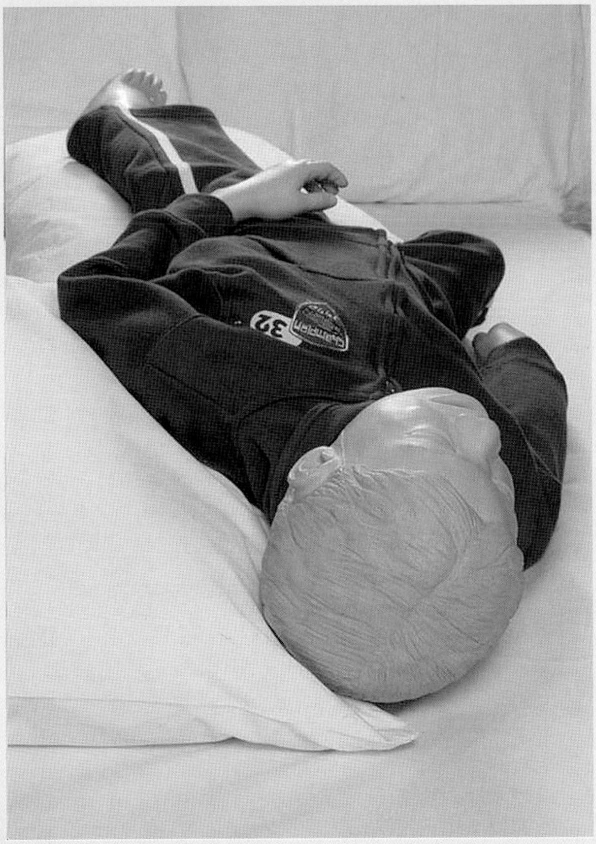

Actions
Regularly change the child's position as care and condition dictate:

- using appropriate moving and handling equipment if required
- by encouraging the child to move position and limbs as able.

Record this in the notes.

Reasons *Prevents constant pressure on one area.*
Prevents formation of pressure ulcers.
Using appropriate equipment allows for the safe moving of the child.
If children are able to move, this allows them to alleviate their own pressure areas.
Documentation in the notes provides evidence that the child's position is changed regularly and when this action has taken place.

Action
Provide care that reduces constant pressure by:

- ensuring that the child is pain-free
- educating the child and parents and family about pressure ulcer prevention.

Reasons *If children are in pain they will not move for fear of hurting themselves.*
Keeps the child and family informed of risks and the procedures that are performed, allowing them to assist in prevention techniques.

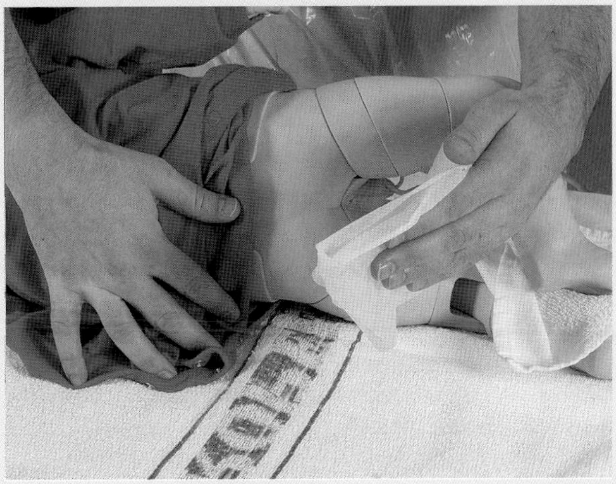

Action
Maintain skin integrity by:

- using soft linen and ensuring that sheets are smooth and dry
- changing an incontinent child as soon as he or she is soiled and ensuing that the child is clean and dry
- ensuring that skin is thoroughly dried after bathing or soiling
- using non-scented wipes for cleaning after incontinence (otherwise use mild soap and water and ensure that the skin is thoroughly dry)
- ensuring optimum fluid and dietary intake and involving a dietician as appropriate.

Reasons *Hard linen can rub on the skin.*
Wrinkled linen will leave marks on the skin, increasing the risk of pressure ulcer formation.
Wet linen will cause excoriation of skin and increase the likelihood of pressure ulcer formation.
Soiled linen and nappies will cause excoriation of skin and increase the risk of pressure ulcer formation.
Wet skin causes excoriation and can lead to pressure ulcer formation.
Scented wipes and soap may sting any broken skin.
Good hydration and nourishment ensure that skin is healthy and will aid in the prevention of pressure ulcers, but they will equally aid in wound healing should there be skin breakdown.

Action
Other considerations include:

- checking all wires, tubes and medical equipment whenever washing or repositioning the child for signs of skin deterioration
- ensuring that these areas are dry and clean
- documenting any changes in skin integrity, repositioning equipment and tubes as required and able
- considering removing any jewellery that the child may be wearing, ensuring that the child's and parent's consent are obtained.

Procedures Box 12.1 Pressure ulcer care in children—cont'd

Reasons *Wires, tubes and medical equipment in contact with the skin can cause pressure areas (more so if wet), leading to formation of ulcers.*
Documenting provides evidence that care has been performed and when.
Jewellery may pose a risk for pressure ulcer development.

Action
Reassess skin integrity and patient risk as the child's care or condition changes or as required, and document in the notes any changes to skin condition, implementing pressure-relieving techniques and/or wound care as appropriate.

Reasons *Allows skin condition to be monitored regularly.*
Documentation of changes to skin integrity provides evidence that skin is checked.
Implementing pressure-relieving techniques provides evidence that action is taken.
Implementing wound care provides evidence that action is taken.

Now test your knowledge

- Take a look at two or three paediatric assessment tools that are available in your work area. Apply each one to an age range of children and also apply all of them to one patient. Consider what the advantages and disadvantages for each tool are, which one works best for your area, and whether one tool can be applied to all age groups and all clinical settings.
- A 10-year-old child with cerebral palsy is admitted to hospital for surgery. He weighs 32 kg. He has limited movement and is mobile in an adapted wheelchair. What would you need to take into consideration when assessing the child for pressure ulcer prevention before and after surgery?

References

Baldwin KM (2002) Incidence and prevalence of pressure ulcers in children. Journal of Advances in Skin and Wound Care 15(3):121–124

Barnes S (2004) The use of a pressure ulcer risk assessment tool for children. Nursing Times 100(14):56–58

Bedi A (1993) A tool to fill the gap. Professional Nurse 9(2):112–120

Bergstrom N, Braden B, Holman V et al (1987) The Braden scale for predicting pressure sore risk. Nursing Research 36(4):206–210

Curley MAQ, Razmus IS, Roberts KE et al (2003) Predicting pressure ulcer risk in pediatric patients. Nursing Research 52(1):32–33

Defloor T, Bale S, Bellingeri A (2005) Statement of the European pressure ulcer panel – pressure ulcer classification. Journal of Wound, Ostomy and Continence Nursing 32(5):302–306

Department of Health (1993) Pressure sores: a key quality indicator. HMSO, London

Gunningberg L (2005) Are patients with or at risk of pressure ulcers allocated appropriate prevention measures? International Journal of Nursing Practice 11:58–67

Huffines B, Lodgson MC (1997) The neonatal skin risk assessment scale for predicting skin breakdown in neonates. Issues in Comprehensive Pediatric Nursing 20:103–114

Muller E, Nordwall A (1994) Brace treatment of scoliosis in children with myelomeningocele. Spine 19(2):151–155

Murdoch V (2002) Pressure care in the paediatric intensive care unit. Nursing Standard 17(6):71–76

National Institute for Clinical Excellence (2003) Pressure ulcer prevention. Clinical guideline 7. Online. Available: http://www.nice.org.uk/pdf/CG7_PRD_NICEguideline.pdf

Nursing and Midwifery Practice Development Unit (2002) Pressure ulcer prevention: best practice statement. NMPDU, Edinburgh

Okamoto G, Lamers JV, Shurtleff DB (1983) Skin breakdown in patients with myelomeningocele. Archives of Physical and Medical Rehabilitation 64(1):20–23

Olding L, Patterson J (1998) Growing concern. Nursing Times 94(38):74–79

Phelan W (1980) Complications of earrings in an infant. Journal of the American Medical Association 243(22):2288

Pickersgill J (1997) Taking the pressure off. Paedaitric Nursing 9(8):25–27

Quigley SM, Curley MA (1996) Skin integrity in the pediatric population: preventing and managing pressure ulcers. Journal of the Society of Pediatric Nurses 1(1):17–18

Royal College of Nursing (2000) Clinical practice guidelines: improving practice, improving care. Pressure ulcer risk assessment and prevention. RCN, London

Samaniego I (2004) A sore spot in pediatrics: risk factors for pressure ulcers. Dermatology Nursing 16(2):153–154,157–159

Silverwood B (2004) Prevention of sore heels: evidence and outcomes. Paediatric Nursing 16(4):14–18

Suddaby EC, Barnett S, Facteau L (2005) Skin breakdowns in acute care paediatrics. Pediatric Nursing 31(2):132–138

Thomas J, James J (2002) Pressure area management: a static-led approach. British Journal of Nursing 11(14):967–968,970,972

Waterlow J (1997) Pressure sore risk assessment in children. Paediatric Nursing 9(6):21–24

Willock J, Maylor M (2004) Pressure ulcers in infants and children. Nursing Standard 18(24):56–58,60,62

Willock J, Harris C, Harrison J et al (2005) Identifying the characteristics of children with pressure ulcers. Nursing Times 101(11):40–43

Zollo M, Gotisha ML, Berens RJ, Schmidt JE, Weigle CG (1996) Altered skin integrity in children admitted to a paediatric. Journal of Nursing Care Quality 11(2):62–67

Further reading

National Health Service Quality Improvement Scotland (2005) Pressure ulcer prevention: best practice statement. Online. Available: http://www.nhshealthquality.org

National Health Service Quality Improvement Scotland (2005) The treatment/management of pressure ulcers. Best practice statement. Online. Available: http://www.nhshealthquality.org

National Institute for Health and Clinical Excellence (2005) The prevention and treatment of pressure ulcers. Clinical guideline 29. Online. Available: http://www.nice.org.uk/page.aspx?o=CG029quickrefguide

Royal College of Nursing (2003) Pressure ulcer risk assessment and prevention: implementation guide and audit protocol. Clinical practice guidelines. RCN, London

Royal College of Nursing (2005) The management of pressure ulcers in primary and secondary care. Clinical practice guidelines. RCN, London

Waterlow J (2005) Pressure ulcer prevention manual. JA Waterlow, Taunton

13 Breastfeeding

Jacqueline Baker

The World Health Organization (2003: 7) states that: 'Exclusive breastfeeding in the early months of life is strongly correlated with increased infant survival and lowered risk of illness, particularly from diarrhoeal disease'.

Breastfeeding also protects against gastroenteritis, urinary tract infections, ear infections, chest infections, heart disease, obesity and diabetes. Babies who are breast fed have increased development of teeth and jaw and improved cognitive development. The benefits for the mother include protection against premenopausal breast cancer, ovarian cancer and osteoporosis (Arulkumaran et al 2004). The Department of Health (2004) and the World Health Organization (2003) recommend that women are supported to breastfeed and offer the following advice:

- Breast milk is the best form of nutrition for infants.
- Exclusive breastfeeding is recommended for the first 6 months of an infant's life, as it provides all the nutrients a baby needs.
- Breastfeeding should continue beyond the first 6 months along with appropriate types and amounts of solid foods (National Health Service 2007).

As professionals we have a duty to provide our patients and clients with the best possible advice. Certainly where breastfeeding is concerned this advice needs to be consistent and evidence based (Findlay et al 2006). We must ensure that we are aware of the latest evidence on the anatomy of the breast (Medela 2006) so that we can be sure that the mother has the best possible chance of exclusively breastfeeding her baby. Education starts before delivery; it is essential to give good breastfeeding advice antenatally, as this is the optimum time to give this information (Netdoctor 2007).

UNICEF and the World Health Organization in 1991 launched the Baby-Friendly Hospital Initiative to ensure that all maternity units become centres of breastfeeding support. This is a global initiative, and in many areas where hospitals have been designated baby-friendly more mothers are breastfeeding their infants and child health has improved (National Health Service 2007).

To become baby-friendly a hospital needs to fulfil the 10 following requirements:

1. Provide a written breastfeeding policy that is communicated to all healthcare staff
2. Provide training for all healthcare staff in the skills necessary to implement the policy
3. Inform all pregnant women about the benefits and management of breastfeeding
4. Help mothers initiate breastfeeding within one half-hour of birth
5. Demonstrate to mothers how to breastfeed and maintain lactation; this should be provided even if they are temporarily separated from their infants
6. Newborn infants should be given only breast milk unless medically indicated otherwise
7. Provide facilities to allow mothers and infants to remain together 24 h a day
8. Encourage breastfeeding on demand
9. Give no artificial teats or pacifiers to breastfeeding infants
10. Encourage the participation of breastfeeding support groups and refer mothers to them on discharge from the hospital or clinic.

In hospital

The majority of babies continue to be born in hospital. Therefore it is not only important to give evidence-based information to the mother but also to get hospital personnel motivated and supportive (Findlay et al 2006). Relevant, up-to-date, evidence-based training should be provided by qualified trainers. For all members of staff, breastfeeding training should be mandatory and supported by management in terms of both time and resources. It is vital that all professionals should be giving the same information. One of the commonest reasons for mothers' frustrations concerning anything to do with baby care, and particularly breastfeeding, is mixed messages from professionals.

There should be adequate privacy in the hospital setting, although this is sometimes difficult to achieve. Professionals should be sensitive to mothers' feelings at this vulnerable time. Hospitals should not be afraid to involve others, such as personnel from the La Leche League, who will come into maternity units to give advice and help to mothers and staff.

At delivery

As long as the delivery is normal and the baby is in good condition at birth there should be skin-to-skin contact and delivery of the baby on to the abdomen, allowing the baby to crawl up and search for the nipple. Contact within 30 min not only promotes bonding and breastfeeding but also helps keep the baby warm and stabilises the baby's heart and respiratory rate (Arulkumaran et al 2004). 'Early breastfeeding enhances bonding, increases chances of breastfeeding success and generally lengthens the duration of breastfeeding' (World Health Organization 2003: 5). It is important that the breasts are stimulated as soon as possible, as the quantity of milk depends on how often the baby suckles (Netdoctor 2007).

There is often a desire to 'get the baby cleaned up', but the mother should be given the option of not bathing the baby straight away so that she can get to know him or her intimately. These are precious moments following delivery and will obviously not be repeated.

General advice

It is vital to ensure correct positioning and attachment of the baby on to the breast (Royal College of Midwives 2002). It is *breast*feeding not *nipple*feeding. Incorrect position or attachment can cause sore and cracked nipples and insufficient milk supply. This can lead to discouragement of the mother, a hungry baby and possibly even the discontinuation of breastfeeding. There should be no use of supplementary or complementary feeds for healthy term infants. The use of pacifiers should be discouraged. The baby should have unhindered and frequent access to the breast; this helps establish and maintain a good milk supply (Arulkumaran et al 2004). There should be no time constraints (e.g. 'four-hourly feeds'). The mother should be reassured that it is normal for her baby to feed frequently, particularly in the early days. The baby should not be moved to the nursery 'so mum can have a rest'. Successful breastfeeding requires 100% commitment and is tiring for the mother, particularly in the first few weeks. Full-term newborns should breastfeed eight to twelve times in each 24-h period (Findlay et al 2006). This equates to feedings 2–3 h apart. As babies grow and their stomachs become larger, they naturally begin to go longer between feeds and develop more regular feeding patterns. During the first few months the baby's feeding pattern may vary through the day, and she or he may 'cluster feed', spacing feeds closer together at certain times of the day (usually during the evening) and going longer between feeds at other times (La Leche League 2006).

At home

The most important people at home who influence the success, or otherwise, of breastfeeding are almost never the professionals but are more likely to be the mother's partner and close female relatives (such as mother and mother-in-law).

The professional must be careful how she handles this situation. She must not be seen to discredit the partner or mother but should continue to encourage the mother to exclusively breastfeed. There is no evidence that test weighing is useful. It is more likely to worry the mother and put her off breastfeeding.

The community midwife, then health visitor and general practitioner, must ensure consistent advice (Arulkumaran et al 2004). There is no reason why breastfeeding cannot continue for many months, even several years if this is what the mother desires.

'To achieve optimal growth, development and health, WHO recommends that infants should be exclusively breastfed for the first 6 months of life' (World Health Organization 2003).

Some problems

Separation of mother from baby at birth, for example admission to a special care baby unit or neonatal intensive care unit, should happen only if it is absolutely necessary for medical reasons. Try to keep mother and baby together if possible, and use transitional care units if available. Encourage the mother to express her breast milk three-hourly. Make sure that all staff are familiar with hand expressing as well as using the breast pump. Put the baby to the breast as soon as is medically possible; even nuzzling and licking at the breast will improve lactation and enhance the mother–baby relationship. Kangaroo care is a lovely way for the mother to enhance the bonding process, and the father can be encouraged to partake in this also (Lang 2005).

Prevention of problems

- Improve training for professionals.
- Committed professionals.
- Keep the mother and baby together unless separation is medically necessary.
- Baby-friendly hospital status for maternity units.
- National Childbirth Trust and local breastfeeding support groups.
- Wider issues: more difficult to control (e.g. the influence of the media portraying breasts as sexual objects).
- Education in schools.

Procedures Box 13.1 The skill of breastfeeding

Actions
Ensure that the mother has the level of privacy she requires.

Provide comfortable surroundings and seating.

Ensure that you have no interruptions.

Reason *Ensures that the mother and baby are relaxed to encourage lactation and allow the baby to feed.*

Action
Assess the mother's level of knowledge and confidence regarding breastfeeding.

Reason *To ascertain if the mother requires any advice or support.*

Actions
If assistance is required this should be verbal only initially.

If the mother is unable to achieve a satisfactory feeding technique more practical help can then be given.

Reason *It is important not to intervene too quickly; observe and encourage the mother's own efforts to maintain her confidence.*

Action
Adopt a comfortable feeding position.

Reason *Ensures that mother and baby are comfortable and relaxed.*

Actions
Sitting up:

- Provide a chair of appropriate height; pillows may be needed at the small of the back
- A footstool to slightly raise the knees helps prevent back strain
- The mother may need to lean forwards a little to facilitate attachment
- The baby's head should be in the crook of the mother's arm and her hand should hold baby's buttocks

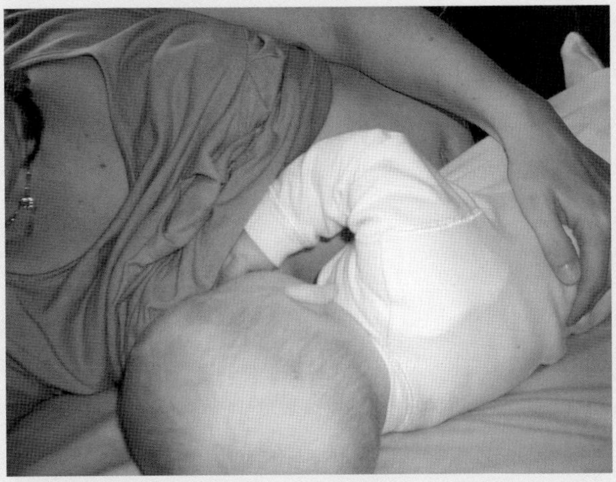

Lying down:

- The mother lying on her side, her head supported by pillows

Actions
The baby should be close to the mother, with his or her head and shoulders turned 'square on' to the breast; this will usually mean that the baby will need to face slightly upwards.

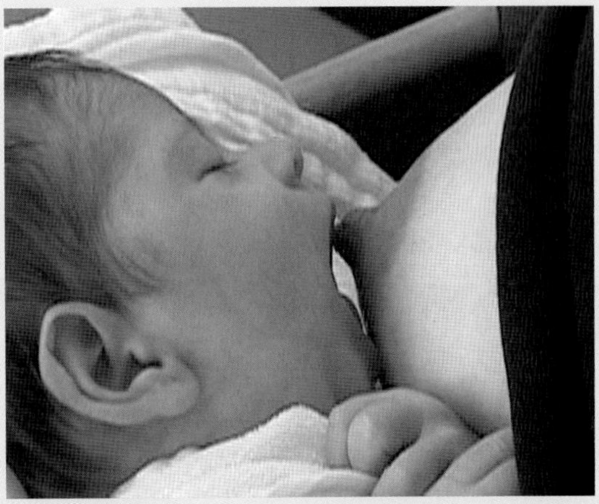

Move the baby against the breast, stroke the baby's lips with the nipple, and when she or he starts to open her or his mouth move the baby on to the breast gently.

Point the nipple to the roof of the baby's mouth (figure courtesy of the Health Education Board for Scotland).

The baby's chin and lower lip should touch the breast first.

It may help to keep the baby's head slightly extended (tipped backwards); this will keep the nose clear and allow the baby to breathe easily, but over-extension will make swallowing impossible.

Reason *The baby must get enough of the breast into her or his mouth so that milk can be squeezed out of the ducts behind the areola with her or his tongue.*

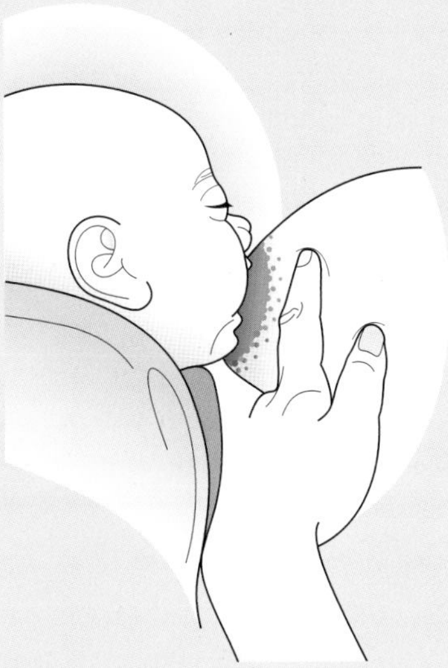

Actions
It is unnecessary to 'ram' the baby on to the breast.

Procedures Box 13.1 The skill of breastfeeding—cont'd

When the baby is attached some of the dark areola tissue will show above the upper lip but the base of the areola will be covered by the baby's lower lip; the baby will have a large mouthful of breast.

The baby's cheeks and chin will be close to the breast and the nose is tipped away.

Reason *Attempting to force the baby on to the breast will be unsuccessful and distressing for mother and baby.*

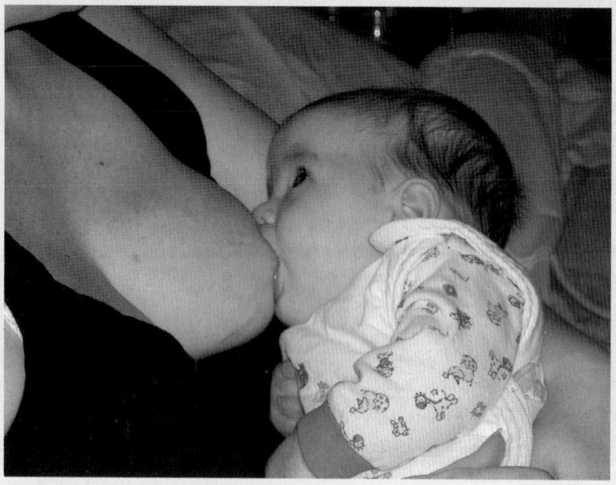

Actions

The mother and baby should be able to look into each other's eyes when well attached.

The mother should be able to hear the baby swallowing.

The baby will release the breast when he or she has had enough (Department of Health 2004).

Now test your knowledge

- A 6-week-old baby is admitted to the children's ward for minor surgery. What advice would you give to the mother to enable her to maintain her lactation during the time when the baby is 'nil by mouth'?
- Describe the physiology of lactation.
- What advice would you give to a mother who asked you about 'giving the baby an occasional bottle of formula'?
- What advice would you give to a mother who asked your opinion about giving her breastfeeding baby a pacifier?
- Describe the actions you would take if a mother complained that she had sore and cracked nipples.

References

Arulkumaran S, Symonds IM, Fowlie A (2004) Oxford handbook of obstetrics and gynaecology. Oxford University Press, Oxford

Department of Health (2004) Good practice and innovation in breastfeeding. Department of Health, London

Findlay L, Stuart R, MacDonald F, Holliday L (2006) Breastfeeding. In Glasper EA, McEwing G, Richardson J (eds) Oxford handbook of children's and young people's nursing. Oxford University Press, Oxford

La Leche League (2006) Online. Available: http://www.lalecheleague.org

Lang S (2005) Breast feeding special care babies. Baillière Tindall, London

Medela (2006) Anatomy of the lactating breast. Medela, Baar

National Health Service (2007) About breastfeeding. Online. Available: http://www.breastfeeding.nhs.uk/in_infoaboutbf.asp Apr 2007

Netdoctor (2007) Breastfeeding. Online. Available: http://www.netdoctor.co.uk/health_advice/facts/breastfeeding.htm Apr 2007

Royal College of Midwives (2002) Successful breast feeding. Churchill Livingstone, London

World Health Organization (2003) Infant and young child feeding. WHO, Geneva

14

Artificial feeding

Doris A.P. Corkin

In the early years of a child's life it is essential to ensure that infants receive optimum nutrition, which is a basic human requirement for their specific needs, in order to allow for normal growth and development (Department of Health 2006, Holden & MacDonald 2000, World Health Organization 2003). Parents should be advised that infants will require frequent feeds, usually every 3–4 h over a 24-h period (averaging six to eight feeds daily); as infants get older they may feed less frequently. Even though there is a wealth of information available on bottle feeding (Ellis & Kanneh 2000, Hockenberry et al 2003, Trigg & Mohammed 2006), much of it may cause confusion and indeed appears to have become a source of tension for new mothers and a negative experience for various healthcare professionals (Hehir 2005).

Bottle feeding is an acceptable method of feeding (Hockenberry et al 2003) that refers to the preparation of artificial feeds using a bottle and teat to feed an infant milk formula instead of using the breast (Corkin 2006). The composition of infant formula is similar to that of breast milk. Infant milk formulas should be continued until 1 year of age (Department of Health 2003) and are intended to replace breast milk when a mother has opted to bottle feed her infant. Therefore it is important that parents are supported in their decision and their choice respected (Hehir 2005). Indeed, when requested, parents should be given accurate and consistent information regarding the preparation and use of infant milk formula, which is based on cow's milk and is the only alternative to breast milk (Department of Health 2006). Furthermore it is recommended that infant milk formulas are made up as required and only used or changed following the advice of an identified health professional (e.g. midwife, health visitor, dietitian, paediatrician or general practitioner). Cow's milk is not safe for infant consumption, as it is too high in some nutrients and too low in others, such as iron (Ellis & Kanneh 2000).

Infant formula

There are *two* main types of infant artificial formula (Box 14.1):

1. *Whey-based* milks, recommended from birth, are easy to digest and have a protein composition and low renal solute load resembling breast milk
2. *Casein-based* milks are similar to cow's milk and are often given to a hungrier baby, but as there is no scientific evidence to support this practice it should not be encouraged.

Infant formula must be prepared as per the manufacturer's instructions, using the measuring scoop provided (the scoop should not be exchanged between brands).

Preterm and low birth weight formula

Infants born prematurely have greater nutritional requirements than infants born at term. Although preterm infants should be encouraged to breastfeed or be fed breast milk this practice may not always be possible, therefore the infant will need to be supplemented after medical recommendation with low birth weight formula (prescription only). Low birth weight formulas tend to provide preterm infants with more protein and energy and a greater weight gain. These formulas are mainly introduced while in hospital because they are available only as 'ready to feed' formula, but they may be continued in the community setting while healthy growth and development are under the clinical review of a consultant paediatrician, paediatric dietitian or general practitioner.

Follow-on milk formula

These milks have a vitamin- and mineral-fortified formula that is aimed at infants who are being weaned, especially when there is concern over the dietary intake of iron (Ellis & Kanneh 2000, Glasper & Richardson 2006).

Examples of follow-on milks are:

- Aptamil Forward (Milupa)
- Cow & Gate Step-up
- SMA Progress
- Farley's Follow-on Milk.

Either infant or follow-on formula should be given as the main milk drink between 6 and 12 months and if the child's diet is inadequate may be continued until 18 months of age. This milk is not available on milk token.

Soya protein-based formula

This formula is based on soya protein, has no milk constituents and is the preferred management for galactosaemia. Indeed, soya formula is no longer considered an

Box 14.1. Main types of infant artificial formula

Whey-based

- Aptamil First (Milupa)
- Farley's First Milk
- Cow & Gate Premium
- SMA Gold

Casein-based

- Aptamil Extra (Milupa)
- Farley's Second Milk
- Cow & Gate Plus
- SMA White

appropriate treatment for the intolerance of lactose or cow's milk protein for infants under 6 months old (More 2003), because these infants who are at risk of allergy may also be sensitive to soya protein (Fiocchi et al 2003). Therefore lactose-free formula has been specially developed for lactose intolerance, and extensively hydrolysed formulas such as Cow & Gate Pepti-Junior are available for the treatment of cow's milk protein intolerance. The chief medical officer has recommended that soya-based formulas be given only in exceptional circumstances, for example to infants of vegan parents, and this is supported by the Paediatric Group of the British Dietetic Association (2004), who highlight the need to protect infant organ systems, which are vulnerable.

Examples of nutritionally complete soya formulas are:

- Farley's Soya
- Cow & Gate Infasoy
- SMA Wysoy.

Elemental formula

Neocate is a special formula (prescription only) that consists of essential amino acids and may be required if the infant has a family history of multiple food allergies or malabsorption problems with protein or milk intolerance. This elemental formula is free of cow's milk protein, soya and lactose; is only available in powder form; and is relatively expensive formula (Hockenberry et al 2003).

Antireflux formula

Enfamil A.R. and SMA Staydown are gastric-thickening feeds that thicken when in contact with stomach acid. These formulas should not be used with an antireflux medication because they will not thicken when the stomach acids have been neutralised. They are currently recommended for reflux management when the addition of a thickener such as Carobel or Nestargel is not appropriate. However, specialist advice must be sought when dealing with gastric reflux.

Goat's milk

This milk is totally unsuitable for infants under 1 year of age because it is not always pasteurised, is a poor source of iron and vitamins, and has an excessively high protein and salt content. Goat's milk may be perceived by some parents as less allergenic; however, this claim has not been substantiated (Hockenberry et al 2003).

The weaning process

The process of weaning should not be introduced before the age of 6 months, to allow the infant's gut time to functionally mature, and only then should the diet be expanded to include foods and drinks other than breast milk or infant formula (Department of Health 2003, World Health Organization 2003). No solid food should ever be added to the infant's bottle. Furthermore drinking from a lidded free-flow cup should be encouraged from 6 months and bottle feeding discontinued by 1 year of age, as spoon feeds should be well established by this stage. Cow's milk must be used only to mix solid foods from 6 months and not as a main drink until after 1 year of age (Department of Health 2006).

Calculating the volume of artificial feed

A children's nurse should be able to give advice on infant formula feeding as well as calculating the appropriate amount of feed an infant is expected to take to ensure adequate protein, vitamins and minerals (see Table 14.1). However, there may be exceptional medical reasons for adjusting calculations, especially when an infant has a history of faltering growth and requires extra calories or, indeed, needs restricted fluids if suffering from cerebral oedema, cardiac problems or renal failure (Trigg & Mohammed 2006).

Table 14.1. Average fluid requirements

Age of infant	Total fluid in 24 h (mL/kg)
Newborn	30
2 days	60
3 days	90
4 days	120
5 days	150
1 week to 8 months	150
9–12 months	120

(After Huband & Trigg 2000)

Procedures Box 14.1 Safe preparation of bottle-feeding utensils and infant formulas

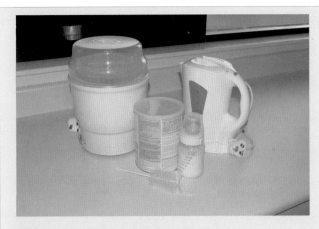

Action

Collect the required equipment:

- Plastic apron
- Steam-sterilising unit and instructions
- Feeding bottle, disc, screw ring, teat and cap
- Kettle with freshly boiled water from the tap
- Tin of infant milk formula with scoop
- Plastic knife with straight-edged back
- Bottle brush for washing utensils.

Reasons *The apron prevents cross-infection.*
The knife is plastic to allow for sterilisation and straight-edged to ensure correct measurement of milk powder.

1 Care of bottle-feeding utensils

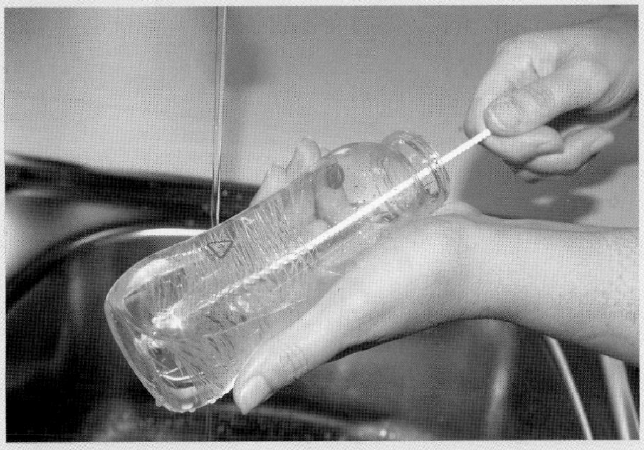

Actions

All the utensils used for bottle feeding need to be thoroughly washed with the aid of a bottle brush in warm soapy water.

Rinse with running water from the tap and then sterilise (until the infant is at least 6 months old).

Use an appropriate bottle brush that is used only for this cleaning purpose.

Then place the brush in the sterilising unit with the teats, discs, screw rings, bottles and caps.

Reason *To protect against infections such as gastroenteritis and oral thrush.*

2 Ensure safety of feeding teats

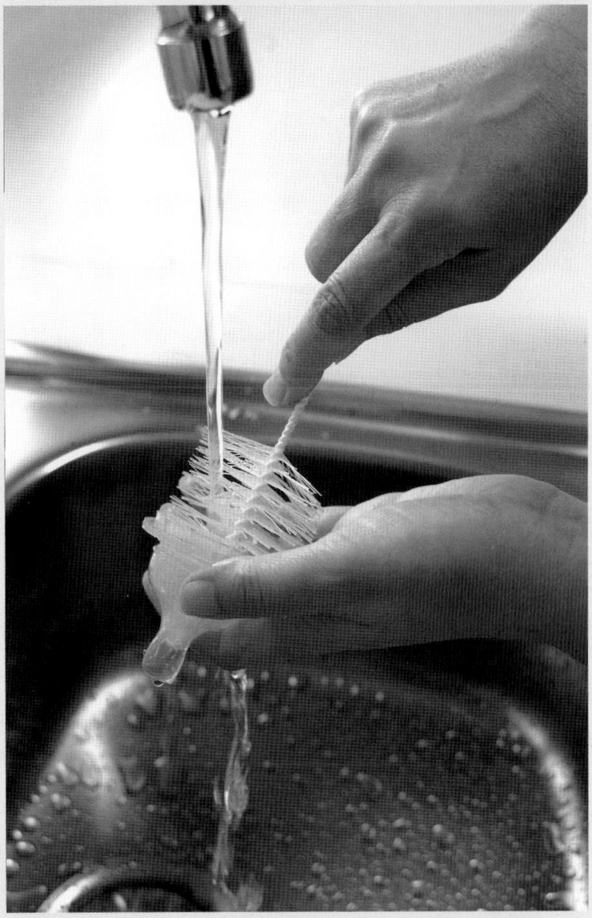

Actions

Clean the teats carefully by squeezing the water through the hole of the teat with the aid of the brush to ensure removal of milk residues and liquid soap (Ellis & Kanneh 2000).

ALERT
Salt is no longer recommended for cleaning teats as this can damage silicone teats (Department of Health 2006). Cracked or split teats must be discarded.

3 Three methods of sterilising

Actions

Steam sterilising is either by electric or microwave; both are quick and efficient.

When steam sterilising follow the manufacturer's instructions and add the recommended amount of water to the sterilising unit.

Cold water sterilising requires a tank and either chemical solution or tablets; ensure that the manufacturer's guidelines are followed.

Reason *Protects against infections.*

Procedures Box 14.1 Safe preparation of bottle-feeding utensils and infant formulas—cont'd

3 Continued

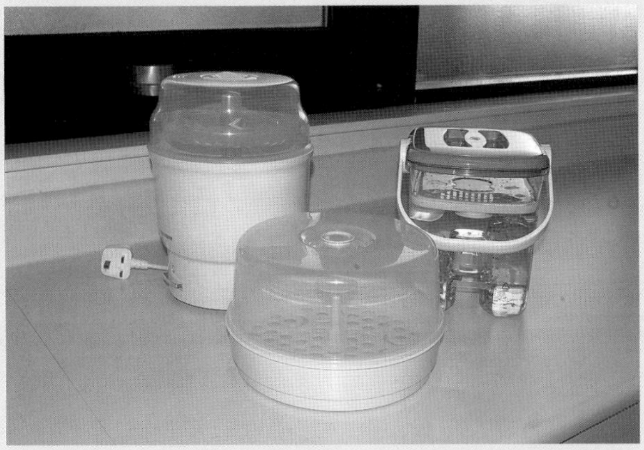

4

Preparing a feed

Actions

Before making up a feed, wipe the work surface with a damp clean cloth and then dry the surface area with a hygienic paper towel.

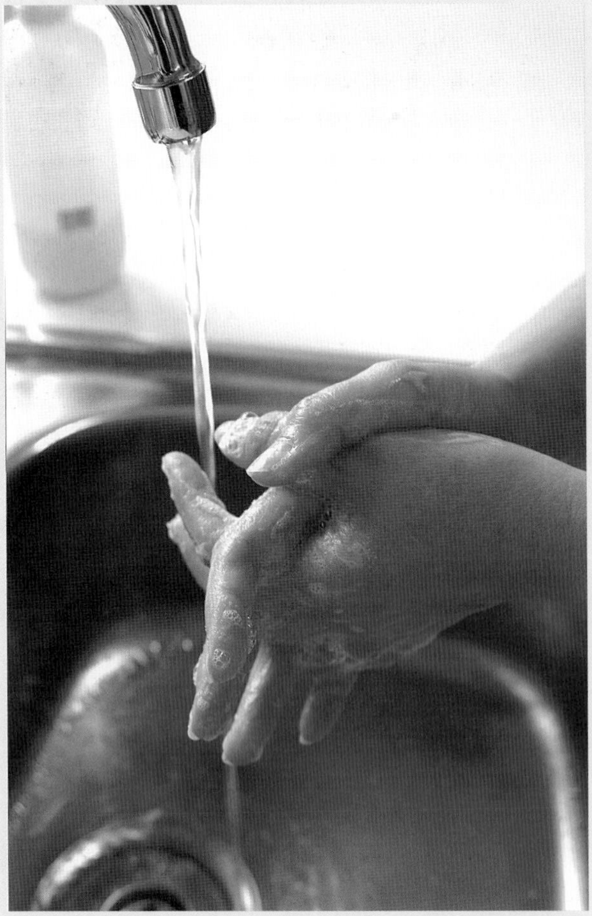

Wet your hands with warm running water then apply liquid soap.

Wash your hands, ensuring that your fingers have been interlaced (Trigg & Mohammed 2006).

Rinse and dry your hands before touching the sterilised utensils.

Reason *Protects against infections.*

5

Making a bottle feed

Actions

Boil in the kettle fresh cold water supplied from the mains tap.

Leave the water to cool for no more than 30 min; meanwhile read the instructions on the formula tin.

ALERT

Bottled mineral water, filtered water and repeatedly boiled water are not recommended, as they may contain high concentrations of salts (Department of Health 2006, Ellis & Kanneh 2000).

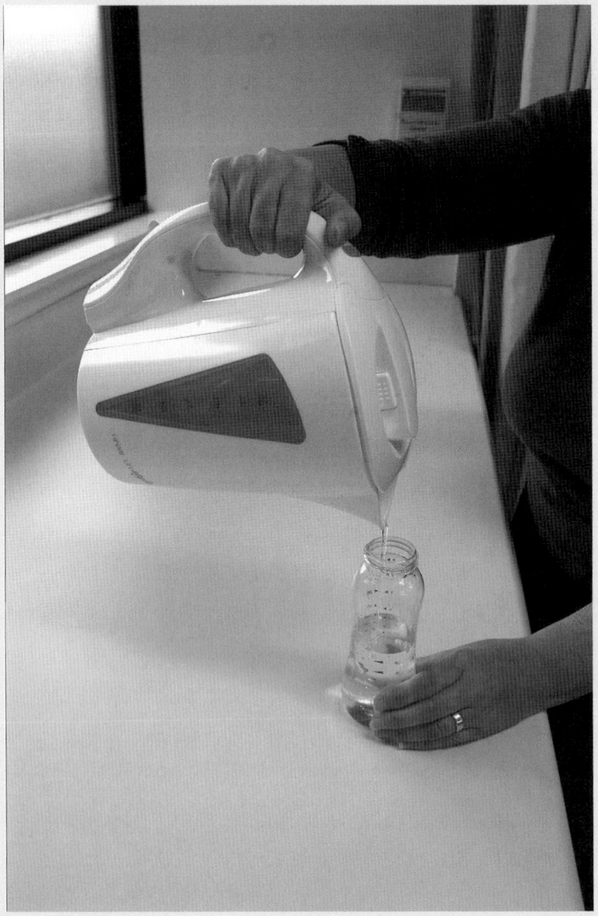

Action

Place the empty bottle on a flat clean surface; always pour the cooled boiled water into the bottle first then check the water level before adding milk powder.

Reason *Ensures accurate measurement of water.*

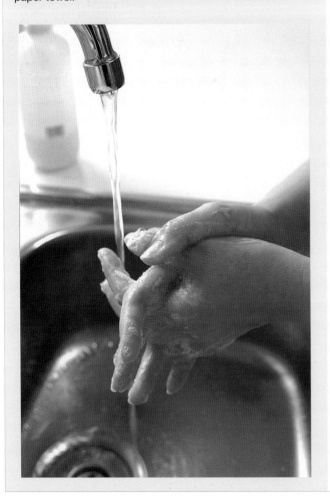

Procedures Box 14.1 Safe preparation of bottle-feeding utensils and infant formulas—cont'd

6

Safe preparation of milk formula

Action
Remember to check the expiry date on the formula tin and use it within 4 weeks of opening.

Actions
Follow the manufacturer's instructions regarding the number of scoops to the amount of water.

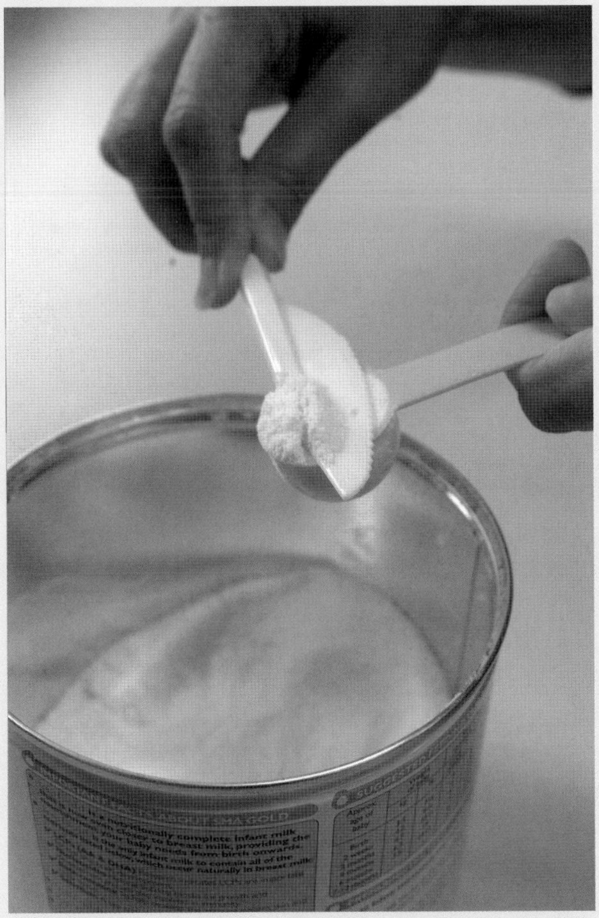

Loosely fill the scoop supplied with milk powder and level it with the sterilised straight-edged back of the plastic knife (Trigg & Mohammed 2006).

Reason *Ensures accurate measurement of milk powder.*

Actions
Add scoops of powder to the bottle of cooled boiled water.

Seal the bottle with the supplied disc, screw ring and cap then gently shake the bottle to dissolve the milk powder.

7

Before bottle feeding the infant

Actions
Remove the disc and secure the sterilised teat with the screw ring provided.

Ensure that the teat has a hole that lets the milk out in regular drops rather than a stream.

Check the temperature of the milk feed by dropping a few

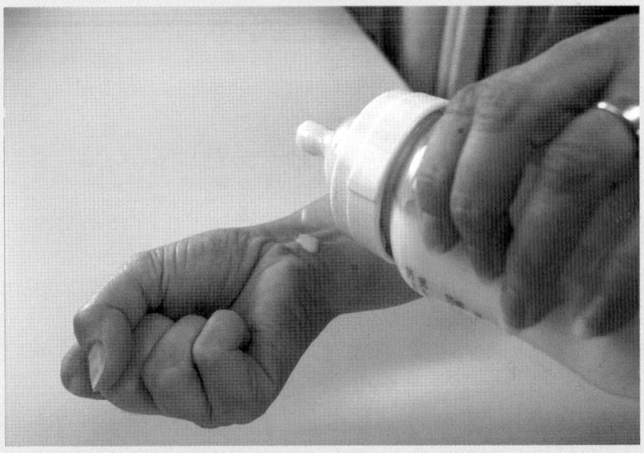

drops on to the inside of your wrist.

Cool the bottle of milk formula under cold running water if necessary.

ALERT
Never reheat a bottle feed in the microwave because the heat is not equally distributed and the milk could scald the infant's mouth (Hockenberry et al 2003) – warming a bottle feed with warm water is sufficient.

It is unsafe practice to reheat a bottle feed more than once, as bacteria can multiply rapidly – discard any remaining milk formula after bottle feeding (European Food Safety Authority 2004).

How to routinely bottle feed an infant

Prior to bottle feeding, promote comfort by ensuring that the infant's nose is clean and clear of mucus and that he or she has a dry nappy:

- Wash your hands thoroughly, as demonstrated in the procedure box.
- A plastic apron may be worn to prevent cross-infection; however, be careful as plastic may be slippery on a carer's knee.
- Feeding bottles and teats are available in various shapes and sizes; choose and sterilise them appropriately prior to use.
- Calculate and prepare the bottle feed as recommended by the manufacturer of the infant formula, ensuring that the milk scoop is used correctly (see procedure box).

- Test the temperature of the milk as demonstrated in the procedure box.
- Should the milk feel hot it can be cooled under cold running water from the tap before it is offered to the infant; this avoids scalding (Hockenberry et al 2003).
- In order to protect clothing it is best for infant to wear a bib, and keep tissues convenient should the infant lose a mouthful.
- The carer should sit down in a comfortable chair with the infant's head supported in the upright position. Relax and enjoy the experience, as bottle feeding is an ideal time to observe development and promote eye contact and verbal stimulation.
- Ensure that the infant does not lie flat when feeding, as there is a danger of choking and possible aspiration of stomach contents into the lungs.
- Offer the bottle feed by gently placing it to the lips of the infant – never force a bottle feed into an infant's mouth.
- Hold the bottle feed at an angle, tilted, so that the teat is always full of milk; this prevents the infant swallowing air (Corkin 2006).
- Should the teat flatten while feeding, gently ease the bottle to release the vacuum in the teat.
- Swallowed air will cause the infant to cry due to discomfort, therefore with her or his head supported position the infant upright two or three times during the bottle feed and gently rub the infant's back to release the trapped air – do not expect a burp each time.
- Clear away the bottle-feeding equipment and wash the bottle and teat thoroughly before sterilising, as highlighted in the procedure box.

Now test your knowledge

- What are the two main types of infant artificial formula and which one is appropriate for the newborn infant?
- When is soya protein-based formula used as an infant feed?
- What is the fluid requirement for a 3-day-old baby weighing 4 kg?
- Discuss the identified risks that a children's nurse should highlight when safely demonstrating how to prepare bottle-feeding utensils and infant milk formula.

References

Corkin D (2006) Bottle feeding. In Glasper EA, McEwing G, Richardson J (eds) Oxford handbook of children's and young people's nursing. Oxford University Press, Oxford, p 692–693

Department of Health (2003) Infant feeding recommendations. Department of Health, London

Department of Health (2006) Birth to five: your complete guide to parenthood and the first five years of your child's life. Online. Available: http://www.dh.gov.uk

Ellis M, Kanneh A (2000) Infant nutrition: part two. Paediatric Nursing 12(1):38–43

European Food Safety Authority (2004) Opinion adopted by the BIOHAZ Panel related to the microbiological risks in formulae and follow-on formulae. European Food Safety Authority Journal 113:1–34

Fiocchi A, Restani P, Gualtiero L, Martelli A (2003) Clinical tolerance to lactose in children with cow's milk allergy. Pediatrics 112(2):359

Glasper A, Richardson J (2006) A textbook of children's and young people's nursing. Churchill Livingstone, Edinburgh

Hehir B (2005) Stop hitting the bottle. Nursing Standard 19(52):28–29

Hockenberry MJ, Wilson D, Winkelstein ML, Kline NE (2003) Nursing care of infants and children, 7th edn. Mosby, Philadelphia

Holden C, MacDonald A (2000) Nutrition and child health. Baillière Tindall, London

Huband S, Trigg E (2000) Practices in children's nursing. Guidelines for hospital and community. Churchill Livingstone, Edinburgh

More J (2003) New guidelines on infant feeding in the first 12 months of life. Journal of Family Health Care 13(4):89–90

Paediatric Group of the British Dietetic Association (2004) Position statement on the use of soya protein for infants. British Dietetic Association, Birmingham

Trigg E, Mohammed TA (2006) Practices in children's nursing. Guidelines for hospital and community, 2nd edn. Churchill Livingstone, Edinburgh

World Health Organization (2003) Global strategy for infant and child feeding. Online. Available: http://www.wh.int/nut/documentss/gs-infant-feeding

15 Enteral feeding

PART A Nutrition via enteral feeding devices

Doris A.P. Corkin • Julie A. Chambers

Issues surrounding enteral feeding will be discussed within the following chapters, highlighting the importance of best practice (Bond & Moss 2003) when undertaking enteral feeding in the hospital and community setting.

Enteral feeding is an artificial method of supplying the child with nutrition and can be via an orogastric (neonate), nasogastric or gastrostomy tube. A multidisciplinary team approach is essential when considering artificial feeding with a child or young person and should be both hospital and community focused, with a key worker identified in the community to coordinate care (Corkin & Chambers 2007, Townsley & Robinson 2000).

The reasons as to why the child or young person may need to be artificially fed can be many, such as inability to swallow, history of faltering growth and/or life-limited and requiring respite care (Corkin et al 2006). Without adequate nutrition a child's growth and development will suffer and illness recovery will be delayed.

Four main groups of children who require enteral tube feeding have been identified:

1. Children with short-term feeding needs for example, due to prematurity, severe burns and cancer treatment (Huband & Trigg 2000)
2. Children with neurological disorders, for example cerebral palsy (Samson-Fang et al 2003)
3. Children with chronic disorders, for example cystic fibrosis, renal failure and inflammatory bowel disease
4. Children with miscellaneous conditions, for example psychological problems such as anorexia nervosa, although this group is considered to be very rare.

The organisation of the essential equipment required for enteral feeding, such as feeding tubes, extension sets, syringes for both feeding and medication, pH indicator strips or paper (National Patient Safety Agency 2005a, Northern Ireland Adverse Incident Centre 2004) and feeding pumps, should be arranged while in hospital prior to discharge. Daveluy et al (2004) reported that 98% of their 416 community-based sample used a feeding pump for enteral feeding. Following discharge into the community setting clear information should be available for both parents and health professionals (Huband & Trigg 2000). Parents will need to know who to contact for further supplies of disposable equipment, as this can vary from community children's nursing team, dietician or local chemist to direct from the feeding company, who can supply complete feeding packages if arranged. Clear feeding pump guidelines, addressing the storage of all feeding equipment, will also need to be supplied.

Discharge planning

To facilitate a safe discharge early planning and a multidisciplinary team approach are essential. This should include coordinated child and parent or carer education, relevant information and organisation of equipment (Stephens 2005).

Once the decision has been agreed to commence a child or young person on enteral feeding, planning for discharge should begin. Information must be accurate and consistent to child and parents from all healthcare professionals.

Information must include:

- the community children's nurse contact name and telephone number
- the community paediatric dietician contact name and telephone number
- verbal and written guidelines on enteral feeding pump operation and the company contact number, should advice or replacement be required
- advice regarding storage, ordering and administration of the feed
- written feeding regimen for the individual child or young person, completed by an identified dietician, with a copy given to parents and other members of the multidisciplinary team
- an agreement made by professionals as to the continual monitoring of the child on enteral feeding
- a written troubleshooting guide given to parents.

A comprehensive detailed assessment is vital to ensure that the individual needs and lifestyle of children, young people and their families are addressed within the context of family life, culture and the community in which they live. At the initial discussion to commence enteral feeding the individual child's needs are paramount and need to remain so. In hospital enteral feeding may appear to be a routine procedure, but it is a major commitment physically, emotionally and psychologically for children and families at home. Therefore the community children's nurse needs to empower the family and child, taking into account individual lifestyles and environments (Fig. 15.1). Continuous needs assessment is ongoing and varies not only with the child's medical condition but also with natural development such as altered body image. Emotional support needs to be at the forefront, and the psychological impact of enteral feeding must not be overlooked. Indeed, referral for further psychosocial support may be required due to the impact of tube feeding (Rollins 2006). Each child and family is unique, so each case has to be planned and managed individually. The care pathway should encompass partnership working, family-centred care (Smith et al 2002) and the formation of a negotiated care plan that is continuously reviewed.

During infancy, oral feeding builds the sensory foundations for future feeding skills and leads to comfort and opportunities for bonding with parents. However, oral feeding should only be maintained provided it has been deemed safe. Nasogastric tube feeding is the most commonly used method of enteral feeding for short-term nutritional support and can offer hydration to the child with gastroenteritis (Fonseca et al 2004).

In order to maintain growth and healing and to avoid malnutrition, feeding via a gastrostomy tube may be needed to provide the child or young person with long-term nutritional support following a period of nasogastric feeding. A gastrostomy is an artificial opening through the abdomen into the stomach. The decision to insert a gastrostomy tube under anaesthetic is not taken lightly. A multiprofessional approach will be required, taking into consideration the complications associated with a gastrostomy tube, such as leakage and hypergranulation tissue around the stoma site (Rollins 2000).

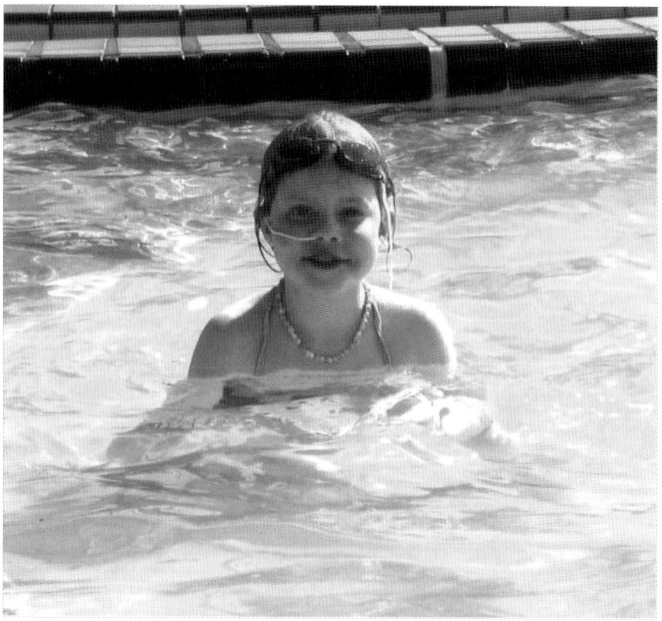

Fig. 15.1 • The care plan for enteral feeding must account for individual lifestyles and environments.

It is possible that enteral feeding may have a negative impact on the child, and this may include hypersensitivity, therefore it is important that pleasurable oral stimulation activities are carried out; these activities can be demonstrated to family by speech and language therapists.

PART B Nasogastric tube insertion and feeding

Janet Kelsey • Gillian McEwing

Choice of tube

The principle considerations when choosing a nasogastric feeding tube should be its size and material. There are two main types commonly used: polyvinyl chloride (PVC) and polyurethane tubes. The PVC tubes quickly lose their flexibility when in contact with gastric secretions; these are, therefore, primarily used for short-term feeding, as they need changing frequently according to the manufacturer's guidance (Hockenberry et al 2003). The polyurethane tubes are more suitable for longer term feeding, as they are softer and more flexible and can remain in situ for up to 1 month. These tubes usually have a guide wire to assist with passing the tube; the wire is removed when the tube has been passed but should be kept in case the tube has to be repassed (National Health Service Quality Improvement Scotland 2003).

Tubes are sized according to their internal lumen; 6, 8 and 10 French gauge (Fg) are most commonly used in children. It has been reported that small-lumen tubes (size 6Fg) may be too narrow to use with thickened feeds (Huband & Trigg 2000).

Tube measurement

Traditionally the NEX measurement (length from nose to earlobe to xiphoid process) has been used to indicate the length of tube required to reach the stomach. However, a study by Klasner et al (2002) suggested that for paediatric gastric tube insertion a graphic method based on height was more accurate than the standard NEX method for determining the depth of tube insertion.

Checking tube position

An important issue regarding the insertion of a nasogastric tube is safe and accurate checking of the tube's position. Errors can include initial mistaken positioning as well as displacement over time. If a tube is located in the airway or the oesophagus, feeding through the tube will result in pulmonary aspiration with subsequent morbidity and mortality. If a tube is placed in the duodenum this can result in malabsorption due to a lack of gastric enzymes required for digestion.

Ellett & Beckstrand (1999) found error rates in tube placement to be between 20.9% and 43.5% in a study of 39 hospitalised children. Children with swallowing difficulty or reduced level of consciousness were found to have an increased risk of tube placement error. The Medicines and Healthcare products Regulatory Agency (2004) advised health professionals on methods used to check the correct placement of nasogastric tubes (MDA/2004/026, 14 June 2004) following a fatality due to the misplacement of a nasogastric tube in a child (Department of Health 2004a).

When to check the position of the tube:

- following insertion
- before administering feeds
- before giving medications
- at least once daily when administering continuous feeds
- following episodes of vomiting, retching or coughing
- following suspicion of tube displacement (National Patient Safety Agency 2005b).

There are many methods reported of how to check the position of a nasogastric tube; these include:

- insufflation (blowing air down the tube via a syringe) and auscultation (listening for gurgling or bubbling in the stomach); this is often referred to as the 'whoosh' test
- holding the end of the tube underwater and observing for bubbles
- examining the colour of any aspirate
- testing the aspirate with blue litmus paper
- measuring the pH, bilirubin, pepsin and trypsin levels
- measuring the CO_2 level at the proximal end of the nasogastric tube
- chest or abdominal X-ray.

Many of the above have no evidence to support their accuracy, and some have been found to be dangerous.

When determining the position of nasogastric tubes, insufflation and auscultation of air into the stomach is an unreliable method of checking tube position, as it has been shown to give false-positive results because bowel or chest sounds can be misinterpreted as evidence of gastric tube placement (Metheny et al 1998a).

Placing the proximal end of the tube underwater and observing for bubbles on expiration runs the risk of aspirating the water on inspiration, particularly when the child is ventilated (Metheny et al 1994, Thomas & Falcone 1998).

Examining the colour of the aspirate alone is not a safe indication of tube placement. Metheny et al (1994) demonstrated that visual characteristics of aspirate improved nurses' predictions of nasogastric tube placement; however, colour can only be considered to be another guide when assessing tube placement. Metheny et al (1998b) reports gastric fluid to be grassy green, tan to off-white, bloody or brown, on rare occasions being clear and colourless. It is also likely to have mucus mixed in with it, and if the tube insertion was traumatic, flecks or streaks of blood; however, aspirate from the bronchial tree was shown to be off-white and heavily tinged with mucus, which may be stained bright red or rust coloured by blood.

In the presence of acid, blue litmus paper should turn pink to red. Therefore it has been assumed that if a tube has been passed and aspirate is obtained that turns blue litmus paper pink to red, then it must be in the acidic environment of the stomach. However, litmus paper does not indicate the degree of acidity present. This point is crucial, as bronchial secretions can be slightly acidic, which will turn the litmus pink.

Testing the pH of aspirate is based on the principle that different organs will produce fluids with a different pH. Pate (1998, cited in Ellett 2004) found pH values between 4.5 and 5.0 in tubes placed in the stomach; those placed in the pylorus all had pH values between 6.0 and 7.5, and the one tube tested that was placed in the oesophagus was found to have a pH of 7.5. Metheny et al (1999) found mean gastric pH to be 4.3 compared with a mean intestinal pH of 7.8; in a study of 56 children Westhus (2004) found mean gastric pH to be 4.1 and intestinal pH 7.5. Bronchial secretions range between a pH of 5.5 and 7 (Metheny et al 1990). Aspirate with a pH of between 0 and 4 is therefore unlikely to be from the respiratory tract.

The National Patient Safety Agency 2005b recommends that feeding can commence if aspirate is below pH 5.5 (Appendices 15.1–15.5). However, care should be taken, as the use of antacids, proton pump inhibitor drugs or H_2 receptor antagonists can elevate the pH of the gastric contents and limit the usefulness of this test in those children receiving such therapies.

A cut-off level of pH 5.5 is also recommended in neonates, with senior advice sought if pH values are 6 or above. The National Patient Safety Agency (2005b) acknowledges that gaining aspirate from fine-bore feeding tubes can be difficult and that factors which may affect results from pH indicator strips or paper include:

- gestation
- postnatal age
- small volumes of aspirate
- the effect of medications on gastric pH
- continuous and frequent feeding.

It recommends that a risk assessment is carried out to consider factors that may contribute to a high gastric pH, particularly:

- the presence of amniotic fluid in a baby under 48 h old
- milk in the baby's stomach if she or he is on 1–2-hourly feeds
- the use of medication to reduce stomach acid.

Despite radiography being recognised as the most accurate method for confirming tube placement it should not be used routinely for the sole purpose of confirming correct tube placement. Tubes with markings to enable accurate measurement of depth and length should, however, be used.

Bilirubin does not normally occur in the lungs. Therefore testing for bilirubin in the aspirate from the feeding tube can assist in determining the tube's position. Absence of bilirubin could suggest that the tube is in the lungs; however, there may be occasions when no bilirubin will be detected in the stomach. Metheny & Stewart (2002) suggest a bilirubin concentration of < 5 mg/dL as a good predictor of gastric tube placement in adults irrespective of fasting, but a bilirubin level of > 5 mg/dL is an indication of intestinal placement. These studies have been carried out on adults; only one study has investigated this in children: Metheny et al (1999) found that comparable bilirubin is found in the gastric fluid of neonates. Metheny et al (2000) suggest that a combination of pH test, colour and bilirubin concentration is useful in predicting tube position.

Inability to aspirate fluid is more likely to occur in children because the tubes used have a smaller diameter and are therefore more likely to collapse; however, Ellet & Beckstrand (1999) showed that injecting air (1 mL in infants and 5 mL in adolescents) into the tube enabled aspirate to be obtained in 88.2% of nasogastric tubes. Guidance from the National Patient Safety Agency (2005b) support injecting 1–5 mL of air using a 20- or 50-mL syringe, waiting for 15–30 min, and then attempting to reaspirate.

Measuring the CO_2 level at the proximal end of the nasogastric tube has been tested only in adults; however, Thomas & Falcone (1998) found that the colometric CO_2 device attached to the nasogastric tube reliably discriminated between tubes placed in the airway or the stomach by demonstrating an absence of CO_2 from the nasogastric tube.

X-ray of tube position is extremely accurate. However, problems include the time taken to get and read the X-ray resulting in lost feeding time, radiation exposure in patients who frequently pull out tubes, inconvenience and discomfort for the child, cost, and the possible displacement of the tube post X-ray and prior to feeding.

There is no 100% reliable bedside test of nasogastric tube placement; however, measuring pH is the recommended method for determining tube position in infants and children. If bilirubin testing can be shown to be accurate in children then the two could be used jointly to discriminate between gastric, intestinal and respiratory placements.

Syringe size

When aspirating the tube the negative pressure created at the tip of the syringe is dependent on the size and type of syringe and the force exerted. It is essential to follow the manufacturers' guidelines when aspirating the tube, in order to prevent damage (Viasys 2000).

Securing the nasogastric tube

Most children benefit from using a barrier product such as hydrocolloid dressings to protect the skin and prevent epidermal stripping under the adhesive tape (Dollison & Beckstrand 1995, National Health Service Quality Improvement Scotland 2003). When possible, alternate nostrils should be used when the tube is repassed, and it should be remembered that if nasogastric tube feeding is initiated in infancy areas around the face may become hypersensitive to touch and taste (Holden et al 1997).

Psychological support

It is well recognised that passing a nasogastric tube is a distressing experience (Holden et al 1997, Penrod et al 1999), therefore all children should be prepared for this procedure in a manner sensitive to both their and their family's needs.

ALERT
Nasogastric tubes should not be inserted into patients with base-of-skull fractures.

Procedures Box 15.1 Passing a nasogastric tube on a child

1

Action
Collect the required equipment:
- Nasogastric tube
- Large-bore syringe according to the manufacturer's guidelines
- pH indication paper
- Tape to secure
- Hydrocolloid dressing
- Oral fluid for an older child or dummy
- Two gallipots
- Water or water-based lubricant
- Disposable gloves
- Scissors
- Plastic apron.

2

Action
Wash and dry your hands and put on the plastic apron.
Reason *Prevents cross-infection.*

3

Action
Explain to the child and parent that you are going to pass the nasogastric tube.
Reason *Promotes psychological support.*

4

Action
Clean the work surface or trolley prior to placement of the equipment.
Reason *Passing a nasogastric tube is a clean procedure.*

5

Actions
Prepare a piece of hydrocolloid dressing.
To prevent epidermal damage this should be three times the width of the tube and cover two-thirds of the child's cheek between the side of the nostril and the child's ear.

6

Actions
Cut the adhesive tape and place it within easy reach.
To secure adequately, this should be wide enough to cover the nasogastric tube and overlap the sides sufficiently to hold it securely in place; however, it should not overlap the hydrocolloid dressing.

7

Action
Wash and dry your hands.
Reason *Prevents bacterial contamination of the tube.*

8

Action
Add water or lubricant to the gallipot.
Reason *Lubricates the tip of the tube.*

9

Action
Place a strip of pH paper in the second galllipot.

10

Action
Open the syringe and place it within easy reach.

11

Action
Put on disposable gloves.
Reason *This is a universal precaution.*

12

Action
Remove the nasogastric tube from its packaging and ensure that it is not damaged.

13

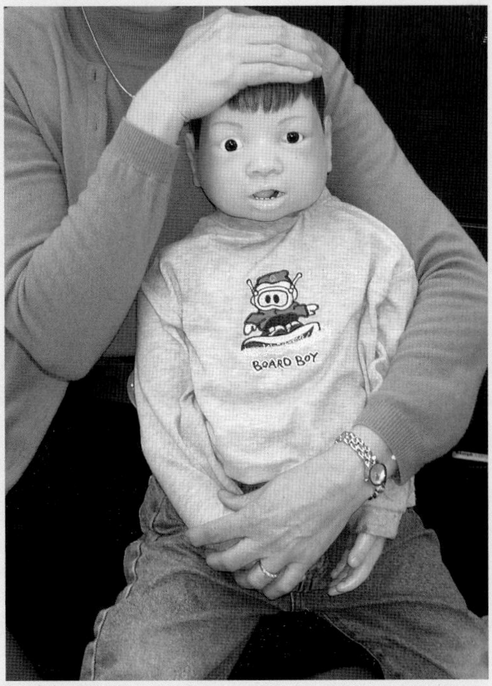

Procedures Box 15.1 Passing a nasogastric tube on a child—cont'd

13 Continued

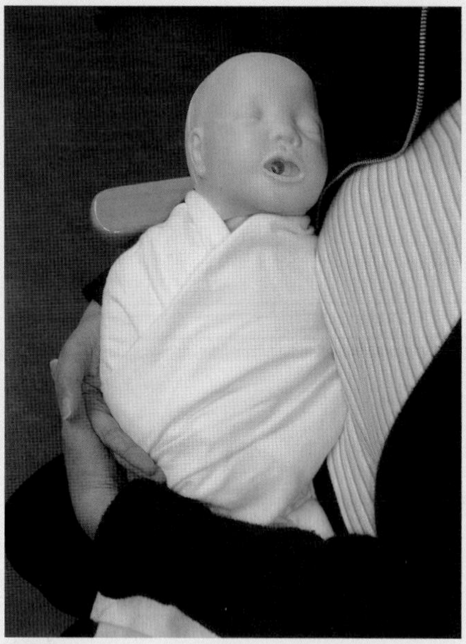

Actions

Ask an assistant (parent) to supportively hold the child as appropriate to age and level of understanding.

Older children may prefer to sit up with their head supported.

Babies can be wrapped in a blanket and encouraged to suck a dummy through the procedure.

Reason *Prevents the child moving during the procedure and provides comfort.*

14

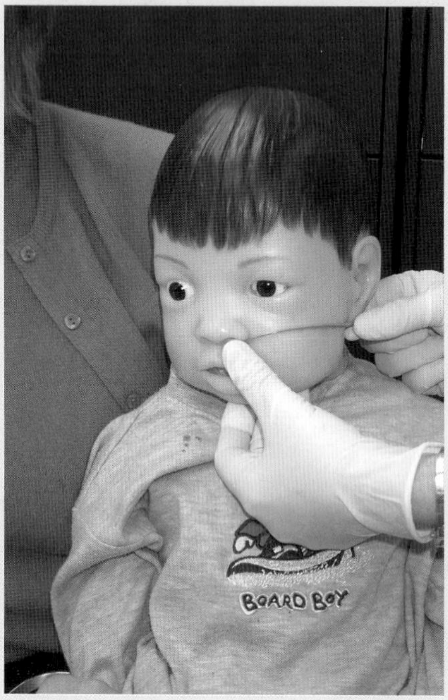

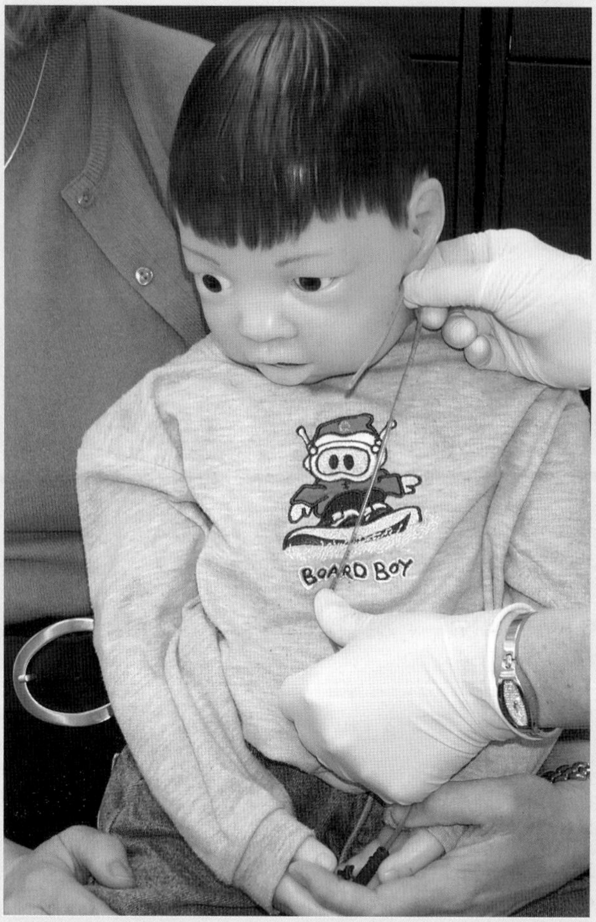

Actions

Measure a length of tube from nostril to ear and then from ear to stomach, just past the xiphoid process.

Note or mark the point on the tube or hold the tube at the calculated point and keep it between the fingers of your non-dominant hand.

Reason *Determines the length of tube required.*

Action

Ensure that the end cap of the tube is in place.

Reason *Prevents leakage of gastric contents.*

15

Action

Select a clear nostril; older children can choose which nostril.

Reason *Consider airway maintenance in infants, who are obligatory nose breathers.*

Action

Lubricate the tip of the tube using a water-based solution; follow manufacturers' guidelines regarding the type of lubrication.

Reasons *Lubrication reduces the risk of friction and tissue damage.*

Procedures Box 15.1 Passing a nasogastric tube on a child—cont'd

15 Continued

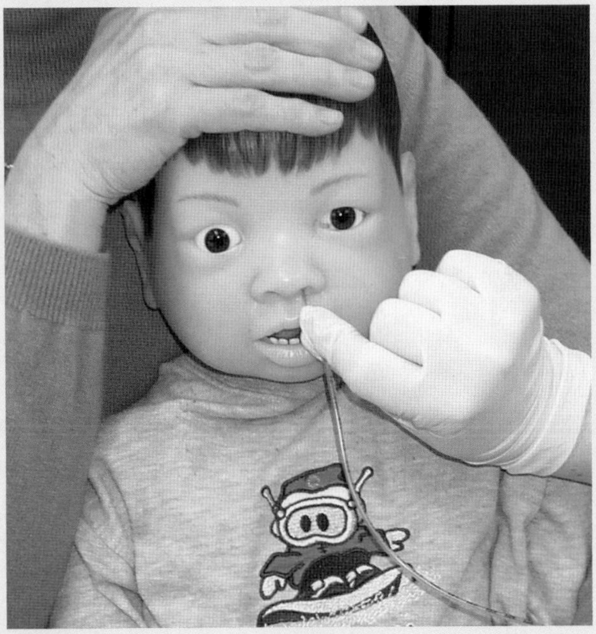

Action
Insert the tip of the tube into the nostril.

Action
Angle the tube slightly upwards and slide it backwards along the floor of the nose into the pharynx.

Reason *Follows the normal contour of the nasal passage.*

16

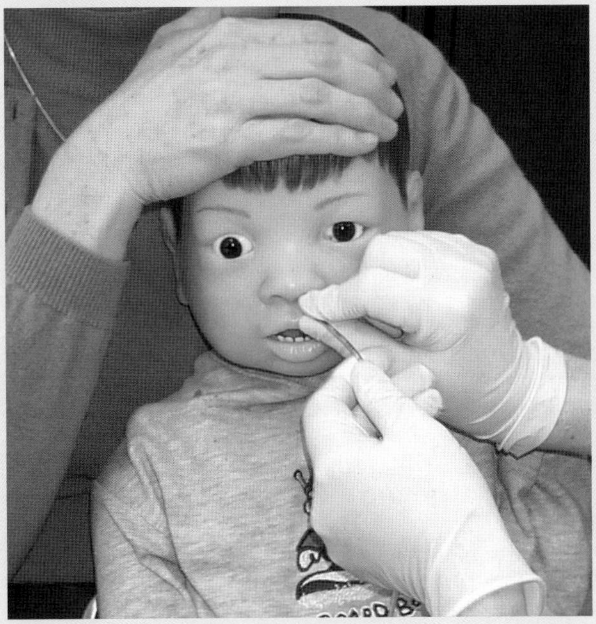

Actions
Continue to gently feed the tube downwards.

As the tube passes to the back of the nose advise the child to take a drink (if appropriate) to help the tube go down or, in the case of babies, offer them a dummy.

In the case of obstruction, pull the tube back, turn it slightly and advance again; if obstruction is felt again try the other nostril.

Actions
A short pause may be necessary for the tube to pass through the cardiac sphincter into the stomach.

The tube should be gently inserted as the child swallows, as this will assist with the movement of the tube and reduce any discomfort.

ALERT
If at any time during this procedure the child starts to cough or his or her colour deteriorates the procedure should be stopped immediately and the tube removed.

17

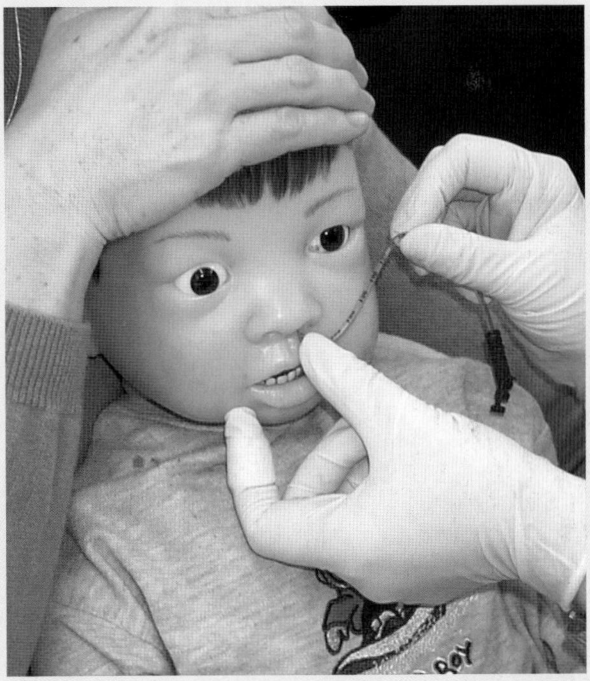

Action
Stop when the point marked on the tube reaches the outer edge of the child's nostril; the tube should be in the stomach.

18

Actions
Ask the person assisting to hold the tube in position.

Check that the nasogastric tube is in the child's stomach.

Remove the end cap.

Using a syringe, aspirate a small amount of gastric contents by gently pulling back on the plunger; detach the syringe and replace the end cap.

Procedures Box 15.1 Passing a nasogastric tube on a child—cont'd

18 Continued

Test the pH of the fluid using pH indicator paper; readings should be less than 5.5.

If any doubt exists on the correct placement of the nasogastric tube then consider repassing the tube or checking the position by X-ray.

Replace the aspirate in infants at risk of electrolyte imbalance.

If there is difficulty obtaining aspirate lie the child on his or her left side and encourage him or her to swallow a small amount of oral fluid, if allowed.

Attempt to push the tube away from the stomach wall by inserting 1–5 mL of *air* down the tube using a 30- or 50-mL syringe.

Try advancing or retracting the tube slightly to alter the position in the stomach.

19

Action
Apply hydrocolloid dressing to the child's cheek and secure the tube using adhesive tape.

Reason *Most children benefit from using a barrier product such as hydrocolloid dressings and transparent films to protect the skin under strong adhesive tapes.*

20

Action
Document the nostril used, size, date and time of insertion.

Reason *PVC tubes lose their flexibility when in contact with gastric secretions and need changing frequently according to the manufacturer's guidance.*

Feeding via a nasogastric tube

Continuous tube feedings are given via an automatic pump to deliver the feed at a specific rate of flow. If the feed is a proprietary brand the full amount of feed should be primed in the administration set to prevent repeated access to the set and reduce bacterial contamination (Patchell et al 1998). If the feed is made locally, i.e. it is not sterile, then the feed bag is filled with formula solution for no more than 4 h at a time (Skipper et al 2003). The enteral pump should be checked to ensure that the alarms are functioning and set to the correct rate and total volume for delivery. Check the nasogastric tube for correct placement every 4 h, and if appropriate aspirate the nasogastric tube to check for formula residual. Refill the formula bag for each 4 h, ensuring that surfaces are cleaned, apron and gloves are worn, and the opening of the administration set and top of the feed container are cleaned using alcohol wipes to prevent bacterial contamination. Observe the child hourly to be sure that the patient is in no distress, the child's abdomen is not distended, the formula is flowing at the correct rate and the tubing connections are secure. Document the amount of feed administered hourly. Refill the bag as necessary or every 4 h. The feeding bag and tubing should be changed according to the local guidelines, usually every 24 h, to prevent bacterial contamination (Anderton 1995).

Procedures Box 15.2 Feeding via a nasogastric tube

Action
Collect the equipment required:

- Plastic apron
- Disposable latex-free gloves
- Cooled boiled water or sterile water for flushing the tube
- Feed of correct type and quantity
- Appropriate size syringe
- Dummy (if appropriate)
- Dishes, spoons, etc., related to feeding for the older infant to play with.

Action
Decontaminate your hands.

Reason *Prevents cross-infection.*

Action
Clean the surface on which the feed is prepared.

Reason *Prevents cross-infection.*

Action
Prepare the feed:

- Check the expiry date
- Check the volume to be given
- Check that the feed is at room temperature
- Shake the feed.

Reason *Ensures safe delivery of feed.*

Action
Explain to the child what is going to happen.

Reason *Promotes psychological support.*

Actions
Ensure that the child is comfortable, with her or his head higher than the stomach either sittng supported for the older infant or, in the younger infant, in a position similar to that of a child being nursed.

If necessary the neonate may be fed lying prone or on the right side (Taylor & Goodison-McLaren 1992).

Reason *Ensures the comfort of the child and prevents aspiration.*

Action
Put on gloves.

Action
Check that the nasogastric tube is correctly positioned according to National Patient Safety Agency guidelines (2005b).

Reason *Ensures safe administration of feed and prevents aspiration of feed into the respiratory tract.*

Actions
Check if it is necessary to assess for residual formula from the last feeding.

Procedures Box 15.2 Feeding via a nasogastric tube—cont'd

Reinstil the gastric aspirate according to the child's care needs.

Reasons *Assesses absorption of previous feed. Prevents acid–base imbalance.*

Actions

Draw up 5–10 mL (depending on the size of the child and fluid status) of cooled boiled or sterile water for flushing the tube in an appropriate size syringe.

Intermittent tube feedings may be given using a large catheter tip syringe or a feeding bag.

Connect the administration set to the nasogastric tube.

Actions

To give the feed using a syringe:

- remove the barrel from the syringe
- open the end of the nasogastric tube and connect it to the end of the syringe
- pour the feeding into the wide end of the syringe and hold to allow the feed to flow by gravity
- top up the barrel of the syringe as the feed empties; do not allow it to empty completely until the feed is completed.

To give an intermittent feed using a feeding bag:

- pour the correct feeding amount into the bag and run it through the tubing connected to the bag down to the tip of the tubing
- clamp the tubing using the roller clamp apparatus
- hang the bag on an intravenous pole just above the child's head
- open the nasogastric tube and connect it to the feeding bag tubing
- open the feeding bag roller clamp apparatus and adjust the flow rate to run the feeding in over a suitable amount of time.

Reason *Prevents air entering the stomach and causing discomfort.*

Action

The feed should take the same amount of time as it would for the child to take the feed orally.

Reason *Prevents discomfort.*

Actions

While feeding, check that the child is comfortable and not showing any signs of discomfort (e.g. retching or vomiting).

Check that the child's breathing and colour are not compromised during feeding.

When the feed is complete clamp the tubing, remove the admistration set, gently flush the nasogastric tube and take the cap off the nasogastric tube.

Clear the equipment and ensure that the child is comfortable.

Replace feeding bags or syringes according to local guidelines to prevent bacterial contamination.

Document the amount, type and time of feed.

Now test your knowledge

- Critically evaluate how you would prepare a 5-year-old child for the insertion of a nasogastric tube. What support and guidance would be required to prepare the parent to assist you in this procedure?
- Carry out a risk assessment for this procedure on a 3-month-old baby with bronchiolitis.
- Consider the consequences of inserting a nasogastric tube into a child following a head injury.

PART C Gastrostomy feeding and tube insertion

Doris A.P. Corkin • Julie A. Chambers

Rationale for gastrostomy feeding

Gastrostomy feeding provides the child and young person with long-term nutritional support in order to maintain good health, growth and healing. Therefore the children's nurse should possess broad knowledge and essential skills in order to facilitate gastrostomy feeding and be competent to teach children, young people and their families the necessary techniques while highlighting the possible effects and risks of gastrostomy feeding (Great Ormond Street Hospital for Children NHS Trust 2000, Green 2005, Hockenberry et al 2003, Huband & Trigg 2000).

Children's nurses are being asked to exercise their clinical judgement when utilising the nursing process to make informed decisions about patient care. However, nutritional care in practice can be inadequate (Grieve & Finnie 2002). Therefore to ensure that a high optimal level of care is achieved, a multidisciplinary approach to care is essential when assessing the special dietary needs of children with different medical conditions such as cerebral palsy and cancer (Goldman et al 2006, Samson-Fang et al 2003). Furthermore the decision to insert a gastrostomy tube is not made lightly, requiring much discussion with the child, family and professionals (e.g. a consultant paediatrician, paediatric surgeon, gastroenterologist, children's nurse, paediatric dietician and clinical psychologist).

A gastrostomy is an artificial opening through the abdomen into the stomach; a gastrostomy feeding tube is then inserted through this opening into the stomach. This procedure can be performed surgically, laparoscopically and endoscopically (Samson-Fang et al 2003) or by radiological techniques (Holmes 2004). Confirmation of gastrostomy tube position using gastric aspirate on a pH indicator strip or paper will continue to be vital for the safe delivery of nutritional supplements and fluids and administration of medications. Generally the introduction to a gastrostomy tube is viewed as a positive event for the child, as the device is hidden under clothing, although there is the possibility that some children can develop a mild irritation and leakage around the gastrostomy tube site, which is uncomfortable for the child and of great concern to the parents.

There are three main types of gastrostomy tube:

1. A percutaneous endoscopic gastrostomy (PEG) tube is a flexible polyurethane tube that is passed down the throat and into the stomach using an endoscope while the child is under a general anaesthetic (Great Ormond Street Hospital for Children NHS Trust 2000). The end of the PEG tube is then brought out through a small incision in the abdomen to allow access for feeding and is secured in place inside the stomach and held against the skin by a fixation device.

   In the first few weeks it is crucial to allow the tract to form, therefore the fixation device or triangle should be moved with caution. However, ensure good care around the site to avoid the fixation device becoming too tight, as this may cause necrosis, and if too loose this may lead to peritonitis. To avoid buried bumper syndrome at 6 weeks the carer may be shown how to open the fixation device and rotate the PEG tube, as cleaning will help prevent the tube from sticking to the surrounding skin. A PEG tube can usually stay in position for about 18 months up to 2 years; however, it must be removed endoscopically and is not suitable for every child. Indications for PEG tube insertion in children include complications of prematurity, faltering growth, cystic fibrosis and administration of an unpalatable diet (Lee et al 2003).

2. A balloon gastrostomy tube is a flexible surgically placed catheter that is inserted through an incision in the abdomen; it is similar to the PEG tube in that it has a long external extension tube, but it has a wider diameter. The main difference is that the section of the tube or catheter that is in the stomach is held in place by an inflatable silicone balloon and may also need to be temporarily secured with sutures to the skin. This tube may be temporary for the first 6–8 weeks and can then be replaced by a balloon device. Surgery is not necessary when removing or changing this tube; however, the doctor or nurse must be trained in the procedure to avoid an admission to hospital (Bunford 2006).

3. A skin-level 'button' device, also known as a balloon retention low-profile gastrostomy tube, is a much shorter tube; the exterior of this device sits flush with the skin, the device has a silicone balloon or mushroom-shaped end that sits inside the stomach, and it is cosmetically pleasing. The child would be measured and the appropriate size of tube fitted by a healthcare professional. Additional attachments are then used for feeding. This device is replaced depending on manufacturers' guidelines and local health policies and is used to replace either a PEG or a balloon gastrostomy tube (Great Ormond Street Hospital for Children NHS Trust 2000). Ensure that there is a replacement device in the child's home or school, as the lifespan of the balloon will vary according to gastric pH, medication, care of the tube and manufacturer's recommendations (e.g. 3–6 months).

Procedures Box 15.3 Replacing a low-profile gastrostomy tube

1

Who will replace the low-profile tube?

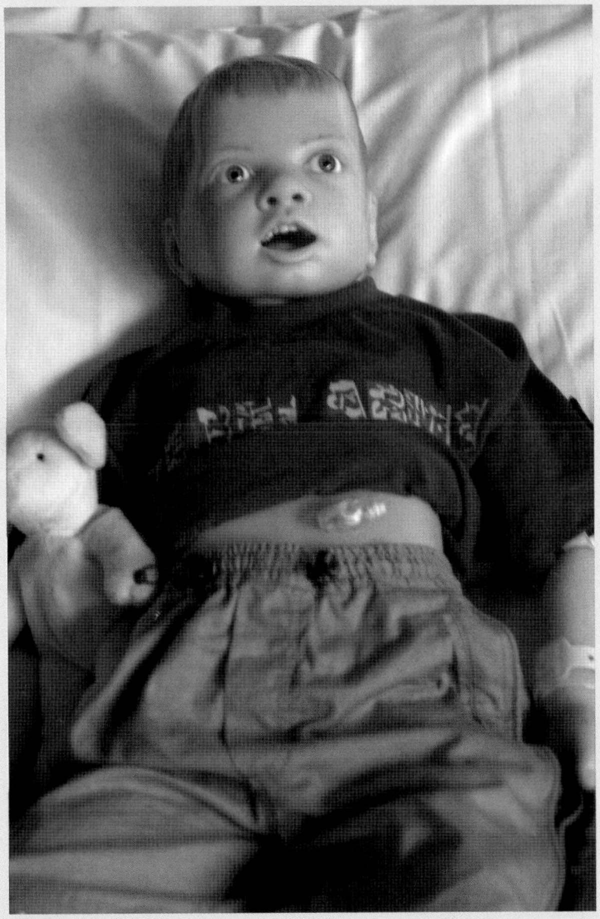

Actions

Generally the nurse specialist/community children's nurse will arrange a suitable time and date with the child and family to replace the low-profile gastrostomy tube (long-term device).

However, should the low-profile tube balloon burst it will need to be replaced within 1–2 h, as the stoma may begin to close; therefore parents may be trained to undertake this procedure in the community setting.

2

Preparing the required equipment

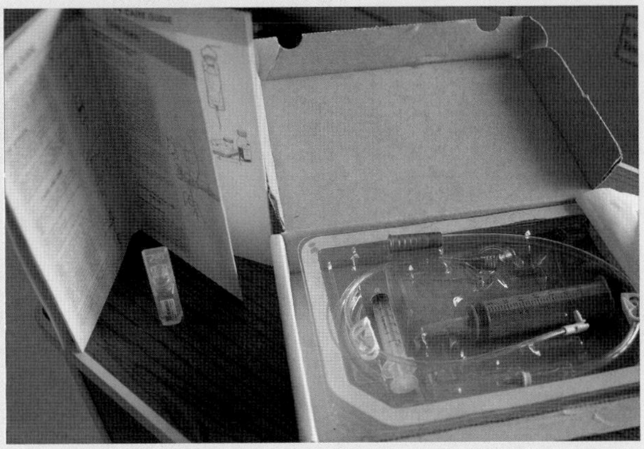

Actions

Put on a plastic apron to prevent cross-infection.

Clean the work surfaces prior to placement of the equipment.

Ensure a suitable low-profile tool kit with manufacturer's instructions.

Use sterile water for the balloon.

Use sterile gloves when handling the tube.

Use sterile water-based lubricant.

Use pH indicator strip or paper.

Use cooled boiled water for the flush.

3

Prior to replacing the low-profile tube

Actions

Explain the procedure to the child and parent in order to obtain their consent and cooperation.

Ensure good hand-washing and drying technique before the application of sterile gloves.

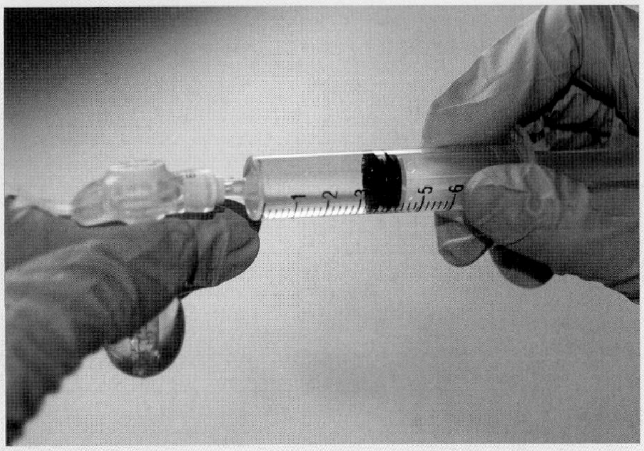

Inflate the balloon of the new low-profile tube with an appropriate amount of sterile water (5–7 mL) as recommended by the manufacturer's guidelines.

4

Checking the low-profile balloon

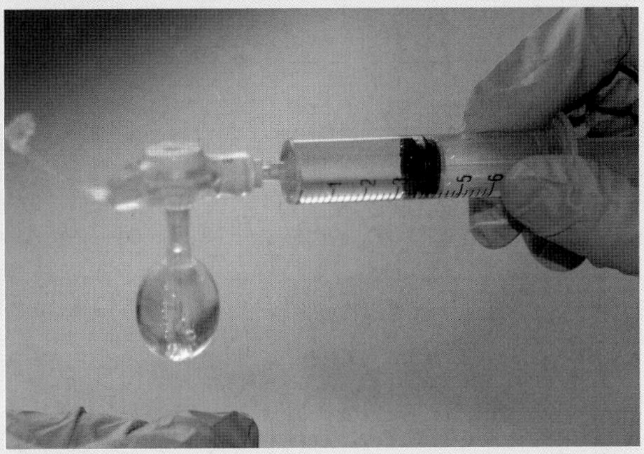

Actions

Remove one hand and observe the balloon for leakage of sterile water.

After checking balloon patency, deflate the balloon by withdrawing water back into the syringe.

Procedures Box 15.3 Replacing a low-profile gastrostomy tube—cont'd

4 Continued

Apply the water-based lubricate to the tip of the new low-profile tube ready for the replacement.

5

Replacing the low-profile tube

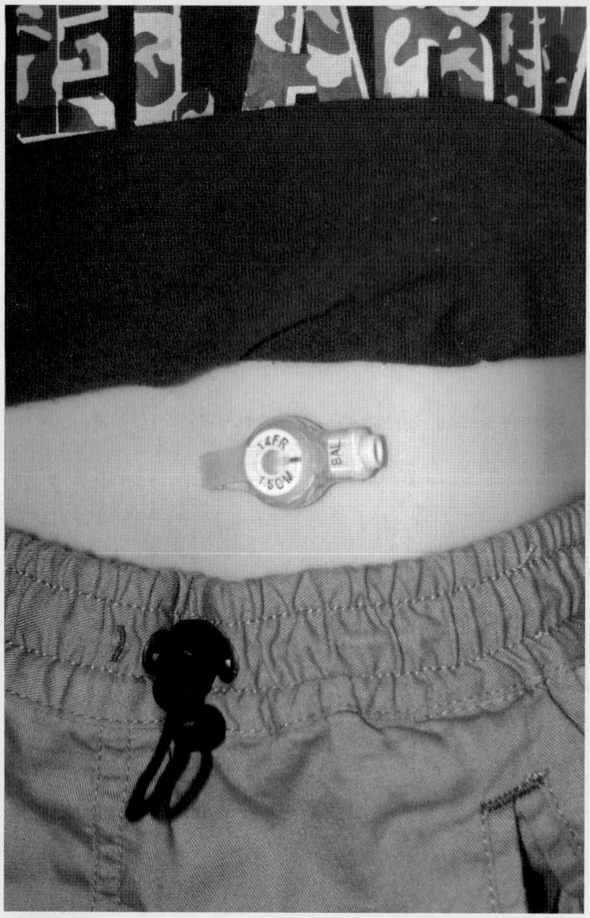

Actions

Attach the Luer tip syringe to the valve that is resting on the child's abdomen.

Pull back on the plunger until all the water is out of the balloon.

Remove the low-profile tube from the child's stomach.

Gently insert the new lubricated tube into the stoma until it is flat against the skin.

6

Securing the new low-profile tube

Actions

Hold the new low-profile tube in place and inflate the balloon with sterile water as recommended, avoiding air.

The balloon device may need to be deflated and inflated weekly to ensure that the correct amount of water remains in the balloon to secure the device.

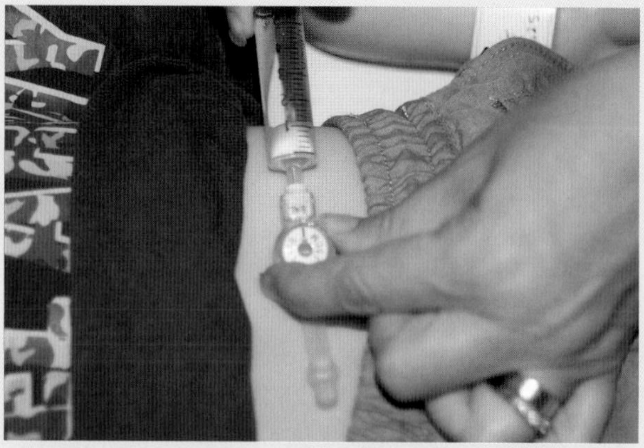

This device may need to be turned daily to help form a healthy stoma and prevent granulation.

7

Checking the tube for correct placement

Actions

Ensure that the new low-profile tube is checked for correct placement.

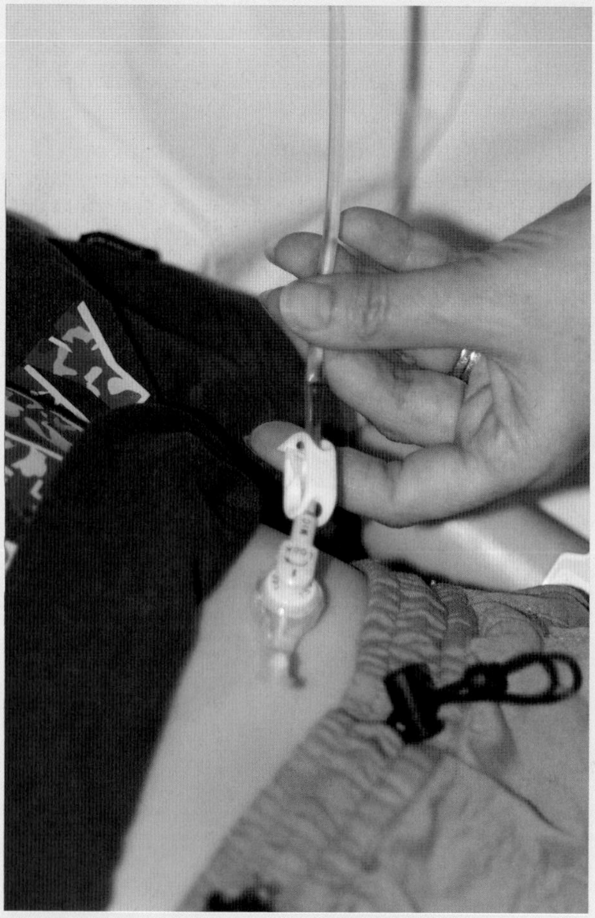

Procedures Box 15.3 Replacing a low-profile gastrostomy tube—cont'd

7 Continued

Choose from the kit an extension set and insert it into the new tube feeding port, align the black lines and rotate the set one-quarter turn clockwise to secure.

Attach a 50-mL syringe to a port at the other end of the extension tube and before feeding obtain 0.5–1 mL of gastric aspirate from the residual stomach contents, then test on a pH indicator strip for pH below 5.5.

8

Preparing a bolus flush via the extension set

Actions

The extension sets have ports to aid bolus flushing, feeding, medications and venting of gas or flatus.

After confirming acceptable pH remove the extension set from the feeding port.

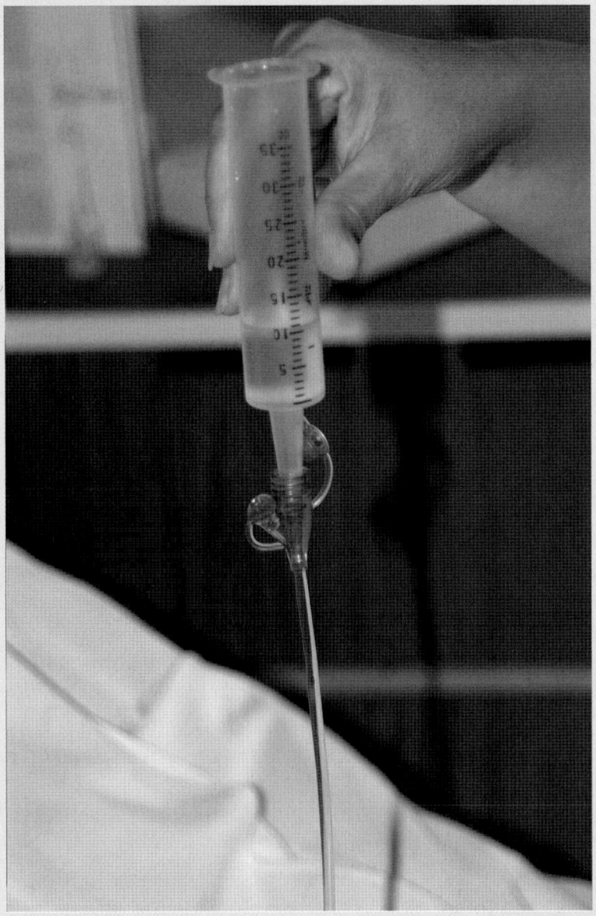

Attach a 50-mL syringe to the extension set and prime the tubing with cooled boiled water, remembering to clamp the extension set next to the locking adapter.

Secure and unclamp the tubing to avoid entry of air into the child's stomach while reattaching into the feeding port of the new tube.

9

Flushing before and after each feed

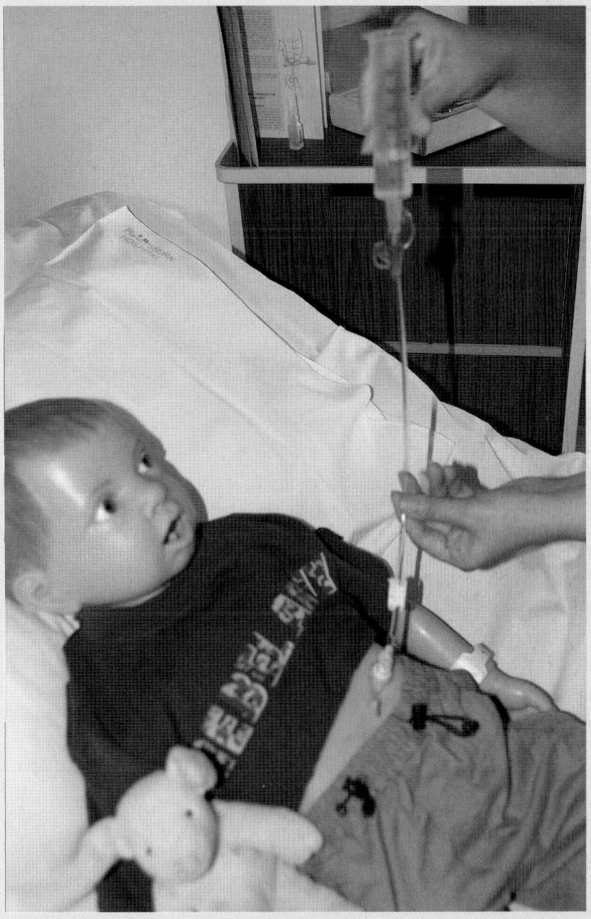

Actions

Ensure at least 10 mL of cooled boiled water flush before and after feed. (This volume must be incorporated into the overall fluid requirements.)

Adjust the flow rate by raising or lowering the attached syringe.

When the syringe is almost empty of water, clamp the extension and either top up with feed or remove the set from the feeding port.

Wash the extension tubing in warm soapy water for reuse as recommended by the manufacturer and organisational policy.

Record the device lot number and expiry date in the child's care plan.

Possible complications of gastrostomy feeding

Complications of PEG tube feeding are infrequent; however, early, local and general problems can occur (Goldman et al 2006). Signs of early complications are haemorrhage, bowel perforation or obstruction, peritonitis, wound separation and local or generalised infection around the stoma site, therefore if blood appears to be mixed with stomach contents call a gastrostomy nurse specialist immediately.

Local problems can be leakage at the stoma site causing skin irritation and superficial skin infection, formation of granulation tissue at the stoma site (Fig. 15.2), tube blockage, accidental tube removal or dislodgement (Fig. 15.3) and discomfort from a migrating internal tube. General issues for discussion with parents are the effects of over-feeding and obesity, the risks of aspiration should vomiting occur, the possibility of diarrhoea, the development of gastro-oesophageal reflux if there is poor gastric emptying, and oral aversion to food.

Leakage of stomach contents

The child may be getting too much feed at one time, causing the stomach to be too full with feed; a build-up of gas may then occur, and this can cause leakage of stomach contents. If the child is being bolus fed consider a trial of continuous feeding and decrease the flow rate on the feeding pump if necessary. Also check the water in a balloon device (5–7 mL), taking care weekly to deflate and inflate the tube, as the tube can be easily pulled out of position.

Over-granulation

Granulation tissue may grow around the gastrostomy site because the body is trying to repair the surgical wound (Fig. 15.2). However, this moist red tissue is not always a sign of infection, and should the stoma site become over-granulated the excess moisture may cause irritation of the surrounding skin and treatment will therefore be required:

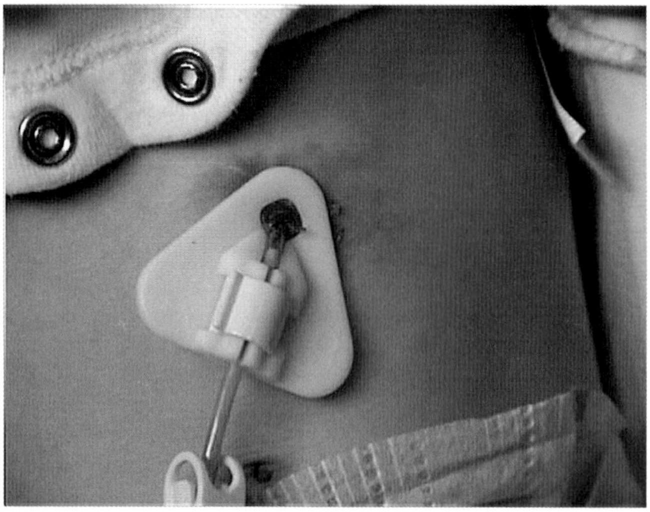

Fig. 15.2 • Granulation tissue at a stoma site.

- Swab the gastrostomy site for the presence of bacteria.
- Control excessive moisture by applying an absorptive dressing around the site, for example Mepilex or Lyofoam (Bunford 2006).
- A steroid-based ointment or antifungal cream may be prescribed for irritated skin (Bunford 2006).
- To reduce the risk of hypergranulation, treatment with silver nitrate sticks may be prescribed (Borkowski 2005, Rollins 2000), for example apply once daily for 5 days; however, care must be taken to protect the surrounding skin with Vaseline.

Tube blockage

Gastrostomy tubes and extension sets can occasionally block with accumulating medicines or feed, therefore great care must be taken to prevent this happening. As the flushing fluid should be water, the type of water will depend on individual risk assessment. Flush before and after each feed as well as before and after giving medications; flushing may indeed be necessary every 4 h.

However, should a tube become blocked first try instilling warm water or fizzy water (Bunford 2006), *but do not use excessive pressure when flushing*. Otherwise use an alkalinised solution of pancreatic enzymes and sodium bicarbonate mix from a pharmacy (Green 2005).

Meticulous care of stoma site

Initially for the first 5 days the stoma site needs to be treated as a wound using an aseptic technique; this is then followed by showering when appropriate. However, the risk of complications will lessen as the skin around the stoma heals:

- Wash your hands thoroughly with soap and water and dry with a clean towel.
- Check the stoma site for signs of leakage, swelling, inflammation, skin breakdown, soreness, movement or lengthening of the gastrostomy tube.
- The stoma site should be cleaned daily with mild soap and warm water and dried thoroughly to prevent excoriation and infection.
- An application of antibiotic ointment may be prescribed to aid healing.
- Securely tape the gastrostomy tube or catheter to the abdomen to prevent an excessive pull on the device, as tension might cause the stoma site to widen, followed by leakage of highly irritating gastric juices.
- The gastrostomy device may need to be rotated daily to help form a healthy stoma and prevent the formation of adhesions.
- Once a stoma site is fully healed, after 2–3 weeks, bathing and swimming are permitted (National Health Service Quality Improvement Scotland 2003).

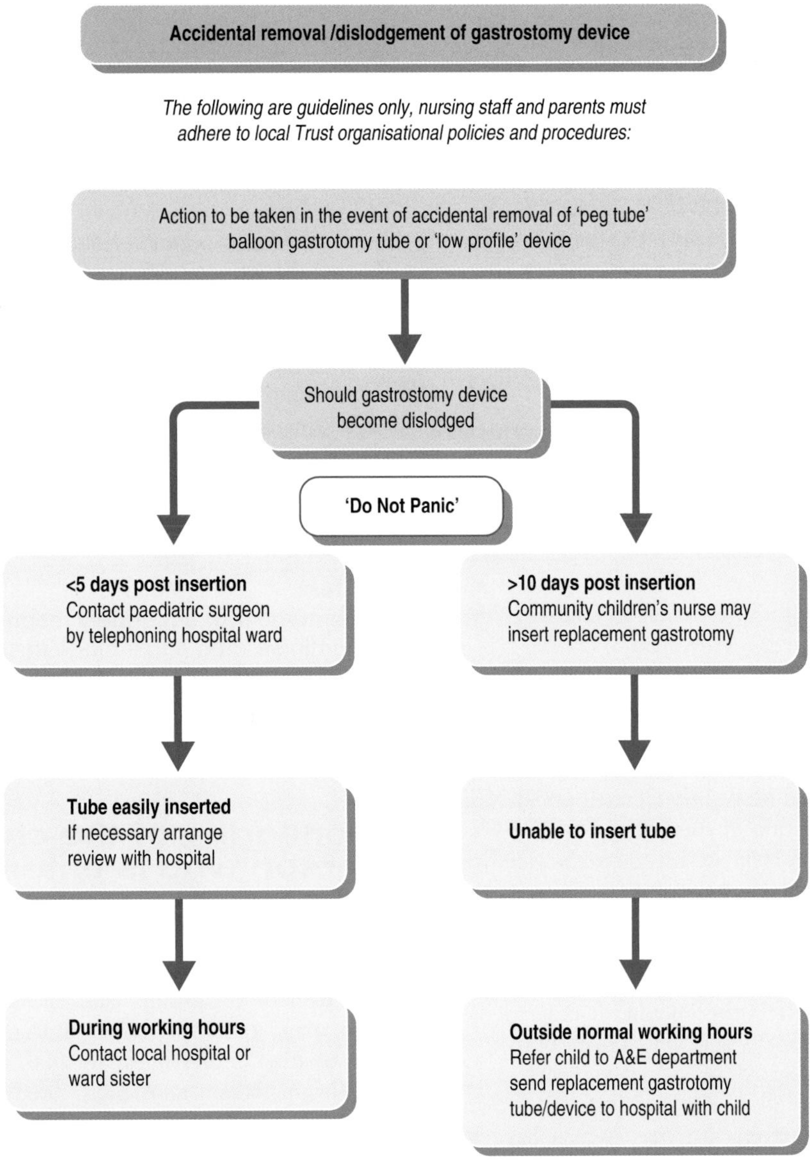

Fig. 15.3 • Algorithm for the accidental removal or dislodgement of a gastrostomy device: guidelines to be used in conjunction with an explanation from a qualified healthcare professional as a pathway of care. These are guidelines only; nursing staff and parents must adhere to local Trust organisational policies and procedures.

Management of enteral feeding

Ensure that the gastrostomy tube is in the correct position before commencing enteral feeding, which can usually be commenced within 12–24 h of tube insertion; however, be sure to check with the surgeon and follow Trust policies and guidelines.

When possible select sterile ready-to-use feeds to which a giving set can be directly attached:

- Feeds should be administered according to the individual enteral feeding regimen, taking lifestyle into consideration (e.g. school routine).
- Feeds may be delivered as a small bolus feed via a 50-mL syringe at set times during the day or as continuous or overnight feeding (e.g. 8–10 h via a feeding pump); a combination of bolus and continuous may even be possible (Bunford 2006, Goldman et al 2006, Green 2005).
- Feeds should be administered at room temperature.

- If the child is being fed while asleep or lying down, the head and shoulders should be raised during feeding and for at to least 1 h after.

LINK CHAPTER 16

Administration of medications via the enteral feeding route

If the child is able to swallow medication orally, then this is the preferred route and the medicine can be administered on a medicine spoon, via an oral syringe or from a medicine cup. However, it is essential that once an oral syringe has been used to administer medication to a child or young person the used oral syringe must not come into contact with the original bottle of medicine again.

At present there are no medications licensed for administration via enteral feeding tubes. Nevertheless, drug administration via this route is often necessary and it is essential to have practical, relevant and authoritative information for those healthcare professionals involved in the drug treatment of children (British National Formulary for Children 2006). Furthermore, children's nurses must be numerically competent in drug calculation, taking the child's weight into consideration, and they should not rely too heavily on calculators; they should also ensure accurate record keeping (Nursing and Midwifery Council 2004, 2005).

Therefore, if administration of medicines is to be via the enteral feeding tube, then it is important to seek advice from a pharmacist to ensure that the most appropriate choice of medicine and formulation is prescribed, as medicines can interact with enteral feeds. A time gap of 1–2 h before and after a feed may be required, as insufficient time between medicine and feed administration can indeed affect the amount of active medicine entering the body (North East Wales NHS Trust 2006).

Medicines that are being administered via enteral feeding tubes should be in liquid or dispersible form and must be measured using coloured oral syringes, which have been designed with a wider neck in order to promote safety. Press-in bungs are also available for medicine bottles to allow easy removal of a dose. Some medicines that cannot be given via an enteral feeding tube are melt and chewable tablets as well as enteric coated or sustained release tablets. Adequate flushing of the enteral feeding tube with water is essential and should be carried out before and after each drug administration to ensure that the full dose of drug is given and that the patency of the enteral feeding tube is maintained.

Children's nurses have a responsibility for assisting in the education of children, young people and their families regarding the safe custody and administration of their medications (Watt 2003). In order to optimise the safe and effective use of medicines it is important that families are given sufficient information to ensure maximum benefit from drug therapy, and this requires a combination of professional competence and best available evidence. The nurse and family should also be aware that medicines require careful labelling and storage in the hospital and home, involving both environment and security factors such as checking the temperature of the fridge and ensuring that the drug cupboard is locked.

Guidelines for the administration of medication via the enteral feeding route are as follows:

- Always check for the correct placement of the feeding tube (pH below 5.5).
- All medicines should have their expiry date checked and be in liquid form when possible, using an elixir or suspension preparation.
- It is important to note the administration time of each medication (i.e. before or after food).
- Medication should be given separately and not mixed or added to the feeding reservoir.
- If administering tablets, crush the tablet to a fine powder and dissolve it in a small amount of sterile water. Never crush enteric coated or sustained release tablets or capsules.
- Avoid oil-based medications because they tend to cling to the side of the tube.

Alert
Remember to accurately record medication administration and include flushing volumes when calculating 24-h total fluid volume to avoid the complication of fluid overload (e.g. in children with cardiac conditions).

Monitoring of the child or young person who is enterally fed

Continuous observation of gastric aspirate, checking for tube misplacement; checking for nausea, for vomiting, for abdominal pain or distension, and the skin condition around the stoma; and recording bowel movements, including history of constipation or diarrhoea, are vital.

Weight, height and length need to be recorded on centile chart as appropriate.

Blood monitoring (urea and electrolytes, full blood count) may be required if the child or young person is feeling unwell, and it is important to ensure communication with the multidisciplinary team.

Dental care

Oral hygiene is an important part of daily living and this should not be overlooked in an enterally fed child or young person, as plaque may build up quickly in the mouth and dental caries will cause pain (Bond & Moss 2003). There is no feeling more uncomfortable than a dry or an unpleasant-tasting mouth, therefore:

- teeth should be cleaned effectively twice a day with a soft toothbrush and toothpaste
- a mouthwash may be used if the child can gargle
- a lubricant such as petroleum jelly can be applied to dry lips
- as with all children, encourage registration with and regular visits to a dentist.

LINK CHAPTER 11

Now test your knowledge

Alice, the youngest of two girls, is now 4 years old and has a history of faltering growth since birth. Following a biopsy she has been diagnosed as having a rare disorder known as multiple allergy to various foods. The dietician has ordered formula elemental Neocate milk, which Alice refuses to drink due to the unpleasant taste. Therefore she was initially fed by an nasogastric tube but now has a gastrostomy button device in situ and is about to be discharged from hospital. Her mum and dad are happy to continue with her care in the home setting with the instrumental support of the community children's nurse:

- Discuss the possible issues for Alice and her family around enteral feeding and the replacement of Alice's gastrostomy button device, highlighting the priorities, management plan and support required from a multidisciplinary perspective.

References

Anderton A (1995) Reducing bacterial contamination in enteral tube feeds. British Journal of Nursing 4(7):368–376

Bond P, Moss D (2003) Best practice in nasogastric and gastrostomy feeding in children. Nursing Times 99(33):28–30

Borkowski S (2005) G tube care: managing hypergranulation tissue. Nursing 35(8):24

British National Formulary for Children (2006) British National Formulary for children 2006. The essential resource for clinical use of medicines in children. BNF, London

Bunford C (2006) Part 2: enteral feeding. In Trigg E, Mohammed TA (eds) Practices in children's nursing: guidelines for hospital and community, 2nd edn. Churchill Livingstone, Edinburgh, p 173

Corkin D, Chambers J (2007) Community children's nursing in Northern Ireland. Paediatric Nursing 19(1):25–27

Corkin DAP, Price J, Gillespie E (2006) Respite care for children, young people and families – are their needs addressed? International Journal of Palliative Nursing 12(9):422–427

Daveluy W, Guimber D, Mention K et al (2004) Home enteral nutrition in children: an 11 year experience with 416 patients. Clinical Nutrition 24(1):48–54

Department of Health (2004a) Chief Medical Officer Update, issue 39. Department of Health, London

Department of Health (2004b) Building a safer NHS for patients: improving medication safety Online. Available: http://www.dh.gov.uk

Dollison EJ, Beckstrand J (1995) Adhesive tape vs pectin-based barrier use in preterm infants. Neonatal Network 14(4):35–39

Ellett ML (2004) What is known about methods of correctly placing gastric tubes in adults and children. Gastroenterology Nursing 27(6):253–259

Ellett ML, Beckstrand J (1999) Examination of gavage tube placement in children. Journal of the Society of Pediatric Nurses 4(2):51–60

Fonseca BK, Holdgate A, Craig JC (2004) Enteral vs intravenous rehydration therapy for children with gastroenteritis. Archives of Pediatrics and Adolescent Medicine 158(5):483–490

Goldman A, Hain R, Liben S (2006) Oxford textbook of palliative care for children. Oxford University Press, Oxford

Great Ormond Street Hospital for Children NHS Trust (2000) Living with a gastrostomy: information for families 13–28. Online. Available: http://www.gosh.nhs.ul/factsheets

Green S (2005) Options and techniques in enteral tube feeding. Clinical Nutritional Update 9(2):6–9

Grieve RJ, Finnie A (2002) Nutritional care: the implications and recommendations for nursing. British Journal of Nursing 11(7):432–437

Hockenberry MJ, Wilson D, Winkelstein ML, Kline ME (2003) Wong's nursing care of infants and children, 7th edn. Mosby, London

Holden C, Sexton E, Lesley P (1997) Enteral nutrition for children. Nursing Standard 11(32):49–54

Holmes S (2004) Enteral feeding and percutaneous gastrostomy. Nursing Standard 18(20):41–43

Huband S, Trigg E (2000) Practices in children's nursing: guidelines for hospital and community. Churchill Livingstone, Edinburgh

Klasner AE, Luke DA, Scalzo AJ (2002) Pediatric orogastric and nasogastric tubes: a new formula evaluated. Annals of Emergency Medicine 39:268–272

Lee ACH, Carter HP, Crabbe D (2003) Percutaneous endoscopic gastrostomy: procedure in practice. British Journal of Perioperative Nursing 13(7):298–305

Medicines and Healthcare products Regulatory Agency (2004) Medical device alert MDA/2004/026. Enteral feeding tubes (nasogastric). MHRA, London

Metheny NA, Stewart BJ (2002) Testing feeding tube placement during continuous tube feedings. Applied Nursing Research 15(4):254–258

Metheny N, Dettenmeier P, Hampton K, Wiersema L, Williams P (1990) Detection of inadvertent respiratory placement of small-bore feeding tubes: a report of 10 cases. Heart and Lung: the Journal of Acute Critical Care 19(6):631–638

Metheny NA, Reed L, Berglund B, Wehrle MA (1994) Visual characteristics of aspirates from feeding tubes as a method for predicting feeding tube placement. Nursing Research 43(5):282–287

Metheny NA, Whrie MA, Wiersama L, Clark J (1998a) Testing feeding tube placement:ausculatation vs pH method. American Journal of Nursing 98(5):37–43

Metheny NA, Wehrle MA, Wiersema L, Clark J (1998b) pH, color, and feeding tubes. Registered Nurse 61(1):25–27

Metheny NA, Eikov R, Rountree V, Lengettie E (1999) Indicators feeding-tube placement in neonates. Nutrition in Clinical Practice 14(5):307-314

Metheny NA, Smith L, Stewart BJ (2000) Development of a reliable and valid bedside test for bilirubin and its utility for improving prediction of feeding tube location. Nursing Research 49(6):302–309

National Health Service Quality Improvement Scotland (2003) Nasogastric and gastrostomy feeding for children being cared for in the community. Best practice statement. Nursing and Midwifery Practice Development Unit, Edinburgh

National Patient Safety Agency (2005a) How to confirm the correct position of nasogastric feeding tubes in infants, children and adults. NHS. Online. Available: http://www.npsa.nhs.uk/advice

National Patient Safety Agency (2005b) Reducing the harm caused by misplaced nasogastric feeding tubes. Interim advice for health care staff. NHS, London

North East Wales NHS Trust (2006) Guidelines for administration of medication to patients with enteral feeding tubes or swallowing difficulties. NEWT, Wrexham

Northern Ireland Adverse Incident Centre (2004) Medical device/equipment alert. Enteral feeding tubes (nasogastric). Online. Available: http://www.dhsspsni.gov.uk/niaic

Nursing and Midwifery Council (2004) Guidelines for the administration of medicines. NMC, London

Nursing and Midwifery Council (2005) Guidelines for records and record keeping. NMC, London

Patchell C, Anderton A, Holden C (1998) Reducing bacterial contamination of enteral feeds. Archives of Disease in Childhood 78:166–168

Penrod J, Morse JM, Wilson S (1999) Comforting strategies used during nasogastric tube insertion. Journal of Clinical Nursing 8(1):31–38

Rollins H (2000) Hypergranulation tissue at gastrostomy sites. Journal of Wound Care 9(3):127–129

Rollins H (2006) The psychosocial impact on parents of tube feeding their child. Paediatric Nursing 18(4):19–22

Samson-Fang L, Butler C, O'Donnell M (2003) Effects of gastrostomy feeding in children with cerebral palsy: an AACPDM evidence report. Developmental Medicine and Child Neurology 45:415–426

Skipper L, Cuffng J, Pratelli N (2003) Enteral feeding infection control guidelines. Infection Control Nurses Association, London

Smith L, Coleman V, Bradshaw M (2002) Family-centred care: concept, theory and practice. Palgrave, Basingstoke

Stephens N (2005) Complex care packages: supporting seamless discharge for child and family. Paediatric Nursing 17(7):30–32

Taylor S, Goodison-McLaren S (1992) Nutritional support – a team approach. Wolfe Publishing, London, p 258–273

Thomas BW, Falcone RE (1998) Confirmation of nasogastric tube placement by colorimetric indicator detection of carbon dioxide: a preliminary report. Journal of the American College of Nutrition 17(2):195–197

Townsley R, Robinson C (2000) Food for thought? Effective support for families caring for a child who is tube fed. Norah Fry Research Centre, Bristol

Viasys (2000) Effect of syringe pressure on Viasys feeding tubes, protocol #170. Viasys, Conshohocken

Watt S (2003) Safe administration of medicines to children: part 1. Paediatric Nursing 15(4):40–43

Westhus N (2004) Methods to test feeding tube placement in children. MCN: the American Journal of Maternal Child Nursing 29(5):282–289

Appendix 15.1 Checking the position of the naso- and orogastric feeding tube in babies under the care of neonatal units

Action
Check for signs of tube displacement (if not initial insertion).

Reasons *The tube may have coiled up in the mouth, or if there is more tube visible than previously documented the tube may have kinked.*
Loose tape may indicate movement.
If the tube has been displaced it will need repositioning or repassing before feeding.

Action
Aspirate 0.2–1 mL of gastric fluid and allow 10–15 s for any colour change.

Reason *Between 0.2 and 1 mL of aspirate will cover an adequate area on single-, double- or triple-reagent panels of pH testing strips or paper.*

Action
Aspirate using a syringe.

Reason *It is safe practice to use gastric tubes and enteral syringes that have non-Luer lock connectors (Department of Health 2004b).*

Action
If the aspirate is pH 5.5 or below, PROCEED TO FEED.

Reasons *Aspirates testing pH 5.5 and below should indicate correct placement in most babies (including the majority of those receiving acid suppressants) and rule out the possibility of respiratory tract placement.*
Always match the pH indicator strip or paper colour change with the colour code chart on the booklet or box; if there is ANY doubt about the position and/or clarity of the colour change on the pH indicator strip or paper, particularly between pH 5 and 6, DO NOT commence feeding.

Actions
If the aspirate is pH 6 or above, CAUTION – STOP THE FEED.

If clinically safe, consider waiting 15–30 min before aspirating again.

Consider replacing and/or repassing the tube and reaspirating.

If the aspirate is still pH 6 or above, seek advice.

IT IS IMPORTANT THAT STAFF FOLLOW THE FLOWCHART, RECORD THE OUTCOMES AND MAKE DECISIONS BASED ON THIS INFORMATION.

Reasons *The most likely reason for failure to obtain gastric aspirate of pH 5.5 or below is the dilution of gastric acid by enteral feed; waiting gives time for the stomach to empty and the pH value to fall.*
If the pH is still 6 and above after waiting and replacing or repassing the tube, seek advice and consider the following questions.

- *Is the baby on medication?*
- *Is the baby only 24–48 h old?*
- *Is the tube in the same position as previously documented on an X-ray?*
- *Is the visible length of the tube the same as previously documented?*
- *What is the trend in pH values?*
- *What is the volume of aspirate?*

It is important that actions and their rationale are documented. Clinical staff should balance the risks of not feeding a baby in the short term with feeding when there is the possibility of the tube being in the lungs.
Consider an X-ray only if timely, for example if the baby is due for an X-ray for other reasons and/or it is clinically safe to do so.
If an X-ray is done, the radiographer should know this advice has been followed and the reason for the request should be documented.

Action
Document all information.

Reasons *Documenting helps the clinical decision-making process.*
The tube size and length should be recorded each time the tube is passed.
A record should also be made each time measurements of the pH level of the aspirate and the length of the tube's advancement or retraction are done.

Actions
Problems obtaining aspirate: suggest using larger size tubes with multiple ports.

Turn the baby on to his or her side.

Reason *This may facilitate the tip of the nasogastric tube entering the gastric fluid pool.*

Action
Inject 1–2 mL of air using a syringe; this is NOT a testing procedure.

Reasons *Injecting air through the tube may dislodge the exit port of the feeding tube from the gastric mucosa.*
Care must be taken when using large syringes on neonates to ensure that the correct amount of air is inserted, i.e. no more than 2 mL.

Actions
Advance or retract the tube by 1–2 cm.

Stop if there is any resistance or obstruction.

Reasons *If the tube is in the oesophagus, advancing it may allow it to pass into the stomach.*
If the tube has been inserted too far, it may be in the duodenum.
Consider withdrawing a few centimetres and reaspirating.

The position of the tube at the nose should already have been recorded and marked if the tube is in situ. *If the mark has not moved then advancing or retracting may not make a difference.* *Document the length of the tube if moved.*	
Action If you still cannot obtain aspirate.	**Reasons** *If this is an initial insertion then consider replacing or repassing the tube.* *If the tube has been in situ already, seek advice.* *Consider whether the length of the tube has changed and discuss options as outlined under the action point on aspirate of pH 6 and above.* *Record all decisions and their rationale.*

(After National Patient Safety Agency 2005b, with permission.)

Appendix 15.2 Reducing the harm caused by misplaced gastric feeding tubes in babies under the care of neonatal units

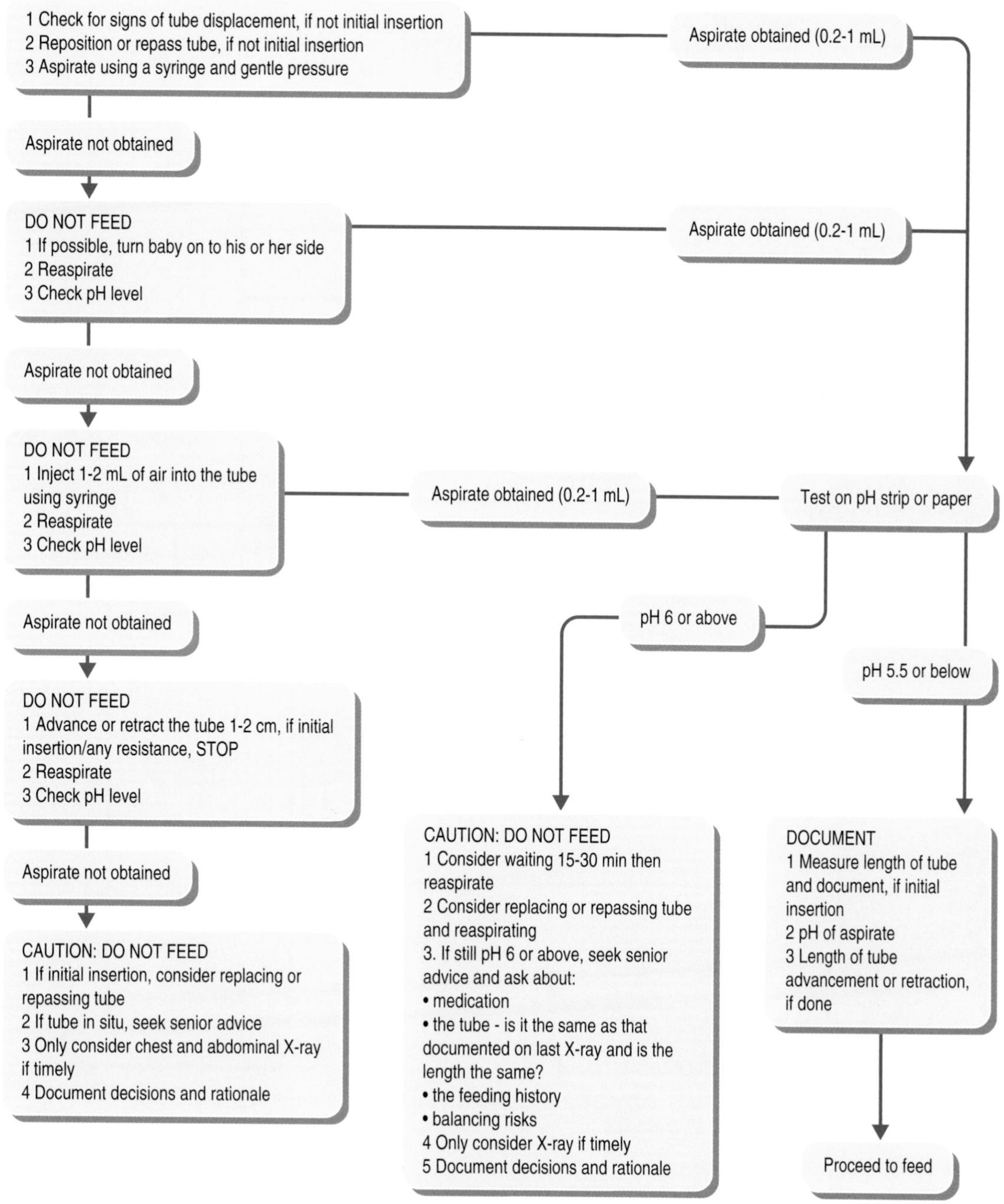

1 Check for signs of tube displacement, if not initial insertion
2 Reposition or repass tube, if not initial insertion
3 Aspirate using a syringe and gentle pressure
Aspirate obtained (0.2-1 mL)
Aspirate not obtained
DO NOT FEED
1 If possible, turn baby on to his or her side
2 Reaspirate
3 Check pH level
Aspirate obtained (0.2-1 mL)
Aspirate not obtained
DO NOT FEED
1 Inject 1-2 mL of air into the tube using syringe
2 Reaspirate
3 Check pH level
Aspirate obtained (0.2-1 mL)
Test on pH strip or paper
Aspirate not obtained
pH 6 or above
pH 5.5 or below
DO NOT FEED
1 Advance or retract the tube 1-2 cm, if initial insertion/any resistance, STOP
2 Reaspirate
3 Check pH level
Aspirate not obtained
CAUTION: DO NOT FEED
1 If initial insertion, consider replacing or repassing tube
2 If tube in situ, seek senior advice
3 Only consider chest and abdominal X-ray if timely
4 Document decisions and rationale
CAUTION: DO NOT FEED
1 Consider waiting 15-30 min then reaspirate
2 Consider replacing or repassing tube and reaspirating
3. If still pH 6 or above, seek senior advice and ask about:
• medication
• the tube - is it the same as that documented on last X-ray and is the length the same?
• the feeding history
• balancing risks
4 Only consider X-ray if timely
5 Document decisions and rationale
DOCUMENT
1 Measure length of tube and document, if initial insertion
2 pH of aspirate
3 Length of tube advancement or retraction, if done
Proceed to feed

CAUTION: if there is ANY query about position and/or the clarity of the colour change on the pH strip, particularly between ranges 5-6, then feeding should not commence.

(After the National Patient Safety Agency 2005b, with permission.)

Appendix 15.3 Confirming the correct position of nasogastric feeding tubes in adults

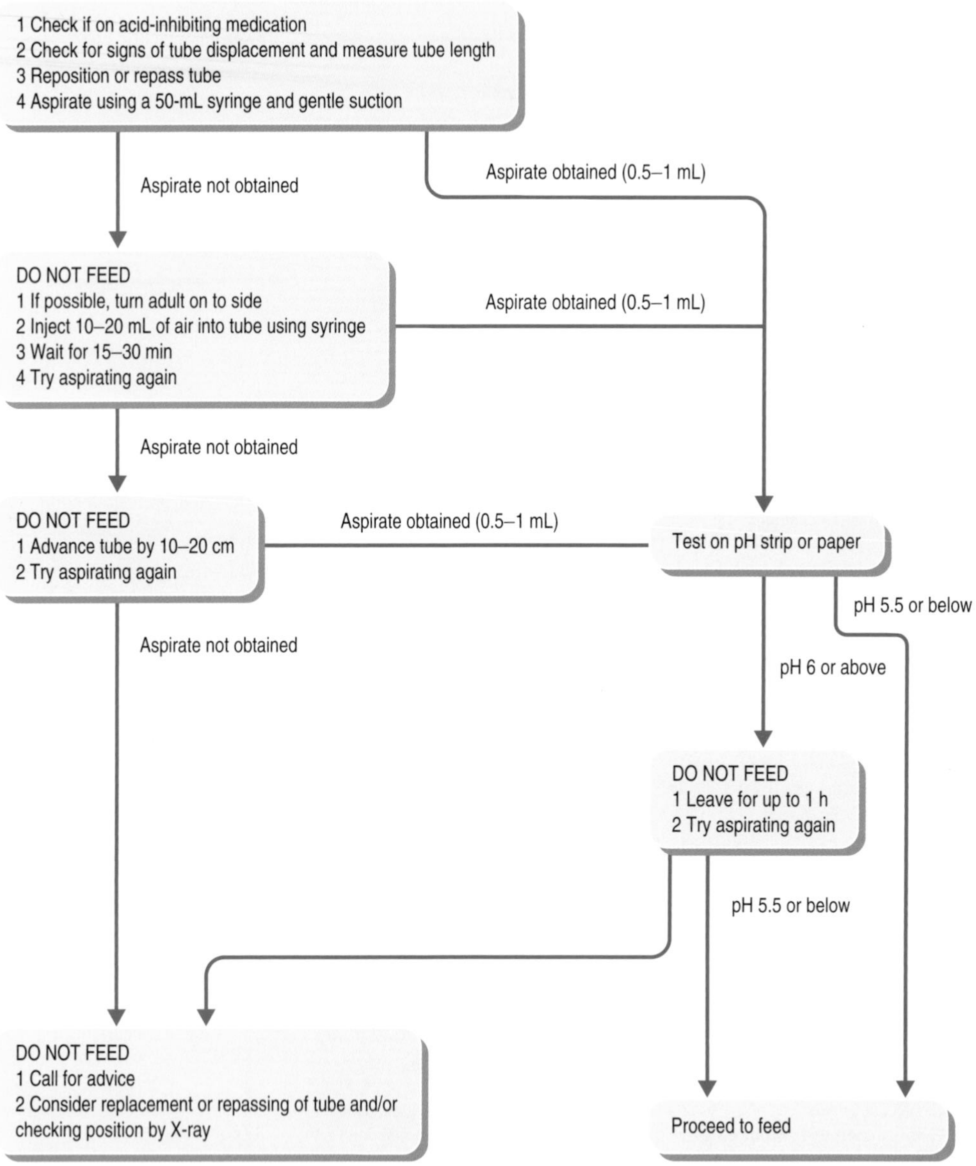
1 Check if on acid-inhibiting medication
2 Check for signs of tube displacement and measure tube length
3 Reposition or repass tube
4 Aspirate using a 50-mL syringe and gentle suction
Aspirate not obtained
Aspirate obtained (0.5–1 mL)
DO NOT FEED
1 If possible, turn adult on to side
2 Inject 10–20 mL of air into tube using syringe
3 Wait for 15–30 min
4 Try aspirating again
Aspirate obtained (0.5–1 mL)
Aspirate not obtained
DO NOT FEED
1 Advance tube by 10–20 cm
2 Try aspirating again
Aspirate obtained (0.5–1 mL)
Test on pH strip or paper
pH 5.5 or below
Aspirate not obtained
pH 6 or above
DO NOT FEED
1 Leave for up to 1 h
2 Try aspirating again
pH 5.5 or below
DO NOT FEED
1 Call for advice
2 Consider replacement or repassing of tube and/or checking position by X-ray
Proceed to feed

CAUTION: if there is ANY query about position and/or the clarity of the colour change on the pH strip, particularly between ranges 5–6, then feeding should not commence.

(After the National Patient Safety Agency 2005b, with permission.)

Appendix 15.4

Confirming the correct position of nasogastric feeding tubes in infants and children

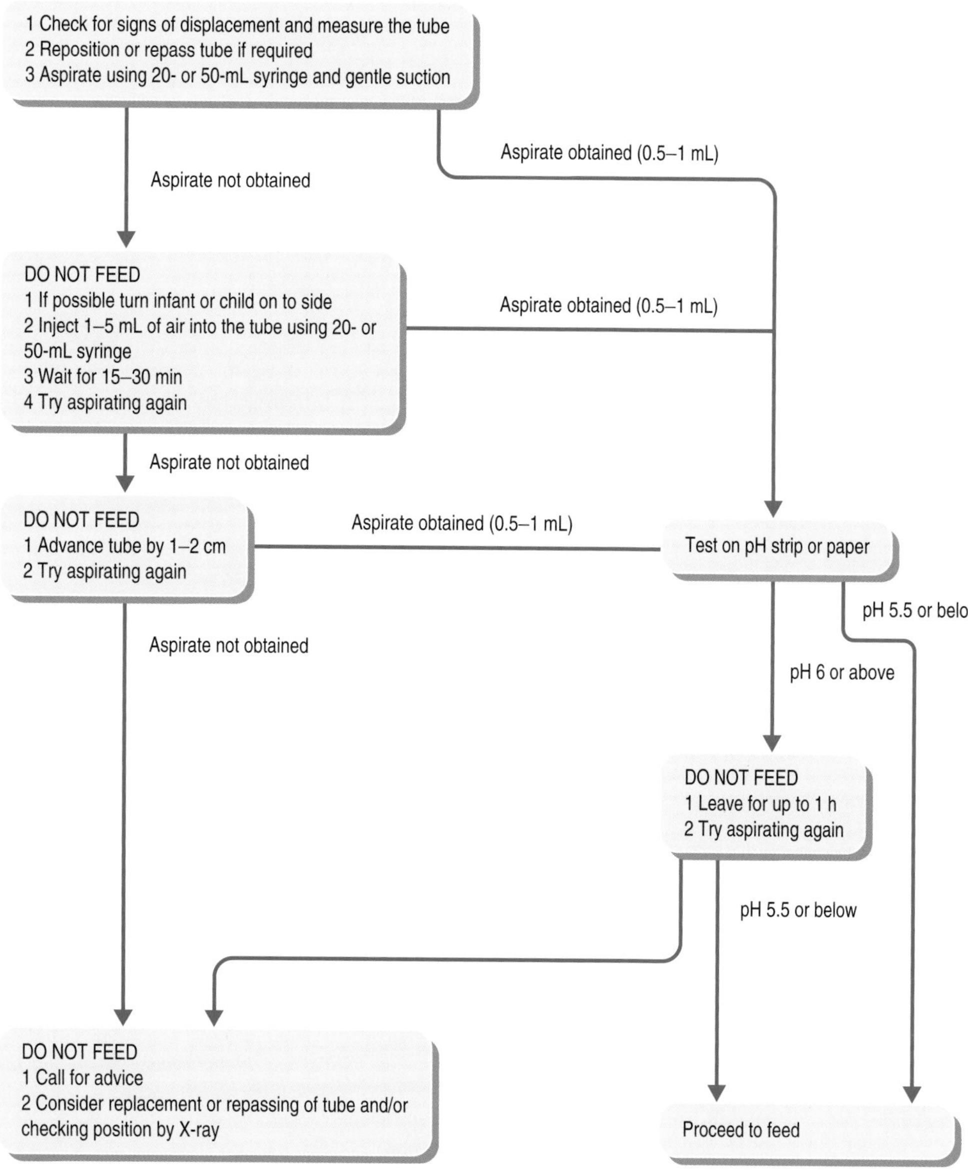
1 Check for signs of displacement and measure the tube
2 Reposition or repass tube if required
3 Aspirate using 20- or 50-mL syringe and gentle suction
Aspirate obtained (0.5–1 mL)
Aspirate not obtained
DO NOT FEED
1 If possible turn infant or child on to side
2 Inject 1–5 mL of air into the tube using 20- or 50-mL syringe
3 Wait for 15–30 min
4 Try aspirating again
Aspirate obtained (0.5–1 mL)
Aspirate not obtained
DO NOT FEED
1 Advance tube by 1–2 cm
2 Try aspirating again
Aspirate obtained (0.5–1 mL)
Test on pH strip or paper
pH 5.5 or below
Aspirate not obtained
pH 6 or above
DO NOT FEED
1 Leave for up to 1 h
2 Try aspirating again
pH 5.5 or below
DO NOT FEED
1 Call for advice
2 Consider replacement or repassing of tube and/or checking position by X-ray
Proceed to feed

CAUTION: if there is ANY query about position and/or the clarity of the colour change on the pH strip, particularly between ranges 5–6, then feeding should not commence.

(After the National Patient Safety Agency 2005b, with permission.)

Appendix 15.5 Checking the position of nasogastric feeding tubes in infants, children and adults

Action
Check whether the patient is on medication that may increase the pH level of the gastric contents.

Reasons *Medication that could elevate the pH level of gastric contents are antacids, H_2 antagonists and proton pump inhibitors.*
For those patients who are regularly on antacids, the initial risk assessment needs to identify actions that staff should take in this scenario and document them in the care plan; the initial pH of the aspirate should also be documented in the case notes.

Action
Check for signs of tube displacement.

Reasons *Documenting the external length of the tube initially and checking external markings prior to feeding will help to determine if the tube has moved.*
The documentation will also assist radiographers if an X-ray is needed.

Action
Sufficient aspirate (0.5–1 mL) is obtained.

Reasons *Between 0.5 and 1 mL of aspirate will cover an adequate area on the single-, double- or triple-reagent panels of pH testing strips or paper.*
Allow 10 s for any colour change to occur.

Action
The aspirate is pH 5.5 or below: COMMENCE THE FEED.

Reasons *There are no known reports of pulmonary aspirates at or below this figure.*
The range of pH 0 to 5.5 balances the risk between increasing the potential problems for clinical staff, for example removing tubes that are actually in the stomach and increased use of X-ray, with the as yet unreported possibility of feeding at pH 5.5 when the tube is in the respiratory tract.

Action
Aspirate is pH 6 or above: DO NOT FEED.

Reasons *There is possible bronchial secretion: leave up to 1 h and try again.*
The initial risk assessment should identify actions for staff to take in this scenario for each patient.
The actions should be documented in the care plan and/or in local policies.
If there is ANY doubt about the position and/or the clarity of the colour change on the pH indicator strip or paper, particularly between the range pH 5 and 6, then feeding should NOT commence – seek advice.

Action
Wait up to 1 h before reaspirating to check the pH level.

Reasons *The most likely reason for failure to obtain gastric aspirate below pH 5.5 is the dilution of gastric acid by enteral feed; waiting for up to an hour will allow time for the stomach to empty and the pH to fall.*
The time interval will depend on the clinical need of the patient and whether or not she or he is on continuous or bolus feeds.

Problems obtaining aspirate?

Action
Turn the patient on to his or her side.

Reason *This will allow the tip of the nasogastric tube to enter the gastric fluid pool.*

Actions
Inject air (1–5 mL for infants and children, 10–20 mL for adults) using a 20-mL or 50-mL syringe.

Wait for 15–30 min and try again.

This is NOT a testing procedure.

DO NOT carry out auscultation of air (the whoosh test) to test tube position.

Reasons *Injecting air through the tube will dispel any residual fluid (feed, water or medicine) and may also dislodge the exit port of the nasogastric feeding tube from the gastric mucosa.*
Using a large syringe allows gentle pressure and suction; smaller syringes may produce too much pressure and split the tube (check manufacturer's guidelines).
Polyurethane syringes are preferable to other syringes.
It is safe practice to use nasogastric tubes and enteral syringes that have non-Luer connectors (Department of Health 2004b).

Action
Advance the tube by 1–2 cm for infants and children or 10–20 cm for adults.

Reason *Advancing the tube may allow it to pass into the stomach if it is in the oesophagus.*

Action
Consider X-ray; all radiographs should be read by appropriately trained staff.

Reasons *X-ray should not be used routinely.*
The radiographer will need to know that this advice has been followed, what the problem has been and the reason for the request; the radiographer should document this.
Fully radiopaque tubes with markings to enable measurement, identification and documentation of their external length should be used.

Action
Additional tip: if the patient is alert, has intact swallow and is perhaps only on supplementary feeding and is therefore eating and drinking during the day, ask her or him to sip a coloured drink and aspirate the tube.

Reason *If you get the coloured fluid back then you know the tube is in the stomach.*

(After National Patient Safety Agency 2005b, with permission.)

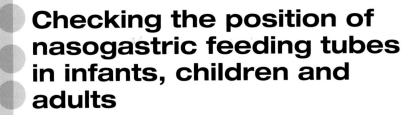

16 Administration of medicines

Louise Holliday • Carla Kierulff

The safe administration of medicines involves five 'rights': the right dose, of the right drug, to the right patient, via the right route, at the right time. This requires the nurse to:

- understand the therapeutic effect and possible side effects of the medicine
- ascertain the recommended dosage range
- be accurate in calculating dosages
- assess the individual patient's condition and any contraindications to him or her receiving the prescribed medicine
- check if the patient has any known allergies, including reactions to any excipients (ingredients used in the formulation to stabilise the active ingredient or to modify its release)
- know what other medicines the patient is receiving and be aware of possible interactions or incompatibilities
- accurately check the patient's identity
- deliver the medicine safely via the prescribed route
- administer the medicine at the prescribed times
- make clear, accurate and immediate records of when any medicine is administered to, intentionally withheld from or refused by the patient
- observe the patient's response during and after drug administration
- act promptly and appropriately if the patient has an adverse reaction (British National Formulary for Children 2007, Nursing and Midwifery Council 2004).

Self-administration

In the community, children and young people generally administer their own medicine with assistance and/or supervision from their parents or carers as required. Similar arrangements are now being introduced into some in-patient units; reported benefits of this practice include more individualised care, empowerment of children and their parents or carers, increased adherence and smoother discharge from hospital to home (Wright et al 2002). The nurse's role in such a setting is more about educating and facilitating and less about actually giving the medicine (Nursing and Midwifery Council 2004).

Obtaining consent and cooperation from children

LINK CHAPTER 1

Many children will be competent to give informed consent to treatment if information is presented to them in an appropriate way (Department of Health 2001, Scottish Executive Health Department 2006). If they are prepared adequately and their preferences are considered, they are more likely to accept the medication (Willock et al 2004). Consent must be obtained without duress, force or fraud (Dimond 1996, Scottish Executive Health Department 2006). When refusal of treatment is consistent, valid and informed but would be likely to result in serious and avoidable damage to a young person's health, legal advice should be sought (British Medical Association 2001).

LINK CHAPTER 1

When the child's safety and well-being may be compromised by delay, holding still may be the preferred option (Royal College of Nursing 2003).

Toddlers and babies who are too young to understand explanations and to cooperate may be held securely but not too tightly (Willock et al 2004). Wrapping a young child or infant in a light blanket (bunny wrapping) may provide comfort as well as effective control.

LINK CHAPTER 6

Dosages for children

There is huge variation from the neonatal period through to adolescence in the way children absorb, metabolise and excrete drugs (Baber & Pritchard 2003). For various commercial, ethical and practical reasons most medicines were designed for adults, until recent legislation encouraged drug companies to conduct more paediatric studies and to seek paediatric marketing authorisations (licenses) for new and existing drugs (Grieve et al 2005). Many children, particularly neonates, are prescribed medicines that are not specifically licensed for use at their age.

If a product is not specifically marketed for paediatric use, it is unlikely to be available in a suitable formulation for children (Nunn & Williams 2005). This could mean that capsules and tablets that were designed to be swallowed whole by an adult need to be split. This could potentially reduce the drug's effect or increase its toxicity when splitting an enteric coating (Baber & Pritchard 2003). A further problem could occur when there is uneven distribution of the drug within the tablet, resulting in dosage errors.

ALERT
There is also a potential risk that errors in dosage calculation might not be detected by the practitioner drawing up the dose if suitable strengths of medications are not manufactured, for example 10-fold errors can occur when an ampoule that contains more than 10 times the required dose is used to draw up an injection for a neonate (Chappell & Newman 2004).

Double-checking complex calculations and administration of high-risk drugs such as cytotoxics are perceived as effective interventions for reducing medication errors within hospitals (Miller et al 2006). It is the practice in many hospitals that two nurses check all drugs for children. However, it is unclear how effective and efficient this is compared with single-nurse administration (O'Shea 1999).

LINK CHAPTER **17**

It is vital to obtain an accurate weight. Checking the correct dosage for a particular child often requires multiplying a standardised dose by the child's weight in kilograms. (Please note there is often a set maximum dose regardless of the child's weight.) The dose may need to be reduced if the child has impaired renal or hepatic function. In overweight children the correct dose for most drugs should be calculated not from their actual weight but from their ideal weight calculated from their height and age (Cheymol 2000).

Surface area is required for calculating some doses, for example in cytotoxic chemotherapy. Body surface area estimates can be made from nomograms published in the *British National Formulary for Children*. In general, developmental differences in physiology between adults and children correlate more closely with surface area than with body weight (Baber & Pritchard 2003).

Accurate identification of patients

Increasing numbers of hospitals are implementing barcoding or radiofrequency identification on wristbands to try to prevent errors in patient identification (National Patient Safety Agency 2005). However, wristband mix-ups may occur and computer systems may have the effect of weakening human vigilance (McDonald 2006). It is recommended that, whenever possible, two forms of identification are used – asking patients their name and date of birth *and* checking the wristband – before any medicine is administered (McDonald 2006, National Patient Safety Agency 2005).

ALERT
Particular vigilance is required in maintaining accurate wristbands on patients who are unable to confirm their own identity (National Patient Safety Agency 2005).

Routes of administration

Oral

Liquid preparations are most appropriate for infants and young children. Doses of 5 mL, or multiples of 5 mL, may be measured using a medicine spoon (Fig. 16.1) or medicine cup (Fig. 16.2) (British National Formulary for Children 2007).

An oral syringe (Fig. 16.3) should be used to draw up other amounts accurately and to administer the medicine in a controlled way.

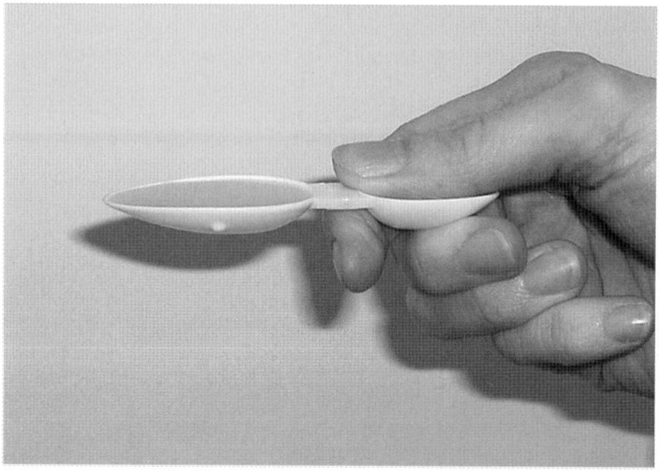

Fig. 16.1 • A medicine spoon.

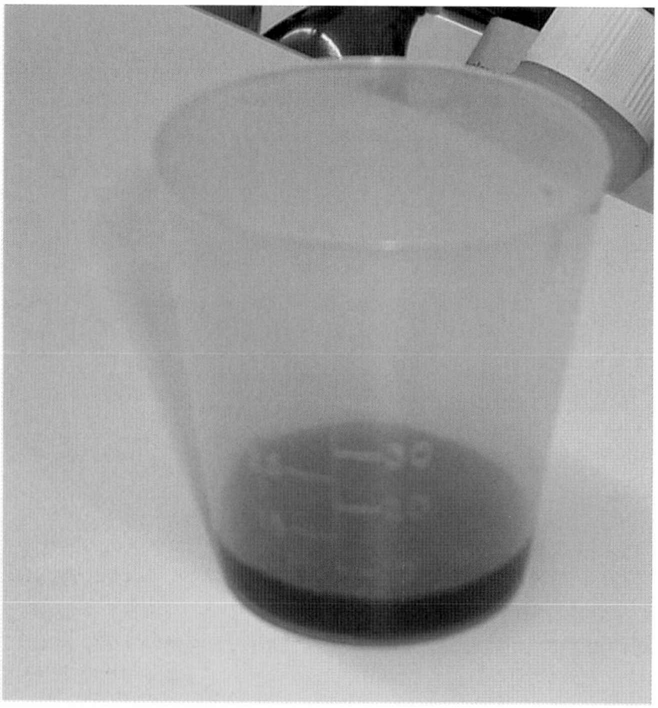

Fig. 16.2 • A medicine cup.

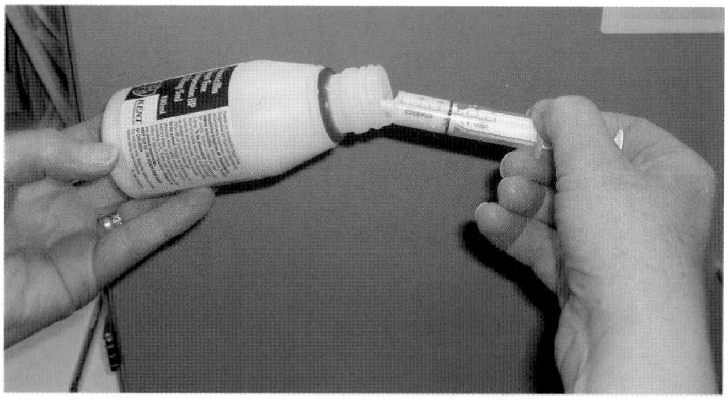

Fig. 16.3 • An oral syringe.

ALERT

Fatalities have occurred when preparations intended for oral administration were mistakenly administered via the intravenous route because they were drawn up into an intravenous rather than a specific oral syringe (Adcock 2001).

In preparing liquid medicine, manufacturers try to mask bitter tastes (Nunn & Williams 2005). Preparations containing fructose, glucose or sucrose may cause dental caries, so it is advised that sugar-free preparations are used, particularly if treatment is required for long periods (*British National Formulary for Children* 2007, Mentes 2001).

Tablets are, however, preferable to liquids whenever they can be taken. They do not contain sugar and are easier to transport and store. Tablets also avoid the risk of spillage, which makes them highly preferable in the case of oral cytotoxic medication. Even preschool children can learn to swallow tablets. There is an increasing variety of other solid dosage forms available, including melts, chewable and orodispersible tablets. Some medicines come as powders, granules or sprinkles, which are usually mixed with a specified food or drink. The drug should be sprinkled on to a small amount (teaspoon) of soft food to ensure that the medicine is taken, not over a bowlful, as the child may not eat all the meal. There is a risk that if medicine is taken in food or drink there will be incomplete digestion and consequently a reduction in the dose given (Nunn & Williams 2005). It could also lead to the child developing an aversion to the food or drink it was added to (*British National Formulary for Children* 2007).

Enteral tube

This route may be used to administer liquid preparations if children are unable to take their medication orally. Fine-bore tubes will be unsuitable for thick liquids. It is advisable to seek pharmaceutical advice before administering any solid-form medicines via this route. The tube should be flushed with water before and after administering any medicine. Sterile water should be used in neonates (*British National Formulary for Children* 2007). Enteral feeds should be interrupted before and after medicine is given, especially if the feed reduces its absorption (e.g. for at least an hour before and after administration of phenytoin). In the event of a blockage, flush using a push–pulling action with at least 10 mL of warm water or soda water in a 50-mL syringe and gently squeeze the tube along its length to relieve the blockage (Nursing and Midwifery Practice Development Unit 2003). Medicines that are absorbed in the stomach should not be given via a nasojejunal tube (Thomson et al 2000).

LINK CHAPTER **15**

Rectal

The administration of rectal medicine is an invasive procedure and should be performed only by a competent practitioner. Whenever possible, two adults should be present during the procedure, one acting as a chaperone for the child (Fuller 2007). Rate of absorption of medication via this route is variable but it may be useful when:

- administration via the oral route results in nausea, vomiting or gastric pain
- patients are uncooperative or have decreased consciousness
- access to the intravenous route is difficult (Bergogne-Bérézin & Bryskier 1999).

The most comfortable position for patients is usually lying on their left side with their left leg straight and right leg bent up (Fig. 16.4).

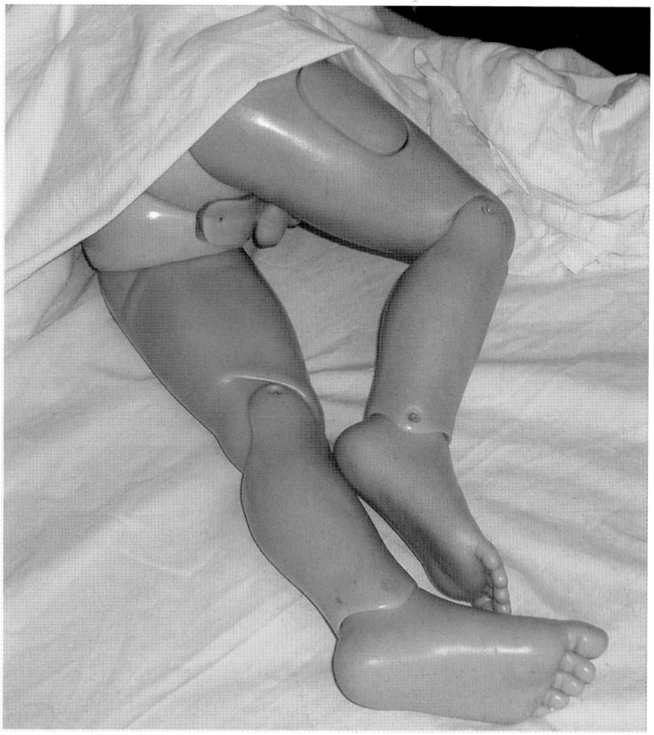

Fig. 16.4 • Patient's position for rectal administration.

The tip of the suppository or enema may be moistened with water or a water-based lubricant prior to insertion. When inserting a suppository the rounded end should be inserted first (Bradshaw & Price 2007).

The rectal route is faster for faecal disimpaction than the oral route but it is invasive and potentially traumatic (Baker et al 1999).

ALERT
Because of the risk of bleeding, the rectal route should be avoided in patients who are thrombocytopenic.

The acceptability of the rectal route varies between cultures. In studies in English-speaking countries, comparing buccal or intranasal midazolam and rectal diazepam for treatment of seizures, midazolam was found to be at least as effective and more socially acceptable and convenient (Harbord et al 2004, Scott et al 1999).

Vulval and vaginal

This route is not commonly used in children. However, there are some occasions when it may be required. Topical oestrogen cream may be prescribed to treat labial adhesions (*British National Formulary for Children* 2007). Fungal infections of the vulva and vagina may be associated with predisposing factors including antibacterial therapy, diabetes mellitus, pregnancy and an infected sexual partner. Oral treatments would normally be prescribed for younger girls, but creams or gels inserted via applicator or pessaries may be prescribed for older girls (*British National Formulary for Children* 2007.). It will usually be appropriate for the patient to self-administer the medication, and instructions about administration should come as a packet insert. However, nurses should not assume that the patient will know where and how to insert the medication and they should check that their patient fully understands what she needs to do.

LINK CHAPTER **4**

Injection

Drugs may be administered via a needle into the body via various routes. These include intravenous, intramuscular, subcutaneous and intradermal (Fig. 16.5).

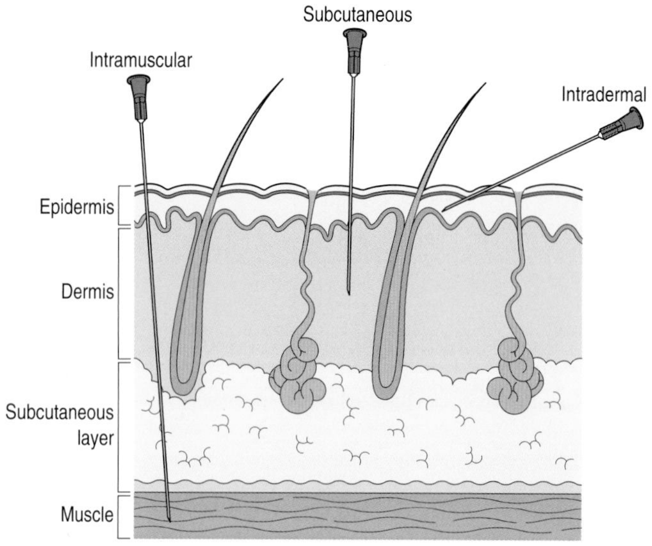

Fig. 16.5 • Subcutaneous needle must reach subcutaneous layer.

Pain reduction for all types of injection

The discomfort of injections may be reduced by various methods including age-appropriate preparation; topical anaesthetic cream; ethyl chloride spray; ice packs; pressing on the skin for 10s before needle insertion (Fig. 16.6); and distraction and relaxation techniques during the procedure, such as singing, blowing bubbles and guided imagery (Chung et al 2002, Duff 2003, Lala & Lala 2003).

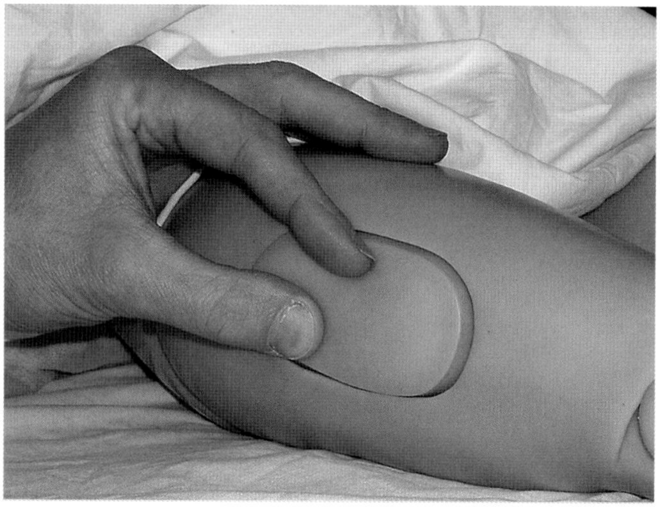

Fig. 16.6 • A patient's discomfort can be reduced by pressing on the skin for 10 s before an injection.

Self-administration of inhaled nitrous oxide may be helpful in school age children and young people (Gerhardt et al 2001).

LINK CHAPTER **18**

Breastfeeding or giving sucrose solution appears to reduce discomfort in infants (Carbajal et al 2003). Occasionally, in non-urgent situations, sedation might be required (Scottish Intercollegiate Guidelines Network 2002, Taxis & Baber 2003).

Procedures Box 16.1 Reducing risks associated with all types of injection

Actions
Use injections in ready-to-use form if possible.

The preparation of injections should be carried out by competent patients, carers or healthcare staff in a suitable environment using safe procedures.

Reason *Reduces the risks of selecting the wrong drug or diluent, the risks of microbial and/or particulate contamination, and risks to the operator and/or the environment.*

Action
Administer any injections prepared in near-patient areas immediately.

Reason *Reduces the risk of contamination and degradation.*

Actions
Wash your hands thoroughly.

Use a no-touch technique: avoid touching syringe tips, vial tops, etc.

Reason *Reduces the risk of microbial contamination.*

Action
Wear gloves and other personal protective equipment as required.

Reason *Reduces the risk of possible contamination with toxic substances and cross-infection.*

Action
Swab vial closures with alcohol wipes.

Reason *Tamper-evident covers to vials do not ensure sterility.*

Action
Allow at least 30 s for the alcohol to dry.

Reason *Decontaminates the surface.*

Actions
Peel wrappers gently from needles and syringes.

Use a filter needle to draw up medicine from glass ampoules and vials with stoppers.

Reason *Reduces particulate contamination.*

Actions
Count needles throughout the procedure.

Never resheath, break or bend used needles.

Use needles with engineered sharps injury protection when available.

Use needle-free self-sealing intravenous access systems.

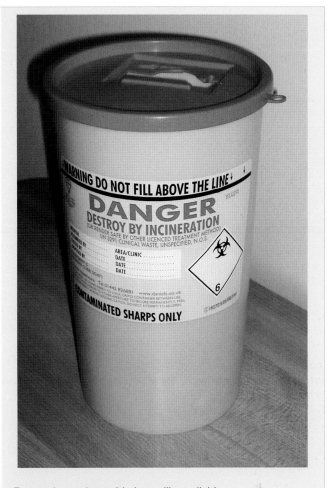

Ensure that a sharps bin is readily available.

Dispose of used needles and syringes into a sharps bin immediately after using them.

Leave used needles and syringes in one piece.

Reason *Minimises the risk of needle stick injury.*

(See Clinical Resource and Audit Group 2002, Cousins et al 2005, Dougherty 2002, Infection Control Nurses Association 2003, Preston & Hegadoren 2004, Royal College of Nursing 2002, Taxis & Baber 2003.)

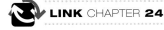

LINK CHAPTER **24**

Intravenous

ALERT
The intravenous route ensures rapid and predictable delivery of medicine but has the highest potential for adverse reactions (Fitzsimons 2001). Risks of using the intravenous route include a higher risk of anaphylaxis than with other routes, speed shock if the medicine is administered too rapidly, extravasation, infiltration, infection and phlebitis (Dougherty 2002).

Extravasation is the inadvertent administration of a vesicant solution or medication into the tissues surrounding a venous access device (Royal College of Nursing IV Therapy Forum 2003). *Infiltration* is the inadvertent administration of a non-vesicant solution or medication into the tissues surrounding a venous access device (Royal College of Nursing IV Therapy Forum 2003). A vesicant is an agent capable of causing injury when it escapes from the intended vascular pathway into the surrounding tissue (Royal College of Nursing IV Therapy Forum 2003).

ALERT
Nurses must never rely on electronic infusion devices to aid the early detection of infiltration or extravasation

but must check the site at least hourly for swelling and skin colour changes (Dougherty 2002).

To allow blood flow around the device, as well as to reduce mechanical irritation, a peripheral venous access device should be the smallest gauge necessary for the vein and therapy. Suitable veins for cannulation are often found in the forearm. As splinting is not required in this area; it is more comfortable for the patient. Veins in the lower extremities should be considered when inserting a peripheral cannula into a baby, in particular the great saphenous vein. However, foot and leg veins should be avoided if possible in older children due to an increased risk of thrombi forming and migrating (Dougherty 2002). A clinician should normally have no more than two attempts at inserting a cannula before referring to a more experienced practitioner (Rothwell & Hegarty 2007). In order to prolong cannula survival time, promote patient comfort and prevent complications, it is important to limit the movement of the cannula within the vein and maintain asepsis. The cannula should be connected to an extension tube (T piece), which allows remote access without movement of the cannula. Use of a transparent, sterile, semipermeable dressing to secure the cannula is recommended (Campbell & Carrington 1999). Areas of flexion should be avoided if possible and should be splinted to reduce the risk of dislodgement (Bravery 1999).

ALERT
Homemade splints must never be used, as they are associated with a greater risk of trauma and infection than custom-made splints.

For example, there were several cases of severe fungal infections associated with tongue depressors being used as splints (Anonymous 1996). The fingers and toes should be visible to check on circulation. If a bandage is used to protect the cannula site it must be removed at regular intervals to allow inspection of the entry site and surrounding tissues (Lane 2007). This needs to be done before using the cannula and at least hourly while an infusion is in progress

LINK CHAPTER **26**

It is recommended that peripheral cannulas are resited every 2–3 days (Royal College of Nursing IV Therapy Forum). However, in children actual practice is often to leave the cannula in situ for as long as it remains patent. A central venous access device is often preferable for children whose treatment involves vesicant drugs or who need to receive intravenous medicines over a long period, as well as for home therapy (*British National Formulary for Children* 2007, Royal College of Nursing IV Therapy Forum 2003).

Any vascular access device requires flushing with 0.9% sodium chloride (or for some acidic medicines, 5% dextrose) prior to use to check it is patent. This needs to be prescribed or may sometimes be given under a patient group direction (patient group directive in Scotland) – a specified written instruction for the supply or administration of named medicines in an identified clinical situation, drawn up locally by appropriate professionals and approved by the employer (Nursing and Midwifery Council 2004).

Infusion devices

Infusion pumps are classified as being suitable for neonatal, high-risk, lower risk or ambulatory infusions depending on their accuracy, consistency, alarm displays and safety features (Quinn 2000). Variable operational requirements between different infusion pumps can lead to errors. This has led many institutions to standardise the pumps used in their respective settings (Allard et al 2002).

The risk of uncontrolled flow (free flow or siphonage) is minimised by using narrow-bore extension lines and antisiphon valves and by positioning the pump as close to the level of the patient's heart as practically possible (Quinn 2000). Delay between starting a syringe pump and delivery of the medicine at the set flow rate (known as mechanical slack or mechanical backlash) is reduced by:

- fitting the syringe tightly into the pump
- using the prime facility on the syringe pump, if this is available
- using a smaller sized syringe, if available and applicable (Amoore et al 2001).

Intramuscular

This route is often used for administering vaccines, and on some occasions may be preferable to intravenous cannulation for single doses of medicines (*British National Formulary for Children* 2007).

ALERT
Potential complications of intramuscular injections are nerve injury, septic or sterile abscesses, muscle fibrosis and contracture, and gangrene. Intramuscular haemorrhage can also occur, so this route must be avoided in people with poor blood clotting such as those with haemophilia (Cook & Murtagh 2005, Hemsworth 2000).

The recommended injection site for infants is the vastus lateralis (Fig. 16.7; Royal College of Nursing et al 2002). For older children the preferred site is the deltoid muscle in the upper arm (Fig. 16.8). This site has a good blood supply so absorption is fast, but it not suitable for repeated injections or

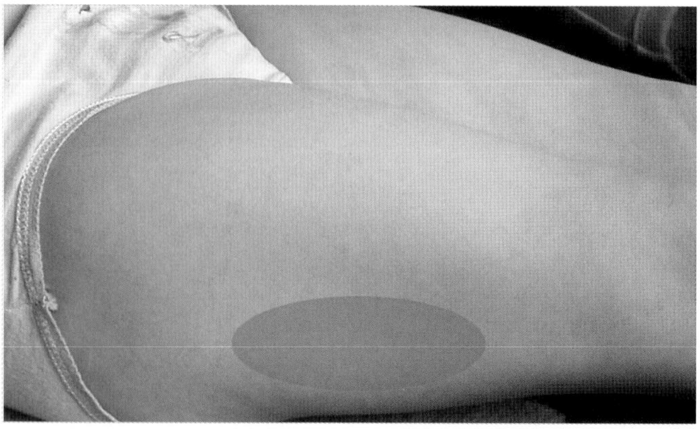

Fig. 16.7 • The vastus lateralis is used for intramuscular injection in infants.

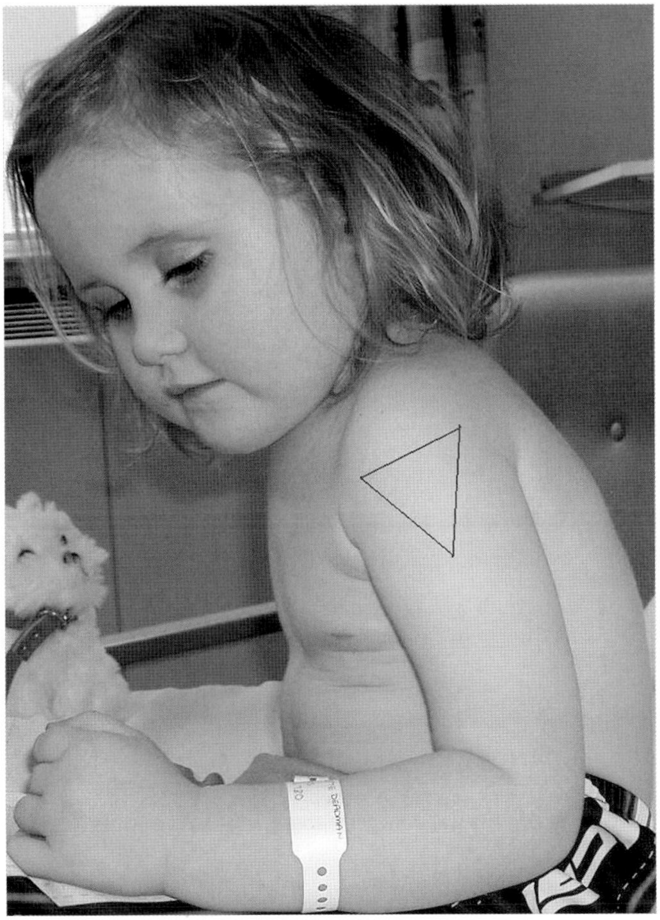

Fig. 16.8 • The deltoid muscle is used for intramuscular injection in older children.

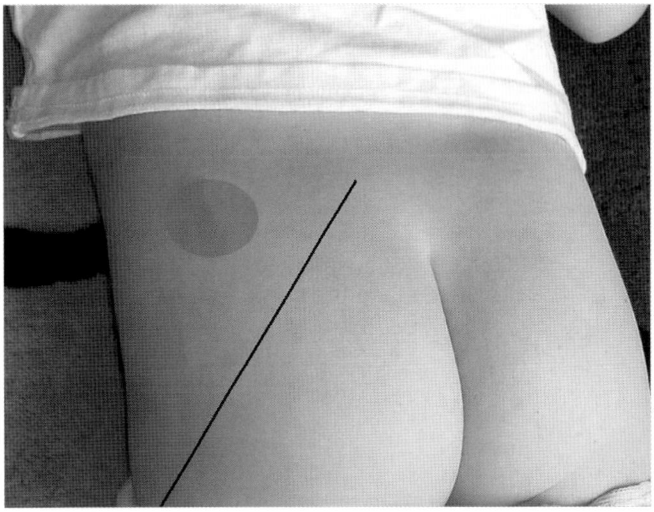

Fig. 16.9 • The dorsogluteal route is not recommended for children.

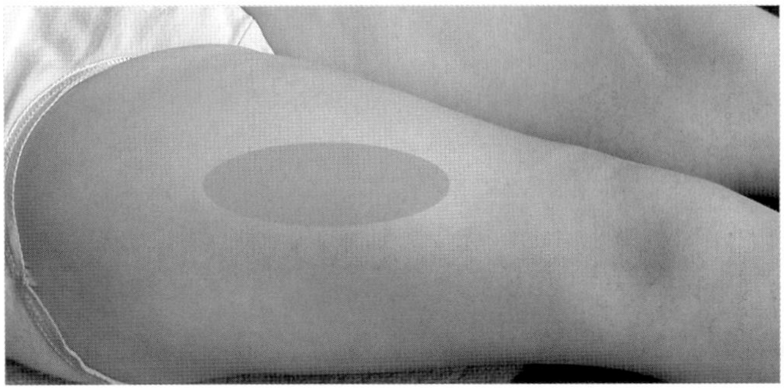

Fig. 16.10 • The rectus femoris muscle may be used for self-injection.

for large volumes of medication. The maximum recommended injection volume for the deltoid site is 2 mL for adults, 1 mL for children and 0.5 mL for infants, compared with 5 mL for adults, 2 mL for children and 1 mL for infants in larger muscles (Hemsworth 2000, Workman 1999).

The dorsogluteal is a possible alternative in children who have been walking for a while (Chiodini 2001, Lala & Lala 2003). However, there is a risk of reduced absorption rate if the injection is deposited into adipose tissue rather than muscle (Workman 1999). When using the dorsogluteal route (Fig. 16.9) there is a danger of the needle hitting the sciatic nerve and the superior gluteal arteries if the child moves, therefore this route is now rarely recommended for children.

The rectus femoris muscle at the front of the thigh is a painful route but may be suitable for self-injection (Fig. 16.10; Fuller 2007).

The ventrogluteal site (Fig. 16.11), which is easily palpable and accessible, is another possible alternative for children and young people and infants over 7 months (Hemsworth 2000).

An intramuscular injection is less painful if the muscle is relaxed. (See the earlier section about pain reduction for injections.) Placing the patient's hand on his or her hip will relax the deltoid muscle. Internal rotation of the femur by flexing the knees will relax the gluteal muscles. An infant or young child may be held securely on an adult's lap with one of the adult's arms holding the child's outside arm, the child's inside arm tucked around the adult's body and the adult's other arm holding the child's legs (Lala & Lala 2003).

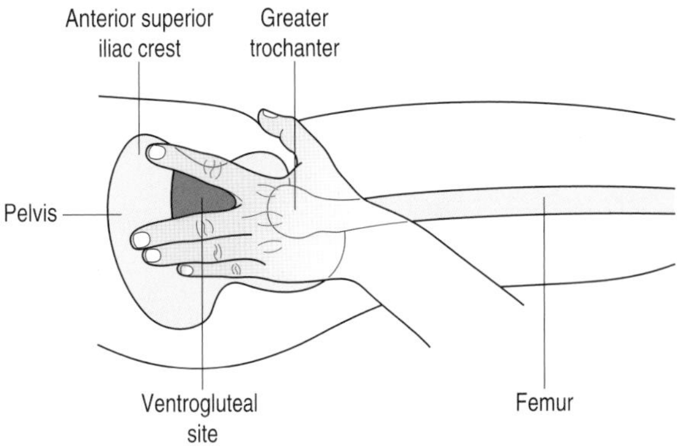

Fig. 16.11 • The ventrogluteal site is accessible and easily palpated. (From: Rodger MA, King L (2000) Drawing up and administering intramuscular injections: a review of the literature. Journal of Advanced Nursing 31(3):574–582. Blackwell Science Ltd, with permission)

Procedures Box 16.2 Technique for administering an intramuscular injection

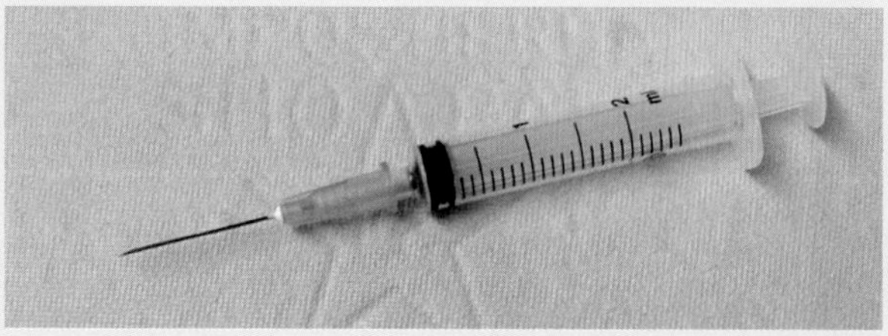

Action
A 23-gauge, 25-mm long needle is usually required (a lower gauge needle may be required for oil-based injections and a longer length for larger children).

Reason *Reduces pain and trauma to the tissue on injection and ensures that the needle reaches the muscle.*

Action
Cleanse the skin (if preferred and in any immunocompromised patients), wiping the skin with an alcohol-impregnated swab in a circular motion and allowing it to dry for at least 30 s.

Reason *Cleansing of the patient's skin prior to injections is not routinely advised.*

Allow drying time to decontaminate the skin effectively and to prevent the stinging of wet alcohol increasing the pain of the injection.

Action
Non-sterile gloves may be worn for the procedure; check employer policy.

Reason *Some employers and individual practitioners may advise the wearing of disposable gloves for this procedure to avoid the risk of contamination from the medicine or the patient's blood.*

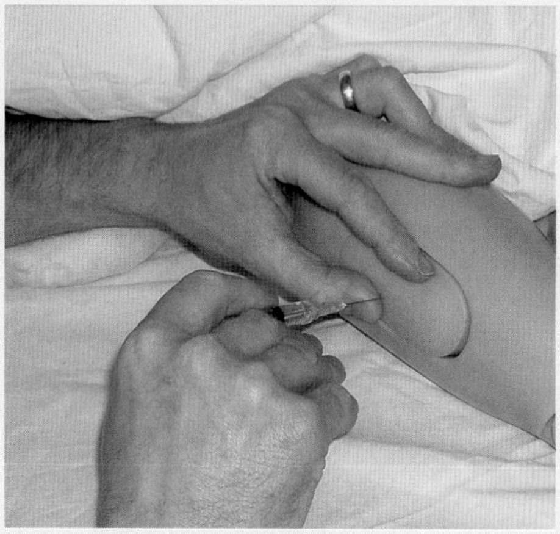

Action
Hold the skin firmly with the free hand (bunch the muscle up in emaciated children) and insert the needle at a 90° angle.

Reason *Ensures that the needle enters the muscle and reduces pain.*

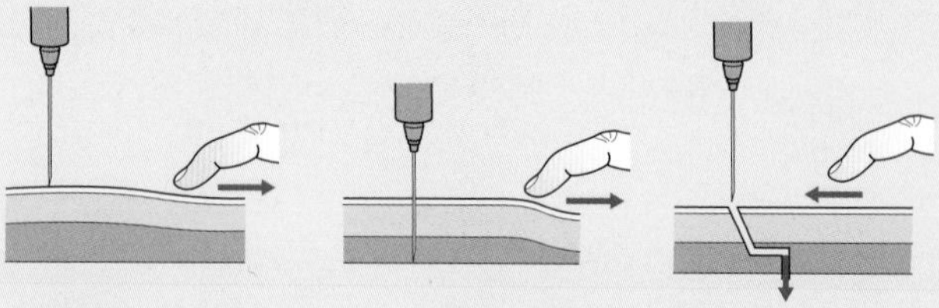

Action
A Z-track technique may be used by pulling the skin and its subcutaneous tissue 2–3 cm sideways prior to insertion of the needle and releasing it back when the needle is withdrawn.

Reason *Creates a disjointed pathway to lock in the medication and may reduce discomfort and complications.*

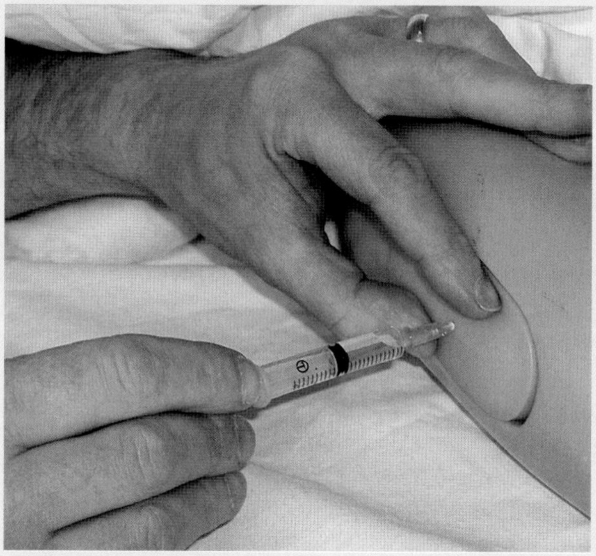

Actions
Aspirate for blood over 5 s.

If blood is aspirated discard the needle and syringe and start again.

Reason *Avoids the risk of giving the drug intravenously by mistake and potentially causing an embolism. (Some guidelines advise that this step is not necessary.)*

Subcutaneous

Potential injection sites are the upper arm, hips, buttocks, abdomen (avoiding the area within a 2.5-cm radius around the navel) and anterior and lateral aspect of the thighs (see Fig. 29.6). Absorption from the subcutaneous route is slower than from the intramuscular route (Workman 1999). Absorption is fastest from the abdomen, then the upper arm, then the thighs, and slowest from the hips and buttocks (King 2003).

ALERT
Repeated injections into the same site can result in lipohypertrophies (fatty lumps).

Procedures Box 16.2 Technique for administering an intramuscular injection—cont'd

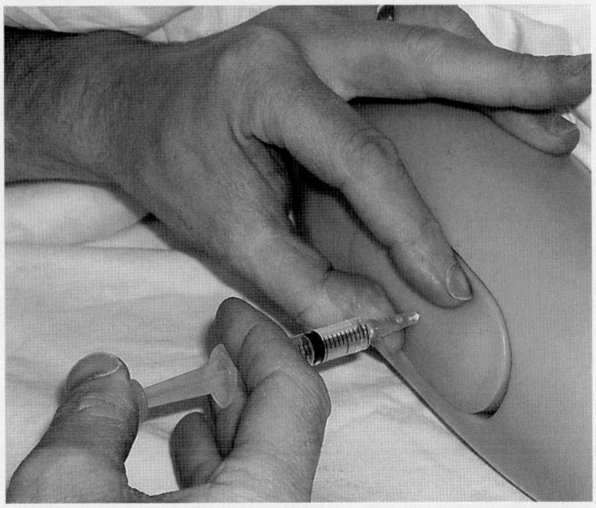

Actions
Inject the medication at a rate that does not exceed 1 mL per 10 s.

Wait for a few seconds.

Reason *To allow the muscle fibres to expand and absorb the solution.*

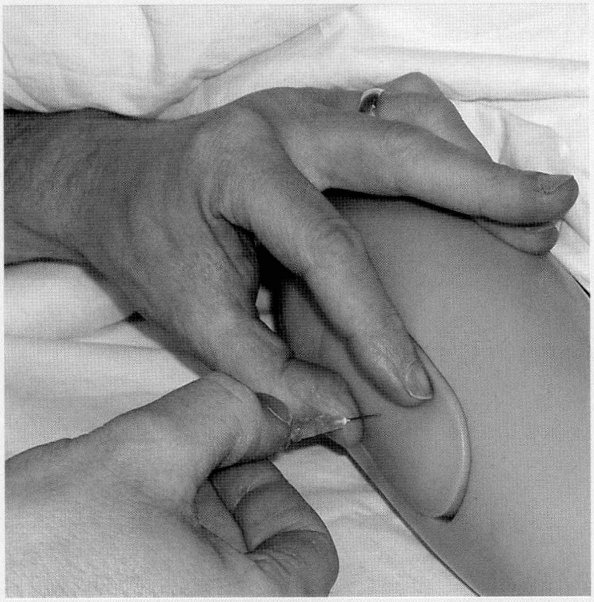

Action
Withdraw the needle smoothly.

Reason *Avoids additional trauma.*

Action
Apply gentle pressure to the site with a cotton wool ball or gauze swab for 30 s.

Reason *Prevents seepage from the site.*

Action
Do not massage the site.

Reason *Massaging might cause the drug to leak from the needle entry site and cause irritation to the local tissues.*

Action
Observe the patient.

Reason *To detect complications.*

Action
Rotate between injection sites if repeated injections are required.

Reason *Avoids repeated trauma to one site, which increases the risk of complications.*

(See Chiodini 2001, Cook & Murtagh 2005, Department of Health 2006, Hemsworth 2000, Lala & Lala 2003, Rodger & King 2000, Royal College of Nursing et al 2002, Workman 1999.)

However, for insulin injections, because of the different absorption rates from different sites, it is recommended that the same body area is always used for injections at the same time each day, for example always in the abdomen in the morning (King 2003).

For administering a subcutaneous injection it is recommended that the same technique is used as for an intramuscular injection, except that:

- a shorter 5-, 6- or 8-mm needle is required (if a longer needle is used the skin may be pinched up and the needle

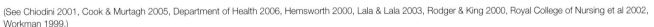

inserted at a 45° angle to avoid injecting into the muscle beneath)
- aspirating for blood is not required (Department of Health 2006, King 2003, Winslow et al 1997, Workman 1999).

LINK CHAPTER 29

Intradermal

This route may be used for vaccinations and allergen tests. Recommended injection sites are the forearm, upper chest, upper arm and shoulder blades (McConnell 2000). To administer an intradermal injection:

- use a 25- to 27-gauge needle (Fig. 16.12)
- stretch the skin with the thumb and forefinger of your free hand
- hold the needle bevel uppermost (Fig. 16.13)
- insert the needle into the skin at a 5–15° angle for about 2 mm (Fig. 16.14)
- inject up to 0.5 mL – a visible blob should form where the medicine is deposited
- withdraw the needle

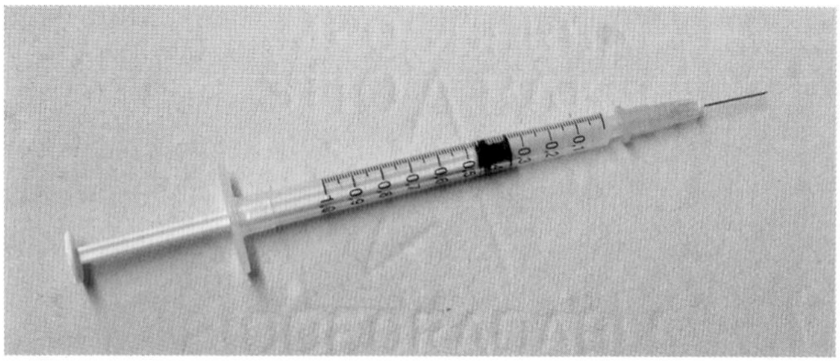

Fig. 16.12 • A needle used for intradermal injection.

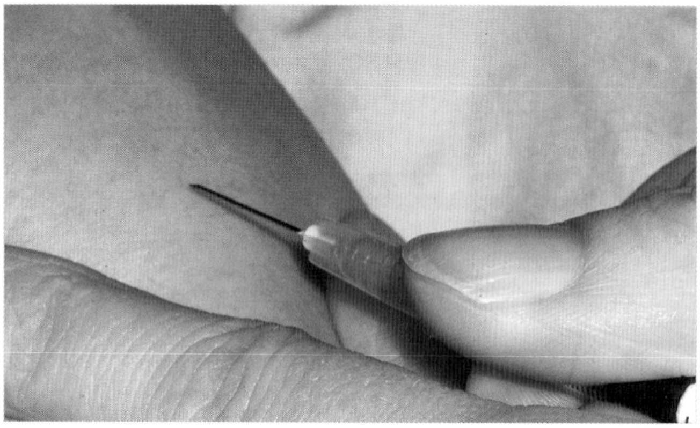

Fig. 16.13 • The needle is held bevel uppermost.

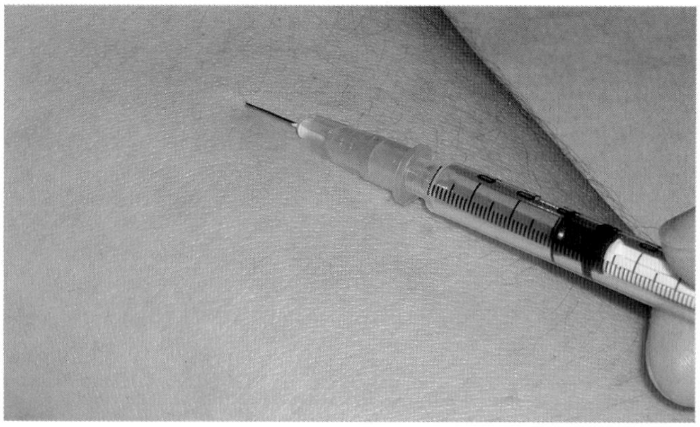

Fig. 16.14 • The injection is made at a 5–15° angle.

- pat dry – do not apply pressure to the site
- draw a ring around the site if it is being used for allergen testing (McConnell 2000, Workman 1999).

Inhalation

This route may be used for systemic treatment and for direct treatment of respiratory diseases (Barry & O'Callaghan 1997). If medication is delivered directly to its site of action it gives a faster response and allows smaller doses of drug to be administered, which reduces systemic side effects (O'Callaghan & Barry 2000).

There are three main types of inhalation device (O'Callaghan & Barry 2000):

1. Pressurised metered dose inhaler (Fig. 16.15)
2. Dry powder inhaler (Fig. 16.17)
3. Nebuliser.

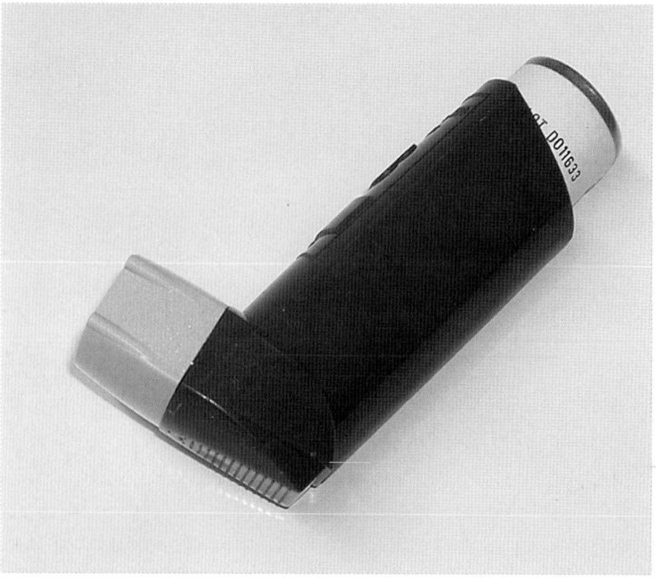

Fig. 16.15 • A pressurised metered dose inhaler.

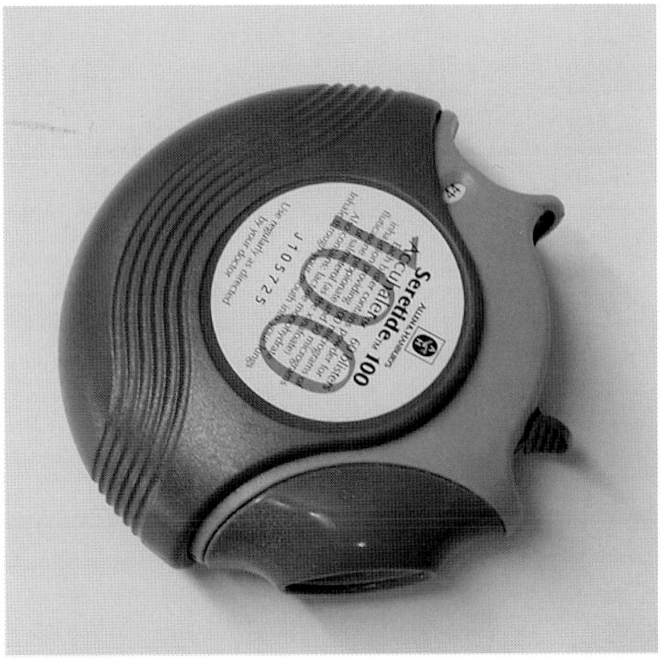

Fig. 16.16 • A dry powder inhaler (Accuhaler).

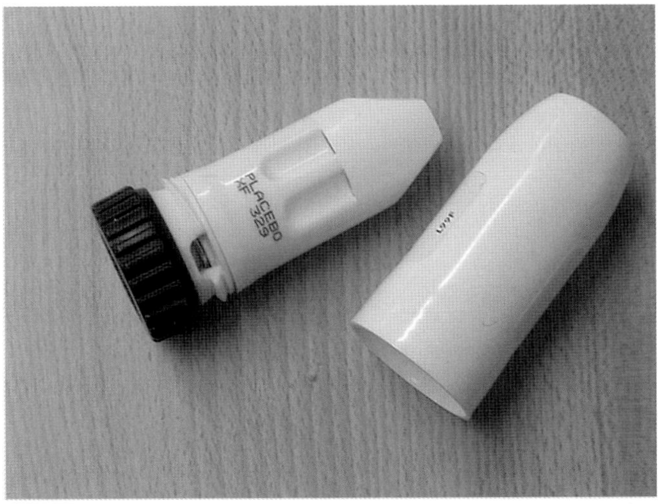

Fig. 16.17 • A dry powder inhaler (Turbohaler).

ALERT
Good inhaler technique is essential for effective treatment.

To achieve good inhaler technique it is important that the most suitable device is chosen for the individual child, and the best method may be trying out a variety of devices with the child to be able to find the correct device (Caldwell 1998). The National Institute for Clinical Excellence (2000) has published a useful review of the use of inhaler systems and devices for children, which can be accessed on their website. Inhaler devices require different levels of skill and coordination to administer effectively. Spacer devices are the best method of delivery for inhaled drugs in young children, as they provide a holding chamber from which the child can repeatedly breathe, increasing the opportunity for the child to inhale the drug (British Thoracic Society & Scottish Intercollegiate Guidelines Network 2005, Jordan & White 2001). Inhaler technique is clearly demonstrated on the website of Asthma UK (2007).

Pressurised metered dose inhaler

This is easy to actuate but difficult to use properly. The drug is emitted at high speed and is mostly deposited in the oropharynx. Use of a valved holding chamber (spacer; Fig. 16.18) with the inhaler allows the patient to breathe tidally from a reservoir of the drug. Face masks can be used with a spacer by children who are too young or who are unable to use a mouthpiece (Fig. 16.19). However, delivery of the drug is more efficient if a mouthpiece is used (O'Callaghan & Barry 2000).

Static electricity can cause output from spacer devices to vary greatly (Vella & Grech 2005). Static can be reduced by washing plastic spacers before use, then every month, with detergent and water and leaving them to drip dry (British Thoracic Society & Scottish Intercollegiate Guidelines Network 2005).

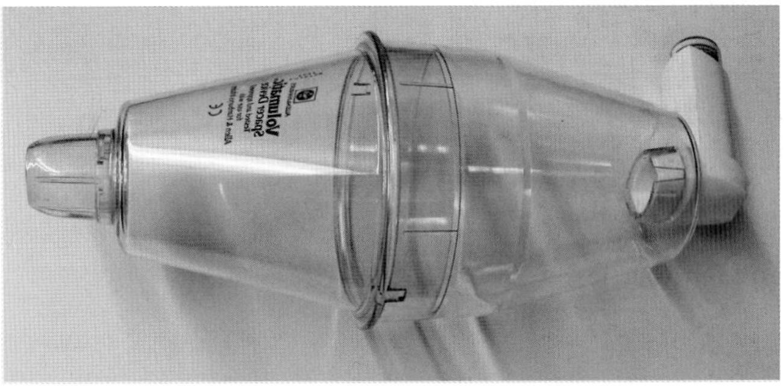

Fig. 16.18 • Inhaler with a valved holding chamber.

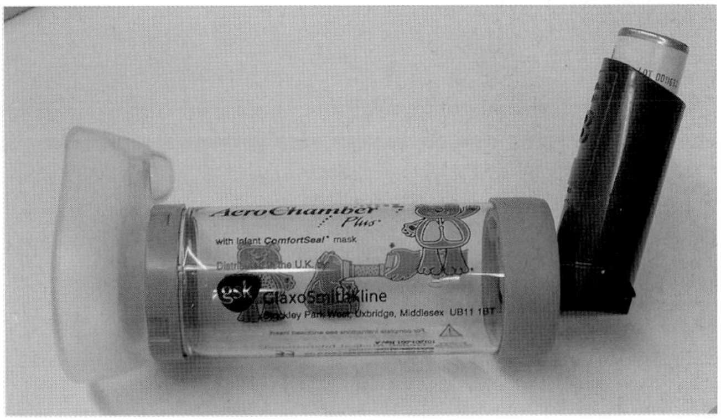

Fig. 16.19 • Inhaler with a spacer and mask.

Procedures Box 16.3 Using a spacer with a face mask to administer medication from a pressurised metered dose inhaler

Action
Remove the inhaler cap, shake the canister and insert it into the device.
Reason *Thoroughly mixes the medication.*

Action
Attach the inverted spacer plus inhaler to the face mask.

Action
Place the facemask over the infant's nose and mouth.
Reason *Ensures a good seal.*

Action
Inverting the spacer, discharge the aerosol into the chamber as prescribed.
Reason *Ensures that the one-way valve falls open.*

Action
The infant inhales during normal tidal breathing for at least six breaths.
Reason *Enables relaxed inhalation of medication.*

Action
Wait 1 min to repeat the sequence if a second dose is required.
Reason *Allows the first dose of medication to be fully absorbed.*

Procedures Box 16.4 Using a spacer device to administer medication from a pressurised metered dose inhaler

Action
Remove the inhaler cap, shake the canister and insert it into the device.
Reason *Thoroughly mixes the medication.*

Actions
The child should stand up and look upwards.
Place the mouthpiece into the child's mouth.
Reason *Enables full diaphragmatic expansion and reduces the pharyngeal angle and therefore minimises depositing the medication in the mouth.*

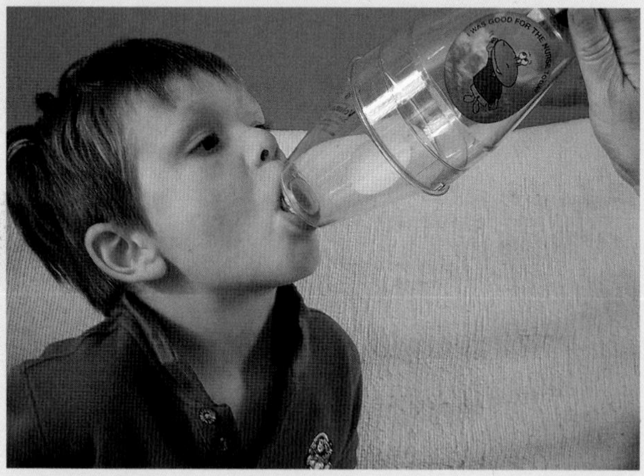

Action
Encourage the child to bite on to the mouthpiece.
Reason *This avoids the child closing the teeth behind it.*

Action
Advise the child to try to keep her or his tongue down.
Reason *Prevents the child occluding the mouthpiece with her or his tongue.*

Action
Encourage the child to breathe in and out gently (tidal breathing).
Reason *This will open and close the valve and a clicking noise will be heard.*

Action
Keeping the device in the same position, depress the canister once to release a dose of the drug.

Action
The child should continue to tidal breathe for five breaths.
Reason *Ensures that the full dose is inhaled.*

Action
Remove the device from the child's mouth.

Action
Wait 1 min to repeat the sequence if a second dose is required.
Reason *Allows the first dose of medication to be fully absorbed.*

Procedures Box 16.5 Administering medication using a pressurised metered dose inhaler

Action
Shake the canister before use.

Reason *Thoroughly mixes the medication.*

Action
The child should stand up and look upwards.

Reason *Enables full diaphragmatic expansion and reduces pharyngeal angle and therefore minimises depositing the medication in the mouth.*

Action
Exhale to functional reserve capacity.

Reason *Allows a full deep breath.*

Action
Activate the inhaler at the start of inspiration.

Actions
Take slow, deep inspiration.

Hold the breath for 10 s.

Reason *Encourages absorption of the medication.*

Action
Take one puff at a time, breaking for 1 min between puffs.

Reason *Allows each dose of medication to be fully absorbed.*

Dry powder inhaler

This type of inhaler requires the patient's inspiratory effort to disperse the medication, and by 5 years children can usually generate enough inspiratory flow to activate dry powder devices. This method may be more convenient than a metered dose inhaler and spacer for day-to-day treatment in school age children (British Thoracic Society & Scottish Intercollegiate Guidelines Network 2005).

Procedures Box 16.6 Using a Turbohaler

Actions
Unscrew and lift off the outer white cover.

Hold the Turbohaler upright.

Action
Twist the grip forwards and backwards as far as you can until you hear the click.

Reason *Releases the medication from the capsule.*

Action
The child should stand up and look upwards.

Reason *Enables full diaphragmatic expansion and reduces the pharyngeal angle and therefore minimise depositing the medication in the mouth.*

Action
Breathe out.

Reason *Allows for a full deep breath in.*

Action
Put the mouthpiece between the lips and breathe in deeply.

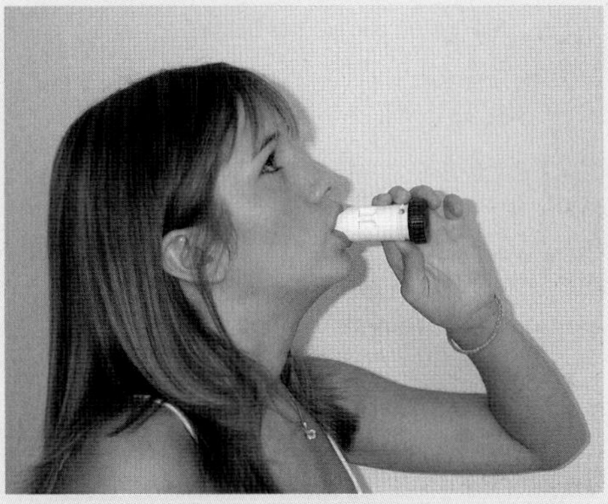

Reason *Generates inspiratory flow.*

Actions
Remove the inhaler from the mouth and hold the breath for 10 s.

Reason *Allows the medication to be absorbed.*

Action
Replace the white cover on the Turbohaler.

Procedures Box 16.7 Using an Accuhaler

Actions
Hold the outer casing of the Accuhaler with one hand while pushing the thumb grip away until a click is heard.
Hold the mouthpiece towards you.

Action
Slide the lever away until it clicks.
Reason *Releases the medication from the capsule.*

Action
Hold the inhaler level.

Action
The child should stand up and look upwards.
Reason *Enables full diaphragmatic expansion and reduces pharyngeal angle and therefore minimises depositing the medication in the mouth.*

Action
Breathe out gently away from the device.
Reason *Allows for a full deep breath in.*

Action
Put the mouthpiece in the mouth and breathe in steadily and deeply.

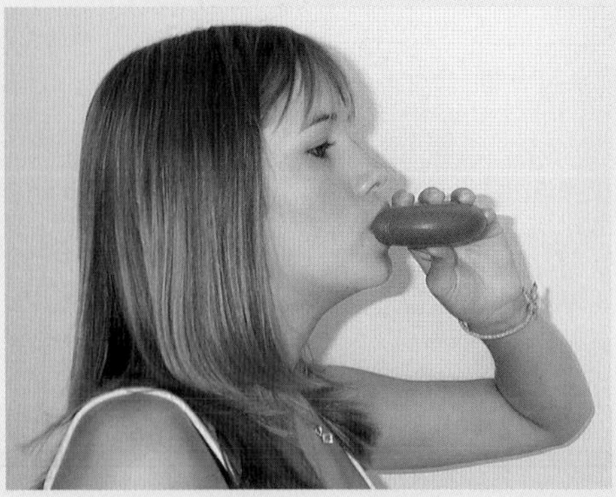

Reason *Generates inspiratory flow.*

Actions
Remove the device from the mouth and hold the breath for 10 s.
Reason *Allows medication to be absorbed.*

Action
Close by sliding the thumb grip back until it clicks.

General points about inhaler use

- Rinse the mouth with water or clean the teeth following inhalation of corticosteroids to prevent oral thrush.
- Leave at least 30 s and up to a minute between each puff for maximum therapeutic effect.

Nebuliser

Nebulisers use compressed gas or the vibration of a piezoelectric crystal to aerosolise liquids (O'Callaghan & Barry 2000). In severe and life-threatening asthma, salbutamol, ipratropium bromide and oxygen can be given together via nebuliser (British Thoracic Society & Scottish Intercollegiate Guidelines Network 2005). Nebulisers are also used to deliver drugs such as antibiotics, which are not available in an inhaler (O'Callaghan & Barry 2000).

Deposition in the lungs is improved by the use of a mouthpiece rather than a face mask, by holding the face mask close to the patient, and by the patient breathing quietly rather than breathing rapidly or crying (Isles et al 1999). Using a nebuliser hood rather than a face mask may result in better drug uptake by infants (Amirov et al 2003). However, ipratropium bromide may trigger acute angle glaucoma, so a face mask must be used with this drug to prevent it entering the eyes (*British National Formulary for Children* 2007).

To reduce the risk of bacterial contamination each patient must have his or her own tubing, nebuliser, and mouthpiece or mask, and drugs must be put into the nebuliser immediately before use. With nebulisers that leave only 0.5 mL of residual fluid after nebulisation, it is sufficient to start with 2–2.5 mL of drug fluid. An oxygen flow rate of 6–8 L/min is required. For bronchodilators 10 min should be sufficient for nebulisation. Antibiotics and steroids may need a longer time to aerolise as much drug as possible (British Thoracic Society 1997).

To avoid growth of microorganisms in the residual fluid the nebuliser should be emptied after each use and washed at least once a day in warm soapy water and dried with clean soft tissue. Special filters prevent antibiotic particles from getting into the atmosphere; these filters need to be dried between use to be effective, so two should be supplied (British Thoracic Society 1997).

Intranasal

This route is used for a range of systemic drugs as well as drugs acting in the nasal area. It is convenient for patients, and the rate of absorption, plasma concentration and pharmacokinetics often compare well to the intravenous route because of the rich vasculature and high permeability of the nasal mucosa (Quraishi et al 1997).

There are three broad methods of nasal administration: drops, pumped aqueous sprays and powered nasal sprays.

Nasal drops

Prior to instilling nasal drops clean away any nasal discharge, crusts and dried secretions using moist cotton wool balls or non-woven swabs. The most effective position for instilling nose drops may be to have the patient lying with her or his

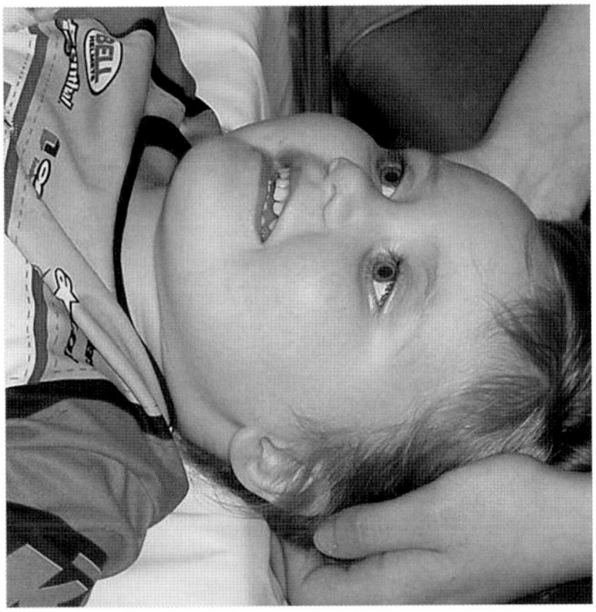

Fig. 16.20 • The child's head is tilted back for nasal drop administration.

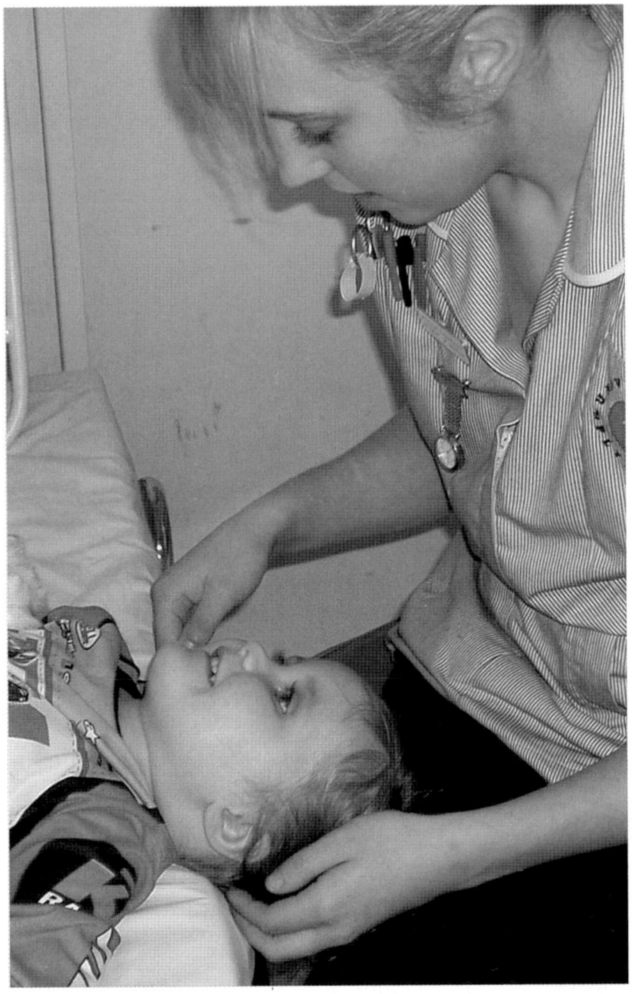

Fig. 16.21 • The carer is now ready to administer the medication.

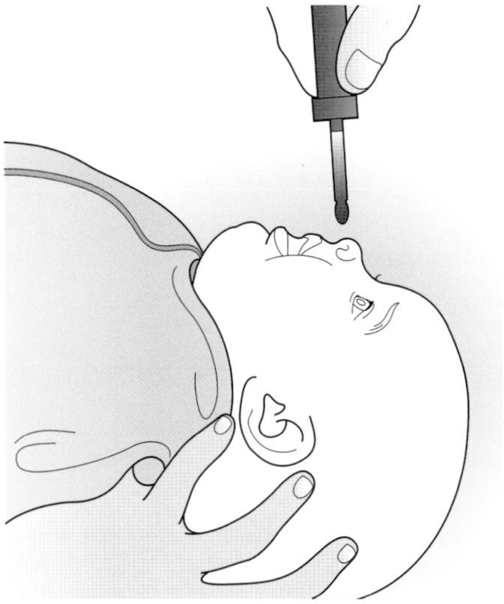

Fig. 16.22 • Administering nasal drops to the back of the nose.

head and neck extended over the side of the bed (Aggarwal et al 2004) (Fig. 16.20). Alternatively a child could lie on the bed with a pillow or folded blanket placed under the child's shoulders so that his or her head is tilted back, or an infant can be held in your arms. The carer can then drip the medication into the nasal passages (Fig. 16.21). As the drops of solution are instilled in the right nostril, the child's head should be turned to the right side and likewise for the left nostril. If the head is not turned to the side on which drops are instilled, the solution may slide directly through the nose and into the back of the throat (Williams 2007a).

Administering nasal drops to infants is best performed by two carers. The infant should be positioned across the carer's knee with the infant's head extended and slightly dipped. The other carer can then drop the required medication into the back of the nose (Fig. 16.22).

Nasal spray

Benninger et al (2004) recommend a seven-step technique for using a nasal spray:

1. Hold the head in an upright position.
2. Clear the nose of any thick or excessive mucus.
3. Insert the spray nozzle into the nostril.
4. Direct the spray away from the septum towards the outer portion of the eye or top of the ear on that side. (If possible use the right hand to spray the left nostril and left hand to spray the right nostril.)
5. Activate the device as recommended by the manufacturer and with the number of sprays prescribed by the doctor.
6. Gently breathe in or sniff during the spraying.
7. Breathe out through the nose.

Procedures Box 16.8 Instilling eye drops and eye ointment

Action
Wash and dry your hands.

Reason *Prevents cross-infection.*

Action
Explain the procedure to the child in a way that is appropriate to the child's level of understanding.

Reason *Promotes partnership and compliance.*

Action
Gently clean sticky lids with cotton wool balls or gauze, non-woven swabs moistened with sterile water or saline.

Reason *There is usually no need to clean the eye itself before drug instillation, as it is self-cleaning.*

Actions
Position the patient lying on her or his back or seated with the head tilted back and neck slightly hyperextended.

Ask the patient to look upwards if possible.

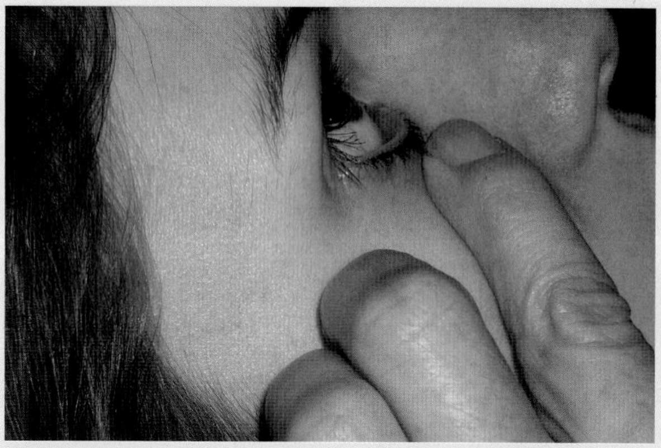

Draw the lower eyelid down and away from the eye.

Actions
Place a ribbon of ointment or allow one drop to fall on to the conjunctival sac behind the eyelid.

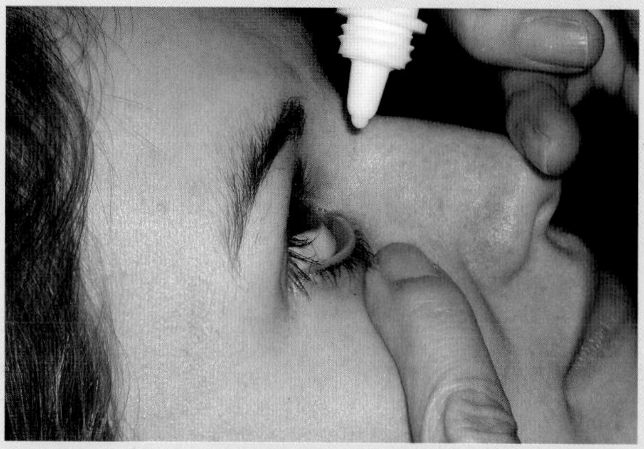

Do not touch the end of the tube or dropper on to the eye.

Reasons *Reduces discomfort and risk of trauma to the eye. Avoids contamination of the medication.*

Actions
Ask older children to close their eyes gently and count slowly to 60 after drop instillation and to avoid blinking if possible.

Reason *Prevents the drop being moved into the nasolacrimal system, where it would be unavailable for absorption.*

Action
Leave ideally 5 but at least 3 min between instilling more drops into the same eye.

Reason *The previous drop will be washed away and not absorbed in a therapeutic amount.*

Action
All drops should be instilled before the eye ointment.

Reason *Ointment 'waterproofs' the eye and prevents absorption of the drops.*

Action
Eye ointment should be applied like the drop but as a 2-cm long strip.

Eye

The technique for delivering medication to the eye via drops and ointment is shown in the procedure box (Marsden & Shaw 2003, McConnell 2001, Ulyatt 2007).

Ear

Medicine may be administered directly into the ears in drops using the method described in the procedure box (Allen 2005, Williams 2007b).

Procedures Box 16.9 Instilling ear drops

Action
Wash and dry your hands.

Reason *Prevents cross-infection.*

Action
Explain the procedure to the child in a way that is appropriate to child's level of understanding.

Reason *Promotes partnership and compliance.*

Action
Warm the drops by holding the container in a hand; if the drops are a suspension shake well.

Reasons *Promotes patient comfort.*
Mixes the suspension to ensure equal distribution of medication.

Procedures Box 16.9 Instilling ear drops—cont'd

Action
Lie the child down with the ear requiring medication uppermost or tilt the head.

Reason *So the affected ear faces up and allows easy access to the ear.*

Action
Gently pull the earlobe.

Reason *Straightens the ear canal.*

Actions
In children under the age of 3 years the pinna should be pulled down and back.

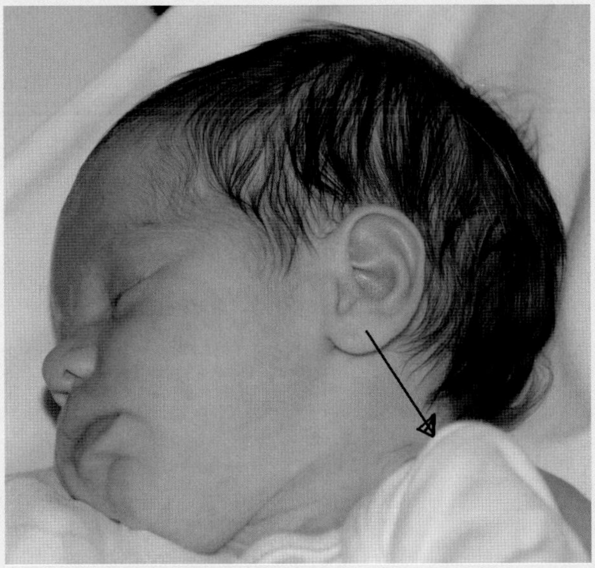

In older children the pinna should be pulled up and back.

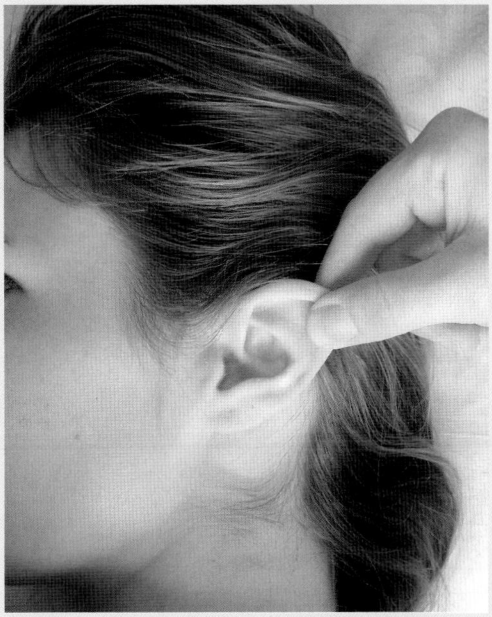

Reason *The internal anatomy of the ear canal changes as the child grows.*

Actions
Place the required number of drops in the ear.

Massage the targus just in front of the ear.

Reason *Helps propel the drops down the ear canal.*

Actions
Keep the ear facing up for 5 min.

Use distraction such as television to help the child maintain position.

Reason *Allows the solution to seep down to the eardrum.*

Procedures Box 16.10 Administration of medicines

1 Check the prescription

Action
Wash and dry your hands thoroughly.

Reason *Prevents cross-infection.*

Action
Check that the prescription chart has the patient's full name, date of birth, identification number and weight.

Reason *These are essential details for checking the correct patient, correct drug and correct dose.*

Action
Check that the prescription is legible and is dated and signed by a doctor.

Reason *These are legal requirements.*

Action
Check which medicine is due and if it has already been given.

Reason *Ensures that medicines are given at the correct time and the child is not overdosed.*

Action
Check if the patient has any known drug allergies.

Reason *Promotes patient safety and prevents allergic reactions.*

Action
Check by which route the medicine is to be given.

Reason *Ensures that the medicine is given via the correct route.*

Action
Check that the dose is appropriate for the child's weight and/or age.

Reason *Maximises therapeutic effects and minimises adverse effects.*

Action
If the prescription appears incomplete or inaccurate contact the appropriate prescriber to amend it before administering the drug.

Reason *Promotes patient safety.*

Procedures Box 16.10 Administration of medicines—cont'd

2 Check the patient

Action
Check that the patient is present in the area before preparing to administer the medicine.

Reason *The patient is immediately available to receive the medicine.*

Action
Check that the patient (and/or his or her parents as appropriate) understands why the medicine is required and how it is to be administered.

Reason *Facilitates informed consent and compliance, concordance and adherence.*

Action
Check any special observations that may be required, such as blood pressure or blood tests.

Reason *To accurately monitor the effect of the medicine.*

3 Check the medicine

Action
Clean any reusable equipment such as trays, drip stands and infusion pumps prior to patient use.

Reason *Prevents cross-infection.*

Action
Put on personal protective equipment as required.

Reason *Prevents contamination by hazardous substances and/or body fluids.*

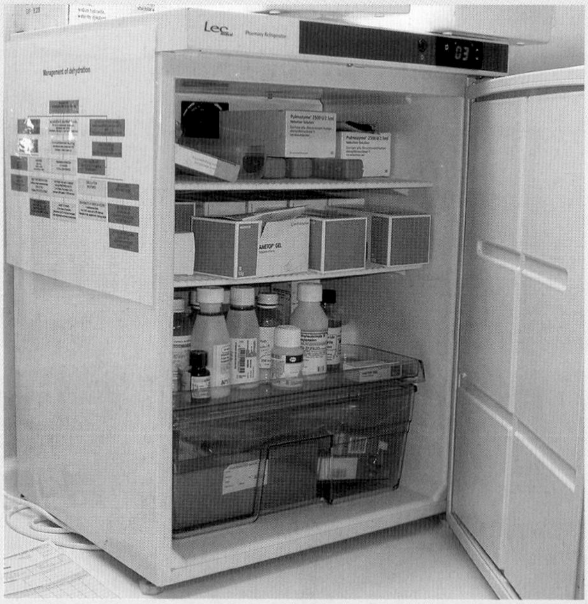

Action
Check that the medicine has been stored in the appropriate place.

Reason *Incorrect storage may lead to degradation of the medicine, resulting in the formation of toxic substances or loss of potency.*

Action
Once a drug container has been removed from its locked cupboard or drug refrigerator you must not leave it unattended.

Reason *Avoids ingestion or tampering by others.*

Action
Check the integrity of all packaging.

Reason *Reduces the risk of potential contamination.*

Actions
Check that drugs are labelled with their name and strength.

If the label is illegible or has become detached the medicine should be returned to the pharmacy.

Reason *Reduces the potential for the incorrect medicine or incorrect dose to be given to the patient.*

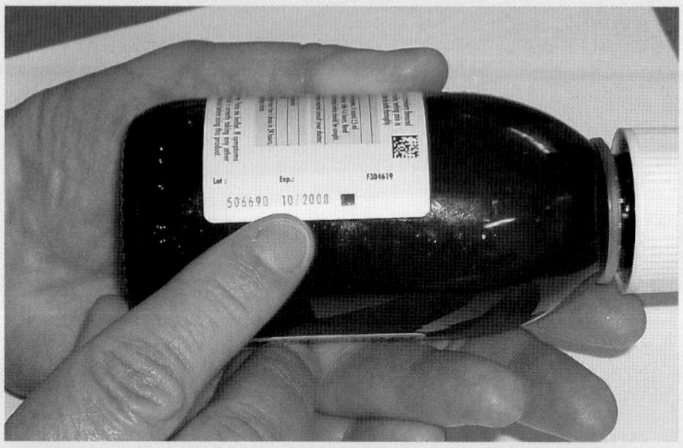

Actions
Check the expiry date of the drug and any diluents or equipment to be used.

Return any drugs exceeding their expiry date to the pharmacy.

Reason *Expired medicine may be less potent or more toxic.*

Action
Check the medicine container against the prescription chart.

Reason *Identifies the correct medication.*

Action
Calculate how much medicine is required.

Reason *To give the prescribed dose.*

4 Administer the medicine

Action
Use a no-touch technique in preparing and administering medicine.

Reason *Reduces exposure to medication and prevents cross-contamination.*

Action
Check the patient's identity using the patient's name band and verbally if possible and against the prescription chart.

Reason *Identifies the correct patient.*

Action
Make sure that the patient actually takes or receives the medicine.

Procedures Box 16.10 Administration of medicines—cont'd

Reason *Promotes patient safety.*

Action
Sign or initial the prescription chart according to local policy.

Reason *To identify when the medicine was given and by whom.*

Actions
Do not resheath, break or bend any used sharps.

Leave any needles and syringes in one piece.

Dispose of all sharp items in a non-permeable, puncture-resistant, tamper-proof container.

Reason *Reduces the risk of exposure to injury and infection.*

Action
Dispose of all hazardous waste (e.g. cytotoxic drugs) in the appropriate containers.

Reason *Reduces the risk of contamination from hazardous waste.*

Action
Wash and dry your hands thoroughly.

Reason *Prevents cross-infection.*

Actions
Observe the patient.

Promptly report abnormal side effects

Reason *To monitor therapeutic and adverse effects.*

Now test your knowledge

Question 1

What two forms of identity check should be used whenever possible before administering any medicine?

Question 2

In what circumstances may it be appropriate to administer rectal medication?

Question 3

What can nursing staff do to reduce the discomfort caused by injection?

Question 4

What actions can be carried out to prevent mechanical backlash or mechanical slack (delay in the patient receiving the prescribed dose) when administering medication via a syringe pump?

Question 5

What are the advantages and disadvantages of giving medication via the intravenous route?

Question 6

What are the possible complications of intramuscular injections?

Question 7

What are the differences in rate of absorption from different subcutaneous injection sites?

Question 8

Why is the use of a spacer recommended when administering an inhaler?

Question 9

After administration of which type of medication via an inhaler should a nurse or carer ensure that children rinse their mouth or clean their teeth, and what is the reason for this?

Question 10

What are the three methods of nasal administration?

Question 11

On which part of the eye should topical drops and ointment be placed, and why is this?

Question 12

For how long, and for what reason, should patients keep their ear facing upwards after ear drops have been given?

References

[Anonymous] (1996) Stop using tongue depressors as splints [editorial]. Paediatric Nursing 8(5):4

Adcock H (2001) Learning from medication errors. Pharmaceutical Journal 267:287–289

Aggarwal R, Cardozo A, Homer J (2004) The assessment of topical nasal drug distribution. Clinical Otolaryngology and Allied Sciences 29(3):201–205

Allard J, Carthey J, Cope J et al (2002) Medication errors: causes, prevention and reduction. British Journal of Haematology 116(2):255–265

Allen S (2005) Outer and middle ear problems. Pharmaceutical Journal 276:83–86

Amirov I, Balanov I, Gorenberg M et al (2003) Nebuliser hood compared to mask in wheezy infants: aerosol therapy without tears! Archives of Disease in Childhood 88(8):719–723

Amoore J, Dewar D, Ingram I et al (2001) Syringe pumps and start up time: ensuring safe practice. Nursing Standard 15(17):43–45

Asthma UK (2007) Demo to help your patients with their inhaler technique. Online. Available: http://www.asthma.org.uk/health_professionals/interactive_inhaler_demo/index.html

Baber N, Pritchard D (2003) Dose estimation for children. British Journal of Clinical Pharmacology 56(5):489–493

Baker SS, Liptak GS, Colletti RB et al (1999) Constipation in infants and children: evaluation and treatment. Journal of Pediatric Gastroenterology and Nutrition 29(5):612–626

Barry PW, O'Callaghan C (1997) Nebuliser therapy in childhood. Thorax 52(suppl. 2):57S–58S

Benninger MS, Hadley JA, Osguthorpe JD et al (2004) Techniques of intranasal steroid use. Otolaryngology – Head and Neck Surgery 130(1):5–24

Bergogne-Bérézin E, Bryskier A (1999) The suppository form of antibiotic administration: pharmacokinetics and clinical application. Journal of Antimicrobial Chemotherapy 43(2):177–185

Bradshaw A, Price L (2007) Rectal suppository insertion: the reliability of the evidence as a basis for nursing practice. Journal of Clinical Nursing 16(1):98–103

Bravery K (1999) Paediatric therapy in practice. In Dougherty L, Lamb J (eds) Intravenous therapy in nursing practice. Churchill Livingstone, Edinburgh, p 401–445

British Medical Association (2001) Consent, rights and choices in health care for children and young people. BMJ, London

British National Formulary for Children (2007) British National Formulary for children. 2007. BMJ, RPSGB, RCPCH, London

British Thoracic Society (1997) Appendix 2: summary of nebuliser guidelines for ward and community staff. Thorax 52(suppl. 2): 18S–19S

British Thoracic Society, Scottish Intercollegiate Guidelines Network (2005) British guideline on the management of asthma, revised edn. Online. Available: http://www.sign.ac.uk/pdf/sign63.pdf

Caldwell C (1998) Management of acute asthma in children. Nursing Standard 92(29):49–54

Campbell H, Carrington M (1999) Peripheral IV cannula dressings: advantages and disadvantages. British Journal of Nursing 8(21):1420–1427

Carbajal R, Veerapen S, Couderc S et al (2003) Analgesic effect of breast feeding in term neonates: randomised controlled trial. British Medical Journal 326(7379):13 Online. Available: http://www.bmj.com/cgi/content/full/326/7379/13

Chappell K, Newman C (2004) Potential tenfold drug overdoses on a neonatal unit. Archives of Disease in Childhood Fetal and Neonatal Edition 89(6):F483–F484

Cheymol G (2000) Effects of obesity on pharmacokinetics: implications for drug therapy. Clinical Pharmacokinetics 39(3):215–231

Chiodini J (2001) Best practice in vaccine administration. Nursing Standard 16(7):35–38

Chung JW, Ng WM, Wong TK (2002) Applied pressure reduced perceived pain at the intramuscular injection site. Journal of Clinical Nursing 11:457–461

Clinical Resource and Audit Group (2002) Good practice statement for the preparation of injections in near-patient areas, including clinical and home environments. Scottish Executive, Edinburgh

Cook IF, Murtagh J (2005) Optimal technique for intramuscular injection of infants and toddlers: a randomised trial. Medical Journal of Australia 183(2):60–63

Cousins DH, Sabatier B, Beuge D et al (2005) Medication errors in intravenous drug preparation and administration: a multicentre audit in the UK, Germany and France. Quality and Safety in Health Care 14(3):190–195

Department of Health (2001) Seeking consent: working with children. Stationery Office, London

Department of Health (2006) Immunisation against infectious disease. 'The green book'. Online. Available: http://www.dh.gov.uk/en/policyand guidance/Healthand Socialcaretopics/Greenbook/DH_4097254

Dimond B (1996) The legal aspects of child health care. Mosby, London

Dougherty L (2002) Delivery of intravenous therapy. Nursing Standard 16(16):45–52,54,56

Duff AJA (2003) Incorporating psychological approaches into routine paediatric venepuncture. Archives of Disease in Childhood 88(10):931–937

Fitzsimons R (2001) Intravenous cannulation. Paediatric Nursing 13(3):21–23

Fuller M (2007) Procedure for the administration of rectal medication to children. In Glasper EA, McEwing G, Richardson J (eds) Oxford handbook of children's and young people's nursing. Oxford University Press, Oxford, p 840–841

Gerhardt RT, King KM, Wiegert RS (2001) Inhaled nitrous oxide versus placebo as an analgesic and anxiolytic adjunct to peripheral cannulation. American Journal of Emergency Medicine 19(6): 492–494

Grieve J, Tordoff J, Reith D et al (2005) Effect of the pediatric exclusivity provision on children's access to medicines. British Journal of Clinical Pharmacology 59(6):730–735

Harbord MG, Kyrkou NE, Kyrkou MR et al (2004) Use of intranasal midazolam to treat acute seizures in paediatric community settings. Journal of Paediatrics and Child Health 40(9–10):556–558

Hemsworth S (2000) Intramuscular (IM) injection technique. Paediatric Nursing 12(9):17–20

Infection Control Nurses Association (2003) Reducing sharps injury: prevention and risk management. ICNA, Bathgate

Isles R, Lister P, Edmunds AT (1999) Crying significantly reduces absorption of aerolised drugs in infants. Archives of Disease in Childhood 81(2):163–165

Jordan S, White J (2001) Bronchodilators: implications for nursing practice. Nursing Standard 15(27):45–55

King L (2003) Subcutaneous injection technique. Nursing Standard 17(34):45–52

Lala KR, Lala MK (2003) Intramuscular injection: review and guidelines. Indian Pediatrics 40:835–845

Lane E (2007) Assisting with cannulation and cannula care. In Glasper EA, McEwing G, Richardson J (eds) Oxford handbook of children's and young people's nursing. Oxford University Press, Oxford, p 148

McConnell EA (2000) Administering an intradermal injection. Nursing 30(3):17

McConnell EA (2001) Instilling eyedrops. Nursing 31(9):17

McDonald CJ (2006) Computerization can create safety hazards: a bar-coding near miss. Annals of Internal Medicine 144(7):510–516

Marsden J, Shaw M (2003) Correct administration of topical eye treatment. Nursing Standard 17(30):42–44

Mentes A (2001) pH changes in dental plaque after using sugar-free pediatric medicine. Journal of Clinical Pediatric Dentistry 25(4):307–312

Miller J, Cross M, Gerrett D et al (2006) A prioritisation of the most effective interventions for reducing medication errors in UK hospitals as perceived by senior pharmacists. European Journal of Hospital Pharmacy Science 12(2):23–28

National Institute for Clinical Excellence (2000) Online. Available: http://www.nice.org.uk

National Patient Safety Agency (2005) Safer practice notice 22 November. 2005. Wristbands for hospital patients improves safety. Online. Available: http://www.npsa.nhs.uk 27 Apr. 2006

Nunn T, Williams J (2005) Formulation of medicines for children. British Journal of Clinical Pharmacology 59(6):674–676

Nursing and Midwifery Council (2004) Guidelines for the administration of medicines. NMC, London

Nursing and Midwifery Practice Development Unit (2003) Nasogastric and gastrostomy tube feeding for children being cared for in the community. Best practice statement. National Health Service Quality Improvement Scotland, Edinburgh

O'Callaghan C, Barry PW (2000) How to choose delivery devices for asthma. Archives of Disease in Childhood 82(3):185–187

O'Shea E (1999) Factors contributing to medication errors: a literature review. Journal of Clinical Nursing 8(5):496–504

Preston ST, Hegadoren K (2004) Glass contamination in parentally administered medication. Journal of Advanced Nursing 48(3):266–270

Quinn C (2000) Infusion devices: risks, functions and management. Nursing Standard 14(26):35–41,42–44

Quraishi MS, Jones NS, Mason JDT (1997) The nasal delivery of drugs. Clinical Otolaryngology and Allied Sciences 22(4):289–301

Rodger MA, King L (2000) Drawing up and administering injections: a review of the literature. Journal of Advanced Nursing 31(3):574–582

Rothwell J, Hegarty A (2007) Venous blood sampling. In Glasper EA, McEwing G, Richardson J (eds) Oxford handbook of children's and young people's nursing. Oxford University Press, Oxford, p 814–815

Royal College of Nursing (2002) Good practice in infection control. RCN, London

Royal College of Nursing (2003) Restraining, holding still and containing children and young people: guidance for nursing staff. RCN, London

Royal College of Nursing IV Therapy Forum (2003) Standards for infusion therapy. Becton Dickinson, Franklin Lakes

Royal College of Nursing, Royal College of General Practitioners, Community Practitioners' and Health Visitors' Association, Royal College of Paediatrics and Child Health (2002) Position statement on injection technique. RCN, RCPCH, London

Scott RC, Besag FMC, Neville BGR (1999) Buccal midazolam and rectal diazepam for treatment of prolonged seizures in childhood and adolescence: a randomised trial. Lancet 353(9153):623–626

Scottish Executive Health Department (2006) A good practice guide on consent for health professionals in NHS Scotland. Scottish Executive, Edinburgh

Scottish Intercollegiate Guidelines Network (2002) Safe sedation of children undergoing diagnostic and therapeutic procedures. SIGN, Edinburgh

Taxis K, Baber N (2003) Ethnographic study of incidence and severity of intravenous drug errors. British Medical Journal 326(7391): 684–687

Thomson FC, Naysmith MR, Lindsay A (2000) Managing drug therapy in patients receiving enteral and parenteral nutrition. Hospital Pharmacist 7(6):155–164

Ulyatt J (2007) Eye care. In Glasper EA, McEwing G, Richardson J (eds) Oxford handbook of children's and young people's nursing. Oxford University Press, Oxford, p 135

Vella C, Grech V (2005) Assessment of use of spacer devices for inhaled drug delivery to asthmatic children. Pediatric Allergy and Immunology 16(3):258–261

Williams J (2007a) Administration of nose medication. In Glasper EA, McEwing G, Richardson J (eds) Oxford handbook of children's and young people's nursing. Oxford University Press, Oxford

Williams J (2007b) Administration of ear medication. In Glasper EA, McEwing G, Richardson J(eds) Oxford handbook of children's and young people's nursing. Oxford University Press, Oxford

Willock J, Richardson J, Brazier CL (2004) Peripheral venepuncture in infants and children. Nursing Standard 18(27):43–50

Winslow EH, Jacobson AF, Peragallo-Dittko V (1997) Rethinking subcutaneous injection technique. American Journal of Nursing 97(5):71–72

Workman B (1999) Safe injection techniques. Nursing Standard 13(39):47–53

Wright A, Falconer J, Newman C (2002) Self-administration and reuse of medicines. Paediatric Nursing 14(6):14–17

17 The use of calculations in the administration of medicines

Theresa Pengelly

Ensuring that each child receives the correct dose of medicine is a vital and integral part of the administration of medicines. The nurse has a responsibility to check prior to each administration that the dose is correct (Nursing and Midwifery Council 2004).

Standard 10: Medicines for Children and Young People (Department of Health 2004) states that all health professionals who are involved must be able to calculate doses of both medicines and infusions. Many nurses find this aspect of care difficult, often due to difficulties with the numeracy skills involved (Stephenson 2005). The number of drug errors continues to rise, with miscalculation being a common cause (Wright 2006). It is thought that the occurrence is similar to that in adults but the consequences are likely to be far more serious (Hutton & Gardener 2005). This is because age and developmental stage will affect the way that medicines are metabolised and excreted. In general an immature system is less able to cope with an excessive amount of medication (Kanneh 2002). The exact figures are not known but it is estimated that this makes a child three times more likely than an adult to suffer adverse effects from a miscalculation (Woodrow 1998).

This chapter explains the principles of accurate calculations and then gives a step-by-step approach to undertaking the different types. The accompanying PowerPoint presentation contains more activities to work through to further develop your calculation skills as an essential part of your professional development as a children's nurse.

Numeracy skills

The understanding of basic numeracy skills is essential (Wilson 2003). It is important that you feel confident in this aspect. Coben & Atere-Roberts (2005) suggest that drawing up a plan that suits your particular learning needs will help to ensure that you are successful in developing calculation skills. Being confident in basic numeracy skills will mean that learning the different ways of calculating will be so much easier. Gatford & Phillips (2002) explain that undertaking a diagnostic numeracy test will help you to identify areas that you find difficult, so that you can ensure that you are competent in all the necessary aspects. The main areas that you need to be confident in are the use of fractions, percentages, decimals and ratios. There are a wide variety of sources of help. The selection of one that you feel suits your learning style and specific needs will be an important part of your future success in achieving calculation skills.

Principles of accurate calculation

Before the calculation is undertaken you have a responsibility to check that it is the correct dose. There should never be reliance that this has already been done by the prescriber. In most circumstances the dose is based on the weight and the age of the child (Hutton 2003). If there is any degree of uncertainty then it is important to check with the current edition of a paediatric formulary, for example the *British National Formulary for Children* (2006; Fig. 17.1).

The metric system is used for calculating all measurements; if the weight is available only in pounds and ounces then it must be converted (see the example later in this chapter). For a small range of medicines, for example in cytotoxic therapy, the calculation is based on the child's surface area. This involves using both the weight and the height of the child. This specialised calculation can be found in a paediatric formulary. In some emergency situations weighing the child may not be possible. In these rare circumstances there are charts available to assist in estimating the weight (Flaherty & Glasper 2006).

Being distracted is likely to increase the risk of miscalculation (Stratton et al 2004). You need to develop the ability to undertake calculations in a busy environment; however, it is always important to be assertive if you feel that you are being interrupted or rushed unnecessarily. If there are two drug checkers then the calculations should be undertaken independently (Dyer et al 2006).

Calculators are now commonplace and have their role, but they are not failsafe and should never be totally depended on. The calculator is reliant on you using it properly. It will be accurate only if used in conjunction with the correct formula. You should only use a calculator that you know how to use. Common sense is also an important factor. Working out a rough dose beforehand and first checking that this is a realistic volume for that particular child is an important step in minimising potential errors associated with the use of calculators.

Straightforward calculations

If the calculation is very easy, mental arithmetic may be sufficient.

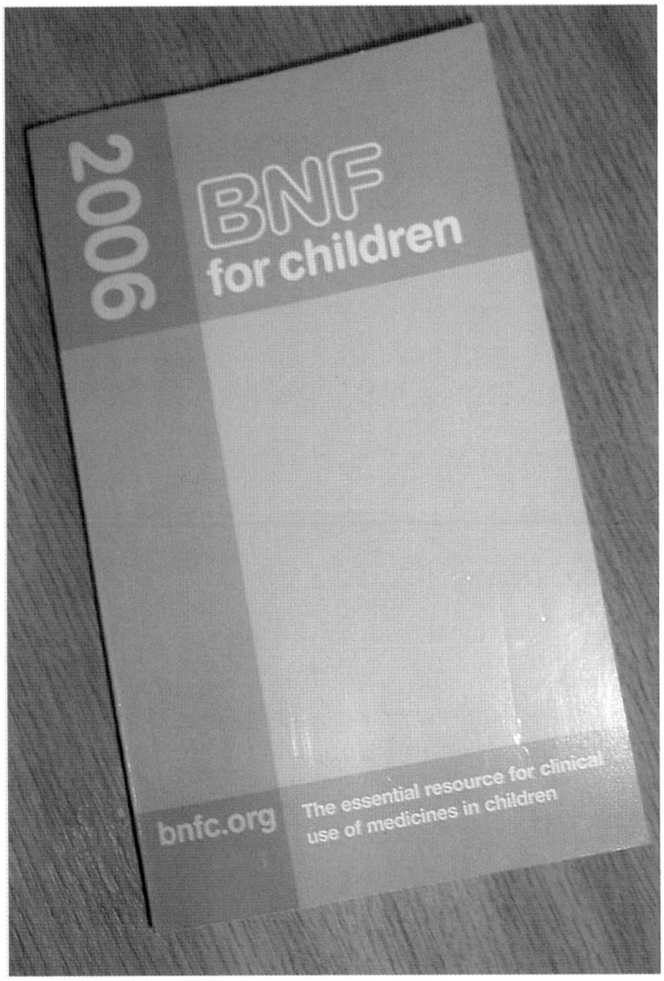

Fig. 17.1 • The *British National Formulary for Children*.

Example

Paracetamol 60 mg is prescribed. You have 120 mg in 5 mL. In looking at the numbers involved you can see that 60 is half of 120. There is 120 mg in 5 mL; you therefore need half of 5 mL, which is 2.5 mL (Fig. 17.2).

This calculation is a familiar one and easy to see; many are more difficult. If the answer is not immediately obvious then it is recommended that you use a formula.

Use of a formula

Once correctly learnt a formula will always work. Before using the formula work out roughly what the answer should be and how much volume that is likely to be, and then check that this is a realistic amount for the child. This is good practice that will help to eliminate errors in using the formula, such as when the decimal point has been wrongly placed. Misplacement of the decimal point can result in 10-fold errors, for example 10 mg being given instead of 1 mg. There are different formulas but the example given is the most common. The consistent use of the

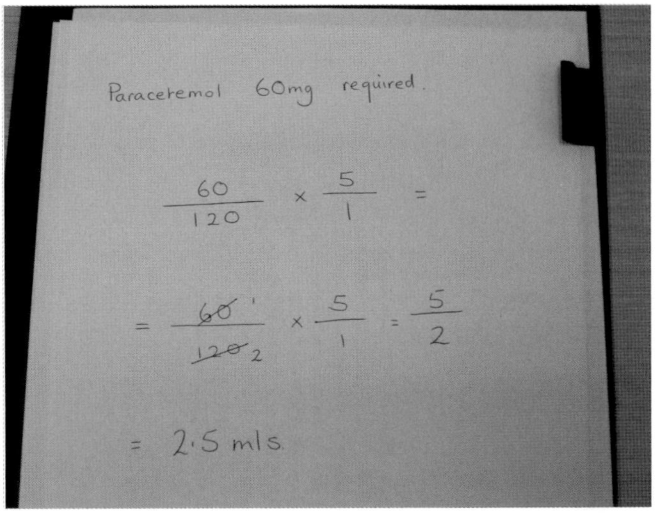

Fig. 17.2 • Calculating the volume needed for paracetamol 60 mg when you have 120 mg in 5 mL.

most common formula will help to standardise practice (Watt 2003). The formula can be used in both the following ways.

Example

This example is quite easy to work out but it is still advised to have rough answer before undertaking the calculation. If this important step becomes part of your everyday practice for all calculations it will play a vital part in minimising errors.

You require flucloxacillin 500 mg. You have flucloxacillin 250-mg capsules. What you require is 500 g divided by 250 mg = 2.

$$\textbf{Dose} = \frac{\textbf{what you want}}{\textbf{what you have}}$$

$$\textbf{500 mg} = \frac{\textbf{500 mg = 2}}{\textbf{250 mg}}$$

Many medicines for children are in suspensions (Fig. 17.3), so then you also need to include the volume that the medicine is in.

Example

You require flucloxacillin 62.5 mg. You have flucloxacillin 125 mg in 5 mL. What you want is 62.5 mg divided by 125 mg multiplied by 5.

$$\textbf{625 mg} = \frac{\textbf{62.5 mg × 5 = 2.5 mL}}{\textbf{125 mg}}$$

The use of a formula requires practice. Below are some examples to try. It is recommended that for all the questions you write down all your workings out. This then means that if you make an error you can work out how it occurred and what areas of numeracy need more development.

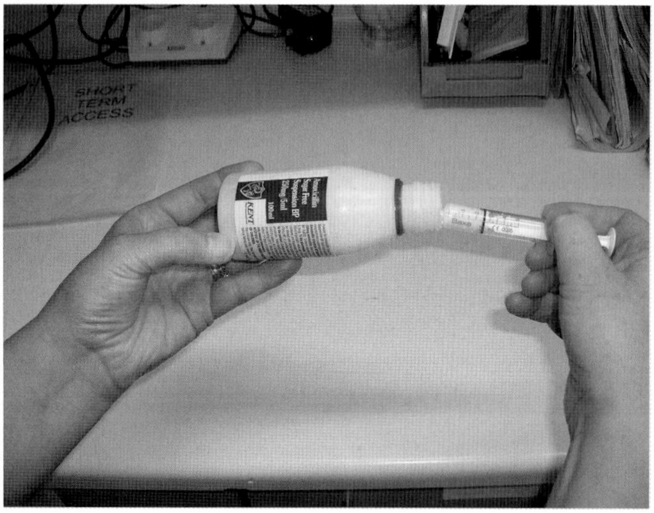

Fig. 17.3 • Medicines often come in suspensions.

Now test your knowledge

Question 1

Calculate the amount needed in the following situations.

1. Ampicillin 500 mg is required. You have 250-mg capsules.
2. Chloral hydrate 100 mg is required. You have 500 mg in 5 mL.
3. Ibuprofen 60 mg is required. You have 100 mg in 5 mL.
4. Digoxin 35 micrograms is required. You have 50 micrograms in 5 mL.

Conversion from metric to imperial units

The weight of the child should be in kilograms, as this is more accurate (Dyer et al 2006). It is recommended that a weight is obtained just prior to the drug being prescribed. There will be the occasional situation in which this may not be possible. Parents often know the weight of their child but sometimes this will be in pounds and ounces. There are weight conversion charts but there also could be occasions when these are not readily accessible (Hutton 2003). The calculation is straightforward but you need to know the following information first:

- 1 stone = 14 lbs
- 1 lb = 16 oz
- 1 kg = 2.2 lbs.

Example

A child is 2 stone, 4 lbs. The weight first needs to be changed to pounds.

28 lbs (2 stone) + 4 lbs = 32 lbs
1 kg = 2.2 lbs
32 lbs ÷ 2.2 lbs = 14.5 kg

Now test your knowledge

Question 2

Use the above calculation to convert these imperial weights to metric weights:

1. 4 stone
2. 1 stone, 7 lbs
3. 8 lbs, 8 oz
4. 7 lbs, 2 oz.

Calculating a dose by body weight

The vast majority of medicines for children are calculated by body weight. In order to check that it is the correct dose you need to be confident in how this is done.

Example

The child weighs 12 kg. The requirement is cefotaxime 50 mg/kg every 8 h.

50 mg × 12 = 600 mg

Therefore 600 mg is the daily dose. To break this down into each dose, 24 h is divided by the hours required.

24 h ÷ 8 h = 3 h

Then the daily dose is divided by this number.

600 mg ÷ 3 = 200 mg

Now test your knowledge

Question 3

What are the doses in the following situations?

1. The child weighs 15 kg. Erythromycin 12.5 mg/kg every 6 h is prescribed. What is the total daily dose?
2. A baby weighs 4 kg. Erythromycin 12.5 mg/kg every 6 h is prescribed. What is the individual dose?
3. A child weighs 4 stone. Paracetamol elixir 20 mg/kg as a single dose is prescribed. Convert the weight to kilograms and calculate the dose.
4. A baby weighs 2 kg. Digoxin 30 micrograms/kg three times a day is prescribed. What is the individual dose?

Conversion between metric units

The metric system is based on decimals and has been the recommended method of describing units of measurement in the National Health Service since 1975 (Coben & Atere-Roberts 2005). There is a base unit with other smaller and larger units. The commonly used base units are the gram (g; Table 17.1), metre (m) and litre (L; Table 17.2). Understanding how the units work and what the different words mean is very important, as you must know how to calculate between the different units. For example, a medicine maybe prescribed in micrograms but only available in milligrams. You therefore need to be competent in converting between the different units to undertake the calculation.

The tables indicate the abbreviations that the *British National Formulary for Children* (2006) states are acceptable to use. There are abbreviations for nanograms and micrograms but as they can easily be misread they are not recommended. For this same reason the use of decimal points is not advised unless it is absolutely necessary. For example it should be 6 mg not 6.0 mg. If a decimal point has to be used it should always have a zero in front, for example 0.6 mg.

Now test your knowledge

Question 4

Now try the following conversions:

1. 0.5 g to mg
2. 2.5 mg to micrograms
3. 6.25 mg to micrograms
4. 45 micrograms to nanograms.

Question 5

Now try the following conversions:

1. 0.5 L to mL
2. 450 mL to L
3. 0.002 L to mL
4. 1.3 L to mL.

Table 17.1. The base unit (gram) and the smaller and larger units

Unit (abbreviation)	Relation to base unit
Kilogram (kg)	Base unit × 1000
Gram (g)	Base unit
Milligram (mg)	Base unit ÷ 1000
Microgram	Base unit ÷ 1000 000
Nanogram	Base unit ÷ 1000 000 000

Table 17.2. The base unit (litre) and the smaller units

Unit (abbreviation)	Relation to base unit
Litre (L)	Base unit
Millilitre (mL)	Base unit ÷ 1000

Reconstitution calculations

There are some drugs that come in powder form and may have to be mixed just prior to use; one example is that of some intravenous antibiotics. They will have what is called a displacement value. This value must be taken into consideration when undertaking the calculation. This is important because otherwise the correct dose will not be administered.

Example

The displacement value of a drug is 0.2 mL. You require 250 mg in 2 mL. You draw up 1.8 mL to reconstitute to the correct strength.

Percentages

There are some times when it is necessary to have solution at a certain strength. There are several everyday solutions that are commercially prepared, for example intravenous fluids such as glucose 5% and also drugs such as lidocaine. There will be times when a specific strength solution has to be made up. In some instances the prescription may be in milligrams or micrograms. It is therefore important to understand how percentages are calculated and to be able to transfer to a metric unit. A percentage is a part of a hundred, therefore 5% is 5 parts of 100 parts. The percentage means the number of grams per 100 mL of solution.

Examples

Five percent glucose means that for every 100 mL of solution there is 5 g of glucose. Broken down further it means that there is 50 mg of glucose per 1 mL of solution.

As another example, 0.5% lidocaine means that for every 1 mL there is 5 mg of lidocaine.

If you are a bit uncertain about transferring within the metric system, you may find it helpful to refer back to Table 17.1 before answering the following questions.

Now test your knowledge

Question 6

Work out the following:

1. How many grams per 100 mL does dextrose 10% contain?

2. How many milligrams per 1 mL does dextrose 10% contain?
3. You require lidocaine 4 mg. You have lidocaine 0.5%. How much do you require?
4. You require lidocaine 4000 micrograms. You have lidocaine 1%. How much do you require?

Ratios

A ratio means a comparison of two quantities using division (Chernecky et al 2006). This can be used for some drugs, for example skin or mouthwash preparations when dilution is required.

Example

A 1:5 solution means that there is one part stock to five parts dilution. This means that overall there are six parts. If your stock solution is 5 mL you will require 25 mL of dilution, giving a total of 30 mL.

Now test your knowledge

Question 7

Calculate the volumes and solution strengths in the following situations:

1. The stock solution is 4 mL. You require a 1:10 solution. What is the total volume?
2. The stock solution is 10 mL. You require a 1:3 solution. What is the total volume?
3. The total volume is 12 mL. The stock solution was 2 mL. What strength is the solution?
4. The total solution is 1 L. The stock solution was 25 mL. What strength is the solution?

Intravenous fluid calculations

As with medicines for children, intravenous fluids need to be calculated. To minimise the risk of the child receiving a fluid overload the use of an infusion pump is always recommended (McIntosh 2006). It is possible to calculate intravenous fluids by working out the drops per minute (not using an infusion pump); however, because of the associated risk it is not recommended for use with children and is therefore not covered in this chapter.

Intravenous fluids may be calculated at an hourly rate, an amount to be administered over a set time. As with all medicines, before undertaking the calculation it must first be checked that this is a realistic amount for that specific child. When making this decision it is important to take into consideration all the fluids the child is receiving and check this against the maintenance fluid requirements. Maintenance fluid requirements are calculated taking into consideration a number of factors regarding the child's condition (Willcock & Jukes 2000). You should check your trust guidelines for the agreed policy regarding maintenance fluids. If the prescription is to run over a set time then this needs to be calculated to an hourly rate.

Example

Five hundred millilitres of intravenous fluids is prescribed over 8 h.

500 mL ÷ 8 h = 62.5 mL/h

Intravenous fluids may also need to be calculated as part of the maintenance requirement. On some occasions you may need to calculate a percentage of the maintenance requirement and also take into consideration other fluids such as intravenous drugs or flushes.

Example

The maintenance fluid requirement is 400 mL/day. The prescription is for 75% of the maintenance requirement, to be given hourly.

75% of 400 mL = 300 mL ÷ 24 h = 12.5 mL/h

Now test your knowledge

Question 8

Provide answers to the following:

1. A child is prescribed intravenous fluids; the volume is 500 mL to run over 6 h. What is the hourly rate?
2. A baby weighs 6 kg. The maintenance fluid requirement is 150 mL/kg in 24 h, and 75% maintenance fluids are prescribed. What volume is this over 24 h?
3. A child weighs 10 kg. He is prescribed an intravenous infusion of glucose 5% with aminophylline 1 mg/kg per h. The concentration required is 1 mg/mL. What will the total volume of this infusion be in 24 h?
4. A baby weighs 1.6 kg. The maintenance fluid requirement is 150 mL/kg per day. You need to give oral feeds 3-hourly and use 75% of the maintenance requirement. What is the volume of each feed?

Recommendations

- Check that your practice adheres to your Trust's administrations of medicines policy.
- Critically evaluate your calculation skills using an SWOT (strengths, weaknesses, opportunities and threats) analysis. Draw up an action plan so you can address these.
- Using your action plan as a guide, keep a reflective sheet of your drug calculation activity. This will enable you to ensure that you are aware of calculations that you rarely use in the clinical area and may need to update by different methods.
- Think of all the associated risks in drug calculation and how you can minimise the risk of these occurring in your own practice.

References

British National Formulary for Children (2006) British National Formulary for children 2006. BMJ Publishing Group, Royal Pharmaceutical Society of Great Britain, RCPH Publications, London

Chernecky C, Infortunata H, Macklin D (2006) Drug calculations and drug administration, 2nd edn. Saunders, St Louis

Coben D, Atere-Roberts E (2005) Calculations for nursing and healthcare, 2nd edn. Palgrave Macmillan, Hampshire

Department of Health (2004) Standard 10: medicines for children and young people. National service framework for children, young people and maternity services. Department of Health, London

Dyer L, Furze C, Maddox C, Sales R (2006) Administration of medicines. In Trigg E, Mohammed T (eds) Practices in children's nursing: guidelines for hospital and community. Churchill Livingstone, London, p 45–82

Flaherty J, Glasper EA (2006) Emergency department management of children. In Glasper EA, Richardson J (eds) A textbook of children's and young people's nursing. Churchill Livingstone, London, p 361–364

Gatford J, Phillips N (2002) Nursing calculations, 6th edn. Churchill Livingstone, London

Hutton M (2003) Calculation skills for new prescribers. Nursing Standard 17(25):47–52

Hutton M, Gardener H (2005) Calculation skills. Paediatric Nursing (suppl.) 17(2):1–18

Kanneh A (2002) Paediatric pharmological principles: an update. Part 3. Pharmacokinetics:metabolism and excretion. Paediatric Nursing 4(10):39–43

McIntosh N (2006) Intravenous therapy. In Trigg E, Mohammed T (eds) Practices in children's nursing: guidelines for hospital and community. Churchill Livingstone, London, p 211–223

Nursing and Midwifery Council (2004) Guidelines for the safe administration of drugs. NMC, London

Stephenson P (2005) Trust brings in maths test to reduce drug errors. Nursing Standard 19(38):5

Stratton KM, Blegen MA, Pepper G, Vaughn T (2004) Reporting of medication errors by pediatric nurses. Journal of Pediatric Nursing 19(6):385–392

Watt S (2003) Safe administration of medicines to children: part 1. Paediatric Nursing 15(4):40–43

Willcock J, Jewkes F (2000) Making sense of fluid balance in children. Paediatric Nursing 12(7):37–42

Wilson (2003) Nurses' maths: researching a practical approach. Nursing Standard 17(47):33–36

Woodrow P (1998) Numeracy skills. Nursing Standard 17(30):48–55

Wright K (2006) Barriers to accurate drug calculations. Nursing Standard 20(28):41–45

18 The management of procedural pain in children using self-administered Entonox

Denise Jonas

Entonox is the brand name for 50% nitrous oxide and 50% oxygen supplied by the British Oxygen Company. Nitrous oxide was discovered by Priestley in 1772; it is a sweet-smelling and colourless gas. The fixed mixture of nitrous oxide and oxygen was introduced by Tunstall in 1961 for use in obstetrics (British Oxygen Company 2000). Entonox is a compressed gaseous mixture of 50% nitrous oxide and 50% oxygen; this combination ensures that the patient receives the benefits of oxygen alongside the pain relief of nitrous oxide without producing unconsciousness.

Entonox is most commonly used in dentistry, in childbirth and by the ambulance service; however, its use in children is steadily increasing (Annequin et al 2000, Bruce & Franck 2000, Cleary et al 2002, Ekbom et al 2005, Pickup & Pagdin 2000). Entonox is an effective method of managing short-term pain while offering the child some control over his or her pain and reduction in anxiety.

Entonox acts as a very potent analgesic agent with a very rapid onset of action and rapid elimination, largely unchanged from the body, via the lungs. Its low fat solubility does not allow it to accumulate within the body and cause toxicity (British Oxygen Company 2000). It has been suggested that Entonox activates the release of noradrenergic substances within the pain pathway; these substances activate receptors in the dorsal horn of the spinal cord, reducing pain signals to the brain (Sealey 2002). Entonox is fully effective within six to eight breaths and wears off rapidly with minimal side effects, making it suitable for outpatient use and dressing clinics. An additional advantage is that it provides pain relief but continues to allow verbal contact and cooperation with the child throughout the procedure.

In most cases Entonox is administered using a patient demand system with either a mouthpiece or a face mask. Continuous flow Entonox is used only by specialist trained personnel, as nitrous oxide is an anaesthetic gas; free flow Entonox can cause deep sedation and requires close monitoring (Bruce & Franck 2000).

The valve on a patient demand system allows gas to flow only when the child inhales through the mouthpiece or mask; a characteristic hissing sound is heard as the Entonox is inhaled. Using such a system ensures that when the child becomes drowsy the mouthpiece or mask drops away from the child's mouth and the Entonox ceases to flow; this prevents loss of protection of laryngeal reflexes and over-sedation (Brody et al 1995). For this reason it is important to ensure that the child holds the demand system and not the health professional or parent.

Entonox can be used alone or in conjunction with other analgesics; however, its use is restricted to short-term procedural pain and it is not an alternative to a general anaesthetic.

Contraindications

Nitrous oxide will diffuse into any air-filled space within the body and expand the area, causing increased pressure within a confined space (British Oxygen Company 2000). Therefore Entonox should not be used in any condition in which air may be trapped in the body:

- Pneumothorax
- Gross abdominal distension or bowel obstruction
- Recent underwater dive or decompression sickness
- Air embolism
- Closed head injury
- Raised intracranial pressure
- Severe bullous emphysema
- Glue ear in children.

Entonox is inappropriate in cases of potential impaired level of consciousness:

- Maxillofacial injuries
- Partial airway obstruction
- Impaired conscious level from head injury, intoxication or sedation.

Use with caution

- Repeated use can interfere with the production of vitamin B_{12} and cause megaloblastic changes in the bone marrow function (Culshaw et al 2003, Peate & Lancaster 2000). Children having Entonox more frequently than every 4 days should have regular monitoring of full blood count (British Oxygen Company 1995). Careful consideration should also be given to use in children with poor nutritional status.
- Patients with acute exacerbation of asthma may develop postinhalation hypoxia following use of Entonox. However, a study by Seddon et al (2005) suggests that Entonox is safe and effective in children with cystic fibrosis.
- Long-term use of Entonox can lead to peripheral neuropathy (Doran et al 2004).

- Exposure of high levels of Entonox for prolonged periods can reduce fertility (Gray et al 1993, Rowland et al 1992). There is no conclusive evidence to suggest that Entonox is harmful to the fetus but staff may wish to avoid exposure in the first trimester of pregnancy (British Oxygen Company 1995).
- With frequent use Entonox drug addiction is a possibility.

Possible adverse effects

- Dizziness
- Dry mouth and nausea
- Children may become giggly or verbally abusive
- Drowsiness
- Euphoria.

These symptoms will resolve once the Entonox administration stops.

Possible indications for use

- Changing dressings
- Removal of wound drains or wound packs
- Removal of Kirschner wires (K wires) or cleaning of pin sites
- Suturing or removal of sutures from painful areas
- Short-term dental treatment
- Physiotherapy and limb manipulation
- Application of splints, traction and plaster of Paris
- Acute trauma
- Invasive procedures such as venepuncture or cannulation in needle-phobic children for whom distraction or local anaesthetic agents have failed.

Staff training

The health professional must be fully qualified and competent in the management of Entonox, according to individual organisational protocols, guidelines and educational training programs. The procedure and administration of Entonox must be carried out using a minimum of two people. The health professional supervising the Entonox administration must not get involved with the procedure but maintain contact with the child at all times. Neither is it sufficient for the care of the child to be handed over to the parent.

Entonox use in children is usually prescribed but this depends on individual organisational policy.

Equipment required

Entonox is normally supplied in cylinders coloured blue with white quarter segments on the collar. The cylinder must be stored above −6 °C. Below this temperature the gas separates; if this occurs a high concentration of oxygen will be delivered first with no analgesic effect, but as the cylinder empties the mixture will become progressively more potent as it approaches 100% nitrous oxide. If the cylinder has been left outside in temperatures below −6 °C then it should be kept at room temperature for 2 h before use (British Oxygen Company 1995). Ideally the cylinder should be stored in a horizontal position; however, it may be stored upright in a cradle or attached to a wall. It is recommended that the demand system should be stored in a separate area to the cylinder to prevent unauthorised use of Entonox. Community staff should seek advice from their organisation on the transportation of Entonox cylinders.

It is important that Entonox administration is undertaken in a well-ventilated room; the occupational exposure standard for nitrous oxide exposure is less than 100 parts per million (British Oxygen Company 1995, Pascoe 2003). Frequent use in the same area should prompt instigation of a gas-scavenging system (Pediani 2003, Robertson 2006).

Assessment of the child

- The child should be assessed to exclude any contraindications.
- The success of Entonox depends on the cooperation of the child, therefore age-appropriate explanation and information are needed.

LINK CHAPTER 3

- The age of the child is only a guide: success will depend on the complexity of the procedure, pain intensity and level of anticipatory anxiety (Liossi 2002). The child should be old enough to trigger the demand valve; often young children are unable to maintain Entonox for a lengthy procedure.

Use of intravenous opiates and fasting

- Children requiring intravenous opiates, large doses of oral opiates or sedative drugs as part of their pain management may need to be starved prior to the use of Entonox. In these circumstances it is suggested that the health professional seek advice from medical personnel. It is recommended that children who have received intravenous opioids have monitoring of oxygen saturations and respiratory rate throughout the procedure.
- Children using Entonox alone or mild oral analgesia do not need to be starved but these children should abstain from food for at least 1 h before the use of Entonox.
- Additional oral analgesia is recommended at least 1 h prior to the procedure, as the analgesic effects of Entonox wear off quickly yet the child may continue to experience residual pain from the procedure.

The use of Entonox is rapidly increasing in children with the recognition that it is safe and effective. It is ideal for children undergoing painful procedures for whom distraction, relaxation and analgesia will be beneficial.

Procedures Box 18.1 Self-administration of Entonox by a child

1 Preparation

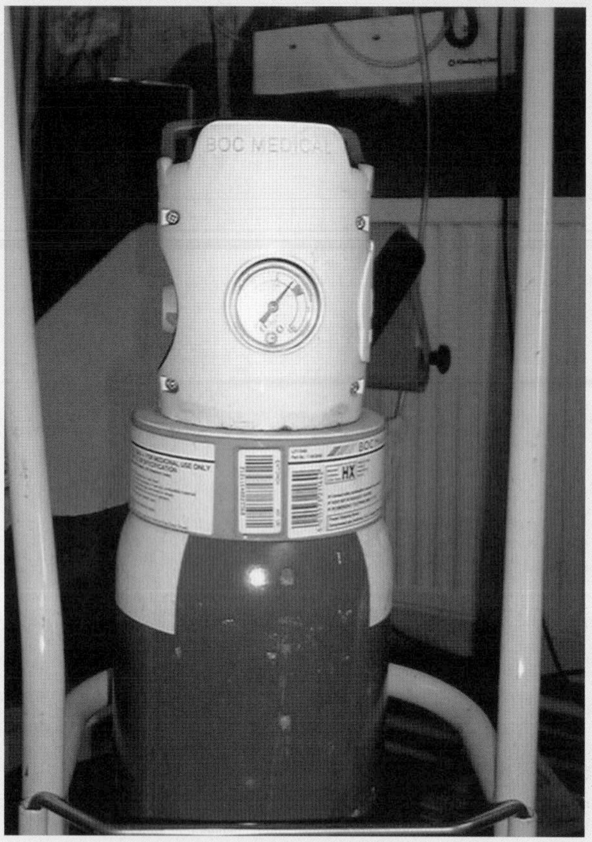

Action
Prepare the equipment and environment.

Actions
Check the cylinder by inspecting the blue and white collar.
Check the expiry date.

Reason *Ensures that the correct cylinder is used.*

Action
Check the level of gas in the cylinder by examining the contents gauge on the cylinder.

Reason *Ensures that there is enough Entonox in the cylinder for the whole of the procedure; if the cylinder is less than one-quarter full, ensure that a new full cylinder is available.*

Action
Check for any signs of oil or grease on the cylinder.

Reason *Entonox is non-flammable but supports combustion in the presence of oil, grease or open flame.*

Action
If the cylinder has been stored in a vertical position the cylinder should be inverted several times before use to mix the gas.

Reason *Ensures that the correct concentrations of analgesia are delivered.*

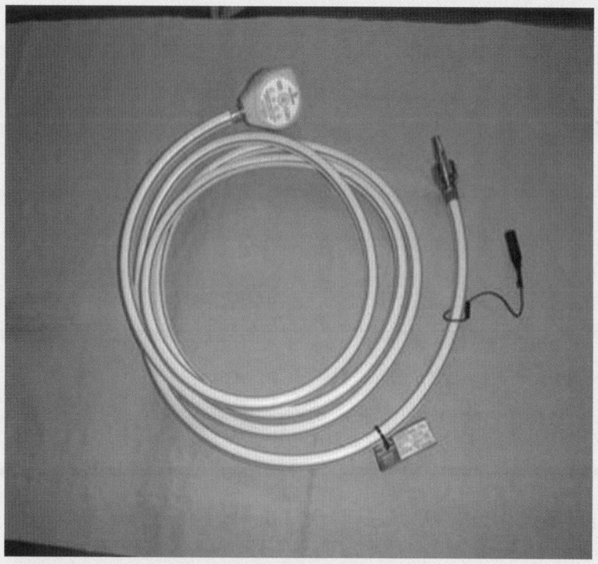

Action
Connect the demand system to the Entonox cylinder.

Reason *Ensures that the system is working correctly prior to commencing the procedure.*

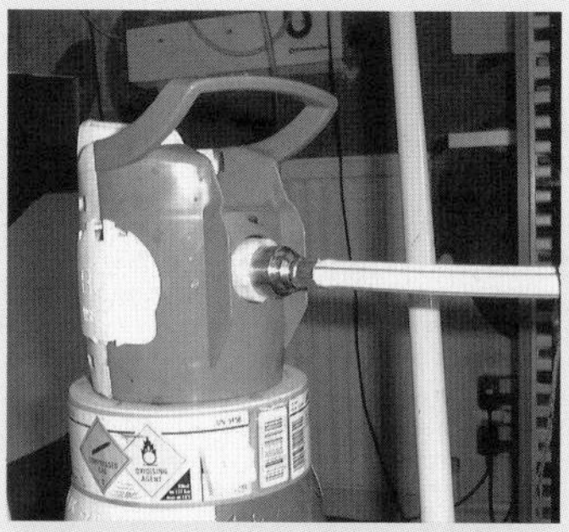

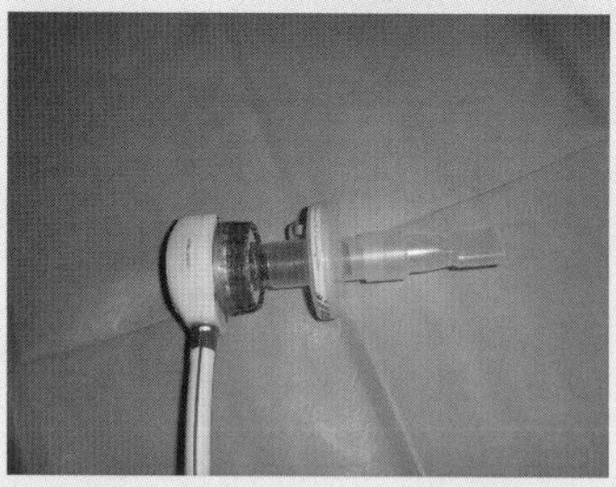

Actions
Apply a single-patient-use filter and single-patient-use mouthpiece.
A mask may also be used in place of the mouthpiece.

Reason *Prevents cross-infection.*

Action
If using a mask, ensure that the mask is the correct size for the child; it should fit snugly on to the child's face over the nose and mouth.

Procedures Box 18.1 Self-administration of Entonox by a child—cont'd

1 Continued

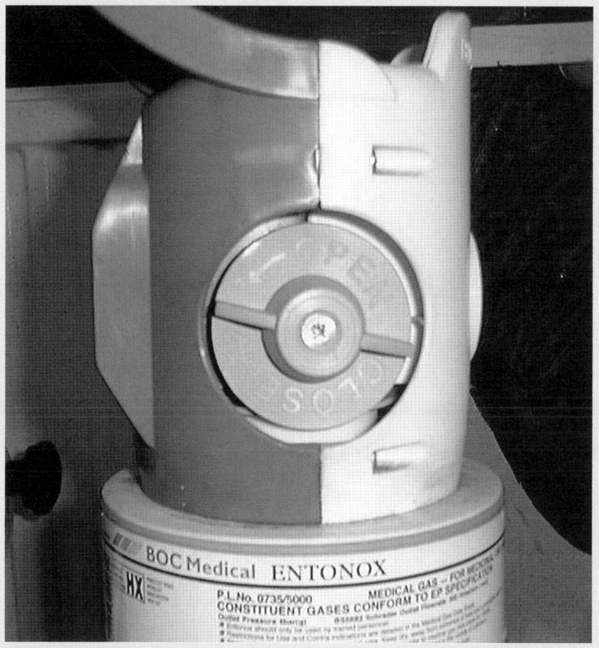

Action
Turn on the gas at the valve on the side of the cylinder.

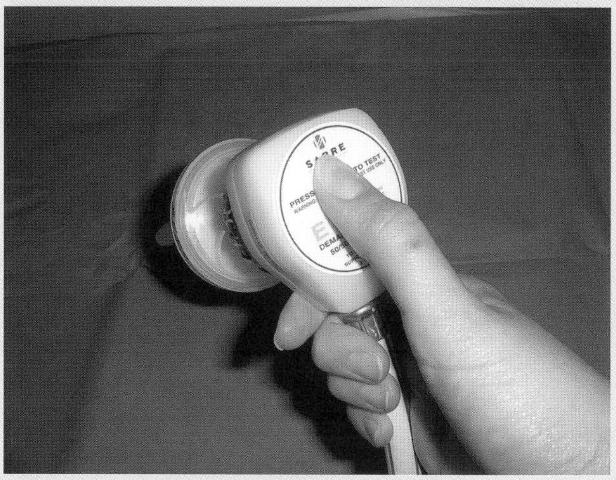

Action
Test that the system is working by depressing the button on the demand system.

Reason *Gas will flow from the system and any stale air or particles of dust will be expelled.*

Action
Ensure that the room is well ventilated.

Reason *Ensures a safe environment for both the patient and the staff by avoiding unnecessary accumulation of ambient levels of nitrous oxide.*

Action
Check that oxygen and suction are readily available and working next to where the child is.

Reason *Ensures that essential equipment is functioning correctly before the procedure commences.*

Action
Ensure that resuscitation equipment is within close proximity to the area the procedure is being carried out.

Reason *Ensures the child's safety should an adverse event occur.*

Actions
If the child has received intravenous opioids or sedation ensure that a pulse oximeter is used.

The child's oxygen saturation and respiration should be recorded every 5 min.

Reason *Ensures the provision of adequate monitoring and documentation.*

Action
Undertake a baseline set of observations before the child uses the Entonox.

Action
Measurement of oxygen saturation should continue for 5 min after the Entonox administration has ceased.

Reason *Observes for postinhalation hypoxia.*

2

Assessment of the child

Action
Assess the child to exclude any contraindications to the use of Entonox.

Reason *Ensures that Entonox is appropriate for the child.*

Actions
Assess the child for the ability to use Entonox appropriately.

Assess the duration and invasiveness of the procedure.

Reason *Self-administration relies on the cooperation of the child for its effective use.*

Actions
Teach and demonstrate the use of Entonox to the child in a manner appropriate to her or his level of understanding.

Involve parents in the education and handling of the equipment.

Reason *Reduces parent and child anxiety.*

Actions
Allow the child to become familiar with the noise the Entonox makes by momentarily depressing the button on the demand system.

Reassure the child that she or he will not lose consciousness.

Offer the child the option of a mask or mouthpiece.

Reason *Ensures that the child gains maximum benefit from the Entonox and assesses if the child will be able to use Entonox effectively.*

Action
The nurse or health professional supervising the Entonox administration will have received training in the use of Entonox and been formally assessed as competent.

Reason *Ensures that staff are trained to undertake Entonox administration and are aware of any potential side effects and contraindications and the safety aspects of the use of Entonox.*

Procedures Box 18.1 Self-administration of Entonox by a child—cont'd

2 Continued

Action
Ensure that there are adequate numbers of staff to undertake the procedure.

Reason *Ensures adequate supervision of the child.*

Action
Ensure that Entonox is prescribed.

Reasons *To conform to the organisational drug policy on medicine administration.*

Action
Check that the child has received no food for 1 h before the procedure.

Reason *Reduces the risk of inhalation of vomit.*

Action
If the child is receiving intravenous opiates or sedation ensure that the child has been fasted for the appropriate period prior to the procedure.

Reason *Sedation and intravenous opiates in combination with Entonox can increase sedation and the incidence of vomiting.*

Actions
Ensure that the person undertaking the procedure prepares the equipment beforehand and away from the sight of the child.

Cover the equipment with a sterile towel.

Reasons *Prevents unnecessary distress to the child caused by witnessing the equipment.*
Prevents delays in undertaking the procedure.
Ensures that Entonox is used for the minimum amount of time.

3

Administration to the child

Action

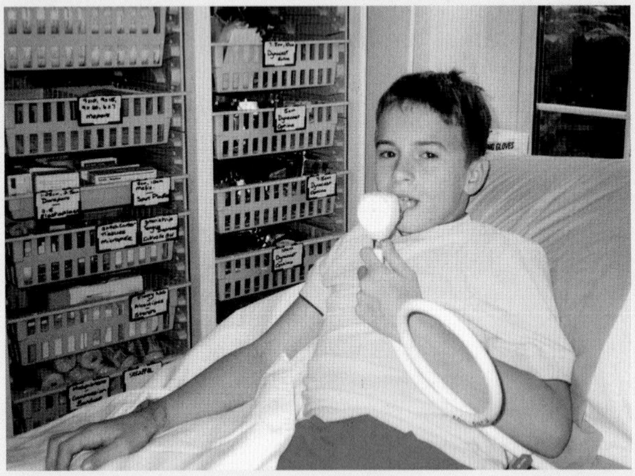

Help the child to achieve a comfortable position prior to commencement of inhalation of the Entonox.

Reason *Promotes relaxation.*

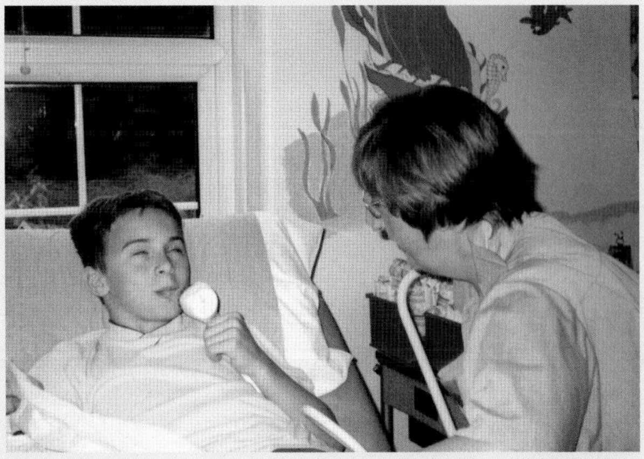

Actions
Encourage the child to breathe for about six to eight breaths before commencement of the procedure.

Do not allow the painful part of the procedure to start until the child is receiving the full effects of the Entonox.

Reason *Allows reasonable levels of nitrous oxide to accumulate in the body prior to the painful stimuli, thus providing optimum analgesia.*

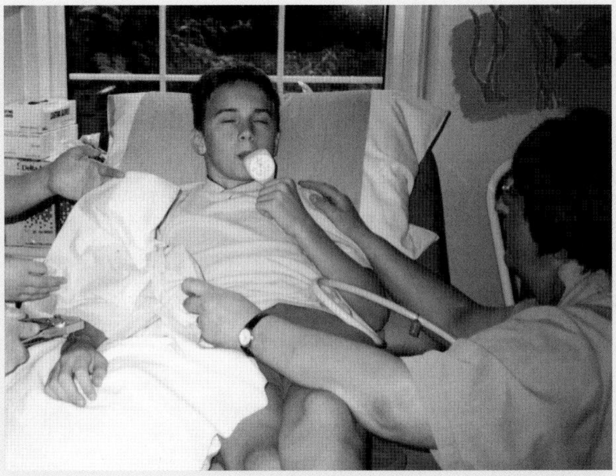

Actions
Observe the child's level of pain consistently throughout the procedure.

Maintain frequent verbal contact, encouraging relaxation and steady breathing.

Encourage deeper breathing if the child experiences pain or suspend the procedure until the pain has reduced.

Reason *Ensures that the child has minimal discomfort throughout the procedure.*

Action
Should the child experience any side effects, reassure the child that they will wear off.

Reason *Reduces anxiety.*

Procedures Box 18.1 Self-administration of Entonox by a child—cont'd

3 Continued

Action
If necessary, stop the procedure and allow the side effects to wear off.

Action
If pain relief is poor then the procedure must be halted until alternative analgesia or sedation can be instigated.

Reason *Entonox may not be effective for everyone; it is better to abandon the procedure than have the child suffer excessive pain and distress.*

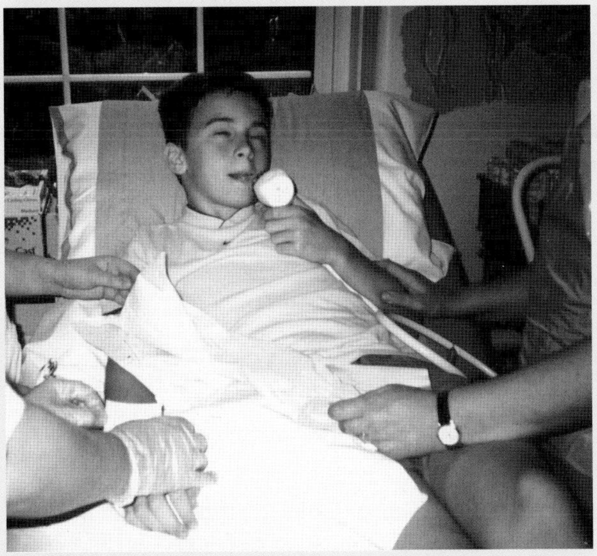

Action
Continue to allow the child to breathe the Entonox until the procedure is completed.

Reason *Ensures that the child has minimal discomfort.*

4 Recovery

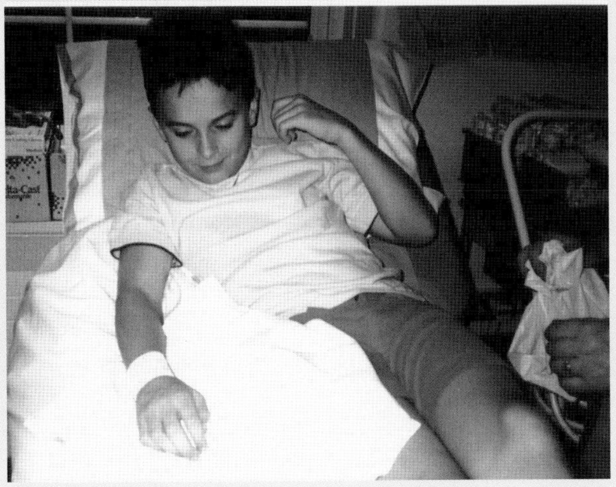

Action
When the child has stopped breathing the Entonox and the procedure is complete, stay with the child until the effects of the Entonox have completely worn off (usually approximately 20 min).

Reason *Protects the child from falls or injury caused by transient dizziness while under the influence of Entonox.*

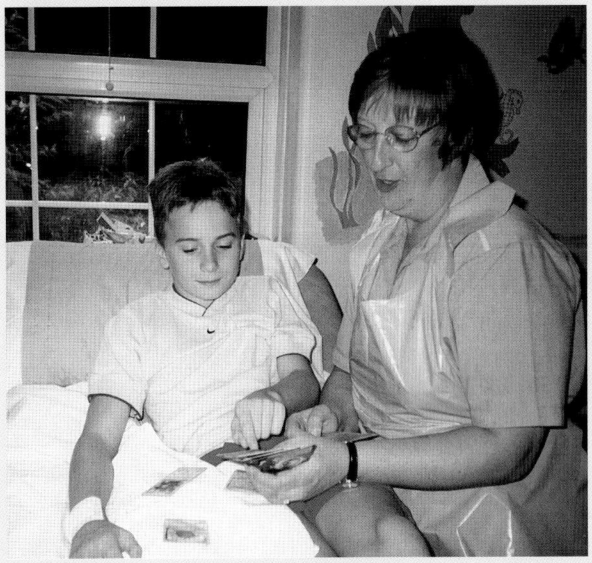

Action
Reward the child with the use of stickers or certificates.

Reason *Increases the child's self-esteem and reinforces the positive aspects of the procedure.*

5 Documentation

Action
Evaluate the procedure and the effectiveness of Entonox in the child's care plan or notes.

Reasons *Ensures accurate documentation of the use of Entonox.*
Ensures that other members of staff are aware of the effectiveness of Entonox for future reference should the procedure need to be repeated.

Action
Sign the Entonox prescription on the child's medication chart.

Reason *To conform to the organisational hospital drug policy on medicine administration.*

6 Dismantling of equipment

Actions
Turn off the Entonox cylinder.

Exhaust the residual gas and depressurise the cylinder by depressing the test button on the demand set.

Procedures Box 18.1 Self-administration of Entonox by a child—cont'd

6 Continued

Dismantle the Entonox equipment.

Reason *Maintains the system in good working order.*

Action

Dispose of the filter and mouthpiece.

Reason *Prevents cross-infection.*

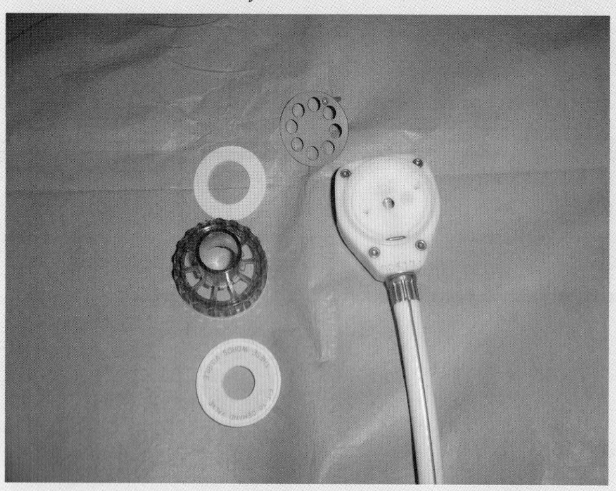

Actions

Clean the system by washing the working parts and mask in soap and water, drying, and then wiping over with an alcohol-based solution or similar.

Wipe the demand system head and length of hose.

Reason *Cleaning should be undertaken according to organisational infection control policy.*

Action

Store the equipment and cylinder in the appropriate manner.

Reasons *Prevents inadvertent misuse of Entonox by leaving the system connected.*
Maintains a safe environment.

(Photographs courtesy of Central Manchester and Manchester Children's University Hospitals NHS Trust.)

Entonox® is a registered British Oxygen Company Group trademark.

Now test your knowledge

- Undertake a risk assessment for the introduction of Entonox use for children in your area.
- List the contraindications that the health professional has to take into account when delivering Entonox to a child.
- Document how you would assess and prepare a 7-year-old child for removal of a wound drain and abdominal sutures using Entonox.

Question 1

What does Entonox gas contain?

Question 2

What are the ideal conditions that the Entonox cylinder and demand system should be stored in?

Question 3

How old must children be before they can use Entonox?

Question 4

List the types of painful procedure that you could use Entonox for.

Question 5

What possible interventions should be considered before using Entonox in a child requiring insertion of an intravenous cannula?

Question 6

What possible adverse effects may the child experience when breathing Entonox?

Question 7

For how long does the child need to breathe Entonox in order for it to be fully effective?

Question 8

While supervising a child aged 8 years self-administering Entonox, the child starts to complain of pain. What do you do?

Question 9

How long does it take for the effects of Entonox to wear off?

Question 10

What measures should you take to minimise infection when undertaking Entonox administration?

References

Annequin D, Carbajal R, Chauvin P, Gall O, Tourniaire B, Murat I (2000) Fixed 50% nitrous oxide oxygen mixture for painful procedures: a French survey. Pediatrics 105:e47

British Oxygen Company (1995) British Oxygen Company medical gases: Entonox data sheet. Online: Available: http://www1.boc.com/uk/sds/ 20 Jun 2006

British Oxygen Company (2000) Entonox. Controlled pain relief reference guide. BOC, Manchester

Brody TM, Larner J, Minneman KP, Nue HC (1995) Human pharmacology, 2nd edn. Mosby, London

Bruce E, Franck L (2000) Self administered nitrous oxide (Entonox) for the management of procedural pain. Paediatric Nursing 12(7):15–19

Cleary AG, Ramanan AV, Baildam E, Birch A, Sills JA, Davidson JE (2002) Nitrous oxide analgesia during intra-articular injection for juvenile idiopathic arthritis. Archives of Disease in Childhood 86:416–418

Culshaw V, Yule M, Lawson R (2003) Considerations for anaesthesia in children with haematological malignancy undergoing short procedures. Paediatric Anaesthesia 13:375–383

Doran M, Rassam SR, Jones LM, Underhill S (2004) Toxicity after intermittent inhalation of nitrous oxide for analgesia. British Medical Journal 328:1364–1365

Ekbom K, Jakobsson J, Marcus C (2005) Nitrous oxide inhalation is a safe and effective way to facilitate procedures in paediatric outpatient departments. Archives of Disease in Childhood 90:1073–1076

Gray RH, Rowland AS, Baird DD, Weinberg CR, Brodsky JB, Baird PA (1993) Nitrous oxide and fertility. New England Journal of Medicine 328:284–285

Liossi C (2002) Procedure related cancer pain in children. Radcliffe Medical Press, Oxford

Pascoe EW (2003) Every precaution has to be taken when using Entonox. Nursing Times 99(1):15

Peate I, Lancaster J (2000) Safe use of medical gases in the clinical setting: practical tips. British Journal of Nursing 9(4):231–236

Pediani R (2003) Patient administered inhalation of nitrous oxide and oxygen gas for procedural pain relief. World wide wounds. Online. Available: http://www.worldwidewounds.com/2003/october/Pediani/Entonox-pain-relief.html 19 Jun 2006

Pickup S, Pagdin J (2000) Procedural pain: Entonox can help. Paediatric Nursing 12(10):33–36

Robertson A (2006) Nitrous oxide – no laughing matter. Online. Available: http://www.birthinternational.com/articles/andrea27.html 19 Jun 2006

Rowland AS, Baird DD, Weinberg CR, Shore DL, Shy CM, Wilcox AJ (1992) Reduced fertility among women employed as dental assistants exposed to high levels of nitrous oxide. New England Journal of Medicine 327:993–997

Sealey L (2002) Nurse administration of Entonox to manage pain in ward settings. Nursing Times 98(46):28–29

Seddon PC, Lenton C, Warde C (2005) Effectiveness and safety of nitrous oxide/oxygen mixture for analgesia during painful procedures in children with cystic fibrosis. Archives of Disease in Childhood 90(suppl. 2):A29

19 Peak flow monitoring

Gilli Lewis

Peak flow monitoring is an example of objective lung function measurements used in the diagnosis and management of respiratory conditions such as asthma (British Thoracic Society & Scottish Intercollegiate Guidelines Network 2005, Global Initiative for Asthma 2005). Asthma is a common chronic respiratory disease that affects as many as 1 in 10 children in the UK (Asthma UK 2004).

Peak expiratory flow (PEF) has been defined as 'the maximum flow of air achieved during an expiration, delivered with maximal force, starting from the level of maximal lung inflation' (Quanjer et al 1997). More simply it measures the fastest rate of air (airflow) that you can blow out of your lungs. It records airflow in litres per minute.

In 1959 Dr BM Wright produced the first peak flow meter. In 2004 a new standard European Union (EU) peak flow meter was introduced (Fig. 19.1). PEF readings obtained on an EU scale meter have been shown to be more accurate than those from a Wright scale meter, because changes in airflow will result in PEF readings changing uniformly for the whole range of the meter. The Wright scale has been previously noted to over-represent changes in airflow in the mid-range and under-represent changes in the low and high ranges (Miles et al 1996).

Until the new standard EU meters are used for all PEF measurements it will be important to note which meter (scale) has been used by each patient.

The peak flow meter is relatively cheap, is portable and does not require the support of a technician. Therefore it can easily be used to measure lung function at home, in consulting rooms and in hospitals. However, it is not a very sensitive instrument and therefore does not replace more sophisticated lung function machines (spirometers).

The most effective way to instruct a child to perform a peak flow correctly is to demonstrate the procedure clearly to the child.

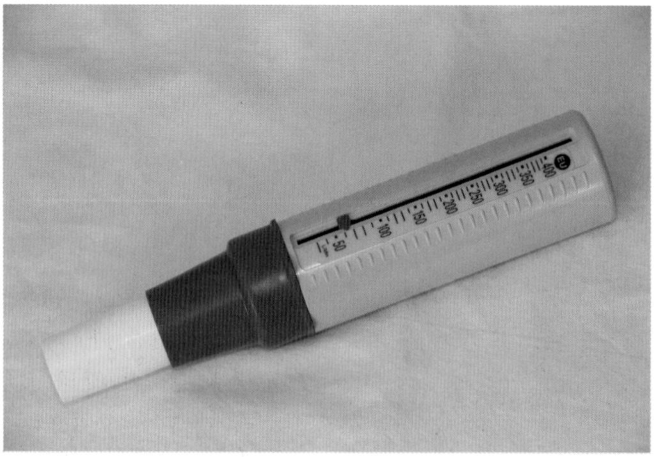

Fig. 19.1 • The new standard EU peak flow meter.

Procedures Box 19.1 Instructing a child to perform a peak flow

1

Action
Ensure that the child is sitting upright or is standing up.

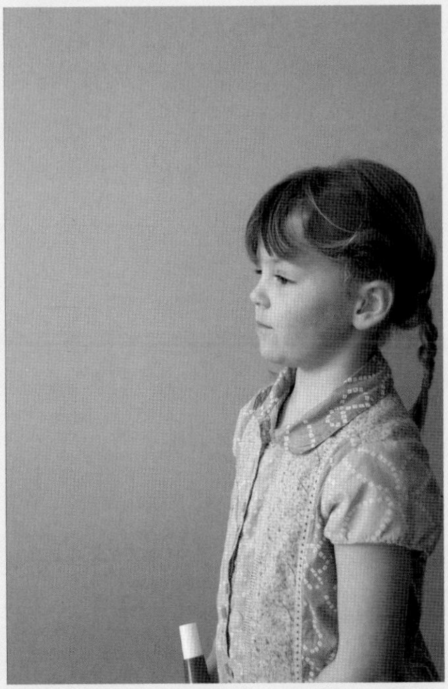

Reason *A larger lung function is achieved when standing.*

2

Action
Ensure that the child holds the peak flow meter level.

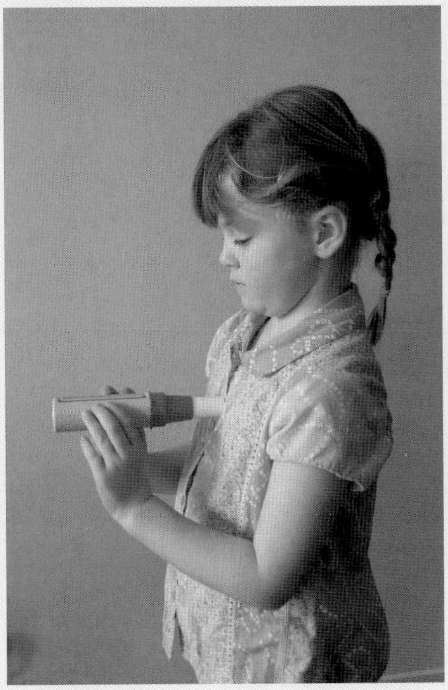

3

Action
Ensure that the pointer on the peak flow meter is pushed to the lowest number on the sliding scale.

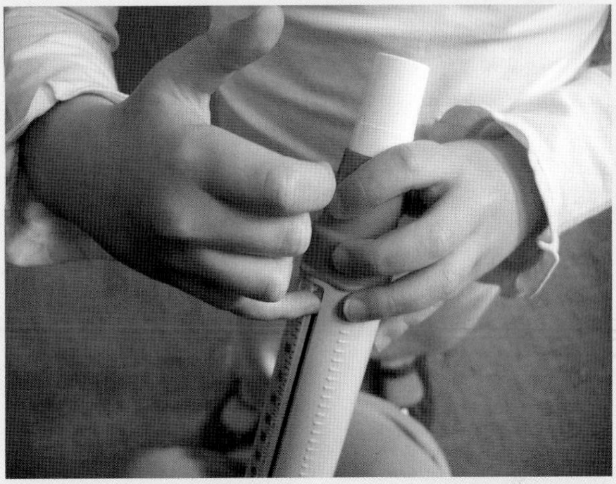

Reason *Prevents a false reading being recorded.*

4

Action
Ensure that the fingers are clear of the pointer and gauge.

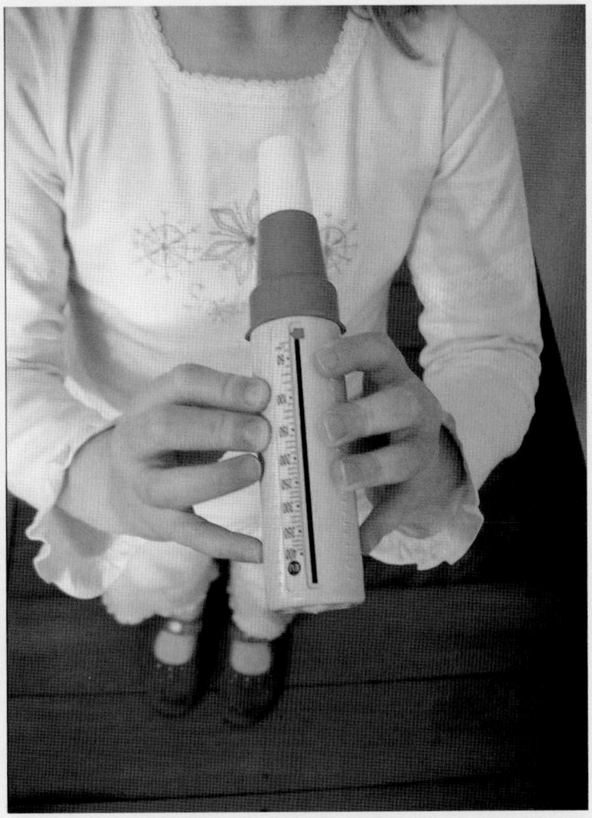

Reason *Allows a clear run for the pointer to move.*

Procedures Box 19.1 Instructing a child to perform a peak flow—cont'd

5

Action
Encourage the child to blow (breathe) out as much as she or he can first.

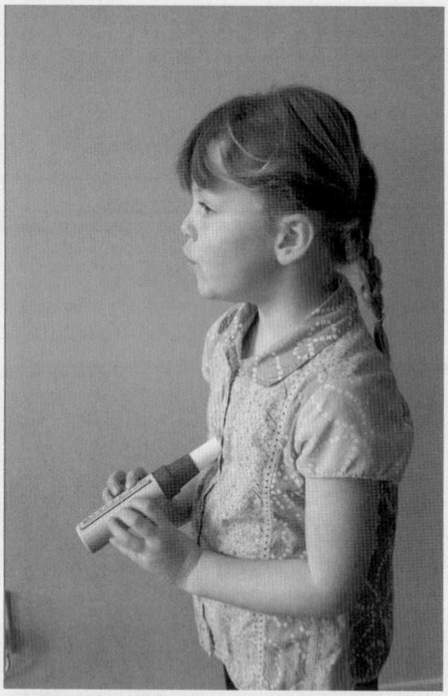

Reason *Helps the child to then take a good deep breath.*

6

Action
Encourage the child to take a deep breath, filling the lungs to their capacity.

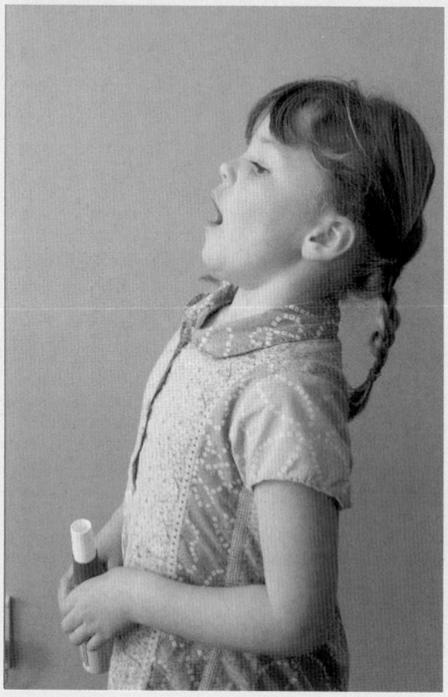

7

Actions
Ensure that the child seals his or her lips around the mouthpiece of the peak flow meter.

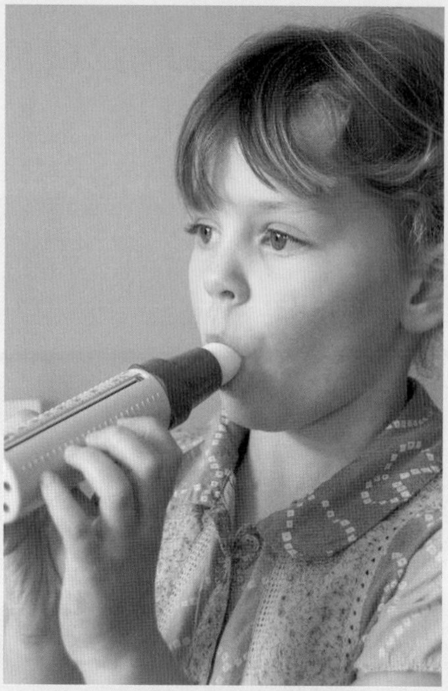

Be sure that the tongue is kept away from the mouthpiece.

Reason *Prevents any air loss, as this can produce a falsely high measurement.*

8

Action
Encourage the child to blow out in one breath as hard and fast as she or he can! (Its sound can be described as a large 'huff'.)

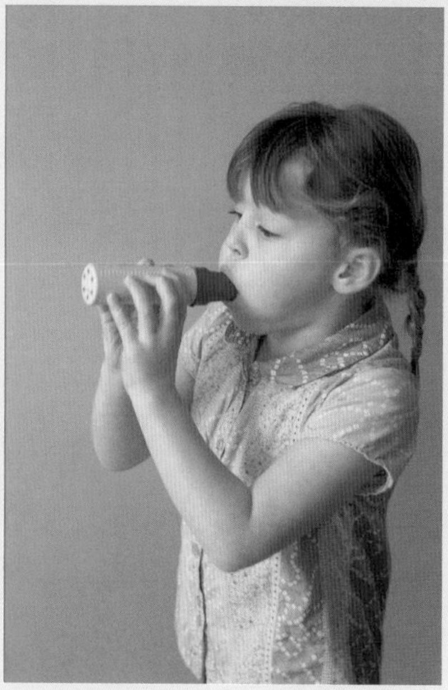

Procedures Box 19.1 Instructing a child to perform a peak flow—cont'd

8 Continued

Reason *A false low reading may be given if maximum effort is not used.*

9

Actions

The force of the air coming out of the lungs causes the pointer to move along the numbered scale.

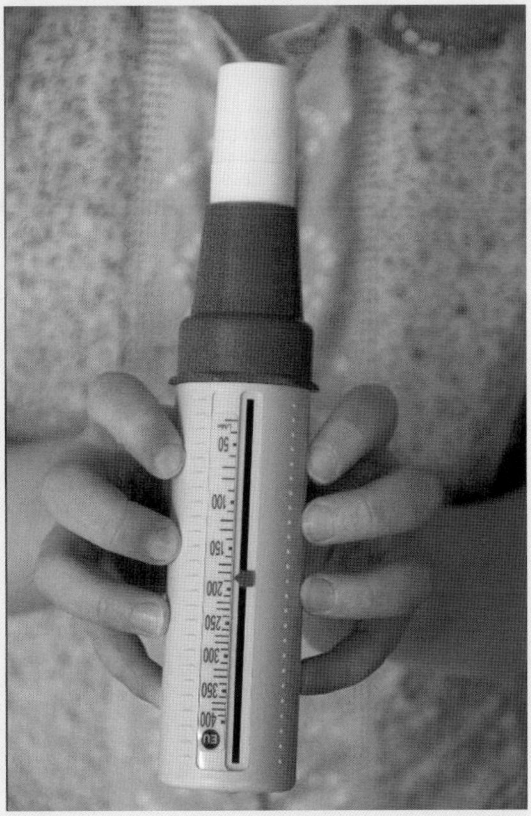

Read out the *peak expiratory flow rate* the pointer reaches and write it down (low flow range, 50–370 L/min; standard range, 80–600 L/min).

Remember that it is the best of three readings, so write each one down before you return the pointer to zero.

10

Actions

Repeat steps 2–9 twice more.

Record the highest of the three readings on the peak flow record sheet or diary.

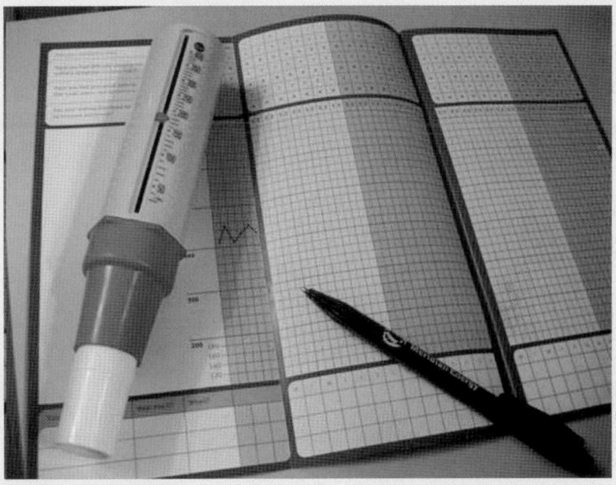

The procedure has been done correctly when the numbers from all three tries are very close together.

Practical points to remember

When observing a child performing a peak flow measurement always do the following:

- Check that the child's technique is correct.
- Make a note if recordings are made less than 4 h after using a bronchodilator or reliever medicine (as the results are likely to be falsely elevated).
- Provide encouragement during exhalation, as the result is effort-dependent.
- Do not allow children to spit into the mouthpiece or flick the mouthpiece with their tongue as they blow (as this will falsely increase the result, as it increases the air pressure).
- Similarly discourage manoeuvres such as throwing the head forwards, as this will affect the accuracy of the result.
- Excess secretions in the throat will affect the reading negatively. The child should perform three blows one after the other. The best of the three is the reading to record; however, they should all be about the same. If they are not then the child may not be blowing into the device correctly. Common errors include not blowing hard enough and not ensuring that the lips are right round the mouthpiece to make sure that all the air blown out goes through the device.

The recording of peak flow measurements

A diary card (Fig. 19.2) can be used to record the morning and evening peak flow values, although more frequent recordings may be done when a more complete assessment of airway status is required.

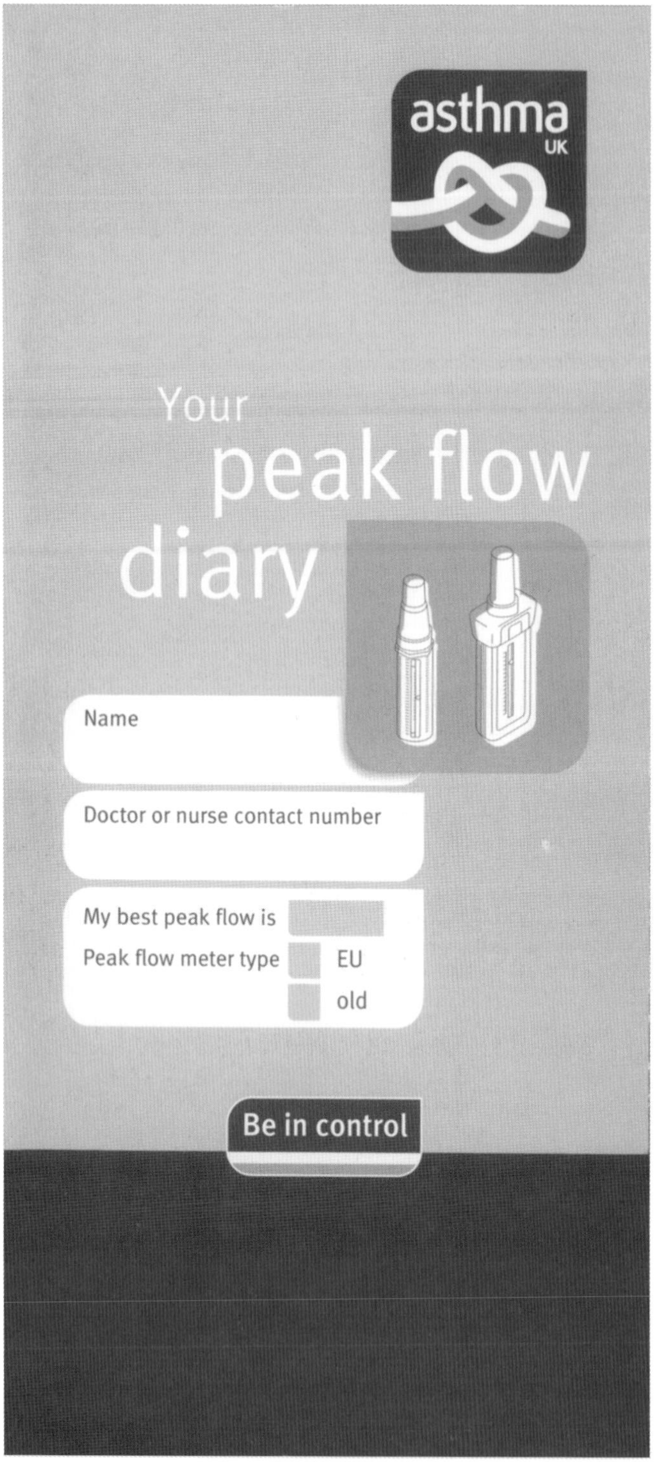

Fig. 19.2 • The Asthma UK peak flow diary card. (Asthma UK, with permission)

- Measure the peak flow rate close to the same time each day, noting when any medication was last taken.
- Measure the peak flow rate twice daily between 7 and 9 a.m. and between 6 and 8 p.m.
- Keeping a record or diary of peak flow rates over a period of time (2–4 weeks; Fig. 19.3) may help monitor lung function.

By recording the peak flow readings together with the frequency of bronchodilator reliever medicines used over a period of time, a profile of the asthma status is obtained. This is valuable:

- in determining the medication needs of a particular patient
- in assessing the benefit of therapy and thereby making appropriate adjustments to a treatment regimen much easier
- as a diagnostic tool in suspected asthma
- as part of a diary to attempt to identify specific triggers (e.g. exercise, differences between school and home).

If asthma is better controlled less rescue medication is needed and there is less chance of the person requiring emergency treatment for asthma, which greatly reduces the personal and financial burden of asthma.

Peak flow readings are higher when patients are well and lower when the airways are constricted. Obstructive airways disease (such as asthma) can lower peak flow or other lung function readings. By knowing the volume per second predicted based on nomograms (normal values for healthy children of lung function related to the physical characteristics of the subject, such as age, gender and height) or, better still, the individual's personal best recording (when well), allows assessment of how relaxed (open) or constricted (narrow) the airways are at the time of testing.

Important practical applications of the peak flow

Early awareness of asthma

A peak flow reading less than 85% of the predicted maximum value is an indicator of early airway narrowing (bronchospasm). This can be recorded before wheezing has developed and therefore gives the advantage of initiating early treatment and thereby often preventing a severe relapse.

Signs of poor control

Variability of peak flow, either spontaneously over time or in response to therapy, is a characteristic feature of poorly controlled asthma. Frequent lower levels and wide variations in morning and evening peak flow recordings (a difference of more than 20%) suggest that a reassessment of the treatment regimen is required. The rationale for using peak flow variability is that it correlates, although weakly, with asthma symptoms and airway hyper-responsiveness (Brand et al 1997, Sly 1997). In addition to peak flow recordings children should be encouraged to become aware of symptoms of poor control.

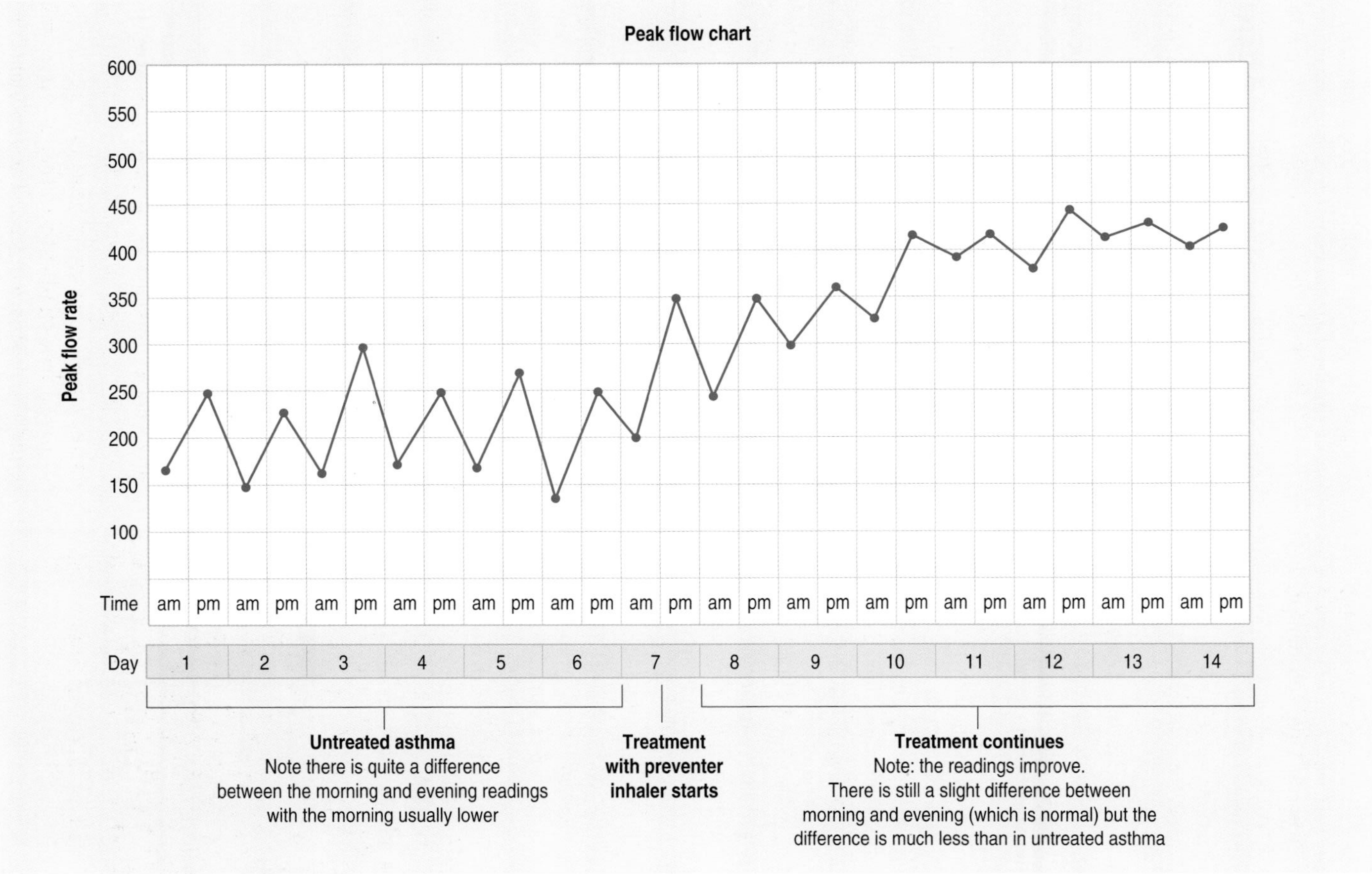

Fig. 19.3 • A completed peak flow diary. In untreated asthma there is quite a difference between the morning and evening readings, with the morning readings usually lower. With treatment the readings improve. There is still a slight difference between morning and evening readings (which is normal), but the difference is much less than in untreated asthma. (Diagram source copyright EMIS and PIP 2006, as distributed on www.patient.co.uk.)

Response to therapy

Recording peak flows before and 10–15 min after the administration of a bronchodilator is an important marker in gauging the efficacy of the administered treatment. Pre- and postbronchodilator (reliever medicine) peak flow measurements are especially valuable when there has been a deterioration in a child's condition.

International guidelines concentrate on self-management of asthma using individualised written action plans based on symptoms and peak flow monitoring (Fig. 19.4) and the use of minimal, appropriate medications to achieve this control (British Thoracic Society & Scottish Intercollegiate Guidelines Network 2005, Global Initiative for Asthma 2005).

According to many randomised controlled trials and a Cochrane review, action plans appear to be one of the most effective interventions available in the routine management of asthma (Beilby et al 1997, Bernard-Bonnin et al 1995, Wolf et al 2003).

The role of peak flow monitoring in the self-management process is unclear. In a recent Cochrane review of self management, outcomes for adults who used action plans based on peak flow measurements did not differ from those who used action plans based on symptom self-monitoring for optimising asthma control (D'Souza et al 1996, Hoskins et al 1996, Lahdensuo et al 1996, Lopez-Vina & del Castillo-Arevalo 2000, Powell & Gibson 2003). Little evidence is available regarding peak flow monitoring in children. Most children under the age of 5 are unable to perform the test reliably. Some who can use a peak flow meter reliably when well may produce low values during a viral illness, and it can be difficult to interpret whether the low values are a result of airway obstruction or poor effort. In older children the role of peak flow monitoring has been evaluated and found to add little to the recognition of symptoms and frequency of bronchodilator use (Clough & Sly 1995). In addition Kamps et al (2001) have shown that the information provided in a peak flow diary by apparently well-motivated children with asthma and their families is unreliable. Not only do patients cheat by inventing peak flow values but they also misreport the readings they have made. However, self-management educational interventions have been shown to improve lung function and decrease some measures of morbidity and healthcare use in children and adolescents with asthma (Wolf et al 2003). Therefore it is advocated that children and their families are educated to use clinical signs and symptoms of deteriorating asthma and/or peak flow recordings, in conjunction with individualised action plans, to self-manage their asthma.

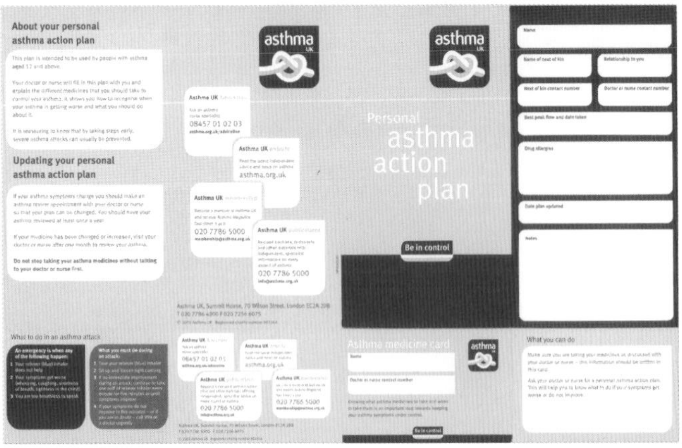

Fig. 19.4 • An asthma action plan. (Asthma UK, with permission)

Now test your knowledge

Question 1

Peter is 9 years old. He arrives for the first appointment at a respiratory clinic. He performs a peak flow but the best of three readings is quite a lot lower than readings he says he has been getting at home. Why might this be?

Question 2

Marie is a 7-year-old who is referred to the local surgery's practice nurse. Her mum explains that she is worried about Marie's activity level. She lags behind the other children walking home from school, often complains of feeling tired and coughs frequently during the night. Marie is quiet and pale. Could she be suffering from asthma? What recordings will the nurse ask Marie to make and for how long?

Question 3

At a school asthma club, children learn to measure their peak flow. A good way to encourage children to blow their hardest is to get a group of similar aged children to line up and perform the peak flow at the same time to see who can blow the hardest. By measuring their peak flow when they have been well, children can establish their personal best recording. Why is this a useful and when is it used?

References

Asthma UK (2004) Where do we stand? Asthma in the UK today. Asthma UK Publications, London

Beilby JJ, Wakefield MA, Ruffin RE (1997) Reported use of asthma management plans in South Australia. Medical Journal of Australia 166:298–301

Bernard-Bonnin AC, Stachenko S, Bonin D (1995) Self-management teaching programs and morbidity of pediatric asthma: a meta-analysis. Journal of Allergy and Clinical Immunology 95:34–41

Brand PL, Duiverman EJ, Postma DS, Waalkens HJ, Kerrebijn KF, van Essen-Zandvliet EE; Dutch CNSLD Study Group (1997) Peak flow variation in childhood asthma: relationship to symptoms, atopy, airways obstruction and hyperresponsiveness. European Respiratory Journal 10:1242–1247

British Thoracic Society, Scottish Intercollegiate Guidelines Network (2005) Guideline 63: British guideline on the management of asthma. Guidelines on the management of acute asthma in children in hospital. Scottish Intercollegiate Guidelines Network, Edinburgh

Clough JB, Sly PD (1995) Association between lower respiratory tract symptoms and falls in peak expiratory flow in children. European Respiratory Journal 8(5):718–722

D'Souza W, Burgess C, Ayson M et al (1996) Trial of 'credit card' asthma self-management plan in a high-risk group of patients with asthma. Journal of Allergy and Clinical Immunology 97:1085–1092

Global Initiative for Asthma (2005) Global strategy for asthma management and prevention: NHLBI/WHO workshop report. National Heart, Lung, and Blood Institute, Bethesda

Hoskins G, Neville RG, Smith B et al (1996) Do self-management plans reduce morbidity in patients with asthma? British Journal of General Practice 46:169–171

Kamps AWA, Roorda RJ, Brand PLP (2001) Peak flow diaries in childhood asthma are unreliable. Thorax 56:180–182

Lahdensuo A, Haahtela T, Herrala J et al (1996) Randomised comparison of guided self management and traditional treatment of asthma over one year. British Medical Journal 312:748–752

Lopez-Vina A, del Castillo-Arevalo E (2000) Influence of peak expiratory flow monitoring on an asthma self-management education programme. Respiratory Medicine 94:760–766

Miles JF, Tunnicliffe W, Cayton RM, Ayres JG, Miller MR (1996) Potential effects of correction of inaccuracies of the mini-Wright peak expiratory flow meter on the use of an asthma self-management plan. Thorax 51:403–406

Powell H, Gibson PG (2003) Options for self-management education for adults with asthma. Cochrane Database of Systematic Reviews (1) CD004107

Quanjer PH, Lebowitz MD, Gregg I, Miller MR, Pedersen OF (1997) Peak expiratory flow: conclusions and recommendations of a Working Party of the European Respiratory Society. European Respiratory Journal 10(suppl. 24):2s–8s

Sly PD (1997) Relationship between change in PEF and symptoms: questions to ask in paediatric clinics. European Respiratory Journal Supplement 24:80S–83S

Wolf FM, Guevara JP, Grum CM et al (2003) Educational interventions for asthma in children. Cochrane Database of Systematic Reviews (1) CD000326 (latest version 2 Aug 2002) Review: self management education improves outcomes in children and adolescents with asthma.

20 Oxygen therapy

Kelly Owens

Oxygen is a clear and colourless gas and constitutes approximately 21% of atmospheric air. Oxygen is necessary for the functioning of all body cells for cellular respiration. Glucose and oxygen are used by the cells to create adenosine triphosphate (ATP); this molecule in turn provides energy for most cell activities (Chandler 2001). Tissues require oxygen for survival, and delivery depends on adequate ventilation, gas exchange and circulatory distribution. Failure of any of these processes will result in tissue hypoxia, which if prolonged can result in cell death. The aim of oxygen therapy is to maintain tissue oxygenation at a functional level and prevent damage to vital organs and tissues. Oxygen requirements vary with each individual. Children have lower pulmonary reserves than adults and can decompensate more quickly (Giles 2006).

LINK CHAPTER **16**

Oxygen should be prescribed by a doctor; it is a drug and is in the *British National Formulary for Children* (2006). Oxygen is prescribed stating the fractional inspired oxygen concentration (F_iO_2), which means the amount of oxygen a child is breathing in. The flow rate required to achieve the prescribed F_iO_2 will be determined by the type of apparatus being used to administer the oxygen (Timby 2005). The amount of oxygen prescribed depends on the circumstances or is in response to careful monitoring of blood gas levels. In a life-threatening situation 100% oxygen may be given; the Advanced Life Support Group (2005) states that in any emergency situation high-flow oxygen should be applied to the child via a non-rebreathe mask, as long as the airway is patent. In the case of carbon dioxide poisoning hyperbaric oxygen may be used, when oxygen is given under a pressure of greater than 1 atm to increase the oxygen perfusion into the blood (Alexander et al 2006).

There are risks related to the administration of oxygen, and therefore only the lowest amount of oxygen should be given for the shortest period of time to maintain required blood levels (Toplis 2006).

Complications of too high a concentration of oxygen include:

- retinopathy of prematurity in preterm neonates (Bateman & Leach 1998); however, there is some suggestion that this is due to wide swings in oxygen saturations rather than high oxygen concentrations (Kotecha & Allen 2002)
- pulmonary oxygen toxicity and permanent lung damage due to lengthy exposure to high levels of oxygen (Giles 2006)
- in children with chronic lung disease, respiratory failure (Toplis 2006).

Identifying the need for oxygen

To ensure that oxygen is administered appropriately it is imperative that the need for oxygen is identified. The initial assessment of the need for oxygen is based on looking at the child; the child's demeanour will be informative, such as if they are restless, confused or lethargic then hypoxia could be present (Casey 2001). Respiratory assessment will inform the practitioner as to how the body is attempting to compensate for any hypoxia. Observing the respiratory rate, depth and any respiratory noises will indicate the level of compensation. Additionally the child, depending on age, may show other signs of respiratory distress, for example recession or nasal flaring. If an older child shows signs of recession then the practitioner should be aware of its seriousness (Casey 2001). Cyanosis is a severe indication of hypoxia. This happens when a large amount of haemoglobin in the blood is poorly saturated. The result is a blue–purple colour being visible in the nail beds, mucosal membranes and skin.

LINK CHAPTERS **7 and 8**

Methods of oxygen administration

The method used to deliver oxygen to the child will depend on the age and condition of the child and the F_iO_2 level required.

Nasal cannula

Prongs or nasal cannulae come in three sizes for neonates, infants and children. At one end is the clear plastic tubing that is attached to the oxygen flow meter; at the other there are two short tapered tubes, approximately 1 cm in length, that sit just inside the nostrils (Fig. 20.1). These can be secured to the cheeks using a suitable adhesive, ensuring that a protective film is placed on the cheeks before securing with tape (Frey & Shann 2003).

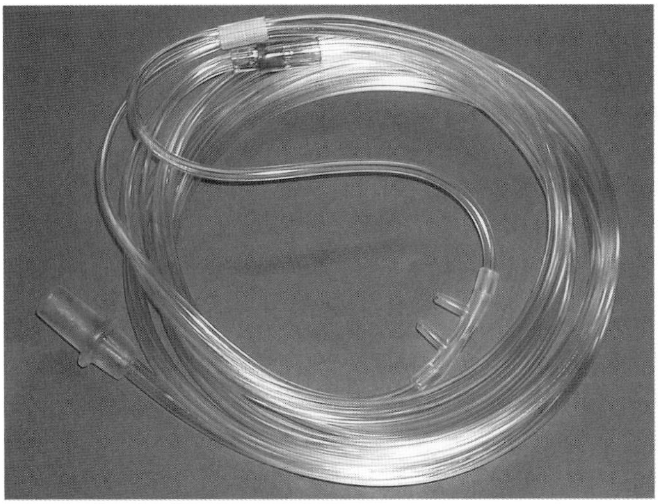

Fig. 20.1 • Nasal cannula.

Humidification is not necessary with nasal cannulae, as this occurs via the natural nasal mechanisms (Toplis 2006). Questions have arisen regarding airway obstruction but there appears to be only a slight risk of obstruction by mucus. Weber et al (1995) observed nasal obstruction in only 8 out of 62 children.

This method of oxygen delivery allows freedom of movement and is usually tolerated well by children. However, it is suitable only for delivering low rates of oxygen up to 2 L, as it would be uncomfortable and humidification would be inadequate with higher flow rates (Chandler 2001).

Procedures Box 20.1 Application of nasal cannulae

Action
Assess the need for supplemental oxygen.

Reason *Oxygen is toxic and should not be administered unless necessary.*

Action
Ensure that the oxygen is prescribed; the prescription should be legible, signed and in accordance with local policy.

Reason *Oxygen is a drug; it can be found in the* British National Formulary for Children *(2006).*

Action
Prepare and collect the equipment:

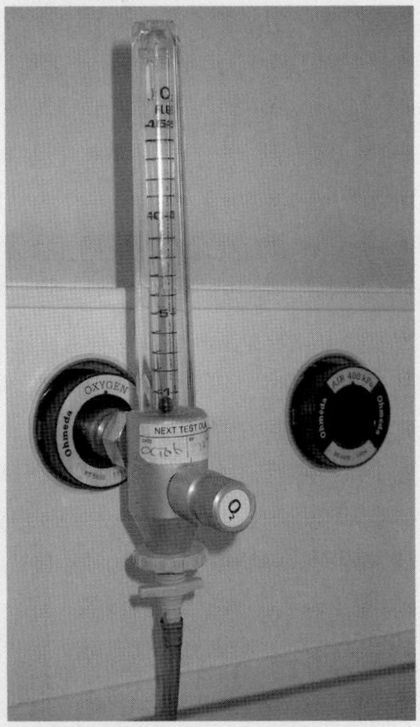

- Oxygen flow meter
- Appropriate size nasal cannula (assess the size of the child's nostrils)
- Protective film to place on the cheeks
- Adhesive to secure the nasal cannula in place.

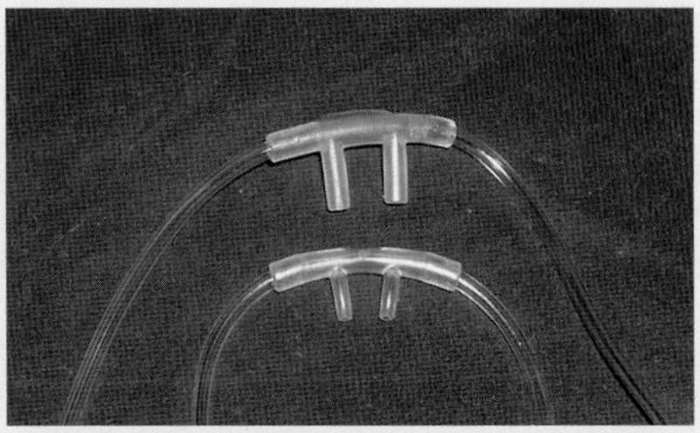

Reason *The placing of tape on young children's skin may cause trauma to the skin.*

Action
In young babies ensure that the prongs of the nasal cannula are not blocking the nostrils.

Reason *Babies are obligatory nose breathers.*

Action
Wash your hands.

Reason *Prevents cross-infection.*

Action
Explain the procedure to the child (if she or he has an appropriate level of comprehension) and parent or carer.

Reasons *Provides an opportunity for the child and parent or carer to ask questions.*
Promotes family-centred care.

Action
Utilise distraction techniques and play as appropriate.

Action
Place a protective film on the child's cheeks.

Reason *Protects cheeks from potential trauma caused by application of tape.*

Action
Place the prongs of the nasal cannula inside the nostrils so that the prongs are pointing downwards, following the shape of the nasal passages.

Procedures Box 20.1 Application of nasal cannulae—cont'd

Reason *If the prongs are pointing upwards they will cause discomfort.*

Action
Once the prongs are in the nostrils secure them to the cheeks with adhesive.

Reason *Keeps the prongs in situ.*

Action
Tighten the tubing around the back of the head, ensuring that it remains comfortable.

Actions
Connect the tubing from the nasal cannula to the oxygen flow meter.

Set to the required or anticipated amount of oxygen.

Reason *Ensures the appropriate flow of oxygen.*

Actions
Observe the child closely.

Document hourly observations.

Inform medical staff of any increase in oxygen requirements or respiratory distress.

Reason *Enables any deterioration to be identified promptly and appropriate action taken.*

Head box

Head boxes are generally well tolerated but not advisable for prolonged periods of time, as they can limit mobility. They come in varying sizes but are suitable only for infants <8 months old. A head box is a clear Perspex box that is placed over the infant's head and sometimes the upper body (Fig. 20.2). Oxygen should be positioned not to blow directly on to the infant's face, and it may be necessary to warm the oxygen to prevent cooling the infant; if therapy is to be prolonged then it should be humidified (Giles 2006). High concentrations of oxygen can be delivered via a head box but the concentration can be variable if the box is opened; F_iO_2 levels of 95% can be achieved (Toplis 2006). A total gas flow of 10 L is advisable or 2–3 L/kg per min to prevent rebreathing of carbon dioxide.

It is important that an oxygen analyser is also placed inside the box to ascertain the oxygen concentration (Fig. 20.3). It is imperative that the analyser is calibrated frequently to ensure its accuracy (Frey & Shann 2003).

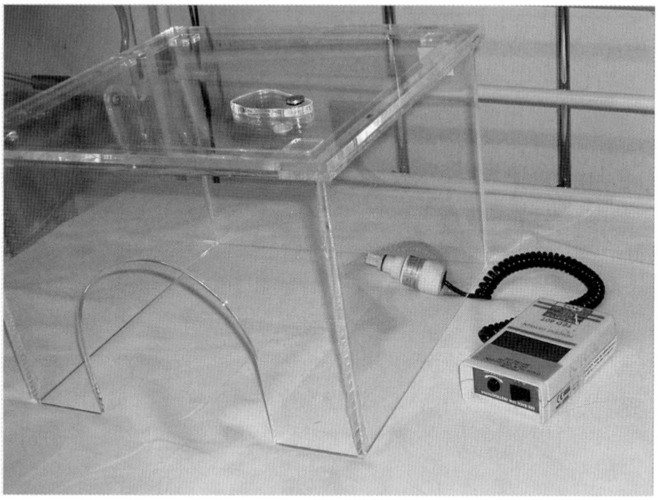

Fig. 20.3 • Head box and oxygen analyser.

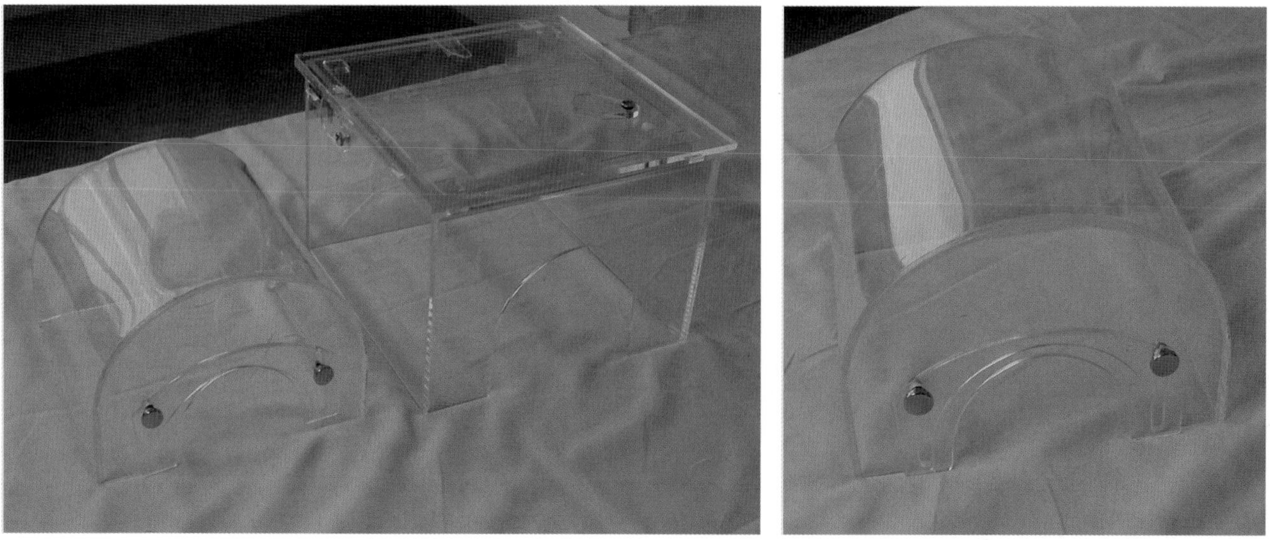

Fig. 20.2 • Head boxes.

Procedures Box 20.2 Using a head box

Action
Assess the need for supplemental oxygen.

Reason *Oxygen is toxic and should not be administered unless necessary.*

Action
Ensure that the oxygen is prescribed; the prescription should be legible, signed and in accordance with local policy.

Reason *Oxygen is a drug.*

Action
Prepare and collect the equipment:

- Appropriate size head box
- Green tubing to connect the humidifier to the flow meter
- Oxygen flow meter

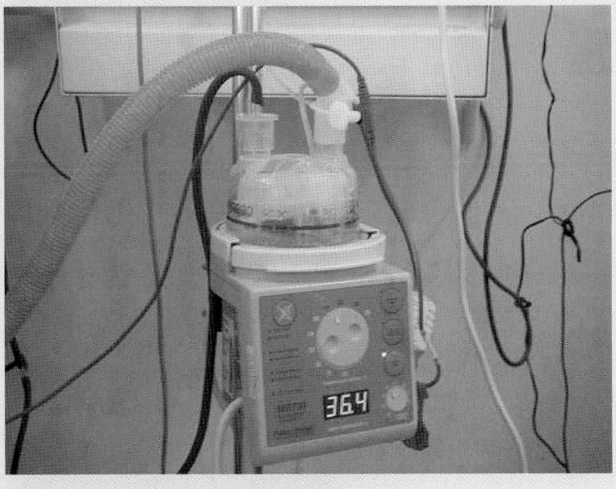

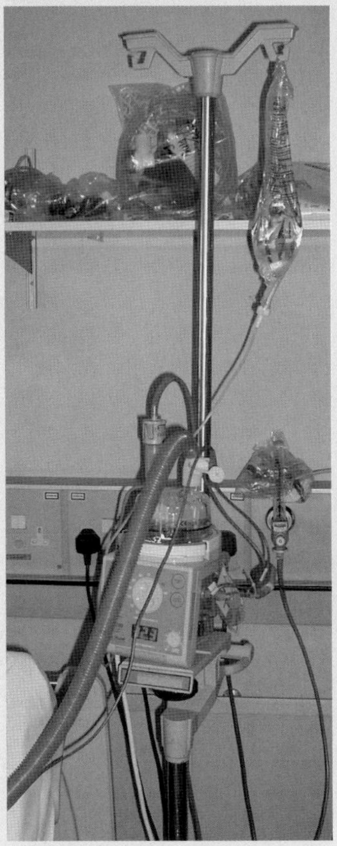

- Elephant tubing to connect the humidifier to the head box

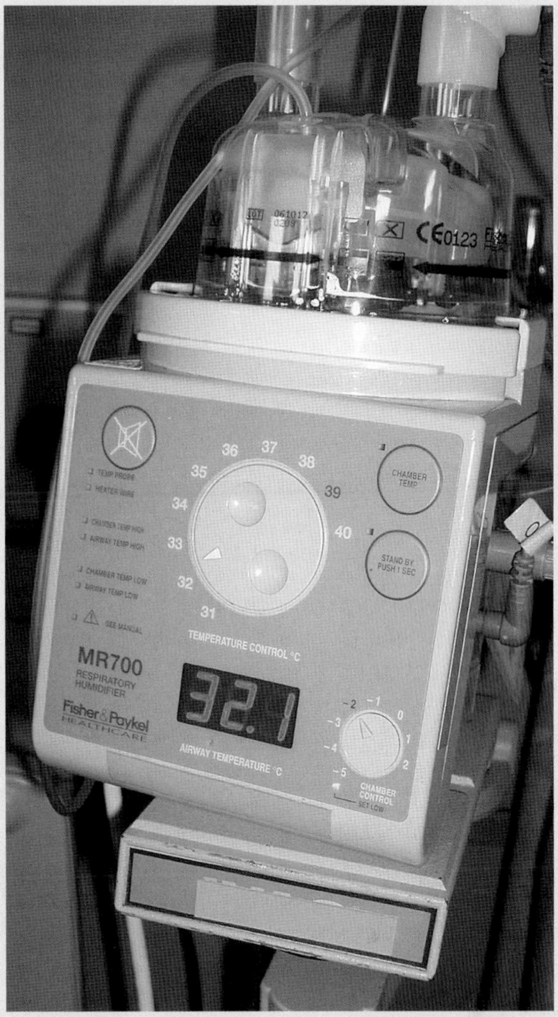

- Humidification system according to manufacturer's guidelines

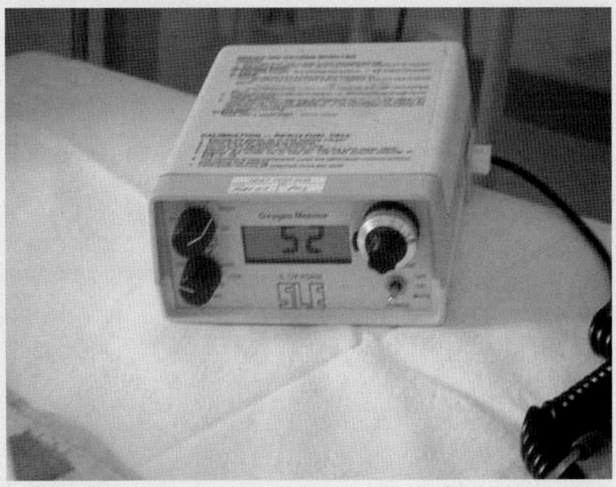

- Oxygen analyser (accurately calibrated in air and 100% oxygen)

Procedures Box 20.2 Using a head box—cont'd

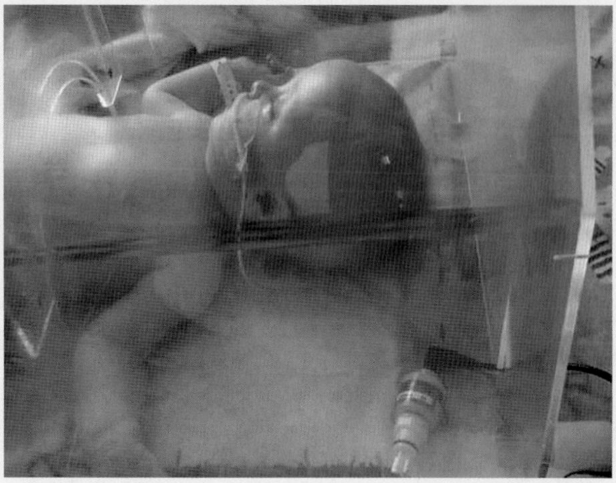

- Oxygen analyser probe (attach through the port in the head box and set the upper and lower limits for assessment of oxygen concentration)

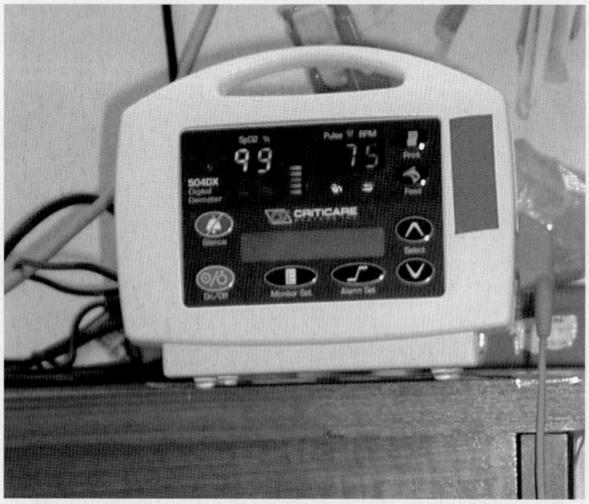

- Oxygen saturation monitor.

Action
Wash your hands.

Reason *Prevents cross-infection.*

Action
Explain to the child and parent or carer that you are going to use a head box to administer oxygen.

Reasons *Keeps the child and parent or carer informed. Promotes family-centred care.*

Action
Connect the green oxygen tubing from the oxygen flow meter to the humidifier.

Reason *Ensures safe and effective functioning of the apparatus.*

Actions
Position the humidifier close to the cot.

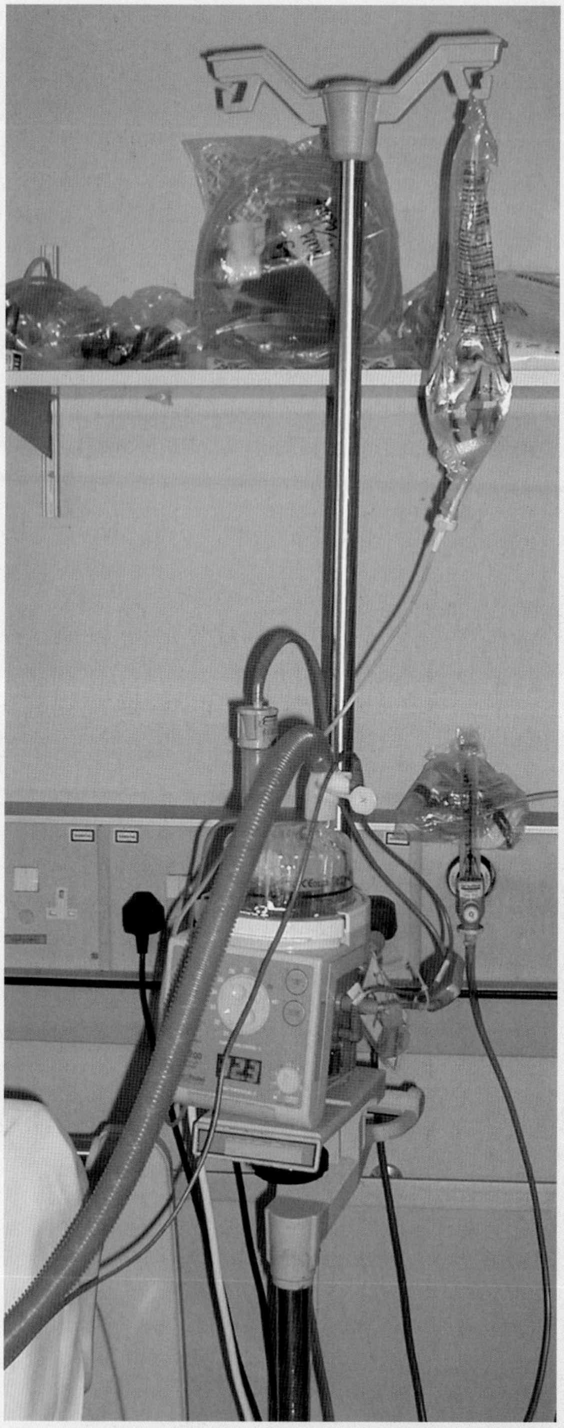

Check the water level in the humidifier and ensure that the water bottle is replaced as required.

Reason *Ensures that water is available to provide humidification.*

Actions
Position the baby on either his or her back or side.

Procedures Box 20.2 Using a head box—cont'd

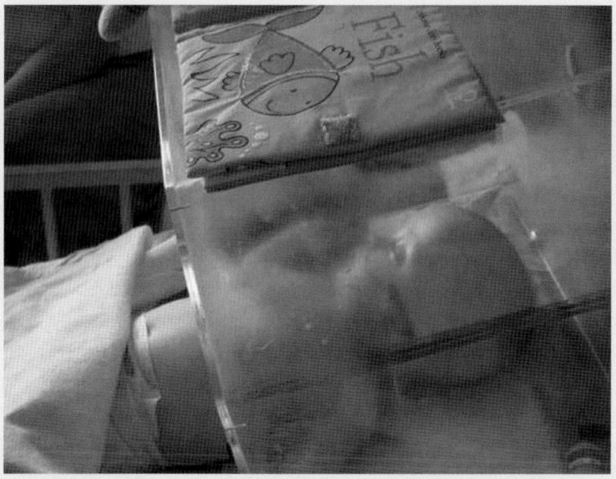

Place the head box carefully over the baby's head with the shoulders outside the box.

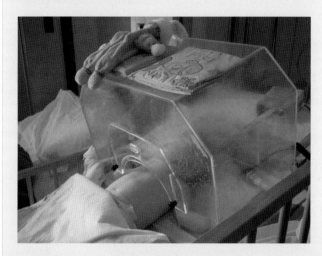

With small infants it may be necessary to position the shoulders inside the box; do not allow the box to exert any pressure on the infant or the shoulders to fill the arch into the box.

Reasons *Provides a safe and comfortable position for the baby. Prevents damage to the skin.*
Allows gases to circulate out of the box and avoids carbon dioxide building up.

Action
Connect elephant tubing through the appropriate port in the head box; the flow from the tube should not be directly into the baby's face.

Action
Position the oxygen analyser probe in the head box; this should not be close to the entry site of the elephant tubing and as close to the baby's face as is comfortable.

Reason *Assesses as accurately as possible the level of oxygen the baby is breathing in.*

Actions
Determine the level of oxygen required from the prescription sheet.

Turn on the oxygen at the flow meter.

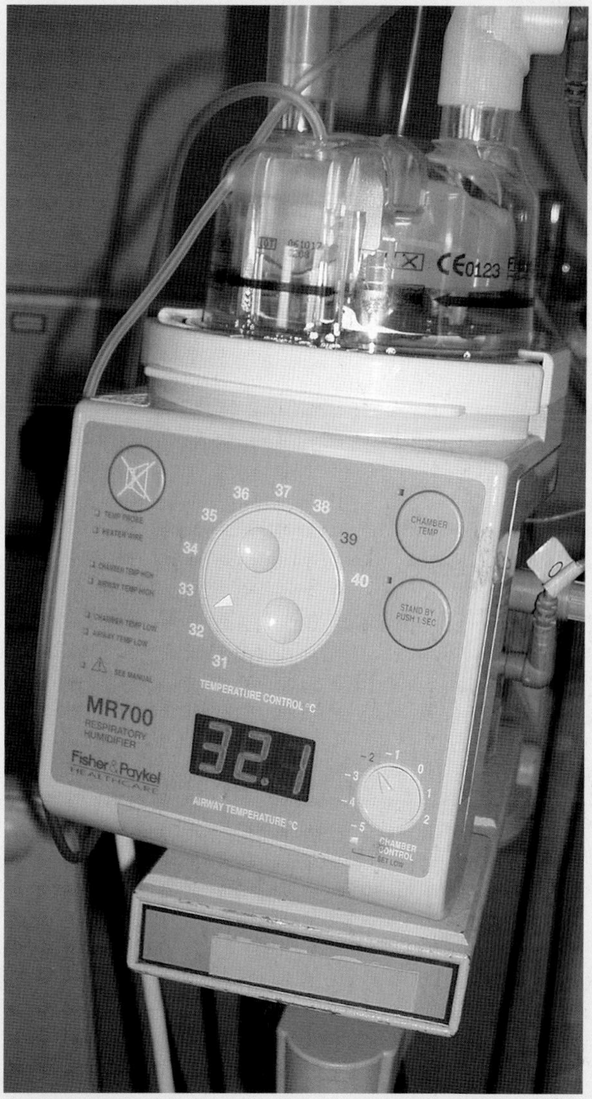

The dial on the humidifier will state the flow rate required to achieve the prescribed concentration of oxygen from the humidifier.

Read the oxygen analyser to determine the oxygen concentration being delivered to the baby.

Adjust the flow rate to provide the correct concentration of oxygen to the baby.

Reason *Ensures that the correct concentration of oxygen is delivered to the baby.*

Actions
Attach the oxygen saturation probe and connect it to the monitor.

Turn on the saturation monitor and set the alarm limits.

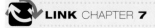

LINK CHAPTER **7**

Procedures Box 20.2 Using a head box—cont'd

Actions

Observe the child closely: oxygen saturations, temperature, pulse, respiratory rate and respiratory effort.

Document the effect of oxygen therapy by recording observations hourly.

Oxygen concentration and the oxygen–air mix need to be recorded hourly.

Reasons *Enables any improvement or deterioration in the child's condition to be identified and dealt with promptly.*

To check that the baby is not becoming too cold.

Enables any increase in oxygen requirement to be identified and acted on.

Action

Position colourful toys within baby's visual field.

Reason *Provides visual stimulation for the baby.*

Face mask

There are many different types of face mask; usually they are rigid with vents within the mask to dilute the oxygen (Fig. 20.4). The oxygen concentration is not set and can be altered by adjusting the flow rate. High concentrations can be given via these types of masks, but if low concentrations are given there is a risk that carbon dioxide will accumulate. The percentage of oxygen inspired will depend on the child's inspiratory rate.

Venturi or Hudson masks are available in 24, 28, 35, 40 and 60% and provide a fixed concentration of oxygen. Although expensive, safety is an important benefit, as the prescribed percentage can be delivered accurately (Bateman & Leach 1998, Chandler 2001).

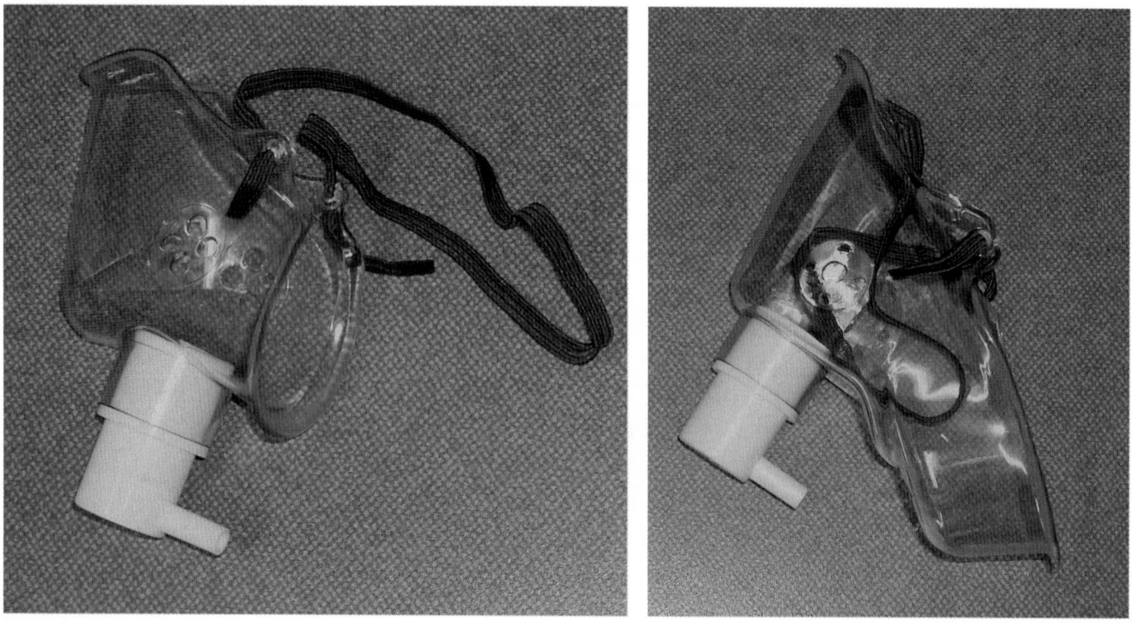

Fig. 20.4 • Face masks.

Procedures Box 20.3 Application of an oxygen face mask

Action
Assess the need for supplemental oxygen.

Reason *Oxygen is toxic and should not be administered unless necessary.*

Action
Ensure that the oxygen is prescribed; the prescription should be legible, signed and in accordance with local policy.

Reason *Oxygen is a drug.*

Action
Prepare and collect the equipment:

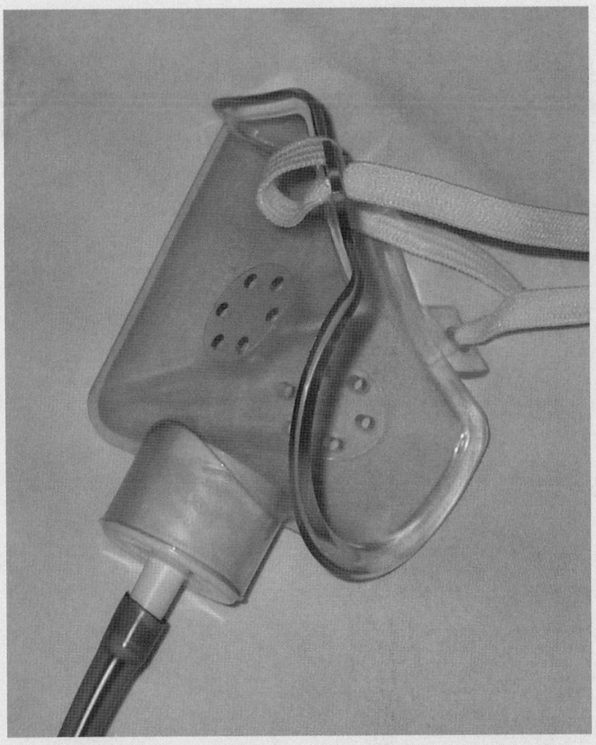

- Appropriate size of oxygen mask
- Green tubing to connect the mask to the flow meter
- Oxygen flow meter.

Action
Wash your hands.

Reason *Prevents cross-infection.*

Action
Explain to the child and parent or carer that you are going to apply an oxygen mask.

Reasons *Keeps the child and parent or carer informed. Promotes family-centred care.*

Action
Use play techniques and toys as appropriate.

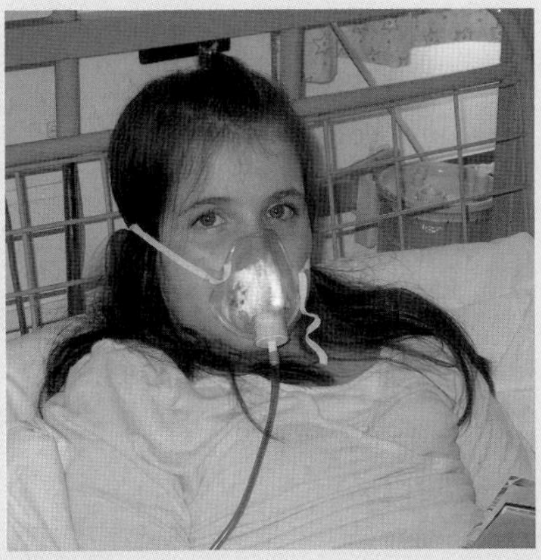

Actions
Place the oxygen mask over the child's face with the elastic placed around the back of the head.

Ensure that the mask is comfortable.

Reason *If the mask is comfortable the child is more likely to tolerate it.*

Action
Connect the green oxygen tubing from the mask to the flow meter.

Reason *Allows oxygen to be transported from flow meter to mask.*

Action
Turn on the dial of the flow meter to the desired amount of oxygen.

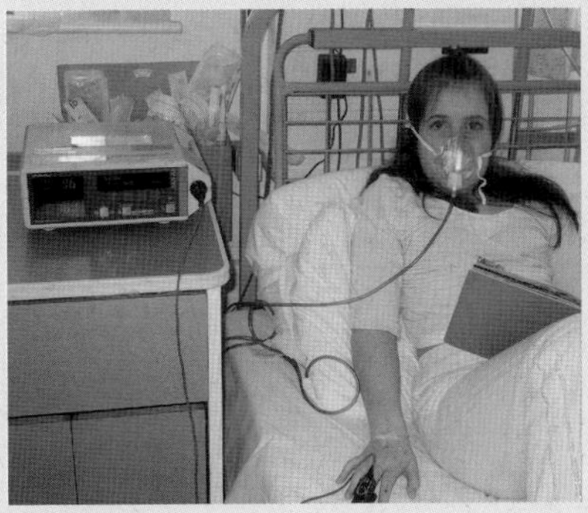

Actions
Continue to observe the child closely.

Document the effect of oxygen therapy by recording observations hourly.

Reason *Enables any improvement or deterioration in the child's condition to be identified and dealt with promptly.*

Non-rebreathing mask

Non-rebreathing masks (Fig. 20.5) are often used in an emergency situation; they have a large reservoir bag attached that enables only oxygen to be inhaled, prevents the mixing of gases and consequently results in high levels of oxygen. The flow should be set at 15 L, ensuring that the bag is inflated before putting the mask on the child (Advanced Life Support Group 2005, Chandler 2001).

The efficiency of any mask is affected by how well it fits the face; without a good seal, oxygen will leak around the mask, reducing the concentration (Fig. 20.6). Face masks are often not tolerated well, because they interfere with communication and can make children feel as though they are being suffocated (Timby 2005).

Other modes of oxygen delivery

'Wafting oxygen' is sometimes used for children who will not tolerate conventional methods of oxygen administration. The term *wafting* refers to aiming oxygen at the patient to give some benefit but without contact. In a study carried out by Davies et al (2002) looking at three methods of wafting oxygen, they found that wafting oxygen administered via a standard paediatric mask can provide significant oxygen therapy. It is important that the mask is placed opposite the sternum in order to achieve maximum concentration. However, oxygen will be diluted with the ambient air and the percentage of oxygen inhaled by the child is unpredictable.

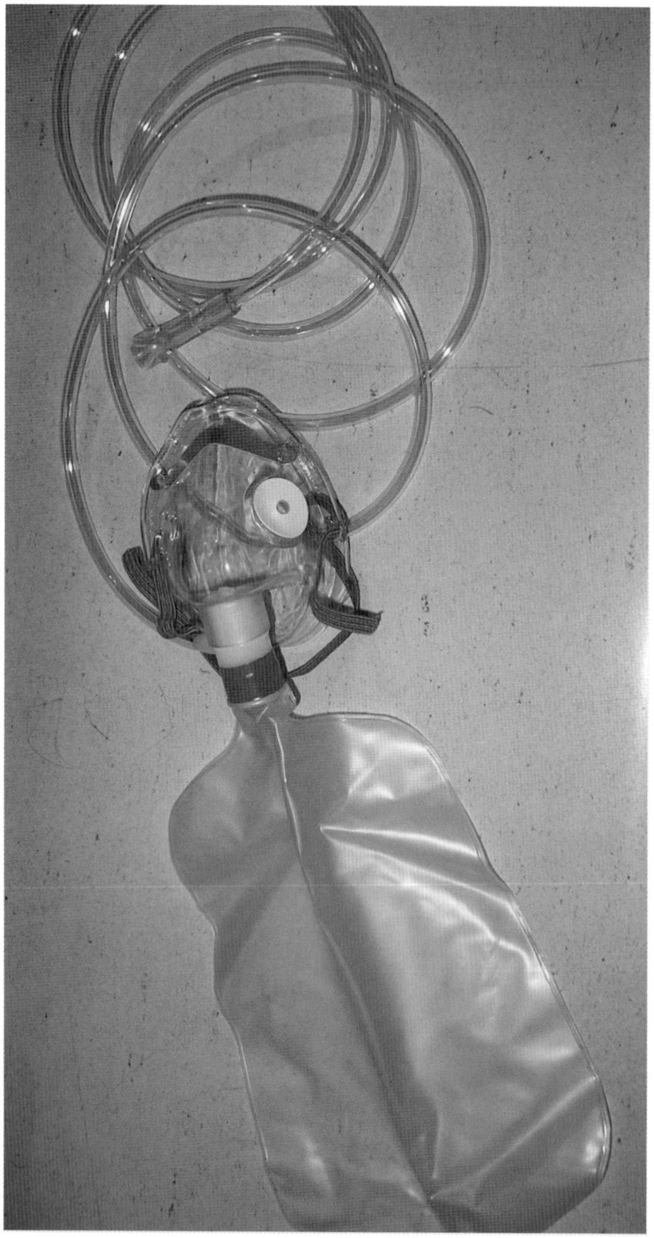

Fig. 20.5 • Non-rebreathing mask.

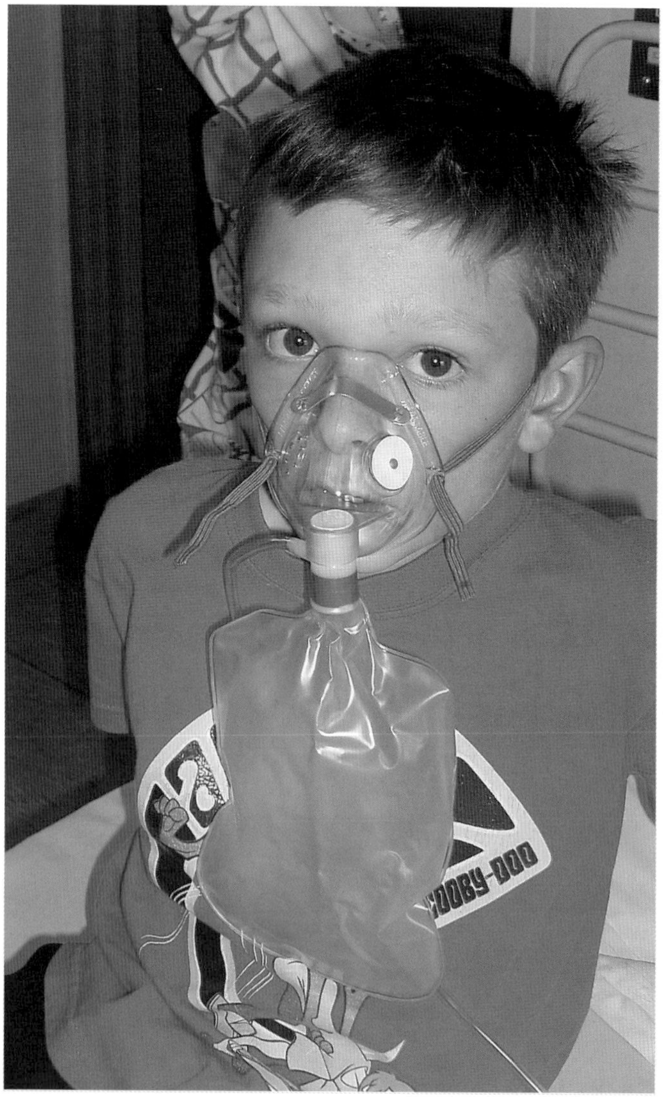

Fig. 20.6 • A face mask in use.

Oxygen-filled self-inflating resuscitators, or 'bag and masks' as they are more commonly known, have been used to deliver oxygen for spontaneously breathing patients. The bag is not compressed but oxygen is assumed to flow freely from the mask positioned loosely near or on the child's face. However, a study carried out by Carter et al (2005) found that self-inflating resuscitators deliver a significantly lower flow of oxygen than the amount provided by the inlet flow and so should not be relied on to provide a precise amount of oxygen to spontaneously breathing patients.

Humidification

During normal breathing inspired air is humidified, heated and filtered via the nasal mucosa. If, however, this process is impaired by, for example, mouth breathing or respiratory tract infections, side effects such as hypoxia, moisture loss and bronchoconstriction can occur.

When administering oxygen, supplementary humidification may be necessary. The method of humidification depends on the method of oxygen administration and the equipment available in the clinical setting. There are numerous adaptors available to supply sterile water for humidification (Pilkington 2004).

Monitoring

Pulse oximetry is a non-invasive method of monitoring the oxygen saturation of haemoglobin of capillary blood. It does not inform the user as to how much haemoglobin is present or how well the oxygen is being transported around the body to the tissues and cells (Casey 2001, Chandler 2000). A falsely high reading occurs in the presence of carbon monoxide, as it has a greater ability to bind to haemoglobin molecules and once in place prevents the binding of oxygen molecules.

The normal level for a newborn is 85–90% and thereafter 95–99% (Bloxham 2006); whenever possible the child's oxygen level should be judged against her or his own 'normal', as many individuals function on lower levels due to chronic cardiac or respiratory conditions.

Pulse oximetry provides useful information but the user must be aware of its inaccuracies and it must be used in conjunction with other clinical information obtained from assessing the patient (Casey 2001).

LINK CHAPTER **7**

Now test your knowledge

Question 1

What is oxygen and why do we need it?

Question 2

Why should oxygen be prescribed?

Question 3

How should nurses identify the need for oxygen?

Question 4

List the various methods of oxygen administration.

Question 5

What information does a pulse oximeter provide?

Question 6

Why should pulse oximeters not be used when carbon monoxide poisoning is suspected?

References

Advanced Life Support Group (2005) Advanced paediatric life support. BMJ, London

Alexander M, Fawcett J, Runciman P (2006) Nursing practice hospital and home – the adult, 3rd edn. Churchill Livingstone, Edinburgh

Bateman N, Leach R (1998) Acute oxygen therapy. British Medical Journal 317:798–801

Bloxham N (2006) Transfer and retrieval. In Glasper E, McEwing G, Richardson J (eds) Oxford handbook of children's and young people's nursing. Oxford University Press, Oxford

British National Formulary for Children (2006) British National Formulary for children. BMJ Publishing Group, London

Carter B, Fairbank B, Tibballs J, Hochmann M, Osbourne A (2005) Oxygen delivery using self inflating bags. Pediatric Critical Care Medicine 6(2):125–128

Casey G (2001) Oxygen transport and the use of pulse oximetry. Nursing Standard 15(4):46–43

Chandler T (2000) Oxygen saturation monitoring. Paediatric Nursing 12(8):37–42

Chandler T (2001) Oxygen administration. Paediatric Nursing 13(8):37–42

Davies P, Cheng D, Fox A, Lee L (2002) The efficacy of noncontact oxygen delivery methods. Pediatrics 110(5):964–967

Frey B, Shann F (2003) Oxygen administration in infants. Archives of Diseases in Childhood: Fetal and Neonatal Edition 88:84–88

Giles R (2006) Oxygen therapy. In Trigg E, Mohammed T (eds) Practices in children's nursing: guidelines for hospital and community, 2nd edn. Churchill Livingstone, Edinburgh

Kotecha S, Allen J (2002) Oxygen therapy for infants with chronic lung disease. Archives of Diseases in Childhood 87(1):F11–F14

Pilkington F (2004) Humidification for oxygen therapy in non-ventilated patients. British Journal of Nursing 13(2):111–115

Timby B (2005) Fundamental nursing skills and concepts, 8th edn. Lippincott Williams & Wilkins, London

Toplis D (2006) Administration of oxygen. In Glasper E, McEwing G, Richardson J (eds) Oxford handbook of children's and young people's nursing. Oxford University Press, Oxford

Weber M, Palmer A, Oparaugo A et al (1995) Comparison of nasal prongs and nasopharyngeal catheter for the delivery of oxygen in children with hypoxemia because of a lower respiratory tract infection. Journal of Pediatrics 127:378–383

21

Suctioning

Matthew Carey • Janet Kelsey

In normal physiology babies and children are able to keep their airways clear through coughing, blowing their noses, sneezing and the protection of the gag reflex. However, when young children become ill due to the immaturity of their respiratory system and the altered physiology of disease processes, secretions may be retained and altered gaseous exchange may occur, thereby adversely affecting the patient's respiratory status. If this continues over time, the secretions retained may damage the cilia and interfere with mucus production, leading to atelectasis (collapse of the alveoli) and infection. Suctioning nonetheless is a traumatic and distressing process, and therefore should be used only after careful assessment and when less invasive treatments are ineffective (Dixon 2006).

In the critically ill child there may be a more prominent need to suction based on the type of patient presenting and the severity of illness. It is therefore important for all healthcare workers to learn how to effectively use suctioning as a measure in preventing respiratory compromise in children. There are many inconsistencies in the use of the procedure in clinical practice and a lack of evidence-based guidance on which to deliver care. It is therefore essential that nurses review and update their practice in relation to local and national guidelines in order to deliver safe and effective care for their patients.

There are two main techniques for suctioning:

1. Oro- and nasopharyngeal suction
2. Endotracheal or tracheostomy suction.

In addition, oral suctioning may be carried out to remove secretions from the mouth; this is usually performed using a Yankauer suction catheter.

Oro- and nasopharyngeal suctioning removes accumulated saliva, secretions and other foreign material from the trachea or nasopharyngeal area that cannot be removed by spontaneous cough. Endotracheal or tracheostomy suction involves suctioning via an artificial airway to remove excessive secretions. In intubated patients there is difficulty clearing the airway of secretions due to the tube in situ. In this instance the suction catheter is passed through the nasopharyngeal or oropharyngeal tube to a required depth to remove the forming secretions (Dixon 2006).

It is important to know the specific indications or signs that point to the build-up of aspirates and the need to suction. Determining when suctioning is needed is decided by nursing assessment of the patient's clinical condition (Swartz et al 1996); this should include the rate and depth of respiration, observing for signs of difficulty in breathing, and chest auscultation before and after suctioning to assist in assessing both the need for and the effectiveness of the suctioning procedure (Day 2000, Glass & Grap 1995).

If the child is able to clear the secretions independently, suction should not be used. Specific clinical signs presenting the build-up of aspirates including all the following:

- Respirations compromised by excessive secretions; these may be visible or audible
- Coarse breath sounds
- Noisy breathing
- Increased or decreased pulse
- Increased or decreased respirations
- Prolonged expiratory breath sounds
- Decreased oxygen saturations associated with obstructed respirations or deteriorating arterial blood values
- Diminished air entry
- Increased airway pressure when ventilated
- Altered chest movement (American Association for Respiratory Care 2004, Thompson 2000).

Effects of suctioning and complications

Suctioning is a potentially harmful procedure that can result in a number of complications:

- Trauma to the tracheal or bronchial mucosa
- Suctioning-induced hypoxaemia (insufficient oxygen reaching the body tissues)
- Raised intracranial pressure
- Cardiac arrhythmias
- Respiratory arrest
- Infection
- Hypertension
- Hypotension
- Pulmonary atelectasis
- Hypoxia (Dixon 2006, Donald et al 2000, James et al 2002, Thompson 2000, White 1997).

ALERT

Suctioning is potentially harmful and should be carried out only after careful assessment, not as a routine procedure.

There are specific potential complications when suctioning patients with head injury due to the cumulative increases reported in mean intracranial pressure, mean arterial pressure and cerebral perfusion pressure with each suction pass, therefore patients should be monitored continuously and suctioning performed only when necessary (Thompson 2000).

ALERT
Suction must never be carried out on a child with suspected epiglottitis.

Determining the correct size catheter to use

When carrying out suctioning it is important to ensure use of the correct-sized suction catheter (Table 21.1). Too small and it will not be sufficient to remove large aspirate; however, too large and the catheter both will obstruct the airway and may cause trauma to the airway, leading to further complications (American Thoracic Society 2006). Multiple-eyed catheters (Fig. 21.1) cause less damage and prevent the need to rotate the catheter (Fiorentini 1992).

For endotracheal tubes or tracheostomy tubes the catheter size should be approximately twice the internal diameter of the endotracheal tube (Fig. 21.2). Using a tube larger than this would occlude the internal diameter of the endotracheal tube, increasing the detrimental effects of suctioning on the child (e.g. for a 3.0-mm tube a size 6-Fg suction catheter should be used).

All disposable equipment (suction tubing and catheters) should be replaced every 24–48 h, although local policy guidelines must be followed for each area (Sole et al 2003).

Table 21.1. Catheter sizes and pressures for suctioning of the non-intubated child

Age	Size of catheter	Pressure *mmHg*	*kPa*
Newborn infant	5–6{1/2}	60–80	8–10
6 months	8	60–80	8–10
1 year	8–10	80–100	10.6–13.3
2 years	10	80–100	10.6–13.3
5 years	12	80–100	10.6–13.3
>10 years	12–14	120 (maximum)	16 (maximum)

(From Hazinski 1999 and Linton 2000, with permission of Blackwell Publishers.)

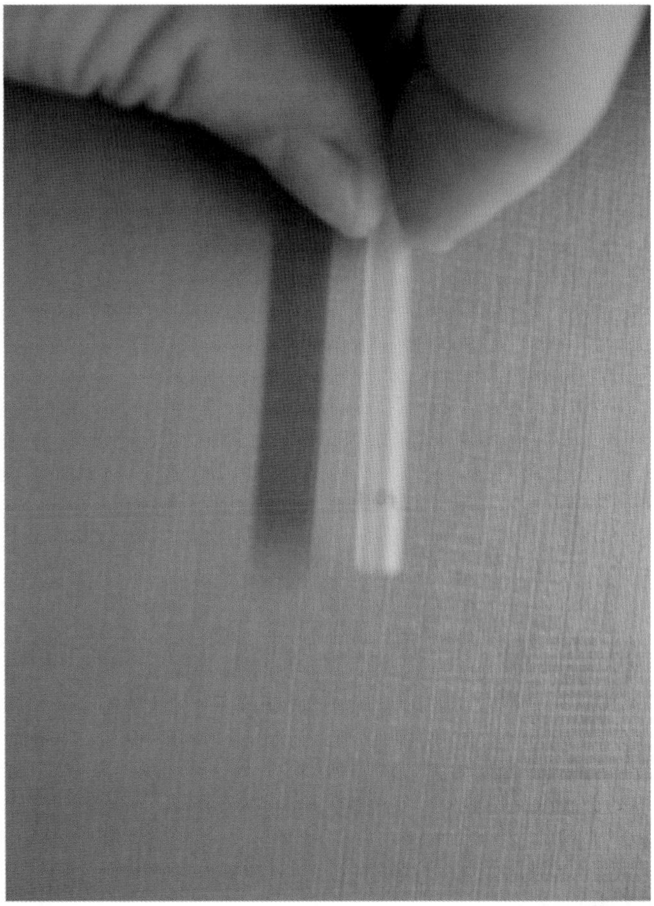

Fig. 21.1 • Multiple eye catheter.

Length of time and frequency

Suctioning should take no longer than 10 s (Mallet & Bailey 2001); patients should be allowed recovery time between each attempt to allow baseline observations to return to normal, and it is suggested that no more than three suction passes are attempted at a time (Glass & Grap 1995).

Depth of suctioning: shallow versus deep

In the case of endotracheal suction (ETS) shallow suctioning refers to the catheter being inserted to the point just past the tip of the nasopharyngeal or oropharyngeal tube. In the child with a tracheostomy, measured or shallow suctioning is recommended to prevent damage to the carina, hence the catheter is inserted only to the length of the tracheostomy tube.

Deep suctioning is when the suction catheter is inserted up to the point when resistance is met, withdrawing the catheter before suction is applied. During the past 10 years, studies using the deep suction technique with animals have shown epithelium damage and inflammation, yet practice records that

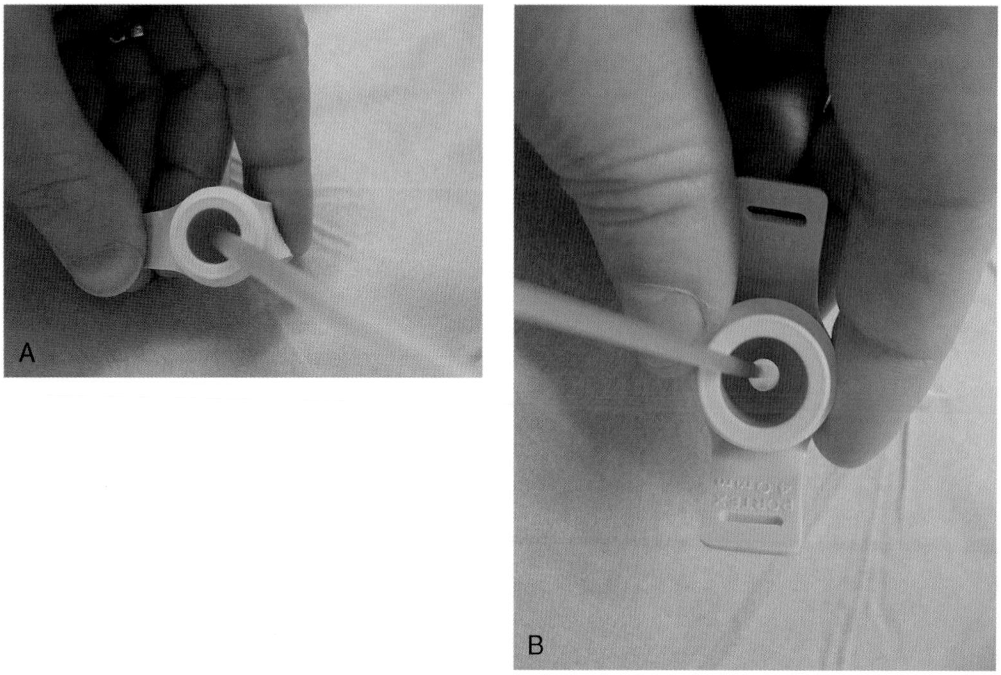

Fig. 21.2 • (a) Incorrect size suction catheter. **(b)** Correct size suction catheter.

many caregivers continue to deep suction (American Thoracic Society 2006). Youngmee & Yonghoon (2003) found that the resistance felt in the case of deep ETS in infants is likely to be as a result of the direct stimulation of respiratory epithelium, or the tracheal bifurcation, rather than a mucus plug from secondary inflammation. They concluded that deep ETS did not appear to have any beneficial effect in improving the oxygenation level, as there were no significant differences in the saturation of peripheral oxygen (S_pO_2) and heart rate responses between deep and shallow ETS in high-risk infants. Ideally a catheter should be premeasured to an appropriate depth that aims to avoid epithelial damage if inserted too deeply. This can be achieved through measuring the length from the mouth to the throat or the length of an unused tracheostomy to the correct size of the patient.

Hyperoxygenation, hyperventilation and hyperinflation

Positive outcomes in the suctioning process derive from the procedure of using hyperoxygenation, hyperventilation and/or hyperinflation of the patient's respiratory system before suctioning (Box 21.1).

Box 21.1. Hyperoxygenation, hyperventilation and hyperinflation

- Hyperoxygenation refers to an increase in the fraction of inspired oxygen (F_iO_2).
- Hyperventilation refers to the technique of increasing alveolar minute ventilation.
- Hyperinflation refers to inflation of the lungs with an increased volume of gas (Thompson 2000).

For self-ventilating patients, hyperoxygenation and hyperinflation are achieved by increasing oxygen intake and asking them to breathe deeply. For ventilated patients this is achieved by increasing the F_iO_2 prior to suctioning. Hyperinflation is achieved by inflating the lungs with a larger than normal tidal volume. In effect these give a high delivery of oxygen to the child's circulatory system to support the body when suctioning. Hyperinflation may have specific clinical implications for patients who have raised intracranial pressure (Thompson 2000) or who are haemodynamically unstable following major surgery.

Positioning

In most cases when the child is conscious the best position for them to be in is lateral, preferably on a parent's or carer's lap, which will give a level of comfort and prevent the inhalation of vomit. The child can also be placed upright, normally for them to see and allowing them to be involved and be aware of the procedure. The unconscious child can be placed in any position for suctioning, normally lateral (on the bed or supine) for better access and removal of vomit (Dixon 2006).

Instillation of normal saline (0.9% NaCl)

Studies on adults have investigated the effectiveness of normal saline instillation as a way to liquefy the secretions before suctioning and to facilitate their removal. It has been shown that normal saline, instead of softening secretions, actually reduces the amount of oxygen that reaches the lungs, increases both arterial blood pressure and intracranial pressure, and increases the risk of nosocomial pneumonia (Acherman 1993, Acherman & Mick 1998). It has been considered useful to help stimulate a cough, loosen or thin secretions, lubricate the catheter, or serve as a vehicle for mucus to be removed from the airway (American Thoracic Society 2006). However, Akgul & Akyolcu (2002) confirm that the use of normal saline negatively affects oxygen saturation levels and arterial blood gas results in adult intensive care patients, and the American Thoracic Society (2006) state that the routine use of normal saline instillation could cause bacteria to grow in the warm environment of the lower airway. Therefore its efficacy is unsupported by current research-based evidence and it is suggested that practitioners should concentrate on ensuring adequate humidification, heat, hydration and the use of mucolytic agents or nebulised saline to maintain airway patency (Akgul & Akyolcu 2002, Blackwood 1999, Griggs 1998).

Equipment

The same equipment is required for all patients requiring both oral and tracheostomy suctioning and those who are intubated:

- Suction catheter: select the correct-sized suction catheter according to the age of the child, the amount of secretions, the size of the airway or nostril, and the condition of the mucosa.
- Suction tubing: connects from the wall or portable suction unit to the suction catheter.
- Collection device: disposable bag and container, or a suction specimen container if obtaining a sample for screening.
- Wall suction or portable suction unit.
- Non-powdered disposable gloves or sterile gloves, goggles and apron.
- Sterile water to be used to clean any build-up of aspirate from the suction tubing, which could cause reduction in pressures.
- Ambu bag and oxygen: emergency equipment will be required if the condition of the child becomes unstable and results in hypoxaemia and respiratory distress (Dixon 2006).

Procedure

Apart from the length of catheter inserted, which will depend on the route selected for suction, the same basic procedure is used for both routes. Children should be observed during the procedure for any signs of discomfort, distress or cardiovascular instability. If these occur then suctioning should be discontinued.

The differences between the two methods are as follows. In oropharyngeal and nasopharyngeal suctioning the suction catheter is gently inserted upwards and backwards into the nostril or mouth of the child, without applying suction, to the point at which either the child coughs or the suprasternal notch is reached (just above the sternum; Figs 21.3 and 21.4); this should be measured from the nose or mouth as appropriate. Once inserted, suction can then be applied and the catheter withdrawn, the whole procedure taking no more

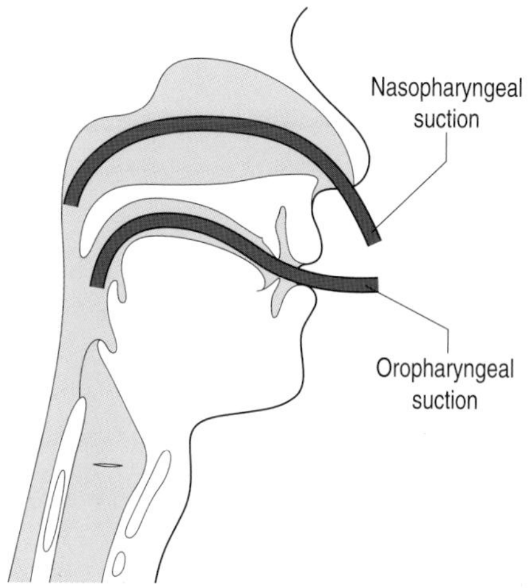

Fig. 21.3 • Nasopharyngeal and oropharyngeal suctioning.

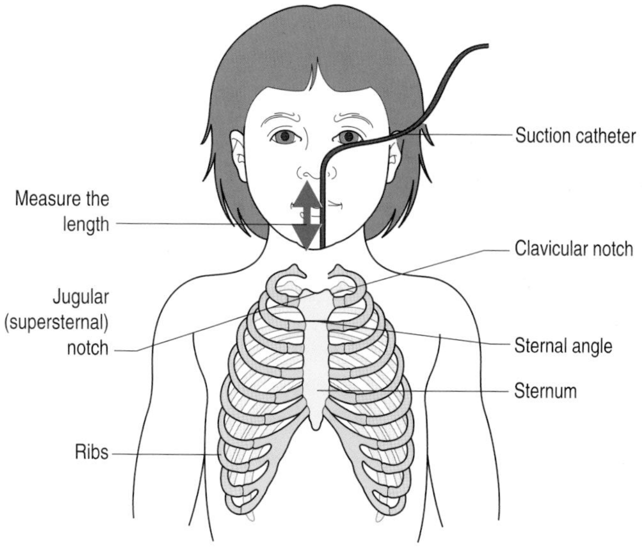

Fig. 21.4 • Measuring the suction catheter in a child with no gag reflex. (After Trigg & Mohammed 2006, with permission.)

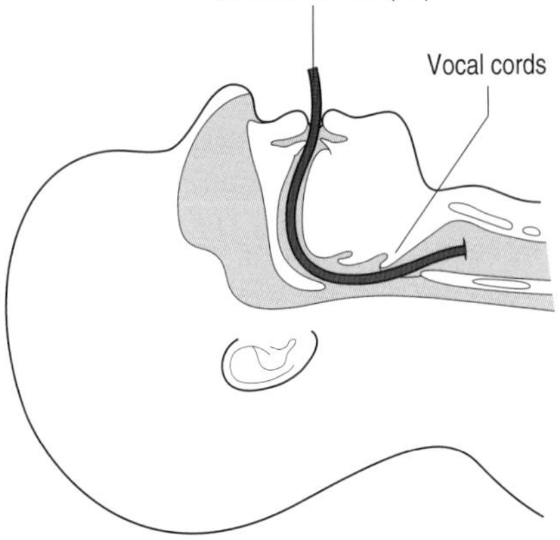

Fig. 21.5 • ETS. Insert the suction catheter just past the tip of the endotracheal tube.

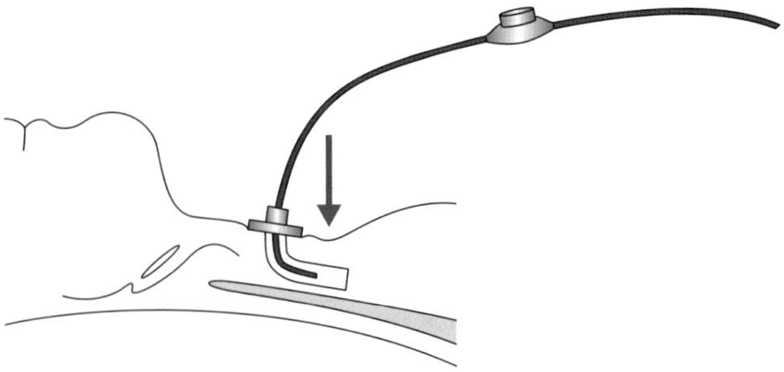

Fig. 21.6 • Tracheal suctioning. Insert the suction catheter the length of the tracheostomy tube.

than 10 s. ETS requires the catheter to be inserted into the endotracheal tube to a point 0.5 cm beyond the end of the tube (Fig. 21.5); suction is then applied and the catheter withdrawn. In tracheal suctioning premeasure the depth of the suction that will be required. Measure the length from the mouth to the throat or the length of an unused tracheostomy to the correct size of the patient. Insert the suction catheter to the tip of the tracheostomy tube before suction is applied (Fig. 21.6) and then withdraw the catheter.

Procedures Box 21.1 Suctioning a child

Actions
Collect all the equipment required for the procedure:

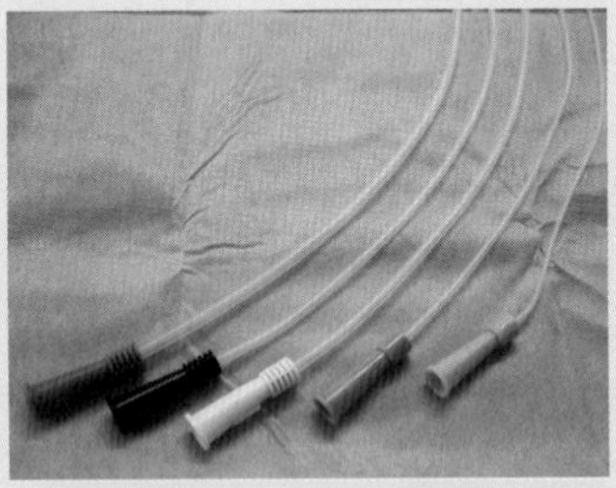

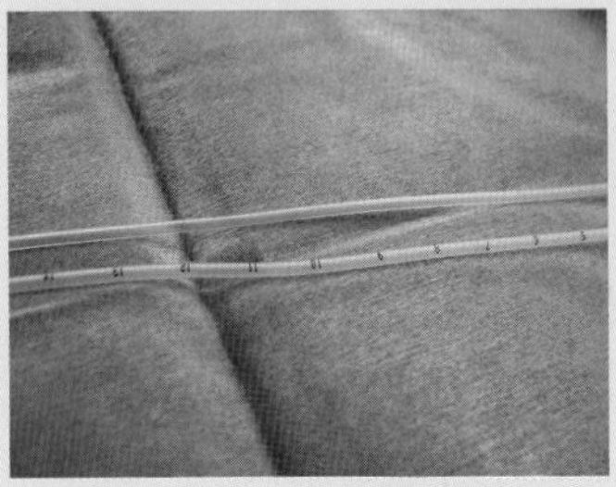

- Suction catheter (appropriate size)
- Suction tubing
- Collection device (disposable bag and container or specimen container)
- Wall suction or portable suction unit
- Disposable gloves, apron, goggles
- Sterile water for cleaning tubing
- Emergency equipment (Ambu bag and oxygen).

Check that the equipment is functioning correctly.

Actions
Tell the patient and family of the procedure, informing them of what you plan to do; if they are new to suctioning then explain each item of equipment and its role.

When suctioning is carried out on an unconscious patient explanations should still be offered.

Reason *Informing patients, either conscious or unconscious, of the procedure will prepare them for the experience; this should aim to reduce any anxiety and uncertainty for both the patient and the family.*

Action
If possible the child should be sitting up.

Reason *If the position is incorrect then the suction procedure will not be as effective and the airway may be prone to increased trauma.*

Action
Wash your hands and then put on non-powdered gloves, apron and goggles.

Procedures Box 21.1 Suctioning a child—cont'd

Reason *These are universal precautions.*

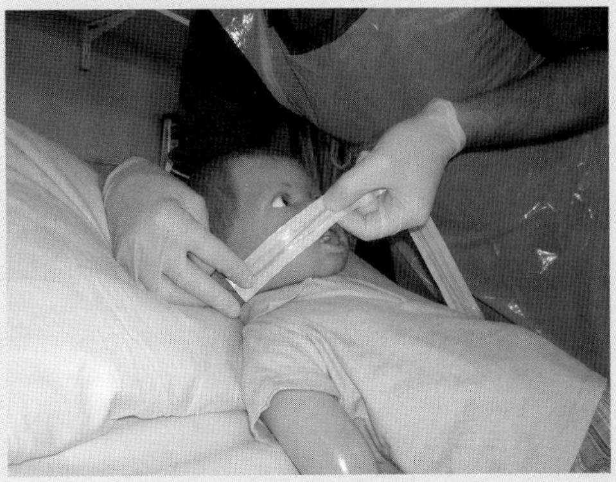

Action
Measure the suction catheter.

Reason *Ensures safe and effective suctioning.*

Action
Hyperoxygenate or hyperinflate before suctioning.

Reason *Minimises postsuction hypoxaemia.*

Action
Without removing it fully, take a suction catheter and open the top, exposing the end; attach this part to the suction tubing.

Reason *Provides a sealed connection to provide adequate suction when applied to the patient.*

Action
Turn on the suction machine and check that it is set to the correct pressure; this should be between 80 and 120 mmHg.

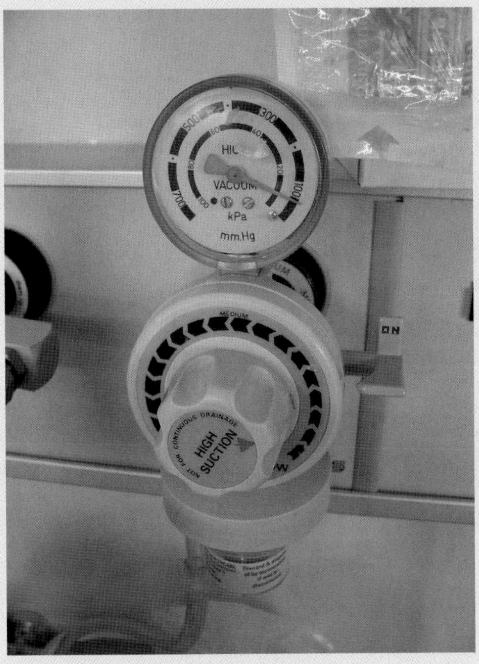

ALERT
Always check the suction pressure; never assume that it has been left at the correct pressure.

Reason *Too much pressure could increase trauma to the airway; too little and the procedure may not be effective.*

Actions
Take out the suction catheter with your dominant hand and approach the patient.

Introduce the suction catheter into the airway.

Action
Do not put apply negative pressure.

Reason *Prevents unnecessary trauma and hypoxia.*

Actions
Once in place, apply negative pressure by placing your thumb over the suction port control and then slowly draw back until the catheter has been removed.

The whole process from insertion to removal of the catheter should take no longer than 10 s.

The secretions should be removed once the suction pressure is applied.

Ten seconds is more than enough time to complete the procedure; longer periods of time can lead to hypoxia and increased risk of trauma to the airway.

Action
Reconnect the oxygen supply as appropriate.

Reason *Minimises hypoxia.*

Action
Wrap the catheter around the gloved hand then pull back the glove over the used catheter and discard according to universal precautions.

Actions
Assess the child after each suction pass.

Allow the child to rest between each suction pass and baseline observations to return to normal.

Repeat the procedure using a clean catheter and glove a maximum of three times.

Reason *To assess the need for further suctioning.*

Action
Clean the suction tubing with sterile water.

Reason *Removes secretions from the tube.*

Action
Decontaminate your hands.

Reason *This is a universal precaution.*

Action
Clean the child's mouth as necessary.

Reason *Removes sticky secretions.*

Action
Document findings, including type, tenacity, consistency, colour and amount of secretions.

Reason *For safe and accurate record keeping.*

Closed suction systems

The closed suction system may be used on patients requiring artificial ventilation. The closed suction system maintains an uninterrupted oxygen supply by reducing ventilator circuit breaks, and it maintains positive end expiratory pressure, thus potentially reducing haemodynamic and gaseous deterioration compared with an open tracheal suction system. It may also reduce the potential for infection.

Minimising the introduction of infection

There is a potential for bacteria to enter the airway during the suctioning procedure. During nasopharyngeal or oropharyngeal suction of the upper airway it has been found that sterile gloves are not necessary; however, we should consider if there is a risk of introducing infection to the child and adapt the technique accordingly. When suctioning the lower airway in patients with artificial airways, aseptic technique with sterile gloves should be used (Thompson 2000). There appears to be little evidence discussing whether to use sterile water or tap water to rinse the suction tubing post procedure; currently American guidelines state that sterile water should be used to rinse the tubing following all types of suctioning. Mallet & Dougherty (2000) also recommend sterile water.

Care of the child in the community

There are an increasing number of children discharged home with tracheostomies, and for these children their parents will be their main caregivers. Parents should have received training in suctioning prior to discharge, and support should be provided by the children's community nursing team. Parents will need to be supplied with appropriate equipment and provision made for the ongoing servicing as well as supply of disposables.

Now test your knowledge

- What size of suction catheter would you use to suction a child with a 3-mm endotracheal tube?
- What suction pressure (kPa) should be used in a non-intubated 10-year-old child?
- How would you explain to parents why they should not carry out deep suctioning?

References

Acherman MH (1993) The effect of saline lavage prior to suctioning. American Journal of Critical Care 2(4):326–330

Acherman MH, Mick DJ (1998) Instillation of normal saline before suctioning in patients with pulmonary infections: a prospective randomized controlled trial. American Journal of Critical Care 7(4):261–266

Akgul S, Akyolcu N (2002) Effects of normal saline on endotracheal suctioning. Journal of Clinical Nursing 11:826–830

American Association for Respiratory Care (2004) Respiratory Care Journal 49(9)

American Thoracic Society (2006) Online. Available: http://www.thoracic.org Jul 2006

Blackwood B (1999) Normal saline instillation with endotracheal suctioning: primum non nocere (first do not harm). Journal of Advanced Nursing 29(4):928–934

Day T (2000) Tracheal suctioning: when, why and how. Nursing Times 96:13–15

Dixon M (2006) Practices in children's nursing. In Trigg E, Mohammed T (eds) Guidelines for hospital and community, 2nd edn. Churchill Livingstone, London, p 273–276

Donald K, Robertson V, Tsebelis K (2000) Setting safe and effective suction pressure: the effect of using a manometer in the suction circuit. Intensive Care Medicine 26(1):15–19

Fiorentini A (1992) Potential hazards of tracheobronchial suctioning. Intensive Critical Care Nursing 8(4):217–226

Glass C, Grap M (1995) Ten tips for safe suctioning. American Journal of Nursing 5:51–53

Griggs A (1998) Tracheostomy: suctioning and humidification. Nursing Standard 13(2):49–53

Hazinski MF (1999) Manual of paediatric critical care. Mosby, London

James S, Ashwill J, Droske S (2002) Nursing care of children: principles and practice, 2nd edn. Saunders, Philadelphia, p 388

Linton M (2000) Endotracheal tube suctioning. In Sinha SK, Donn SM (eds) Manual of neonatal respiratory care. Futura, New York

Mallet J, Bailey C (eds) (2001) The Royal Marsden NHS Trust manual of clinical nursing procedures, 5th edn. Blackwell Science, Oxford

Mallet J, Dougherty L (2000) The Royal Marsden NHS Trust manual of clinical nursing procedures, 5th edn. Blackwell Science, Oxford

Sole M, Byers J, Ludy J, Zhang Y, Banta C, Brummel K (2003) A multisite survey of suctioning techniques and airway management practices. American Journal of Critical Care 12(3):220–230

Swartz K, Noonan DM, Edwards-Beckett J (1996) A national survey of endotracheal suctioning techniques in the pediatric population. Heart Lung 25(1):52–60

Thompson L (2000) Suctioning adults with an artificial airway. Systematic review no. 9. Joanna Briggs Institute for Evidence Based Nursing and Midwifery, Adelaide

Trigg E, Mohammed T (eds) (2006) Guidelines for hospital and community, 2nd edn. Churchill Livingstone, London

White H (1997) Suctioning: a review. Paediatric Nursing 9(4):18–20

Youngmee A, Yonghoon J (2003) The effects of the shallow and the deep endotracheal suctioning on oxygen saturation and heart rate in high-risk infants. International Journal of Nursing Studies 40:97–104

22 Tracheostomy care

Sara Raftery • Imelda T. Coyne

Tracheostomy is an artificial opening in the cartilage of the trachea via the neck that is required when normal respiration through the mouth or nose is ineffective. Except for emergency situations this surgical procedure is usually performed in an operating theatre. It can be a temporary or permanent measure. Tracheostomy is used to relieve respiratory distress caused by a variety of congenital abnormalities, trauma, infection or foreign body airway obstruction (Box 22.1). It is also performed in children who require long-term mechanical ventilation.

Tracheostomy tubes

The artificially created airway is maintained using a suitable tracheostomy tube selected by a specialist surgeon. A variety of tube types are available (Fig. 22.1), and these vary in length and diameter. They may be rigid or flexible silicone or polyvinyl chloride or, less frequently, silver. Tracheostomy tubes may be cuffed or uncuffed. Infants and children are usually fitted with uncuffed tubes, as their airway lumen is narrow with soft membranes that may become damaged by a cuffed tube, resulting in further airway stenosis (Fiske & Gracey 2004).

A tracheostomy tube has three parts: a cannula, which is inserted into the stoma and maintains the airway; a flange, which sits against the neck and has securing ties attached to it; and a hub, which provides direct connection to ventilator tubing and other equipment (Wilson 2005). Neonatal and paediatric tubes are available to ensure that the child has a comfortable and anatomically appropriate fit. One of the most common makes of tracheostomy tube used is the Shiley Mallinckrodt. Neonatal Shiley Mallinckrodt tubes have a lower flange angle than paediatric tubes. Both neonatal and paediatric tubes have a soft flange that provides a comfortable fit against the neck for infants and children. Tubes are available in sizes 3.0–6.5 (this usually refers to the internal diameter of the tube in millimetres) and vary in length to suit the neonate, child and older child.

Tracheostomy tubes are individually packaged and sterile. They are almost always disposable and are inserted for a specified period (often a week) and then changed and discarded. Many are supplied with a smooth, rounded obturator (introducer) that facilitates insertion (Abraham 2003).

Nursing the child with a tracheostomy requires competency in tracheostomy management, astute observation and excellent communication skills. Nurses should be appropriately educated and trained in all aspects of tracheostomy care and deemed competent prior to caring for the child and family. Essential aspects of tracheostomy care are suctioning, administering oxygen, humidification, care of the stoma, changing the tube ties, changing the tracheostomy tube and emergency care.

Equipment required for the child with a tracheostomy

When a child has a tracheostomy there is a constant risk that the tube may become dislodged or blocked. Therefore it is essential that equipment is always readily available to deal with such situations. This equipment must be easily accessible at the child's bedside in hospital and in the home and should also travel with the child at all times.

Essential equipment is as follows:

- Suction equipment:
  - suction machine
  - suction tubing
  - suction catheters of correct size for the child's tracheostomy (the catheter should be half the internal diameter of the tracheostomy tube, e.g. a size 3 tracheostomy tube requires a 6-Fg suction catheter)
  - a bottle or bowl of water to clean tubing
- Oxygen equipment:
  - oxygen tubing
  - tracheostomy mask
- Tracheostomy equipment:
  - spare tracheostomy tube (child's usual size)
  - spare tracheostomy tube (one size smaller)
  - tracheal dilators (as per local policy)
  - scissors
  - tracheostomy ties
  - K-Y Jelly (as per local policy)
- Stoma-cleaning equipment:
  - dressing pack
  - 0.9% sodium chloride
  - non-shedding gauze or cotton buds
  - tracheostomy dressing (if in use)
- Disposable gloves (powder-free)
- 2-mL syringes of 0.9% sodium chloride for emergency use (renew every 24 h)
- Neck roll (roller towel or small blanket)
- Hazardous waste disposal bag.

Box 22.1. Examples of congenital abnormalities that may require a tracheostomy

- Laryngeal abnormalities: laryngeal webbing, laryngeal papilloma, laryngeal haemangioma
- Vocal cord paralysis
- Choanal atresia
- Tracheo-oesophageal anomalies
- Subglottic stenosis
- Micrognathia

(From Phipps et al 2006, with permission.)

It is essential that nurses caring for children with tracheostomies are trained in emergency care including resuscitation of the child. Training should be provided in mouth-to-tracheostomy resuscitation and in the use of an Ambu bag. The child's parents and carers must also be proficient in these skills before the child is discharged from hospital.

Suctioning a tracheostomy

Suctioning the tube is likely to be one of the most frequent procedures required when caring for a child with a tracheostomy. The rationale for suctioning and the related procedure are discussed in detail in Chapter 21. Suctioning should be dictated by the child's needs rather than being a routine procedure; for example, to maintain a clear airway some children may require frequent suctioning because of copious secretions.

Humidification

When air is inhaled through the upper airway (nose, oropharynx and trachea) it is filtered, warmed and moistened. These structures are bypassed in the person with a tracheostomy. This results in inadequate humidification and warming of air, which can cause thickened secretions, loss of ciliary action and damage to mucous glands (American Thoracic Society 2000). This can lead to decreased pulmonary function and predisposes the child to infection (Griggs 1998). Therefore every effort should be made to warm and humidify air inspired via a tracheostomy. Humidification prevents secretions becoming thick and tenacious, thus reducing the risk of tube blockage. It can be provided in a number of ways depending on the individual child's requirements. Humidification may be heated, cold or provided via a heat moisture exchanger (often termed a 'Swedish nose' or *Thermovent*; Edgtton-Winn & Wright 2005). Ideally, warm humidification should be used when delivering supplementary oxygen to the child. Cold humidification can be used to keep secretions mobile and thus increase tracheobronchial clearance. It may be provided via a nebulising humidifier.

The most common method of providing humidity to the child who does not require oxygen is via a heat moisture exchanger (Fig. 22.2). This small device is fitted directly to the child's tracheostomy tube (Fig. 22.3); it captures exhaled heat and moisture and returns it to the cool, dry air of the next inspiration. It should be changed every 24 h, or more frequently if it becomes contaminated with secretions or waterlogged.

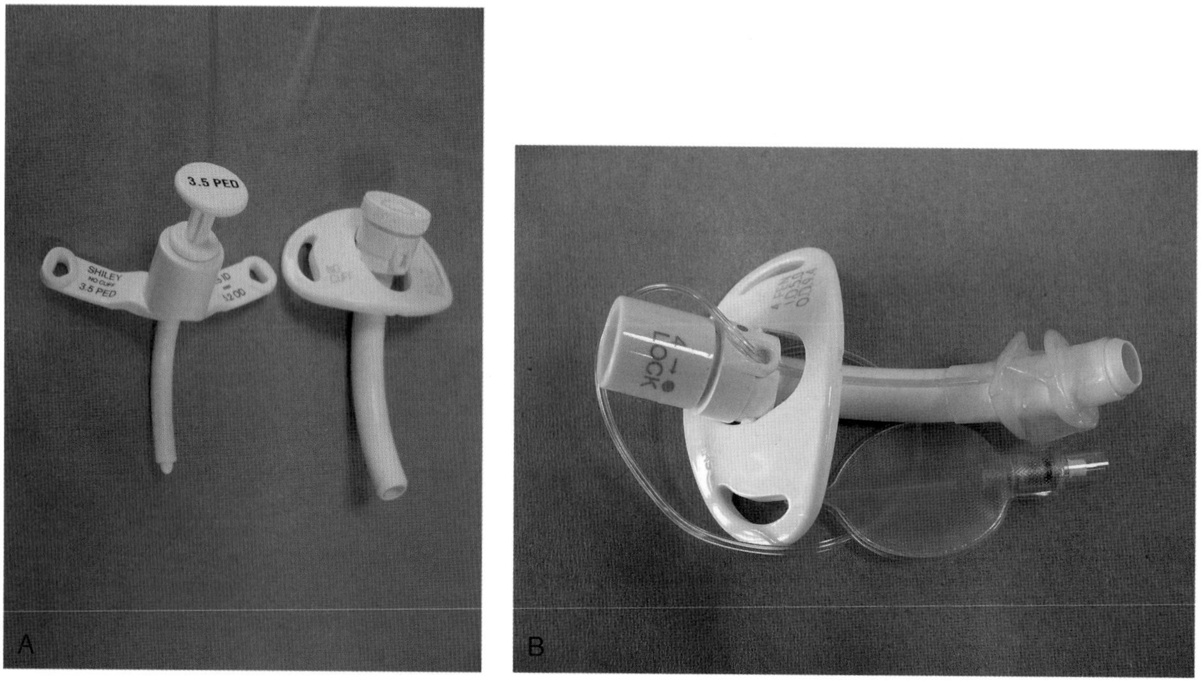

Fig. 22.1 • Tracheostomy tubes.

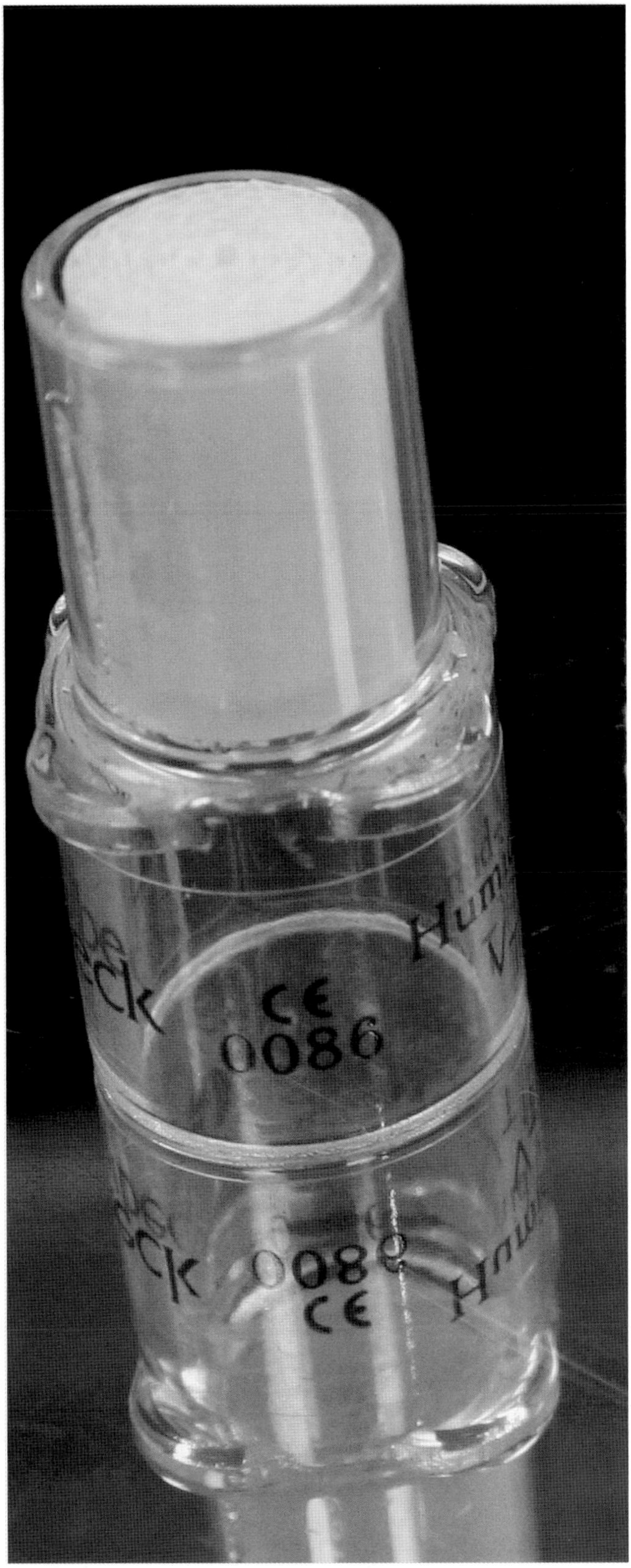

Fig. 22.2 • A heat moisture exchanger.

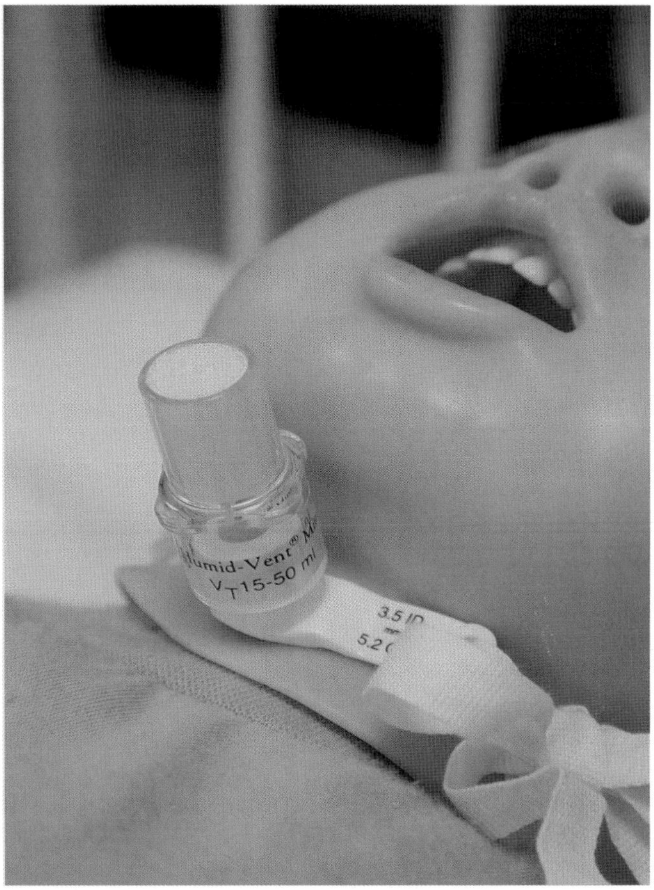

Fig. 22.3 • A heat moisture exchanger in place.

Stoma care

Tracheostomy stoma sites can become soiled by secretions, and this can predispose the child to infection and skin irritation. In order to minimise this risk the stoma site should be cleaned at least daily, or more frequently if there are increased secretions. Daily stoma care facilitates inspection of the underlying skin, which is essential as redness or chafing may lead to granulation and unnecessary discomfort. The flange of the tracheostomy tube should also be cleansed. Depending on local policy either a clean or an aseptic technique is used, with many healthcare providers favouring a clean technique. The recommended agent for cleaning the site is 0.9% sodium chloride and this should be warmed to maintain body temperature at the stoma. Cotton wool or dressings that shed fibres should be avoided, as these can be inhaled or trigger an inflammatory response in the stoma (Parker 2000). Dressings at the tracheostomy site are not used routinely, as this may lead to accidental tube displacement. However, depending on individual need a dressing may be indicated and this decision can be discussed with the surgeon.

The ties securing the tracheostomy tube should be changed daily, or more frequently if they become soiled. The options for securing the tube in situ are Velcro tapes or cotton ties. Velcro tapes are rarely indicated, as infants and children have an inquisitive nature that may result in them opening the tape and causing accidental decannulation. Cotton ties should be used and tied securely to the side of the neck so that the child is not lying on the knot and to avoid confusion with other ties such as those for bibs (Wilson 2005). The ties must be snug against the neck so that when the child is sitting comfortably only one finger should be able to be placed under the tie (Fig. 22.4).

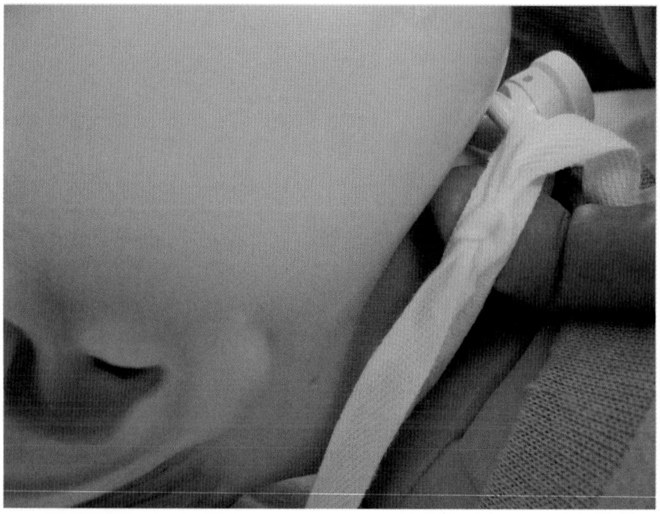

Fig. 22.4 • It should be possible to place only one finger under the tie securing the tracheostomy tube.

Procedures Box 22.1 Cleaning the tracheostomy stoma site and changing the ties

Action
Clean the stoma site and change the ties at least once daily, or more frequently if the ties become soiled by copious secretions.

Reasons *To observe the stoma and skin for signs of irritation. To keep the stoma, skin and tapes clean and dry, and minimise the risk of irritation or infection.*

Action
Collect the equipment required for the procedure:

- Disposable gloves (non-powdered)
- Dressing pack with gallipot
- Non-shedding cotton buds or gauze
- 0.9% sodium chloride
- Scissors
- Tracheostomy tapes
- Tracheostomy dressing (if required; not generally used routinely)
- Neck roll.

Action
Two persons should perform the procedure.

Reason *One person holds the tracheostomy tube in situ while the other person performs the procedure and changes the ties.*

Action
Explain the procedure to the child and carer and gain verbal consent.

Reason *Gains cooperation and minimises anxiety.*

Action
Position the child with a small neck roll under the shoulders (if not contraindicated); the infant may require swaddling in a blanket.

Reason *Provides access to the stoma site.*

Action
Wash your hands.

Reason *This is a universal precaution.*

Action
Pour the 0.9% sodium chloride into the gallipot (or other cleansing agent as per surgeon or local policy).

Action
Apply gloves.

Reason *This is a universal precaution.*

Action
Remove the dressing if in situ.

Actions
Dip the gauze or cotton bud into the sodium chloride and cleanse under the flange outwards from the stoma.

Dispose of the gauze or cotton bud and repeat the procedure until the stoma site, surrounding area and flange are clean.

Reapply tracheostomy dressing if indicated.

Reason *Minimises the risk of infection.*

Action
One person holds the tracheostomy tube in situ while the other removes the tapes.

Reason *Minimises the risk of tube dislodgement.*

Action
Thread the new ties into the flange and tie securely using a reef knot on the opposite side of the neck to the soiled ties removed from the tube; ties should be tight enough so that only one finger can be placed underneath but not so tight as to cause skin damage.

Reason *Prevents accidental decannulation and minimises the risk of skin breakdown.*

Action
Reposition the child appropriately.

Reason *Promotes comfort.*

Action
Dispose of all equipment appropriately.

Reason *This is a universal precaution.*

Action
Document the procedure, including the condition of the skin.

Reason *Provides documentary evidence of the procedure and a record of skin condition.*

Changing the tracheostomy tube

In order to prevent a build-up of secretions that could block a tracheostomy tube, regular tube changes are necessary (Russell 2005). Under normal circumstances it is generally agreed that tubes should be changed weekly. However, there may be occasions when a tube change is not advisable, particularly when a child is unwell, tired or irritable (Great Ormond Street Hospital for Children NHS Trust 2005). Likewise the tube change may need to be performed more frequently if secretions are very tenacious and the child is showing signs of respiratory distress that is not resolved by suctioning. The nurse should be vigilant for signs of respiratory distress such as increased respiratory rate with laboured breathing and/or stridor, tachycardia, increasing anxiety, cyanosis and decreased oxygen saturations. If there are signs of tube obstruction the tube should be changed without delay. Once the tube has been changed the child should be closely observed to ensure that the problem has been resolved.

It is normal for the first tube change to be carried out by the surgeon to ensure that the stoma has healed sufficiently. During the tracheostomy surgery the child will have had sutures inserted on either side of the tracheal opening (stay sutures). If an emergency tube change is required in the first few days postoperatively, these sutures can be pulled on to open the stoma and the new tube inserted. These stay sutures are usually removed by the surgeon at the first tube change.

Routine tube changes should be performed when two persons are present. Tube changes should be avoided when the child has just eaten, as the procedure can sometimes cause the child to cough, which could lead to vomiting (Wilson 2005). All equipment should be prepared and the child made comfortable before beginning. A small rolled towel may be placed under the shoulders to slightly extend the head and improve visibility of the tracheostomy.

Procedures Box 22.2 Changing a tracheostomy tube

Actions
Collect all the equipment required for the procedure:

- Tray or trolley
- Oxygen unit with flow meter and tracheostomy mask
- Ambu bag and oxygen tubing
- Suction unit
- Suction catheters of appropriate size
- Dressing pack
- Disposable gloves (non-powdered)
- Tracheostomy tube (the correct size for the child)
- Tracheostomy tube (one size smaller)
- Tracheostomy ties
- Scissors
- Tracheal dilators (as per local policy)
- Tracheostomy dressing (if required)
- Normal saline 0.9% ampoules
- Non-shedding gauze or cotton buds
- K-Y Jelly (as per local policy)
- Neck roll.

Action
Two nurses should carry out the procedure.

Reason *Ensures that immediate assistance is available in the event of complications.*

Action
Explain all aspects of the procedure to the child and carer and gain verbal consent.

Reason *Gains cooperation and minimises anxiety.*

Action
Time a routine tube change appropriately – avoid changing immediately after the child's meal.

Reason *Minimises the risk of vomiting and aspiration during the procedure.*

Action
Position the child appropriately: older children may wish to sit up; the younger child may lie with a small neck roll under the shoulders (if not contraindicated); and the infant may require swaddling in a blanket.

Reasons *Promotes easy insertion of the tube.*
Extends the neck.

Action
Wash your hands.

Reason *This is a universal precaution.*

Action
Attach the tracheostomy ties to the flange of the new tube.

Reason *So that the tube can be secured immediately following insertion to prevent accidental decannulation.*

Action
If changing a tube with an inner tube ensure that the inner tube fits easily into the outer tube.

Reason *Ensures ease of tube change.*

Action
Ensure that the introducer is properly inserted into the new tracheostomy tube and apply a small amount of K-Y jelly to lubricate the tip (as per local policy).

Reason *Prevents trauma to the trachea.*

Action
If a dressing is in situ remove the dressing and clean the site appropriately.

Reason *Prevents cross-infection.*

Action
Cut the tracheostomy ties and remove the old tube in an outward and downward direction.

Reason *Prevents resistance and trauma.*

Action
Insert the new tube and immediately remove the introducer.

Reason *The child is unable to breathe with the introducer in situ.*

Action
Secure the tracheostomy ties on the opposite side of the neck to the old tube.

Procedures Box 22.2 Changing a tracheostomy tube—cont'd

Reason *Prevents accidental decannulation and minimises the risk of skin breakdown.*

Action
Suction the child if required.

Reason *Coughing often occurs during a tube change and secretions should be cleared.*

Action
Observe the child for any respiratory difficulties and reposition the child appropriately.

Reason *Ensures that the tube change has been successful and the airway is clear.*

Action
If a dressing is in situ this should be renewed.

Reason *Prevents cross-infection.*

Actions
Dispose of all equipment appropriately.

Plastic tracheostomy tubes are single use only and silver tubes are resterilised for use on the same child.

Reason *These are universal precautions.*

Action
Document the tube change in the appropriate patient notes, including details of any problems encountered during the procedure.

Reason *Provides documentary evidence of the procedure and identifies the date for the next tracheostomy tube change.*

Communication

Having a tracheostomy will affect a child's speech and language development. Instead of passing through the larynx and producing speech, air is passed out of the tracheostomy tube, which is placed below the level of the larynx. It is recommended that all children with a tracheostomy are referred to a speech and language therapist. The speech and language therapist, in conjunction with the child, family and multidisciplinary team, will identify communication options and methods of developing language skills (Woodnorth 2004). A number of communication methods can be used.

Communication options for the child with a tracheostomy are as follows:

- Facial expression
- Mouth shapes and early sounds (kisses, blowing raspberries)
- Speaking valves (not all children are candidates): a one-way valve that is attached to the tracheostomy tube (Hull et al 2005); it closes over as the child exhales and passes air through the larynx and out of the mouth
- Pseudovoice: speech is created by using air trapped in the mouth or throat; this can be difficult to understand
- Sign language
- Electrolarynx: this can be suitable for older children; an electronic device is held against the neck as the child talks and it produces an artificial voice.

Now test your knowledge

- Consider how you would prepare a 3-year-old child for the changing of a tracheostomy tube. What support and equipment would be required to ensure satisfactory management of this procedure?
- Identify the respiratory complications that will require urgent medical attention.

References

Abraham SS (2003) Babies with tracheostomies. ASHA Leader 8(5):4–5,26

American Thoracic Society (2000) Care of the child with a chronic tracheostomy. American Journal of Respiratory and Critical Care Medicine 161:297–308

Edgtton-Winn M, Wright K (2005) Tracheostomy: a guide to nursing care. Australian Nursing Journal 13(5):1–4

Fiske E, Gracey K (2004) Effective strategies to prepare infants and families for home tracheostomy care. Advances in Neonatal Care 4(1):42–53

Great Ormond Street Hospital for Children NHS Trust (2005) Living with a tracheostomy: information for parents. Great Ormond Street Hospital NHS Trust, London

Griggs A (1998) Tracheostomy: suctioning and humidification. Nursing Standard 13(2):49–53

Hull EM, Dumas HM, Crowley RA, Kharasch VS (2005) Tracheostomy speaking valves for children: tolerance and clinical benefits. Pediatric Rehabilitation 8(3):214–219

Parker L (2000) Applying the principles of infection control to wound care. British Journal of Nursing 9(7):394–404

Phipps LM, Raymond JA, Angeletti TM (2006) Congenital tracheal stenosis. Critical Care Nursing 26(3):60–69

Russell C (2005) Providing the nurse with a guide to tracheostomy care and management. British Journal of Nursing 14(5):428–433

Wilson M (2005) Tracheostomy management. Paediatric Nursing 17(3):38–44

Woodnorth GH (2004) Assessing and managing medically fragile children: tracheostomy and ventilatory support. Language, Speech, and Hearing Services in Schools 35:363–372

23

Chest drain care

Colleen O'Neill • Imelda T. Coyne

Chest tubes

A chest tube or chest drain is a flexible plastic tube that is inserted through the side of the chest into the pleural space (Fig. 23.1). The purpose of a chest tube is to evacuate air or fluid that has accumulated in the pleural space. Fluid or air that accumulates in the pleural space will reduce lung expansion and lead to respiratory compromise and hypoxia. Insertion of a chest tube enables drainage of air or fluid from the pleural space, allowing negative intrapleural pressures to be re-established, leading to lung re-expansion. The insertion of a chest drain (thoracotomy) may not only provide symptomatic relief but may also prove to be a life-saving intervention for the child.

Indications

The chest tube is commonly placed to resolve the following conditions: pneumothorax, haemothorax, pleural effusion, and the prevention of cardiac tamponade after open heart surgery. A pneumothorax is the collection of air in the pleural space. Pneumothoraces may present with features of pleuritic chest pain, dyspnoea, pallor or tachycardia. Clinically significant signs include reduced breath sounds, hyper-resonant percussion notes and mediastinal deviation away from the side of the lesion. A pneumothorax may be termed spontaneous, tension or open.

The effective drainage of air or fluid from the pleural space requires an airtight system to maintain subatmospheric intrapleural pressure. There are many systems available but all follow the underwater seal principle and consist of a suitable chest drain and tubing, a collection chamber and suction. The underwater seal acts as a one-way valve through which air is expelled from the pleural space and prevented from re-entering during the next inspiration. Retrograde flow of fluid may occur if the collection chamber is raised above the level of the patient, therefore the collection chamber should be kept below the level of the patient at all times to prevent fluid being siphoned into the pleural space.

Pleural effusion

Pleural effusion is the accumulation of fluid within the pleural cavity, which often occurs as a complication of surgery or a pre-existing illness (e.g. cystic fibrosis). Normally, pleural fluid is produced by the parietal pleura and absorbed by the visceral pleura, maintaining a minimal amount of fluid within the pleural space. When this fine balance is upset a pleural effusion develops. If significantly large amounts of fluid are allowed to accumulate, lung tissue becomes compressed and respiratory function distorted.

Cardiac tamponade

Cardiac tamponade is a condition in which the accumulation of blood or fluid in or around the pericardial sac causes a compression of the heart muscle. Cardiac tamponade can result in cardiac arrhythmias and asystole, which can cause death. The use of a chest tube will prevent this condition after thoracic and/or heart surgeries.

Evidence-based practice in relation to chest drains

Currently, chest drains are used in many different clinical settings, particularly in intensive care. Therefore children's nurses must possess the necessary skills and knowledge needed to care for children with a chest drain. However, there appears to be a lack of consensus on the major principles of chest drain management. The literature revealed a limited number of research articles to advise the nurse on the specific care needs of this patient group. Charnock & Evans (2001) conducted a systematic literature review on the nursing management of chest drains and concluded that there is limited research in this area of nursing care, with most of the literature focusing on the adult patient. The British Thoracic Society (Laws et al 2003) issued guidelines for physicians on the care of the patient with a chest tube, and although these guidelines do not relate specifically to children they do provide some guidance on the general care of chest tubes. Subsequently the following content is based on research from general practice and the British Thoracic Society guidelines.

Chest drain 'milking' and 'stripping'

'Milking' and 'stripping' are two practices that traditionally were used in clinical practice and may still be seen in some healthcare organisations. Milking refers to a drainage technique in which the chest tubing is either milked by hand or using

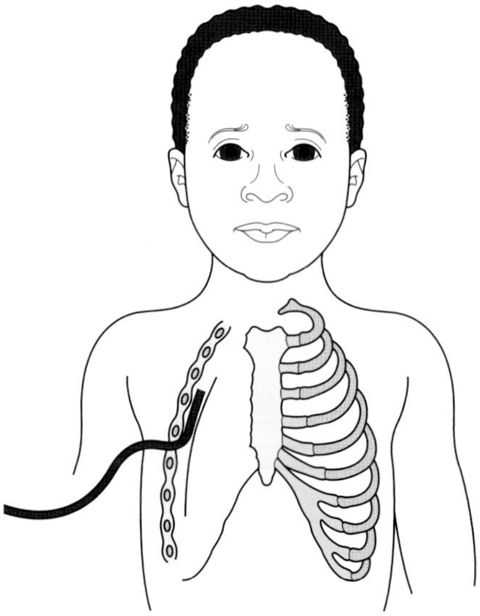

Fig. 23.1 • A chest tube or chest drain.

a specialised roller to compress the tube down its length of tubing. Stripping is executed by running two pieces of alcohol gauze along the length of the tubing, each in their own turn, from top to bottom. The assumption is that if a chest tube is milked or stripped regularly it will extricate or prevent the development of clots in the chest tubing (Trigg & Mohammed 2006). However, research has shown that milking has no consequence on clot formation, as pleura have a defibrinating effect on blood (Carroll 1995). Milking chest drains may cause lung damage, because excessively high intrathoracic pressures may be created (Welch 1993). Therefore stripping and milking of chest tubes is not recommended (Carroll 1995, Welch 1993).

Clamping chest drains

Drain clamping prior to mobilisation is another habitual nursing practice. The belief is that a child who is moving may unintentionally disconnect his or her drainage bottle. If it is clamped, air cannot enter the lung via the tube (Trigg & Mohammed 2006). Conversely, others argue that if there is an air leak within the lung, clamping the drain may cause a tension pneumothorax (Godden & Hiley 1998, Harris & Graham 1991). Furthermore, clamping a chest drain in the presence of a continuing air leak may lead to serious complications such as tension pneumothorax (Laws et al 2003). This risk outweighs the potential risk of the system becoming accidentally disconnected during patient mobilisation (Godden & Hiley 1998). Rather than clamping before mobilisation, attention should be directed at ensuring that all the connections are secured before movement. According to Parslow & Sandell (2005) the only justification for clamping underwater seal drains is to permit bottle changes. However, recent British Thoracic Society guidelines (Law et al 2003) state that although the practice of drain clamping is generally not advised for safety reasons it is acceptable under the supervision of nursing staff who are trained in the management of chest drains and who have received instructions from medical staff.

ALERT

Chest drains should not be clamped for safety reasons. If a drain is clamped air cannot enter the lung via the tube. The only justification for clamping underwater seal drains is to permit bottle changes.

Pain

Pain and the use of analgesia throughout chest drain management remains poorly studied, particularly in children (Henry et al 2003). Most of the research in relation to pain and chest drains has been conducted with the adult population. Chest drain insertion and removal have been reported to be painful procedures. Corbo-Richert (1994) researched the coping strategies and behaviour of 24 children (aged 3–7 years) during a range of chest drain procedures, including removal of the drain. Data regarding the type (but not the dose) of analgesia given before and immediately after the procedure were provided. Seven children (29%) received no analgesia, while the remaining 71% received morphine, fentanyl, paracetamol, midazolam or diazepam. The children displayed a variety of coping behaviours, predominantly self-protection, reaching out, and controlling and information-seeking behaviours. Although the researchers did not collect data regarding pain intensity or sensation, they concluded that chest drain removal was both frightening and painful for children. These claims were inferred from the children's coping behaviours and not from direct measurement of pain, anxiety or fear.

Regular pain assessments using an appropriate pain score assessment tool should be utilised while a chest drain remains in situ (Parslow & Sandell 2005). Regular oral analgesia reduces the development of severe pain from the chest drain site significantly (Miller & Harvey 1993). Additional pain medication should be administered during the insertion and removal of chest drains to ensure adequate pain control. Continued pain at a chest drain site must be investigated to ensure that it is not a symptom of an underlying condition or other local problem.

Psychological support

The insertion of a chest drain can be a traumatic event for the child and family, consequently nurses should provide adequate preparation and explanation prior to and during the procedure. It is essential to explain the procedure in simple, easily understandable terms to the child and parents beforehand. Children can feel less anxious and scared when they know what to expect.

Procedures Box 23.1 Insertion of a chest tube

1

Action
Collect all necessary equipment:

- Dressing trolley
- Sterile gloves and gown
- Skin antiseptic solutions
- Sterile drapes
- Gauze swabs
- A selection of syringes and needles
- Local anaesthetic (e.g. lidocaine)
- Small scalpel and blade
- Suture
- Chest tube
- Connecting tubing
- Closed drainage system (including sterile water if an underwater seal is being used)
- Chest drain clamps
- Dressing.

2

Action
Assist in the correct location and insertion of the drain.

Reason *The fifth intercostal space is the most pre-eminent location for chest drain insertion (Mackway-Jones et al 2001).*

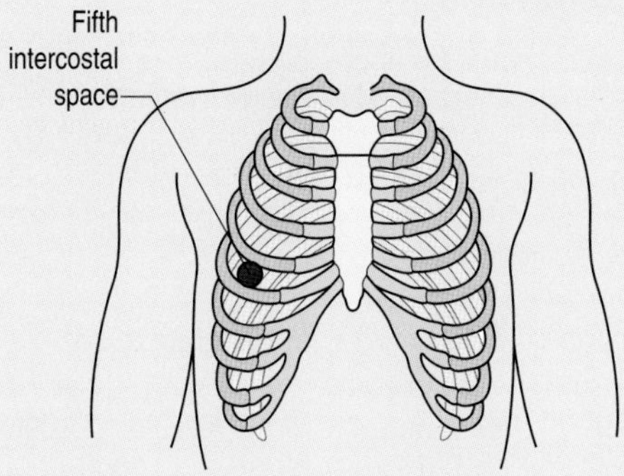

3

Actions
Assess vital signs post insertion.

Record temperature, pulse and respirations.

Record oxygen saturation levels.

Reason *Assessment of vital signs ensures early detection of deterioration in a patient's condition and allows early identification of complications.*

4

Actions
Nurse the child in a high-visibility area and ensure that suction and oxygen are available at the bedside.

Ensure that an extra drainage collection system is readily available.

Reason *Any deterioration in the child's condition can be monitored and equipment is readily available if required.*

5

Action
Ensure that a chest X-ray is obtained after insertion.

Reason *Following insertion a chest X-ray should be taken to confirm the correct location of the chest tube and to exclude complications and determine whether the collection of air or fluid is being drained.*

6

Action
Assess the drainage collection system every 4 h while the chest tube is in place for fluctuations and air bubbles in the air leak indicator.

The frequency of observation will depend on the patient's condition and local hospital policy.

7

Actions
Check for drainage amount, colour and consistency.

It is common practice to mark the level of fluid on the collecting chamber, along with the time and nurse's initials; the level should be recorded on the fluid balance chart in accordance with local policy.

Reason *A change in the colour, consistency or amount of drainage may be significant and should be reported to the doctor.*

8

Action
In a pleural drain observe the swings of fluid in the chest tube bottle; with inspiration the water will rise up into the chest tube and with expiration the water will fall.

Reason *If the swing is less than 2 cm the lung is not likely to be fully expanded and therefore suction may need to be increased.*

9

Action
Check the suction level, if applicable.

Reason *Where suction is required it may be performed via the underwater seal at a level of 10–20 cm of water (Laws et al 2003).*

10

Action
Monitor the water seal chambers for the appropriate level of water.

Reason *The water level in the water seal chamber should be maintained at the 2-cm level with sterile water or sterile saline.*

11

Action
Check the bottle at least every shift and change the chest drainage system if it breaks or it becomes full.

Reason *Frequent changes are unnecessary and may introduce infection.*

Procedures Box 23.1 Insertion of a chest tube—cont'd

12

Action
Position the drainage system in an upright position below the level of the heart; the drainage systems should at all times be at least 30 cm beneath the child's chest (Allibone 2003).

Reason *Retrograde flow of fluid may occur if the collection chamber is raised above the level of the patient.*

13

Action
The tubing should be securely attached to the child's skin with adhesive tape.

Reasons *Taping the connection secures it, thus avoiding potential disconnection.*
Accidental disconnection of tubing may lead to air entry and hence some lung collapse.

Action
Do not tape the chest tube flat to the chest.

Reason *This causes kinking at the tube as it goes through the intercostal space.*

ALERT
Do not tape the chest tube flat to the chest, as this causes kinking at the tube.

14

Action
Check the chest tube for kinks; the tubing should be free and unkinked.

Reasons *Small soft drains are prone to kinking as the drain exits the skin, especially in young mobile children.*
Excess tubing should not be suspended from the bed, as this can amplify resistance and minimise effective drainage (Tang et al 2002).

15

Action
Dressings shall be monitored at least every shift and changed as per local policy.

Reason *Dressings should be monitored to detect drainage or air leakage.*

16

Actions
Assess for pain post insertion and thereafter as indicated and administer analgesia as prescribed.

Non-pharmacological techniques such as distraction and comforting should also be employed.

Reason *Chest drains are uncomfortable and therefore frequent assessment of pain and discomfort is important so that adequate measures can be taken to provide comfort and reduce the child's pain.*

17

Action
Encourage the child to cough and deep breathe frequently.

Reason *Helps drain the pleural space and expand the lungs.*

18

Action
Instruct the child to sit upright.

Reason *This will promote optimal lung expansion and, according to Owen & Gould (1997), it is the most comfortable position for the patient.*

19

Action
Parents and the child should be encouraged to take responsibility for the chest tube and drainage system.

Reason *Helps promote family-centred care, which may reduce the child's anxiety and parental anxiety.*

20

Action
Document all nursing care and report any changes to the medical team.

Reason *Ensures that an accurate record of nursing care of the chest drain has been maintained.*

Removing chest drains

The timing of removal is dependent on the original reason for insertion and clinical progress of the child. Extracting the chest drain can be traumatic and painful (Bruce et al 2006), therefore sedation and analgesia are required. Clamping of the drain before removal is generally unnecessary (Laws et al 2003). If the timing can be coordinated the drain is removed on expiration. Removal of the drain is best carried out while the child performs a Valsalva manoeuvre or else during expiration (Parslow & Sandell 2005). A smooth, quick removal of the drain is preferred to a slow withdrawal. The wound should be closed by the application of Steri-Strips (Parslow & Sandell 2005). Twenty-four hours after removal, a repeat chest X-ray should be performed – sooner if the child's condition deteriorates. Position the child comfortably and monitor for recurrence.

Conclusion

The insertion of a chest drain has significant implications for nursing staff, because it is the responsibility of nursing staff to ensure that the patient and drain are closely monitored.

Now test your knowledge

- List the indications for chest tube placement.
- Explain the process of chest tube insertion and the nursing responsibilities during the insertion process.
- Identify the components of a physical assessment of the patient with chest tubes.

References

Allibone L (2003) Nursing management of chest drains. Nursing Standard 17(22):45–54

Bruce E, Howard RF, Franck LS (2006) Chest drain removal pain and its management: a literature review. Journal of Clinical Nursing 15:145–154

Carroll P (1995) Chest tubes made easy. Registered Nurse 58(12):46–56

Charnock Y, Evans D (2001) Nursing management of chest drains: a systematic review. Australian Critical Care 14:156–160

Corbo-Richert BH (1994) Coping behaviors of young children during a chest tube procedure in the pediatric intensive care unit. Maternal Child Nursing Journal 22:134–146

Godden J, Hiley C (1998) Managing the patient with a chest drain: a review. Nursing Standard 12(32):35–39

Harris DR, Graham TR (1991) Management of intercostal drains. British Journal of Hospital Medicine 45(6):383–386

Henry M, Arnold T, Harvey J (2003) BTS guidelines for the management of spontaneous pneumothorax. Thorax 58(Suppl II):ii39–ii52

Laws D, Neville E, Duffy J (2003) British Thoracic Society guidelines for the insertion of a chest drain. Thorax 58:53–59

Mackway-Jones K, Molyneux E, Phillips B, Wieteska S (2001) Subcutaneous emphysema associated with chest tube drainage. Respirology 6(2):87–89

Miller AC, Harvey JE (1993) Guidelines for the management of spontaneous pneumothorax. British Medical Journal 307:114–116

Owen S, Gould D (1997) Underwater seal chest drains: the patient's experience. Journal of Clinical Nursing 6:215–225

Parslow PM, Sandell JM (2005) Paediatric chest drains: past, present and percutaneous. Trauma 7:163–170

Tang A, Velissaris TJ, Weeden DF (2002) An evidence based approach to the drainage of the pleural cavity: an evaluation of best practice. Journal of Evaluation in Clinical Practice 8(3):333–340

Trigg T, Mohammed T (2006) Practices in children's nursing: guidelines for hospital and community. Churchill Livingstone, London

Welch J (1993) Chest tubes and pleural drainage. Surgical Nurse 6(5):7–12

24 Peripheral intravenous therapy

Janet Kelsey • Neil Bloxham

An intravenous infusion is the process by which an infusion device is used to deliver fluids or drugs in solution to the patient by the intravenous route. Children and young people undergo intravenous therapy for any number of reasons. They may be critically or acutely ill with a requirement for fluid volume, support of cardiac or renal function, or antibiotic or antimicrobial therapy. Alternatively they may require treatment or management of cancer or leukaemia, with all or part of this therapy taking place in the home environment.

Devices

The Medicines and Healthcare products Regulatory Agency (MHRA) has classified infusion devices into three categories according to the potential risks involved. The aim is to enable users to make an appropriate choice of device for the therapy and patient group. Pumps suited to category A can be used for the other categories B and C, pumps in category B can be used for B and C, and pumps in category C can be used only for therapies in this category (Medical Devices Agency 2003; Table 24.1). Hospitals are required to label pumps with their category to enable the correct pump to be chosen for the proposed therapy (Fig. 24.1).

Requirements of devices

The pattern of delivery of fluid from an infusion pump is very dependent on the type of pump used; some have the capacity for variable pressure, maximum flow rate and flow rate increments. It is therefore essential that pumps are configured correctly for their required use. Devices should always be chosen in accordance with MHRA categories to enable suitable accuracy of infusion rate (measured over 60 min) and satisfy short-term minute-to-minute requirements that determine smoothness and consistency of flow (Fig. 24.2). They should also meet the requirements for pressure occlusion, alarm delay time and size of bolus; this should ensure that most problems associated with infusions are prevented or addressed. Further information on the suitability of devices can be obtained from the website of the MHRA (Medicines and Healthcare products Regulatory Agency 2007). Staff should be educated and competent in the use of infusion devices (Table 24.2) and have regular updates when new devices are introduced (Medical Devices Agency 2003).

Gravity flow devices

These depend entirely on gravity to drive the infusion and are dependent on a number of variables including patient movement and height of infusion container. The optimum height is 1 m above the patient to overcome venous pressure; however, alterations in the patient's position may alter flow rate and necessitate changing the speed of the infusion (Medical Devices Agency 2003, Perucca 2001). The system consists of an administration set containing a drip chamber and a roller clamp to control the flow of fluid. Roller clamps should be placed on the upper third of the infusion tubing away from the patient, and the clamp should be repositioned to prevent 'cold creep'; this is when the tubing tries to retain its round shape, pushing the clamp open, but pinched tubing does not apply the same pressure (Medical Devices Agency 2003, Perucca 2001). Inclusion of other in-line devices (e.g. filters) may also affect flow rate (Perucca 2001).

The nurse chooses the appropriate administration set according to need. Neonates should always be infused via a category A infusion pump; children normally require the use of either an infusion pump or an administration set with a burette. Specific administration sets are required for the transfusion of blood or blood products (see Ch. 25). Administration sets will deliver different numbers of drops per millilitre. This has to be taken into consideration when calculating the drip rate of infusions delivered without an infusion device. The drip rate should be checked on the packaging prior to administration to ensure an accurate calculation of flow rate.

Calculating intravenous infusion flow rates

To calculate how to set the infusion at the prescribed rate you need to know the amount to be infused and the length of time the infusion is to take. To calculate how much fluid will be infused in 1 h, divide the total volume by the time the infusion is to take:

$$\text{Number of millilitres per hour (mL/h)} = \frac{\text{total volume (mL)}}{\text{duration (h)}}$$

For example, for 500 mL of fluid transfused over 8 h:

$$\text{mL/h} = \frac{500\text{ mL}}{8\text{ h}}$$
$$= 62.5\text{ mL}$$

Table 24.1. Therapy categories and performance parameters

Therapy category	Therapy description	Patient group	Critical performance parameters
A	Drugs with narrow therapeutic margin Drugs with short half-life[a] Any infusion given to neonates	Any Any Neonates	• Good long-term accuracy • Good short-term accuracy (see below) • Rapid alarm after occlusion • Small occlusion bolus • Able to detect very small air embolus (volumetric pumps only) • Small flow rate increments • Good bolus accuracy • Rapid start-up time (syringe pumps only)
B	Drugs other than those with a short half-life Total parenteral nutrition Fluid maintenance Transfusions Diamorphine[b]	Any except neonates Volume-sensitive except neonates Any except neonates	• Good long-term accuracy • Alarm after occlusion • Small occlusion bolus • Able to detect small air embolus (volumetric pumps only) • Small flow rate increments • Bolus accuracy
C[c]	Total parenteral nutrition Fluid maintenance Transfusions	Any except volume-sensitive or neonates	• Long-term accuracy • Alarm after occlusion • Small occlusion bolus • Able to detect air embolus (volumetric pumps only) • Incremental flow rates

[a]The half-life of a drug cannot usually be specified precisely and may vary from patient to patient. As a rough guide, drugs with half-lives of the order of 5 min or less might be regarded as 'short' half-life drugs.
[b]Diamorphine is a special case. The injected agent (diamorphine) has a short half-life, while the active agent (the metabolite) has a very long half-life. It is safe to use a device with performance specifications appropriate to the half-life of the metabolite.
[c]Not all infusions require a pump. Some category C infusions can appropriately be given by gravity.

The prescribed rate is 62.5 mL/h.

Therefore you know to fill the burette with at least 62.5 mL or program the infusion pump to deliver the nearest whole equivalent to 62.5 mL depending on local policy as to whether it is rounded up or down.

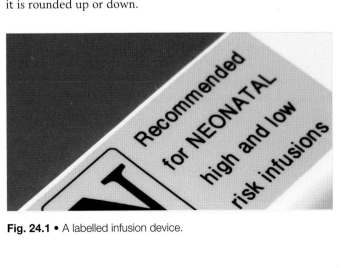

Fig. 24.1 • A labelled infusion device.

To calculate drip flow rate for the same fluid prescription of 500 mL over 8 h use the following algorithm:

$$\frac{\text{Volume of fluid (mL)} \times \text{drops per mL of administration set}}{\text{duration of infusion (min)}}$$

$$\frac{500\text{ mL} \times 20\text{ drops/mL}}{480\text{ min}}$$

= 20.8 drops/min (round up or down according to local policy)

Syringe pumps

These are low-volume high-accuracy devices aimed to infuse at low rates (Fig. 24.3); the volume of the infusion is limited to the size of syringe used in the device. When using syringe pumps the flow delivered at the start of an infusion may be considerably less than that set, and at low flows it can take some time before the drug is delivered to the patient at a

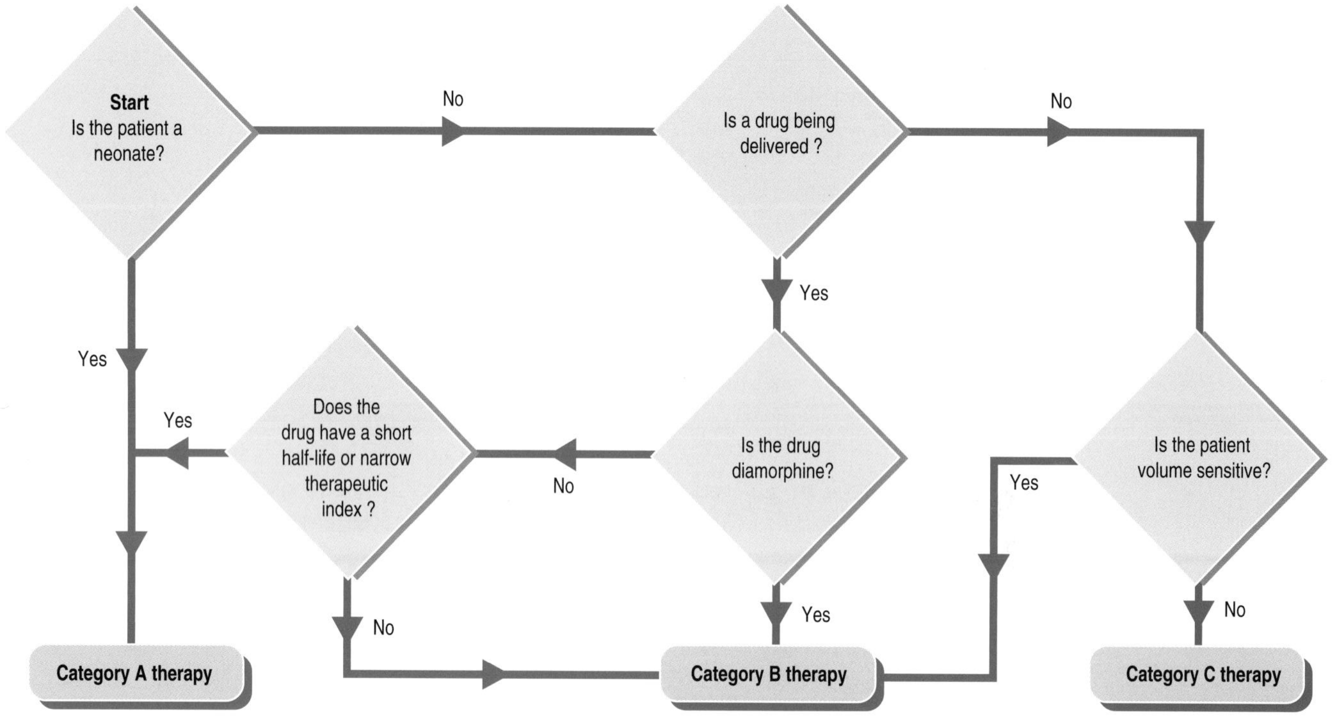

Fig. 24.2 • Decision tree for selection of an infusion device. (Courtesy of the Medicines and Healthcare products Regulatory Agency, 2007)

Table 24.2. Action required by infusion pump users

When	Actions
Before use	• Check that leads, administration sets, bags and cassettes or syringes are in good working order and properly assembled and loaded. • Carry out relevant functional and calibration checks (start-up checks). • Note results. • Check control settings. • Check that the correct flow rate has been set.
A problem occurs	• Stop the infusion. Make sure that all clamps on the giving sets are closed. • Seek technical advice. • Record problems and action taken. • If necessary withdraw the device from service.
At specified intervals	• Check that the observed flow rate corresponds to the rate displayed on the infusion pump. • Inspect fusion site. • Note results. • If tests fail withdraw the device from service.
After use	• Clean. • Safely dispose of single-use devices and other accessories that cannot be reused.
When sending an infusion system to be repaired or serviced	• Include all the leads and accessories needed to operate the device. • Enclose a full account of any problems and faults. • Decontaminate. • Fill in decontamination form.

Table 24.2. Action required by infusion pump users—cont'd

When	Actions
When an infusion device has undergone service	• Carry out all standard preuse inspections. • Check the set-up of protocols and programs, as these may have been altered during servicing.
When an adverse incident has occurred	First take steps necessary for the well-being of the patient and/or staff, then: • do not alter settings or remove administration sets • leave any fluids in the infusion system • note details of all medical equipment attached to the patient • note details of the device (type, make, model and serial number) • retain packaging for details of consumables • note settings of controls and limits of alarms • note the content volume remaining in the set or syringe • if relevant, record the contents of computer memory logs of the infusion pump; seek the assistance of the electrical biomedical engineering department if necessary • if possible, contact the Medical Devices Agency before moving or dismantling the equipment.

(From Infusion systems device bulletin DB 2003(02), with permission of MHRA.)

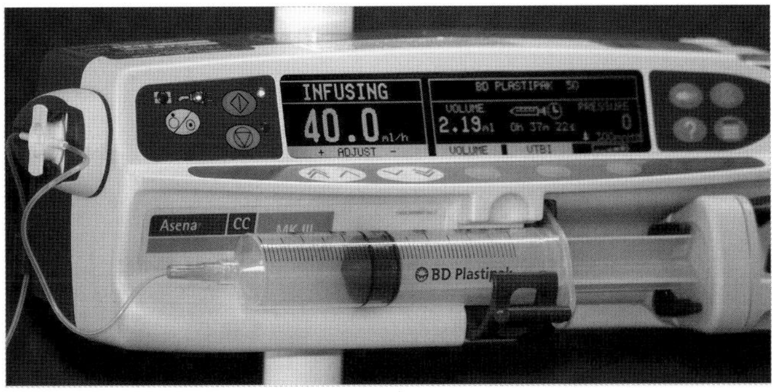

Fig. 24.3 • Loaded syringe pump.

therapeutic level; also, the initial backlash pressure must be overcome before a steady flow is achieved. Care must be taken not to allow free flow of infusion into the child; this is achieved by correct loading of syringe and correct connection of the administration set and syringe. The pump should always be situated as close as possible to the infusion site height, otherwise siphoning may occur, resulting in a bolus dose of the infusion being delivered to the patient.

The MHRA makes the following recommendations for using syringes in infusion pumps:

- 'Always check that the syringe is of the brand and size recommended by the pump manufacturer.
- Check that the syringe barrel clamp is secured over the syringe.
- Do not place tape on the syringe barrel where the barrel clamp is positioned.
- Make sure that the syringe plunger clamp is correctly secured.
- Check that the syringe finger grips are secure within the recess located on the pump body.
- Inspect the syringe before use, checking in particular for signs of damage around the syringe plunger. **NEVER** use a damaged or defective syringe.
- Use the prime or purge facility on the pump to reduce mechanical backlash. **NEVER** prime or purge the line with the extension set attached to the patient' (Medical Devices Agency 2003: 31).

Preparation of the intravenous infusion

Procedures Box 24.1 Priming and connecting the administration set

Action
Decontaminate your hands.

Reason *Maintains universal precautions.*

Action
Two registered nurses check the intravenous fluid (as per local policy) against the prescription.

Reason *According to local policy.*

Action
Check that the outer wrapper is not damaged.

Reason *All medical equipment, dressings and solutions used during invasive proceedures must be sterile (Royal College of Nursing 2005b).*

Action
Open the outer wrapper and remove the bag.

Procedures Box 24.1 Priming and connecting the administration set—cont'd

Action
Check the intravenous fluid bag for:

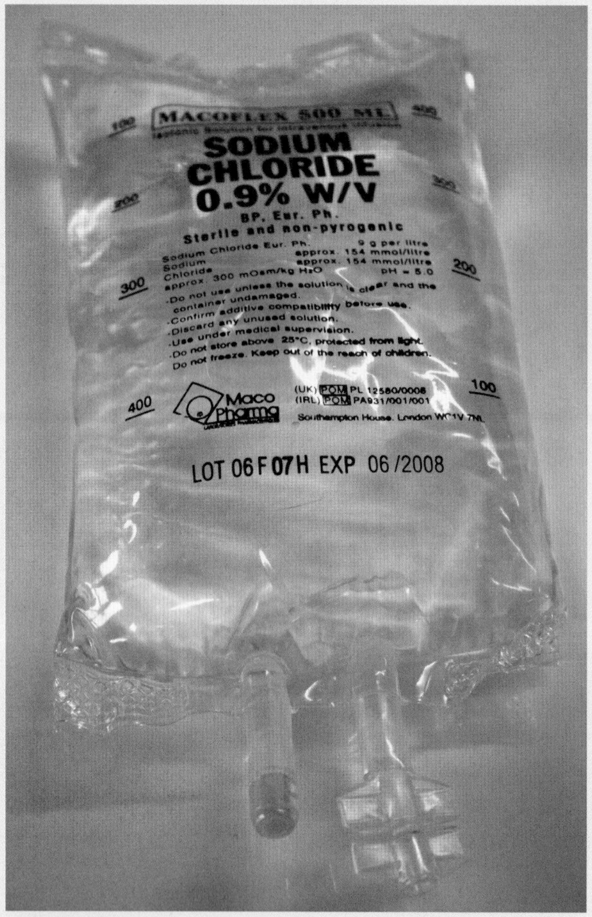

- expiry date
- leakage
- particles
- cloudiness
- batch number.

Reason *Medications, products and equipment must not be used beyond their expiry date (Royal College of Nursing 2005b).*

Actions
Check that the outer wrapper of the administration set is not damaged and that the contents are sterile.

Check the expiry date or date of sterilisation.

Open the wrapper and remove the administration set.

Close the roller clamps on the administration set.

Remove the protective cap from the insertion port on the intravenous fluid bag, maintaining sterility.

Action
Remove the protective cover from the administration set spike, maintaining sterility; note the ridge at the base of the spike – the spike should always be inserted into intravenous fluid up to this ridge.

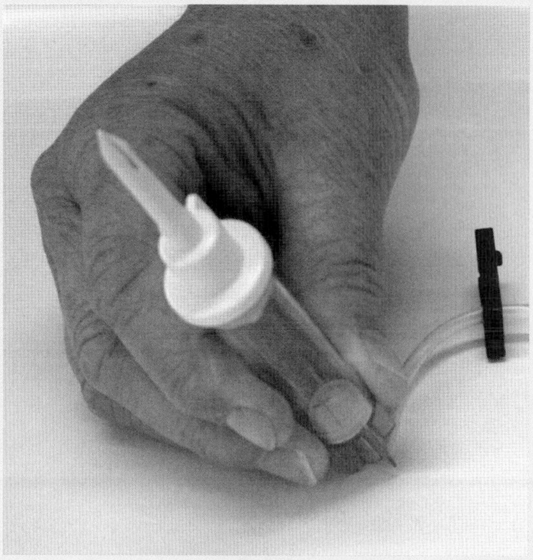

Reason *Prevents contamination of the giving set.*

Actions
Maintaining sterility, insert the spike into the intravenous fluid insertion port, pushing and twisting until fully inserted.

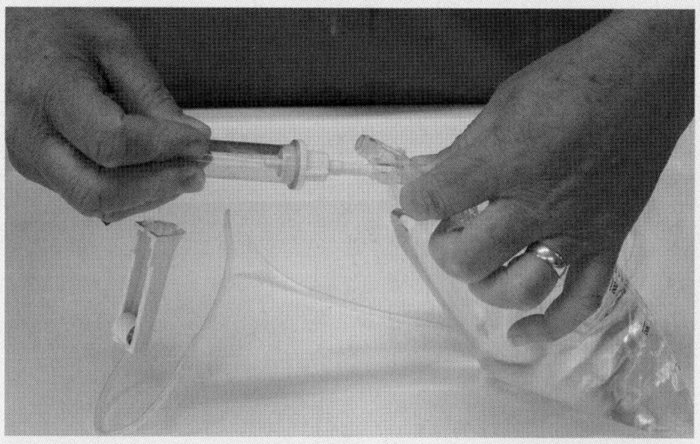

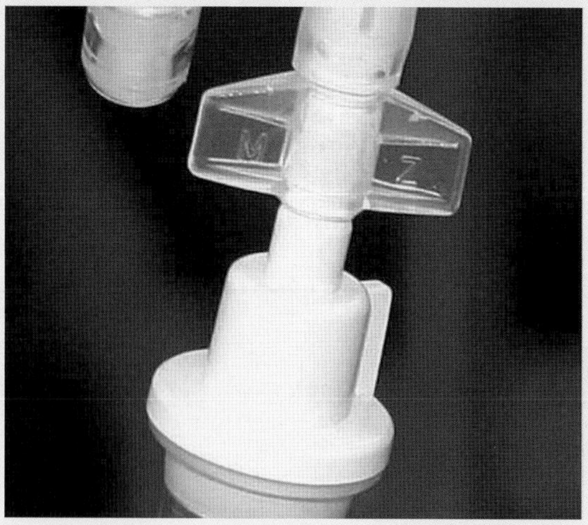

Procedures Box 24.1 Priming and connecting the administration set—cont'd

Hang the intravenous fluid on the intravenous stand.

Release the upper roller clamp and half fill the on-line bubble of the admistration set by squeezing.

Slowly open the lower roller clamp and allow the fluid to run into the administration set, expelling the remaining air.

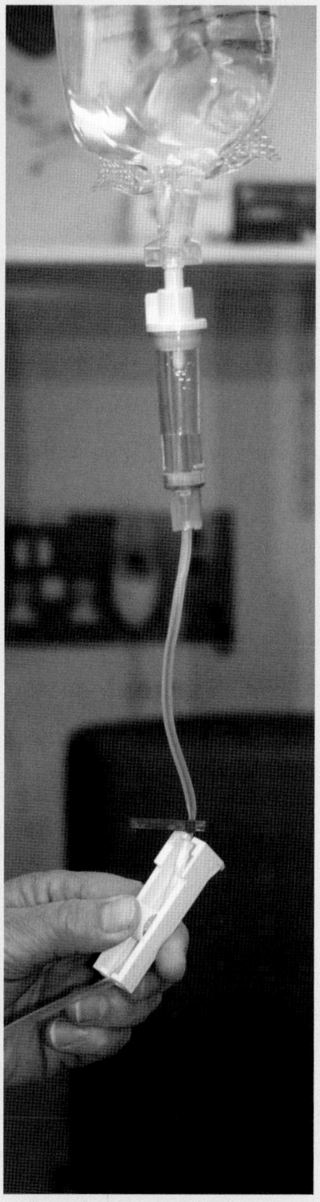

When all air has been expelled close the lower roller clamp.

When using an administration set with a burette, release the upper roller clamp and fill the burette with 20–30 mL of fluid then close the clamp and half fill the on-line bubble of the admistration set by squeezing; fill the burette to the prescribed fluid dose prior to infusion.

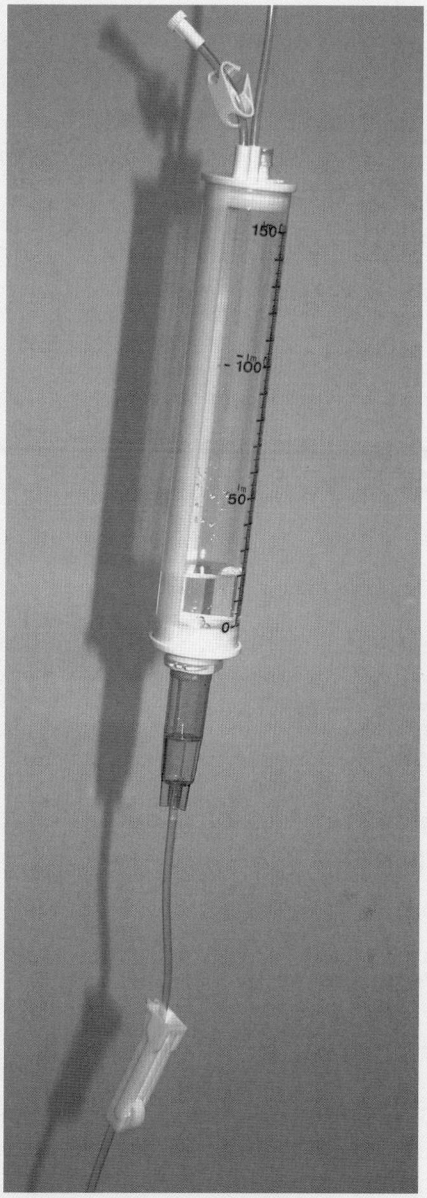

When using an infusion pump place the adminstration set in the pump as per the manufacturer's instructions.

Maintaining sterility, remove the protective cap from the administration set and intravenous cannula.

Action
Put on disposable gloves.

Reason *Reduces the risk from cross-contamination to both patients and staff of organic matter, micro-organisms and toxic substances (Department of Health 20001).*

Action
Put on a disposable plastic apron.

Procedures Box 24.1 Priming and connecting the administration set—cont'd

Reason *Prevents contamination of clothing by blood or body fluids (Department of Health 2001, Royal College of Nursing 2005a).*

Actions

Connect the admistration set to the intravenous cannula.

Secure an intravenous infusion suitable to the child's age and activity level.

Reasons *The dressing should be sterile and allow visual inspection of the site (Department of Health 2001, Royal College of Nursing 2005b).*
Securing of the infusion should not interfere with the assessment or monitoring of the site or impede the infusion (Royal College of Nursing 2005b).

Actions

Set the rate of infusion as prescribed.

Open the lower roller clamp and commence the infusion.

Document the expiry date and batch number of intravenous fluid, time infusion commenced, names of people checking the prescription and commencing the intravenous infusion.

Document the serial number of the pump used.

If not already in place commence fluid balance observations.

Care of the peripheral intravenous site

ALERT
Always ensure that asepsis is maintained.

All care of the peripheral site must be performed using aseptic technique and observing universal precautions (National Institute for Clinical Excellence 2003). The peripheral intravenous site should be covered with a dressing that is sterile (Royal College of Nursing 2005b) and semipermeable to enable the site to be regularly inspected (Healthcare Infection Control Practices Advisory Committee 2002). Intravenous sites should be treated as a surgical wound and the dressing changed if it is wet, is bloodstained or has haemoserous fluid collecting around the site. The infusion site should be checked regularly for and each time an intravenous drug is administered for signs of phlebitis, infiltration and extravasation.

ALERT
Intravenous sites must be checked regularly.

In infants and young children catheter security may be a problem with subsequent infiltration, extravasation and potential infection; neonates are particularly at risk of extravasation injuries, as they often receive high concentrations of glucose and calcium (MacQueen 2005). Preventing catheter dislodgement by securing with tape is common practice; however, Oldman (1991) clearly demonstrated bacterial contamination with subsequent risk of infection following use of non-sterile tape kept in the drawer or pocket of nursing staff. Catheters should therefore be secured with sterile tape or wound closures. Bandaging of the intravenous site may inhibit the moisture permeability of transparent dressings and increase the temperature of the area, providing warmth that may encourage bacterial growth (Nicol 1999). However, children may prefer the site bandaged, preventing them from seeing it and reducing the possibility of it catching on clothing or bed linen. If a bandage is applied it should be a light cling bandage and not a crepe bandage, which may apply pressure and interfere with the infusion. Bandages must be removed every time a drug is administered and at regular intervals to allow visual inspection of the site (Dougherty & Lamb 1999). Movement of limbs may be minimised by splinting; however, this should be carried out only using suitable manufactured devices or locally made thermoplastic splints. Limbs must be splinted correctly to reduce the risk of trauma, nerve or circulatory damage and infection. Using wooden tongue depressors is contraindicated, as they have been found to harbour fungal spores that can result in sepsis (Mitchel et al 1996); the Medical Devices Agency issued a hazard warning preventing the use of wooden splints in 1996.

ALERT
If the child complains of pain always check the infusion.

Infiltration

Infiltration is the inadvertent administration of non-vesicant medication or solution into the surrounding tissue instead of the intended vascular pathway; it occurs when the cannula moves out of the vein so the fluid is delivered into the surrounding tissues (Perdue 2001). The clinical symptoms of infiltration are coolness, leakage at the site and swelling. Infiltration should be identified and assessed, and care planned to minimise the effect of the infiltration. Infiltration should result in immediate discontinuation of the infusion (Lamb 1999). The event should be documented using a grading scale (Table 24.3) and, if necessary, photographic records taken.

Extravasation

Extravasation is the leakage of vesicant medication or solution into the surrounding tissue instead of the intended vascular pathway (Stanley 2002). Extravasation requires immediate assessment and discontinuation of the infusion by the nurse. The incident should be documented in the patient's medical and nursing notes and on a clinical incident form (Intravenous Nurses Society 2000).

In neonates the incidence of extravasation is reported to be 38 per 1000 (Wilkins & Emmerson 2004).

Table 24.3. Infiltration scale

Grade	Clinical criteria
0	No symptoms
1	• Skin blanched • Oedema 2.5 cm in any direction • Cool to touch • With or without pain
2	• Skin blanched • Oedema 2.5–15 cm in any direction • Cool to touch • With or without pain
3	• Skin blanched, translucent • Gross oedema 15 cm in any direction • Cool to touch • Mild to moderate pain • Possible numbness
4	• Skin blanched, translucent • Skin tight, leaking • Skin discoloured, bruised, swollen • Gross oedema 15 cm in any direction • Deep pitting tissue oedema • Circulatory impairment • Moderate to severe pain • Infiltration of any amount of blood product, irritant or vesicant

(From Journal Infusion Nursing 2006, with permission.)

Table 24.4. Phlebitis scale

Signs	Grade	Action
Intravenous site appears healthy	0	No signs of phlebitis
One of the following is evident: • slight pain near intravenous site *or* • slight redness near intravenous site	1	Possibly first signs of phlebitis
Two of the following are evident: • pain at intravenous site • erythema • swelling	2	Early stages of phlebitis: • RESITE CANNULA
All the following signs are evident: • pain along path of cannula • erythema • induration	3	Medium stage of phlebitis: • RESITE CANNULA • CONSIDER TREATMENT
All the following signs are evident and extensive: • pain along path of cannula • erythema • induration • palpable venous cord	4	Advanced stage of phlebitis or the start of thrombophlebitis: • RESITE CANNULA • CONSIDER TREATMENT
All the following signs are evident and extensive: • pain along path of cannula • erythema • induration • palpable venous cord • pyrexia	5	Advanced stage of thrombophlebitis: • INITIATE TREATMENT • RESITE CANNULA

(From Jackson 1998.)

Phlebitis

Phlebitis is the inflammation of the wall of the vein. There are three types identified: chemical caused by infusate damaging the vein wall, mechanical caused by irritation of the venous endothelium by the catheter and infective caused by bacteria causing irritation to the vein wall (Dougherty & Lister 2004). Panadero et al (2002) report that 20–80% of patients receiving peripheral intravenous therapy develop phlebitis. Evaluation of the site for signs of phlebitis should be documented using a standard scale (Table. 24.4) and action taken accordingly.

Use and replacement of cannulae and equipment

It is recommended that in adults peripheral cannulae are replaced every 72–96 h depending on cannula type and therapy; however, in children peripheral catheters should not be replaced unless it is clinically indicated or the cannula has not been placed aseptically, as it has not been demonstrated to reduce the incidence of catheter-related infections (Centers for Disease Control and Prevention 2002, Stenzel et al 1989).

Extension sets can be used to reduce the risk of movement of the cannula when manipulating the administration set, thus reducing the risk of trauma to the vein wall and mechanical phlebitis. Three-way taps may utilised to allow more than one infusion to be administered at the same time. All add-on devices should be changed at the same time as the administration set. Administration sets and connections for non-blood products should be replaced every 72 h unless a cannula-related infection is suspected (Healthcare Infection Control Practices Advisory Committee 2002). Administration sets for blood or blood products and lipid emulsions should be changed every 24 h or after completion of the infusion. There is no strong recommendation made for using in-line filters for infection prevention purposes (Healthcare Infection Control Practices Advisory Committee 2002).

Procedures Box 24.2 Removal of peripheral intravenous cannulae

Action
Explain the procedure to the child.

Reason *Prepares the child for the procedure.*

Action
Decontaminate your hands.

Reason *Maintains universal precautions.*

Action
Put on disposable gloves.

Reason *Reduces the risk from cross-contamination to both patients and staff.*

Action
Put on a disposable apron.

Reason *Prevents contamination of clothing by blood or bodily fluids (Department of Health 2001, Royal College of Nursing 2005a).*

Action
Remove the dressing.

Action
Hold a piece of sterile gauze over the insertion site and remove the cannula carefully using a slow steady movement; keep the hub parallel to the skin.

Reason *Prevents damage to the vein.*

Action
Apply gentle pressure for at least 1 min or as long as necessary, elevating the arm if bleeding persists.

Reason *Prevents haematoma formation.*

Actions
Apply a sterile dressing over the cannula site.

If the insertion site appears infected (score of 3 or more) the tip of the cannula should be sent for culture and sensitivity.

It is easy to contaminate the cannula tip on removal by wiping across the surface of the skin; therefore when sending a cannula tip for culture, first swab the surrounding skin and any pus and send to the laboratory then clean the surrounding skin with a 70% isopropyl alcohol wipe and allow to dry fully.

Remove the cannula and, with sterile scissors, snip 1 cm of cannula into a sterile container and send it to the laboratory.

Dispose of the cannula, unused intravenous fluid and dressing according to local clinical waste disposal guidelines.

Remove your apron and decontaminate your hands.

Document the date of removal of the device in the clinical record.

Now test your knowledge

- What is the current practice for infection control regarding peripheral intravenous therapy in your clinical area?
- What is your local policy on extravasation?
- How would you explain to a junior nurse the importance of choosing the correct infusion pump?
- What steps should you take to avoid extravasation or infiltration in a 3-year-old child?
- What are the advantages and disadvantages of using infusion pumps rather than gravity-fed infusions?

References

Centers for Disease Control and Prevention (2002) Guidelines for the prevention of intravascular catheter-related infections. Morbidity and Mortality Weekly Report 51(RR-10):S35–S63

Department of Health (2001) Standard principles for preventing hospital-acquired infection. Journal of Hospital Infection 74(Suppl.):S21–S37

Dougherty L, Lamb J (eds) (1999) Intravenous therapy in nursing practice. Churchill Livingstone, London

Dougherty L, Lister S (2004) The Royal Marsden Hospital manual of clinical nursing procedures, 6th edn. Blackwell, Oxford

Healthcare Infection Control Practices Advisory Committee (2002) Guidelines for the prevention of intravascular catheter-related infections. American Journal of Infection Control 30(8):476–489

Intravenous Nurses Society (2000) Standards for infusion therapy. Intravenous Nurses Society and Becton Dickinson, Cambridge

Jackson A (1998) Infection control – a battle in vein: infusion phlebitis. Nursing Times 94(4):68–71

Lamb J (1999) Local and systemic complications of intravenous therapy. In Dougherty L, Lamb J (eds) Intravenous therapy in nursing practice. Churchill Livingstone, Edinburgh, p 163–194

MacQueen S (2005) The special needs of children receiving intravenous therapy. Nursing Times 101(8):59,61–62,64

Medical Devices Agency (1996) Hazard notice MDA:HN 9604. Department of Health, London

Medical Devices Agency (2003) Infusion systems device bulletin. DB 9503. Medical Devices Agency, London

Medicines and Healthcare products Regulatory Agency (2007) Online. Available: http://www.mhra.gov.uk

Mitchel SJ, Gray J, Morgan ME, Hocking MD, Durhing GM (1996) Nosocomial infection with *Rhizopus microsporus* in preterm infants: association with wooden tongue depressors. Lancet 348(9025):441–443

National Institute for Clinical Excellence (2003) Infection control prevention of healthcare-associated infections in primary and community care (clinical guidelines 2). NICE, London

Nicol M (1999) Safe administration and management of peripheral intravenous therapy. In Dougherty L, Lamb J (eds) Intravenous therapy in nursing practice. Churchill Livingstone, Edinburgh, p 141–161

Oldman P (1991) A sticky situation: a microbiological study of adhesive tape used to secure IV cannulae. Professional Nurse Feb:265–269

Panadero A, Iohom G, Taj J, Mackay N, Shorten G (2002) A dedicated intravenous cannula for postoperative use: effect on incidence and severity of phlebitis. Anaesthesia 57(9):921–925

Perdue MB (2001) Intravenous complications. In Hankin J et al (eds) Infusion therapy in clinical practice, 2nd edn. Saunders, Philadelphia, p 418–445

Perucca R (2001) Types of infusion therapy equipment. In Hankin J et al (eds) Infusion therapy in clinical practice. Saunders, Philadelphia

Royal College of Nursing (2005a) Good practice in infection control. RCN, London, p 111

Royal College of Nursing (2005b) Standards for infusion therapy. RCN, London

Stanley A (2002) Managing complications of chemotherapy administration. In Allwood M et al (eds) The cytotoxic handbook, 4th edn. Radcliffe Medical Press, Oxford, p 119–194

Stenzel JP, Green TP, Fuhrman BP, Carlson PE, Marchessault RP (1989) Percutaneous central venous catheterization in a pediatric intensive care unit: a survival analysis of complications. Critical Care Medicine 17:984–988

Wilkins CE, Emmerson AJ (2004) Extravasation injuries on regional neonatal units. Archives of Disease in Childhood: Fetal and Neonatal Edition 89(3):274–275

25 Safe administration of blood and blood products

Hermione Montgomery • Jay Kumar

Indications for blood transfusions for infants, children and young people are the clinical need (Desmet & Lacroix 2004, McIntosh 2006, Nohum et al 2002). Blood transfusion could be indicated for a number of reasons, including anaemia, acute haemorrhage, haematological disease, and acute and chronic conditions, as well as during and following surgery.

All blood products will be discussed under one heading and include red cells, cryoprecipitate, platelets, fresh frozen plasma (FFP) and any other blood product, such as albumin, specifically required for transfusion. Infants and children are rarely given whole blood.

Errors in the blood transfusion process can occur at any stage from sampling to the actual administration of blood. The Serious Hazards of Transfusion (SHOT) Committee was established as a voluntary anonymised system in order to collate information relating to adverse reactions, provide feedback about near misses and produce recommendations for good evidence-based practice (Provan 1999). Serious Adverse Blood Reactions and Events (SABRE) is a more recent reporting system, which allows electronic submission of reports of serious adverse reactions and events to the Medicines and Healthcare products Regulatory Agency. The Medicines and Healthcare products Regulatory Agency is a government agency responsible for ensuring that medicines and medical devices are appropriately used or operated in a safe manner.

Consent to the receipt of a blood product should be carried out, as 'Patients have a fundamental legal and ethical right to determine what happens to their own bodies ' (Department of Health 2001). The individual trust policy and appropriate information relating to the indications, benefits, risks and expected outcomes of transfusion should be given to the parents or carers and, when appropriate, to the child. There must be an opportunity to discuss and agree to the proposed treatment and, when possible, the young person should be involved in this process (Department of Health 2003). Gaining consent is not solely about acquiring a signature on a consent form, as there is no legal requirement to seek written consent for transfusion. However, it is essential that you document and record the patient's verbal consent in the patient's health records. It must be noted that consent issues should not delay necessary transfusions in an emergency (Scottish National Blood Transfusion Service 2006). If the child or parents are Jehovah's Witnesses, alternative treatments to the receipt of a blood product should be considered and the local policy needs to be followed.

As healthcare professionals we have a duty to undertake safe practice, and therefore this chapter shall be addressing:

- the checking procedure to prevent incompatibility
- care and management of the transfusion
- other considerations
- future developments in preventing incompatibilities.

ALERT
All personnel who prescribe, collect and administer blood products must have the appropriate training as per local policy.

Checking procedure to prevent incompatibility

ABO incompatibility can lead to acute haemolysis, which may be life threatening. Thorough patient identification, sample labelling, laboratory testing, collection and the administration of blood products can help to minimise this risk.

Compatibility errors can occur when blood is taken for sampling, cross-matching in the laboratory, collection of the unit of blood, safe receipt into the ward or department and the bedside checking of the unit.

Blood sampling and cross-matching

There are a number of sites from which a sample can be taken, and the specific local policy must be adhered to. Avoid taking blood from a site above an existing intravenous cannula, as contamination could occur (West Midlands Regional Transfusion Committee 2005).

The following guidelines reduce the risk of error:

- Ensure that you have the right patient by checking the wristband (Nursing and Midwifery Council 2004, Royal College of Nursing 2005) and see that the surname, first name, date of birth and hospital registration number match the details on the cross-match request form. It is good practice to ensure that you have the correct patient by confirming with the patient, the family or the patient's named nurse (Birmingham Children's Hospital NHS Trust 2003).
- The sample must be taken before completing the details on the cross-matching sample bottle.
- The details on the sample bottle label must be handwritten legibly by the person taking the blood at the patient's

bedside. *Preprinted labels must never be used.* In order to ensure safety, specimens that are incorrectly labelled are not accepted by blood banks and a fresh sample and a new request form are requested.

- Blood should be taken from only one patient at any one time to avoid mixing up blood samples from patients bled at the same time.
- A cross-match request form must be sent with each sample (West Midlands Regional Transfusion Committee 2005). If the sample is not cross-matched by the person requesting the blood then the person taking the blood must also sign the request form in order to verify the sample and the patient (Birmingham Children's Hospital NHS Trust 2003).
- Ensure that the sample is delivered safely according to local policy.
- Document in the patient's health record that a blood sample has been sent for cross-match, giving the time, date, location of the site and amount of blood sent (Nursing and Midwifery Council 2005).

Preparation of blood

The National Blood Service tests donated blood for human immunodeficiency virus, hepatitis B and C, human T-cell leukaemia virus and syphilis (McIntosh 2006). Prior to blood being distributed to the various healthcare settings it is leucodepleted, which is the removal of white cells in order to prevent variant Creutzfeldt–Jakob disease (West Midlands Regional Transfusion Committee 2005).

In some clinical situations gamma-irradiated blood is used in order to prevent graft-versus-host disease. This would apply to children with Hodgkin's disease, those receiving purine analogue drugs (Boulton 2004). Please refer to your local guidelines for further clinical indications. Irradiated product information cards are supplied to all recipients of irradiated blood products giving details of this procedure.

Blood will be tested for cytomegalovirus, as some patients, such as those who are immunocompromised or those having stem cell transplants, and children below the age of 1 year, must receive cytomegalovirus-negative blood products (Desmet & Lacroix 2004).

Compatibility in the blood bank

Serological tests are performed on donated blood to identify the ABO blood group and rhesus group. Incompatibility can lead to acute intravascular haemolysis, therefore when blood is requested the blood bank tests the patient's blood to determine his or her blood group and rhesus factor. The risk of error at this stage is significant, so careful checking is essential (Stainsby et al 2005b).

As you can see from Table 25.1, children whose blood group is O (universal donor) can be transfused with blood from group O only. They can, however, be given A or O platelets and O, A, B or AB FFP. Those with A blood group can be given A or O red blood cells and platelets and A or AB FFP. Those whose blood group is B can be infused with B or O red blood cells and B, O or A platelets but only B or AB FFP. Children with blood group AB (universal recipient) can be given AB, A, B or O red blood cells and AB or A platelets or FFP.

To explain high titre (HT), when group O blood and platelets are given to a patient of another group it should not have HTs of anti-A or -B, otherwise there may be a reaction between the plasma portion of the product and the patient's own red cells.

Table 25.1. Choice of ABO group for blood products for administration to children

Patient's ABO	Red cells	Platelets	FFP
O			
First choice	0	0	0
Second choice	–	A	A or B or AB
A			
First choice	A	A	A
Second choice	0 (HT–)	0 (HT–)	AB
B			
First choice	B	B	B
Second choice	0 (HT–)	0 (HT–) or A	AB
AB			
First choice	AB	AB	AB
Second choice	A or B	A	A
Third choice	0 (HT–)	–	–

(From Boulton F, Transfusion Guidelines for Neonates and Older Children. British Journal of Haematology, 124, 433–453, with permission of Blackwells Publishers.)

Collection of blood from the blood bank

All staff (regardless of experience or grade) who collect blood or blood products must have appropriate training as per their local policy (Provan 1999) and be authorised to undertake this procedure in order to minimise the risk of incompatibility through the error of removing the incorrect blood:

- Check that the blood or blood products have been prescribed before collection takes place.
- The collection of blood should be timed to within 10 min of it being required unless it is to be stored in a satellite fridge such as in intensive care, theatres or the accident and emergency department.

- A request form with the patient's name, hospital number, date of birth and blood products required (West Midlands Regional Transfusion Committee 2005) must be completed by the ward or department nurse and given to the person collecting the blood (an example of a blood-collecting request form is shown in Fig. 25.1). This information must be taken from the patient's hospital record. If subsequent units of blood or blood products are required the top copy of the blood transfusion report form may be sufficient.
- Check to see which fridge and drawer or shelf the blood is located in; every blood bank will have its individual method.
- After removal of the requested labelled product (take out in order as listed by the blood bank) locate the blood transfusion report form (Fig. 25.2), which will be found on the first unit of blood. It is usual to collect only one unit of blood per time; however, in an emergency follow the local policy.
- The following checks must be made to identify the correct unit (Murphy et al 1999).
    - Patient details are identical on the label on the blood or blood product, blood transfusion report form (blood bank–generated compatibility report) and ward- or department-generated request form (Fig. 25.3).
    - Check the expiry date on the blood or blood product (expires at midnight on identified date).
    - Check the barcode number (donor number or batch number for human albumin and anti-D) on the blood bag or product label against the unit number on the blood transfusion report form.

The birmingham Children's Hospital Trust
Blood Transfusion Department
TO THE BLOOD BANK
Please supply compatible blood for the following patient:

Surname (BLOCK CAPITALS) ______________________

Christian names ______________________
____

Registration number ______________________

Date of Birth ______________________

Ward/Theatre ______________________

Signed ______________________

Blood cannot be issued except on presentation of this form with ALL particulars completed.

BCH 171

Fig. 25.1 • Request for supply of blood. This form should be filled in at the ward prior to collection of the blood. The patient details are taken from the patient's notes and are a substitute for the patient's note at the point of blood issue. (From West Midlands Regional Transfusion Commitee (2005). With permission.)

Contact the blood bank staff immediately if any discrepancies are found as a result of these checks.

- If all the checks are correct, record the removal of the blood or blood products on the appropriate laboratory documentation, confirming and recording the following:
    - confirm that the patient's details are correct, including the location of the patient
    - confirm the barcode (donor number or batch number)
    - record the name and signature of the person collecting the blood or blood products
    - record the date and time of collection.

If blood is required in an extreme emergency and the patient has not been able to be cross-matched, O rhesus D negative blood can be given.

Blood and blood products must be stored only in a blood fridge or freezer and **never in a ward fridge or freezer**. If platelets are being collected for a satellite area the bag must be placed on the platelet agitator until required.

If the transfusion is delayed, blood and platelets must be returned to the blood bank fridge if less than 30 min have lapsed (follow local policy). The time returned must be noted and the staff in the blood bank informed. Defrosted FFP must never be returned to the freezer.

Table 25.2 summarises storage conditions for blood components.

Transporting the blood or blood products

If different blood products are being transported at the same time, care must be taken to prevent them touching each other. Contact with frozen or partially thawed bags of FFP or cryoprecipitate can damage blood cells or platelets, which would be harmful to the patient. Also avoid putting blood and platelets in the same container (West Midlands Regional Transfusion Committee 2005).

Platelets should be slightly agitated but not shaken when transporting them, to keep the platelets from clumping together.

Safe receipt of blood into the department

If the blood has not been collected by the person administering the product a qualified member of staff, usually the receiving nurse, must check that the correct blood or component has been delivered (Murphy et al 1999). The time between removing the unit from the blood fridge and actual administration to the patient should not exceed 30 min (West Midlands Regional Transfusion Committee 2005).

ALERT
Transfusion must be commenced within 30 min after blood is taken out of the fridge.

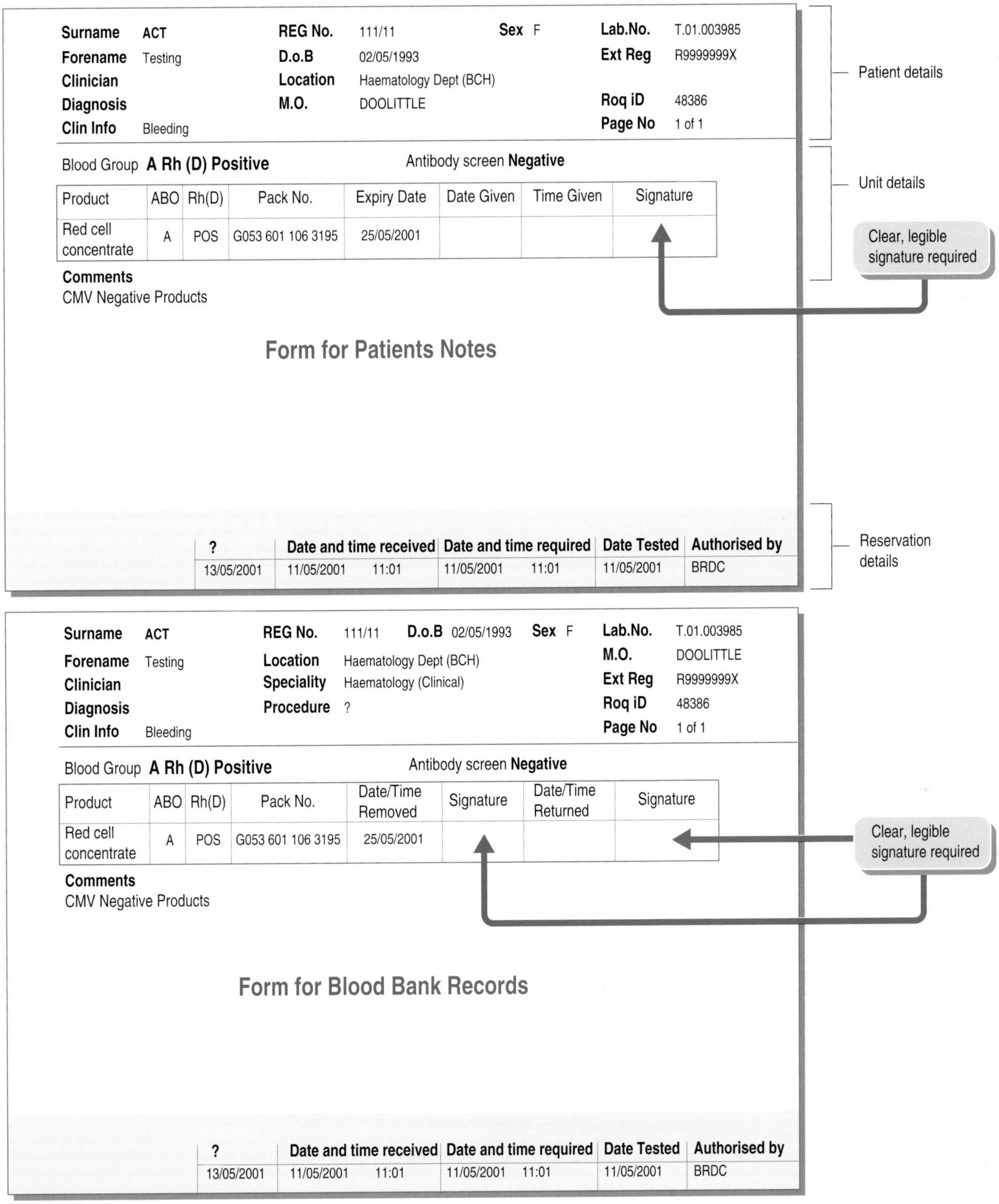

Surname ACT | REG No. 111/11 | Sex F | Lab.No. T.01.003985
Forename Testing | D.o.B 02/05/1993 | Ext Reg R9999999X
Clinician | Location Haematology Dept (BCH)
Diagnosis | M.O. DOOLITTLE | Roq iD 48386
Clin Info Bleeding | Page No 1 of 1

Blood Group **A Rh (D) Positive** Antibody screen **Negative**

Product	ABO	Rh(D)	Pack No.	Expiry Date	Date Given	Time Given	Signature
Red cell concentrate	A	POS	G053 601 106 3195	25/05/2001			

Comments
CMV Negative Products

Form for Patients Notes

?	Date and time received	Date and time required	Date Tested	Authorised by
13/05/2001	11/05/2001 11:01	11/05/2001 11:01	11/05/2001	BRDC

Surname ACT | REG No. 111/11 | D.o.B 02/05/1993 | Sex F | Lab.No. T.01.003985
Forename Testing | Location Haematology Dept (BCH) | M.O. DOOLITTLE
Clinician | Speciality Haematology (Clinical) | Ext Reg R9999999X
Diagnosis | Procedure ? | Roq iD 48386
Clin Info Bleeding | Page No 1 of 1

Blood Group **A Rh (D) Positive** Antibody screen **Negative**

Product	ABO	Rh(D)	Pack No.	Date/Time Removed	Signature	Date/Time Returned	Signature
Red cell concentrate	A	POS	G053 601 106 3195	25/05/2001			

Comments
CMV Negative Products

Form for Blood Bank Records

?	Date and time received	Date and time required	Date Tested	Authorised by
13/05/2001	11/05/2001 11:01	11/05/2001 11:01	11/05/2001	BRDC

Blood Bank Report Forms
It is vital to check the details of the report match those details on the unit of blood.
The pack number on the form should be checked against the bag number on the unit,
NOT the one on the Blood Bank Label (as this is a copy of the form)

Fig. 25.2 • Blood bank report forms. It is vital to check that the details of the report match those details on the unit of blood. The pack number on the form should be checked against the bag number on the unit, NOT the one on the blood bank label (as this is a copy of the form). Note: the patient's name has been fabricated.

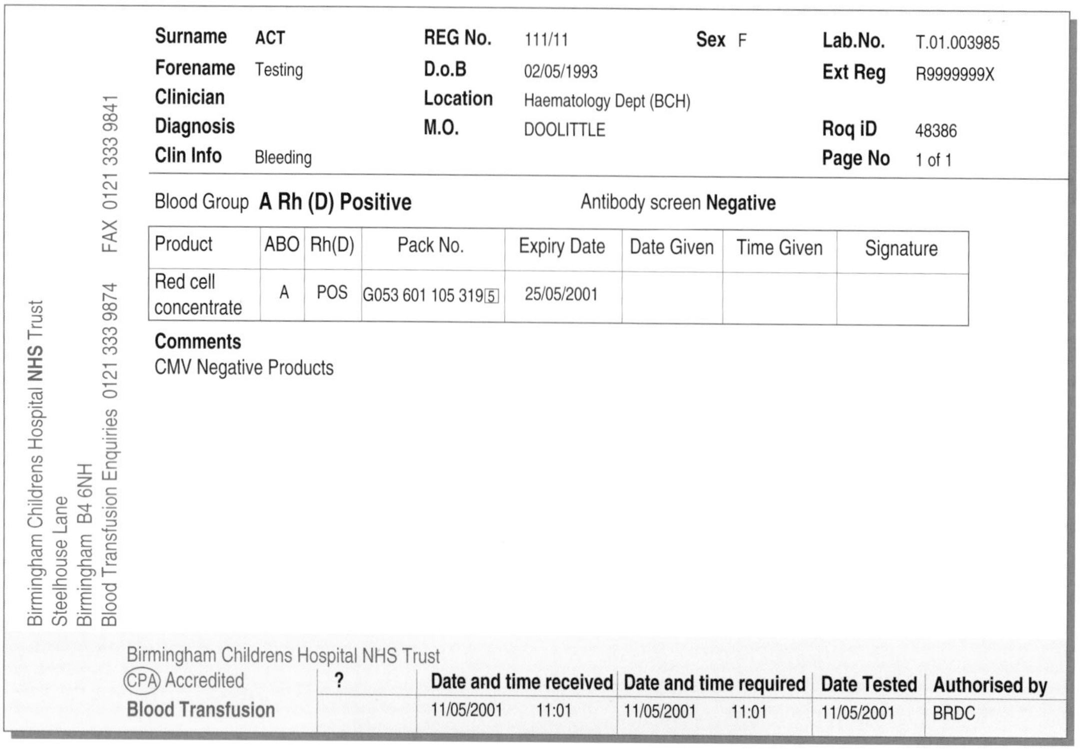

Birmingham Childrens Hospital NHS Trust
Steelhouse Lane
Birmingham B4 6NH
Blood Transfusion Enquiries 0121 333 9874 FAX 0121 333 9841

Surname	ACT	**REG No.**	111/11 **Sex** F	**Lab.No.**	T.01.003985
Forename	Testing	**D.o.B**	02/05/1993	**Ext Reg**	R9999999X
Clinician		**Location**	Haematology Dept (BCH)		
Diagnosis		**M.O.**	DOOLITTLE	**Roq iD**	48386
Clin Info	Bleeding			**Page No**	1 of 1

Blood Group **A Rh (D) Positive** Antibody screen **Negative**

Product	ABO	Rh(D)	Pack No.	Expiry Date	Date Given	Time Given	Signature
Red cell concentrate	A	POS	G053 601 105 319 5	25/05/2001			

Comments
CMV Negative Products

Birmingham Childrens Hospital NHS Trust
CPA Accredited
Blood Transfusion

?	Date and time received	Date and time required	Date Tested	Authorised by
	11/05/2001 11:01	11/05/2001 11:01	11/05/2001	BRDC

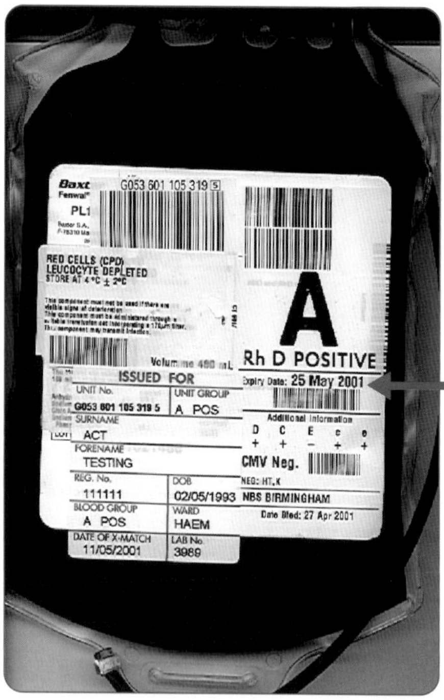

Check expiry date

Check unit details from the report form against the bag unit number, **not** against laboratory sticker. Check the expiry date of the unit

Fig. 25.3 • Blood bank form checked against the unit of blood. Check the unit details from the report form against the bag unit number, NOT against the laboratory sticker. Check the expiry date of the unit. (From West Midlands Regional Transfusion Commitee (2005), with permission.) Note: patient's name has been fabricated.

Table 25.2. Summary of storage conditions for blood components

Product	Storage temperature (°C)	Points to note
All red cells	2–6	Temperature-controlled blood bank fridges ONLY
Platelets	20–24	On agitator
FFP	−30	Thawed at 37°C
Cryoprecipitate	−30	Thawed at 37°C

Checking of blood at the point of administration (bedside check)

ALERT
This is the last opportunity for ensuring that this is the correct unit of blood or blood products for the correct patient: check the patient's full name, date of birth and hospital number.

This is the last opportunity to ensure that the correct unit of blood is administered to the correct patient (West Midlands Regional Transfusion Committee 2005, Williamson et al 1999). Staff responsible for the checking and administration of blood must be qualified and trained for this purpose.

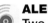

ALERT
Two qualified and trained staff must check the blood product independently.

For each unit administered two people must independently carry out the following checks:

- The unit of blood is correctly prescribed, including the medical officer's signature.
- The patient's identity details match the unit of blood, the blood transfusion compatibility form, the patient's identification wristband and the intravenous prescription chart for the following details (Wallis 2005):
  - First name
  - Surname
  - Date of birth
  - Hospital registration number.

  Also, the National Blood Service barcode number must match the unit number on the blood transfusion report form.
- The expiry date on the unit.
- The unit to be transfused complies with any special instructions, such as irradiated blood, and this must be clearly stated on the intravenous fluid prescription chart.
- The physical state of the blood must be examined for discolouration, for evidence of haemolysis (clumping) and for clots or air in the bag.
- Leaks must also be excluded by applying firm pressure to the bag.

Although the checks appear to be repetitive it is the last chance to check that the correct unit is administered to the correct patient, thereby reducing the risk of error. Murphy et al (1999) suggest five pieces of evidence in the process of ensuring the final check at the point of administration. These are as follows:

1. The National Blood Service label matches all appropriate details
2. The hospital blood bank compatibility label has the correct details
3. The blood bank compatibility form confirms all the correct details
4. The patient's health record matches the details on the blood product to be administered
5. The blood prescription chart must be correctly written.

Transfusion times

Platelets must be transfused as soon as possible on receipt to the department and within 1 h. FFP must be administered as soon as it is defrosted in order for the patient to have the full benefit of the platelets and coagulation factors (Murphy et al 1999).

Blood transfusion should be completed within 4 h after being collected from the blood bank (Royal College of Nursing 2005). FFP and platelets are usually given over 30–60 min.

Procedures Box 25.1 Checking procedure to prevent incompatibility

1

Blood sampling and cross-matching

Actions
Identify the patient by checking the wristband before taking the blood.

ALERT
Accurate wristbands must be maintained on patients who cannot confirm their own identity.

Check that the child or young person and/or parent have given permission for the transfusion.

Ensure that the patient's details correspond with the patient's health records and request form.

Reason *Ensures that the blood has been taken from the correct patient and that he or she and/or the parents have consented.*

Actions
Bleed only one patient at a time and label at the bedside.

Write out the sample label by hand at the patient's bedside.

Procedures Box 25.1 Checking procedure to prevent incompatibility—cont'd

ALERT
Preprinted labels must NEVER be used.

Ensure that the sample is sent according to local policy.

Reason *Prevents errors from occurring.*

2

Preparation of blood

Action
The National Blood Transfusion Service tests donated blood for ABO compatibility, human immunodeficiency virus, hepatitis B and C, human T-cell leukaemia virus, syphilis and cytomegalovirus.

3

Compatibility in the blood bank

Action
Serological tests are performed on donated blood to identify the ABO and rhesus group.

Reasons *Checks for abnormalities and ensures the safe use of blood. Reduces the risk of incompatibility, which can lead to acute intravascular haemolysis.*

4

Collection of blood from the blood bank

Action
All personnel who collect blood must have blood training as per local policy.

Reason *Ensures that staff have the knowledge and skills to safely collect blood from the blood bank.*

Action
Ensure that the blood collection form has been completed.

ALERT
Check that the blood has been prescribed prior to collection.

Reason *Checks that the correct unit of blood is collected from the blood bank.*

Action
Check that the patient's identity details all match on the collection, blood label and request forms.

Reason *Checks that the correct blood is collected for the correct patient.*

Action
Document the removal of the blood from the blood fridge.

Reason *Creates an audit trail of blood removed from the blood bank.*

Action
Collect only one unit of blood at a time unless there are satellite fridge facilities to store the remaining units.

5

Transporting the blood

Actions
If you are collecting more than one type of blood product ensure that they have no contact with each other.

ALERT
Blood products when transported must not come into contact with each other.

Platelets should be slightly agitated but not shaken when transporting.

Reason *Prevents destruction of blood cells and wastage.*

6

Safe receipt of blood into the department

Actions
If the blood has not been collected by the person administering it a qualified member of staff must check that the correct blood has been delivered.

The blood must be transfused within 30 min or returned to the blood fridge.

ALERT
Blood transfusion must be commenced within 30 min of removal from the blood fridge.

Reasons *Contact with partially thawed bags of FFP or cryoprecipitate can damage blood cells or platelets, which would be harmful to the patient.*
Prevents the platelets from clumping together.

7

Checking of blood at the point of administration

ALERT
This is the last opportunity for ensuring that this is the correct unit of blood or blood products for the correct patient: check the patient's full name, date of birth and hospital number.

Action

ALERT
Two qualified and trained staff must check the blood product independently.

For each unit to be administered two trained staff must independently check:

- identity details
- the prescription sheet
- the National Blood Transfusion Service barcode, which must match the details on the blood request form and the blood label
- compatibility
- the expiry date of the unit of blood
- special instructions
- the blood for discolouration, haemolysis (clumping) and evidence of air or clots in the bag
- for leaks, by applying firm pressure to the bag.

Reasons *Ensures that the blood is correct for the patient.*
Prevents destruction of blood cells and wastage.
Checks that the correct unit of blood is administered to the correct patient, therefore reducing the risk of error.

Procedures Box 25.1 Checking procedure to prevent incompatibility—cont'd

8

Transfusion times

Actions

Platelets must be transfused as soon as possible and within 1 h.

FFP must be administered as soon as defrosted.

Platelets and FFP must be given over 30–60 min.

Reason *Ensures that patients receive the full benefit of the blood product.*

Care and management of the transfusion

Prior to giving blood

- Equipment check: ensure that you can easily access functioning oxygen and suction and be within reach of the call bell and the resuscitation trolley in case of incompatibility, allergic reaction or haemolysis occurring during the administration of the transfusion and the patient requiring emergency intervention.
- Spillage kit: this should be within the department in case blood is accidentally spilt when setting up the transfusion. You should be familiar with your local health and safety and infection control policies.
- Where nursed: the patient should be positioned in the department where she or he can easily be observed during the transfusion in case of a reaction (McIntosh 2006).
- The equipment required is as follows:
  - A blood administration set that has a 170- to 200-micron screen filter must be used (Boulton 2004). Do not use a separate filter unless specified by the blood bank. Often the screen filter is within the burette of the giving set. If platelets are transfused a dedicated platelet-giving set can be used if available, or use a new blood administration set if transfusing platelets after any other blood products. The British Committee for Standards recommends that the blood-giving set be changed after administering blood continuously for more than 12 h (Murphy et al 1999, Royal College of Nursing 2005). If intravenous fluids are required following completion of the transfusion the giving set must be changed (McIntosh 2006, Murphy et al 1999, West Midlands Regional Transfusion Committee 2005).
  - Infusion pumps must have the manufacturer specifications confirmation that they can be used for the administration of blood products.
  - Blood warmers are not routinely used except if clinically indicated, such as if a large transfusion is to be administered in a short duration, during exchange transfusions in infants, if specified by the blood bank for patients who have cold agglutinins or for patients at risk of hypothermia (McIntosh 2006, Murphy et al 1999, West Midlands Regional Transfusion Committee 2005). Dedicated blood warmers must only be used for this purpose, as damage can be caused to the red blood cells, which may result in severe transfusion reactions if the temperature is not controlled.

During transfusion

Information and education of the patient

- Although the child and parents or carers would have been given information when they consented to the transfusion, they may have additional questions or concerns that would now need addressing.
- Explain the transfusion procedure to the child and parents or carers and ask them to inform a nurse if any symptoms are experienced (as detailed under *Observations* below) such as feeling hot, feeling shivery, shortness of breath, pain in the extremities, being itchy, having a rash or having a change in the colour of the urine.

Connecting blood

- As previously discussed the final identity and compatibility check will be carried out at the bedside prior to commencing the transfusion.
- Prior to connecting the blood-giving set primed with blood, flush the patient's peripheral or indwelling intravenous cannula to check that it is patent. This should be done as per local policy.
- Reinspect the appearance of blood before starting the infusion (Stainsby et al 2005a) for any irregularity, which may be indicative of infected blood.

Observations

- Prior to commencing the transfusion a set of baseline observations of temperature, pulse, respiration and blood pressure are taken. These are repeated 15 min into the transfusion and then 15 min post transfusion if only one unit of blood or blood product is being administered. These observations are performed 15 min after the commencement of each further unit (Royal College of Nursing 2005). However, do follow local policy. If an allergic reaction or haemolysis occurs it is usually within 15 min of commencement of a transfusion. Continue to visually monitor the child regularly (Murphy et al 1999), and if his or her condition is unstable more frequent observations will be necessary.
- Observe hourly for signs of extravasation if blood is being administered through a peripheral cannula.

Adverse reactions

Administration of blood or blood products may result in adverse reactions, which would be detected through observation (Boxes 25.1–25.6). These reactions can manifest during or

Box 25.1. Acute haemolytic reaction

This is due to an incompatibility reaction that is a result of an immune response between antibodies in the recipient's blood and antigens on the donor's red cells.

Signs and symptoms

- Severe lumbar pain
- Haemoglobinuria and haemoglobinaemia
- Agitation and feeling fearful
- Hyperkalaemia and cardiac arrhythmias
- Chills
- Fever
- Rigor
- Pain at the intravenous site
- Dyspnoea
- Shock
- Haematuria
- Renal failure

Management

- Stop the transfusion
- Medical emergency: ABC resuscitation
- Inform medical staff
- Retain a sample of the donor blood and the child's blood

Box 25.2. Severe reaction

Increased capillary permeability leads to constriction of the smooth muscle, resulting in progressive shock and respiratory alkalosis. The progressive stage can lead to irreversible shock caused by renal tubules being blocked, resulting in precipitation (clumping) of haemoglobin, no urine output and hyperkalaemia. Mechanisms begin to result in multiorgan failure and a rise in levels of waste products. This leads to the irreversible shock.

Signs and symptoms

- Facial flushing
- Pyrexia
- Bradycardia
- Bronchospasm
- Respiratory arrest
- Hyperventilation
- Hypotension

Management

- Stop the transfusion
- Medical emergency: ABC resuscitation
- Monitor vital signs
- Blood gases
- Drug administration: antihistamines, hydrocortisone, bronchodilators, adrenaline (epinephrine)
- Dialysis

Box 25.3. Allergic response

This may have a slow onset and get progressively worse if left untreated. It is less severe and local than severe reaction but may occur at any time during the transfusion. It is an immune response whereby there is recognition that the blood is foreign. Cells form clumps that attach to and bind cells, which then send off chemicals to attract mast cells and basophils into the area. Chemotaxis causes mast cells to rupture and spill out histamine, while basophils activate the release of substances to destroy the allergen.

Signs and symptoms

- Local blood vessels dilate: pruritus and urticaria
- Capillaries more permeable: local swelling or hives
- No fever or mild temperature rise ($<1.5°C$ above baseline)

Management

- Deal with symptoms as they arise
- Stop the transfusion temporarily
- Drug administration: antihistamine and paracetamol if needed
- Continue the transfusion if there is no progression of symptoms

Box 25.4. Anaphylaxis

This is rare and the onset is sudden, early in the transfusion. Immunoglobulin A and immunoglobulin E involvement results in widespread histamine release, leading to shock.

Signs and symptoms

- Dyspnoea
- Pain
- Nausea
- Hypotension
- Bronchospasm
- Oedema
- Erythema
- Urticaria

Management

- Stop the transfusion immediately
- Medical emergency: ABC resuscitation
- Drug administration: antihistamine, hydrocortisone, paracetamol, bronchodilators, prepare adrenaline (epinephrine)
- Consider future care: pretransfusion loading dose of antihistamine, select donors by specific antigens and washed red cells

Box 25.5. Bacterial contamination

This can manifest during or post transfusion. It is usually from an infected donor and it requires only a few millilitres of blood to have an impact. Endotoxins and exotoxins from the bacteria trigger a response that activates the immune response.

Signs and symptoms

- Septic shock
- Fever
- Hypotension
- Tachycardia
- Rigors

Management

- Careful monitoring
- Blood culture
- Appropriate antibiotic therapy
- Drug administration: antihistamine, hydrocortisone and bronchodilators

Box 25.6. The investigation of transfusion reaction

All transfusion reactions will be investigated as follows:

- Recheck the labelling of the blood unit against the details on the blood report form and against the patient's identification details.
- A venous blood sample from a vein away from the transfusion site should be obtained and sent for the following investigations:
  - Full blood count
  - Coagulation screen
  - Antibody investigation
  - Urea and electrolytes
  - Blood culture.
- In discussion with the blood bank return the unit of blood and all previously transfused units.
- Send the first sample of urine for urobilinogen estimation.

Reporting and documentation of adverse reactions

- Inform the blood bank
- Complete the local clinical incident form
- Ensure that the patient's family or carer are aware of the reaction
- Complete and send off the reporting form to SHOT and SABRE

post transfusion. The practitioner needs to be aware of the signs and symptoms and the appropriate treatment (Fig. 25.4).

Documentation during a transfusion

- Record the time the blood transfusion commences on the fluid balance chart.
- Make an entry in the patient's health records that the transfusion has commenced and what product is being given.
- Record baseline and other observations on the appropriate observation chart, ensuring that either a new chart is used or that it is clear that these observations are being recorded during the transfusion. Ensure that the commencement and completion of each transfusion is recorded clearly on the observation chart (Murphy et al 1999) so that if there is a reaction this can be easily seen.
- If the child has any reaction to the blood or blood products this must be recorded in the health records with the action taken.

Completion of transfusion

Disposal of blood

- Follow local policy; however, it is customary to keep the blood or product bag in either a clinical waste bag (yellow) or in another receptacle for 24 h before disposing of it.

Documentation

- Record the amount transfused on the fluid balance chart and on the intravenous prescription chart.
- Document that the transfusion has been completed with no apparent side effect (or with a reaction as appropriate) in the patient's health records.

Observations

- As stated earlier the observation of temperature, pulse, respiratory rate and blood pressure will be recorded 15 min after completion of the transfusion.

Other considerations

Reporting near misses

- As reported by the Department of Health (2002) it is a requirement that near misses relating to transfusion of blood and blood products must be reported.
- SHOT and SABRE compile data of errors and adverse events, undertake surveys and make recommendations to make transfusions safer.

Training and education

- Staff members who undertake venepuncture for blood sampling should be trained and be deemed to be competent.
- Training in the collection, transportation, administration and storage of blood or blood products in satellite blood bank fridges must be provided to staff (Stainsby et al 2005a).
- Staff should be trained to use the storage equipment in the satellite blood bank areas.

Adverse reactions

↓

Acute	Delayed
Acute haemolytic reaction	Graft verses host disease
Allergy and anaphylaxis	Delayed haemolysis
Febrile non-haemolytic	Infection (including viral)
Transfusion related acute lung injury (TRALI)	Iron overload
Circulatory overload	Alloimunisation
Hypothermia	Biochemical changes in stored blood
Anticoagulant reactions	Post transfusion purpura
Potassium changes	
Sepsis	

↓

PHYSIOLOGICAL CHANGES involving the Complement Cascade during a reaction:

- A sequential series of reactions of plasma proteins – C1 to C9
- Activates the classical pathway which begins at C1
- Each stage results in a variety of cell destruction process – chemotaxis, phagacytosis and cytolysis
- Collectively complement activation is an inflammatory response
- On completion of the cascade total cell lysis occurs

↓

Acute Transfusion reactions: Severe or Non-severe?

Will be determined by an assessment of:

- If temperature < or > 1.5 degree centigrade
- If there is presence or absence of urticaria
- The speed and severity of the progression of symptoms

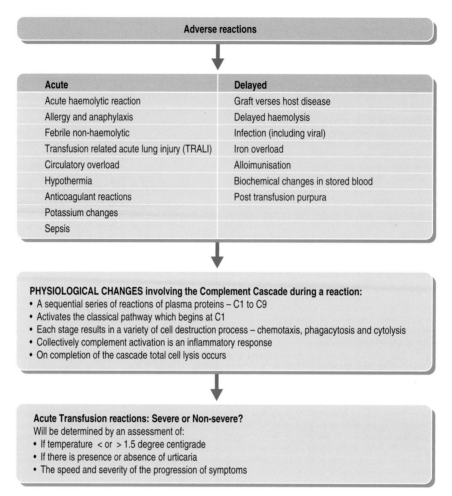

Fig. 25.4 • Adverse reactions flow chart.

Procedures Box 25.2 Care and management of the transfusion

1 Prior to administration

Action
Equipment check: ensure that the call bell, oxygen, suction and resuscitation trolley are accessible and functioning.

Reason *Ensures that emergency equipment is accessible and functioning.*

Action
Spillage kit: ensure that one is available.

Reason *Minimises infection risk.*

Action
The child needs to be nursed in an easily observed and accessible locality.

Reason *Makes it easy to observe the child.*

Action
Ensure that the equipment used, such as giving set, filter, infusion pump and blood warmer (if indicated), is specific for the use of blood products.

Reason *Ensures that the equipment is appropriate for the administration of blood.*

2 During transfusion

Action
Explain the blood transfusion procedure to the child and parent, ensuring that they know what side effects, if any, to look out for.

Reason *Ensures that the child has sufficient information.*

Action
Prime the giving set with blood, check the patency of the cannula and connect the blood.

Reason *Ensures that the cannula is patent.*

Action
Reinspect the blood prior to starting the infusion.

Reason *Irregularity can be an indication of infected blood.*

Action
Observations to be carried out during blood administration:

- Prior to commencing the blood transfusion, baseline observations of temperature, pulse, respiration and blood pressure should be recorded
- These should be repeated every 15 min after commencement of the transfusion

Procedures Box 25.2 Care and management of the transfusion—cont'd

- These observations should be repeated for subsequent units of blood administered
- Hourly observation for signs of extravasation.

Reasons *The child's normal observations need to be compared with the observations performed during the transfusion in order to detect any reaction or incompatibility.*
Detects early signs of extravasation injury.

Action
Administration may result in adverse reactions that may be detected through meticulous observations; these reactions can manifest during or post transfusion, and the practitioner needs to be aware of the signs and symptoms and the appropriate treatment.

Reason *Ensures patient safety during the administration of blood.*

Action
Document the following during the transfusion:

- Time and date of commencement of the transfusion on the fluid balance chart and in the patient's health records
- Baseline and recurrent observations
- Any reactions that manifest themselves.

Reason *It is best safe practice to maintain up-to-date records, which will also act as an audit trail.*

3

Completion of transfusion

Action
Dispose of the blood bag and giving set as per local policy; it is usual to retain these for 24 h.

Reasons *Maintains safety.*
If a post-transfusion reaction occurs the blood bag and giving set will be required by the blood bank in order to ascertain the cause.

Action
Documentation post transfusion should include the recording of the volume of blood administered and the condition of the child or young person.

Reason *Ensures that the patient's health records are up to date.*

Action
Observations of temperature, pulse, respiration and blood pressure must be recorded 15 min post transfusion.

Reason *Detects any reaction or incompatibility post transfusion.*

Procedures Box 25.3 Other considerations

1

Reporting near misses

Action
Report near misses; this is a requirement of the Department of Health.

Reason *SHOT and SABRE compile data of errors and adverse events in order to make recommendations to make transfusions safer.*

2

Training and education

Action
Staff who undertake venepuncture for blood sampling should be trained.

Training in the collection, transportation, administration and storage of blood must be provided to staff.

Reasons *Ensures that they are competent for the role.*
Minimises the risk of errors occurring, thereby safeguarding the patient.

Future developments in preventing incompatibilities

In the SHOT annual report in 2004 (Stainsby et al 2005a,b) it was suggested that the following initiatives could be evaluated and rolled out nationally: barcode technology, whereby the wristband, blood forms and blood bag labels are all barcoded; specific wristbands for patients who are being transfused; patients being given blood or blood products regularly could have photograph identification; and standardisation of training for those people who handle blood.

Both the Department of Health (2002) and SHOT (Stainsby et al 2005a) recommend that each hospital should employ a specialist transfusion practitioner. The role would include implementing staff training, developing local transfusion guidelines and reporting systems for blood ordering, administration and prescribing (including monitoring of wastage and error rates).

Now test your knowledge

- O (universal donor) patients can be transfused with blood from which group? Which groups can they receive platelets and FFP from? Blood group A patients can be given red blood cells, platelets and FFP from which groups? Blood group B patients can be infused with which red blood cells and which platelets and FFP? Children with blood group AB (universal recipient) can be given red blood cells, platelets and FFP from which donors?
- What checks must be carried out before commencing a blood transfusion?
- How would you explain to a 10-year-old the checks carried out by the National Blood Service on blood prior to it being distributed to healthcare settings?

References

Birmingham Children's Hospital NHS Trust (2003) Blood Administration Document. Birmingham Children's Hospital NHS Trust, Birmingham

Boulton F (2004) Transfusion guidelines for neonates and older children. British Journal of Haematology 124:433–453

Department of Health (2001) Good practice in consent implementation guideline. Online. Available: http://www.doh.gov.uk/consent

Department of Health (2002) Better blood transfusion – appropriate use of blood. Health service circular HSC2002/009

Department of Health (2003) Getting the right start: the National Service Framework for Children, Young People and Maternity Services – Standard for Hospital Services. Department of Health, London

Desmet L, Lacroix J (2004) Transfusion in pediatrics. Critical Care Clinics 20(2):299–311

McIntosh N (2006) Intravenous therapy in practices. In Trigg E, Mohammed TA (eds) Children's nursing: guidelines for hospital and community, 2nd edn. Churchill Livingstone, London

Murphy MF, Atterbury CLJ, Chapman FLJS et al (1999) The administration of blood components and the management of transfused patients. Transfusion Medicine 9:227–238

Nohum E, Ben-Ari J, Schonfeld T (2002) Blood transfusion practice indicated by paediatric intensive care specialists in response to four clinical scenarios. Critical Care and Resuscitation 4:261–265

Nursing and Midwifery Council (2004) The NMC code of professional standards for conduct, performance and ethics. Nursing and Midwifery Council, London

Nursing and Midwifery Council (2005) Guidelines for records and record keeping. Nursing and Midwifery Council, London

Provan D (1999) Better blood transfusion. British Medical Journal 318:1435–1436

Royal College of Nursing (2005) Right blood, right patient, right time. RCN guidance for improving transfusion practice. Royal College of Nursing, London

Scottish National Blood Transfusion Service (2006) Better blood transfusion – level 2: blood component use. Effective use of blood group. Scottish National Blood Transfusion Service, Edinburgh

Stainsby D, Jones H, Knowles S et al (2005a) Series hazards of transfusion. SHOT annual report 2004. Series Hazards of Transfusion, Manchester

Stainsby D, Russell J, Cohen H, Lilleyman J (2005b) Reducing adverse events in blood transfusion. British Medical Journal 131:8–12

Wallis JP (2005) Preventing ABO incompatible blood transfusion. British Journal of Haematology 132:530–532

West Midlands Regional Transfusion Committee (2005) Training package for safe transfusion practice. Version 1. West Midlands Regional Transfusion Committee, Birmingham

Williamson LM, Lowe S, Love EM et al (1999) Series Hazards of Transfusion (SHOT) initiative: analysis of the first two annual reports. British Medical Journal 319:16–19

26

Central venous lines

Janet Kelsey

Long-term central venous lines provide vascular access for children with a variety of acute or chronic illnesses. They enable children to undergo treatments such as parenteral nutrition, chemotherapy, immunotherapy and haemodialysis without repeated venepuncture.

There are three types of lines used in children, all of which may have single, double or triple lumens:

- A short-term non-tunnelled long line used in intensive care or high-dependency situations can be inserted under local anaesthetic and held in place with skin sutures.
- Long-term lines include the Broviac or Hickman tunnelled cuffed line and the implanted port line known as Port-a-Cath, Vascuport or totally implantable venous access device. Both are inserted under general anaesthetic into the subclavian or jugular vein (Fig. 26.1). The Groshong is also a tunnelled catheter but does not require an external clamp.

The Broviac or Hickman line is tunnelled under the skin with a cuff around the tube just under the skin surface to help prevent infection tracking along the line (Figs 26.2 and 26.3). The advantage of these lines is that it is not necessary to have needles pushed through the skin; however, the ends of the catheter emerge from the skin, can be seen, require to be covered with a dressing, and care is required with their everyday care to prevent infection. Implanted port catheters end in a rubber bulb or reservoir. The catheter is placed in the vein and the reservoir is buried under the skin. The advantage is that when not in use it cannot be seen very easily and nothing is visible coming through the skin; however, such catheters do require a straight or angled Huber non-coring needle to be inserted through the skin into the reservoir for treatment to take place (Fig. 26.4), although local anaesthetic cream should be used to minimise discomfort.

Principles of care

Quality assurance and continuing education

Reports demonstrate that the risk of infection is reduced with standardisation of aseptic care and education of healthcare personnel (O'Grady et al 2002). However, it increases when nursing staff:patient ratios are reduced below a critical level (Fridkin & Jarvis 1996). All healthcare personnel, including community teams, involved in caring for children with central lines should be included in education and training and assessed as competent before caring for the children (National Institute for Clinical Excellence 2003). In addition, before discharge from hospital patients and their carers should be taught any techniques they may need to use to prevent infection and safely manage their central venous catheter.

Asepsis

The majority of catheter-related bloodstream infections (CRBSIs) in children are caused by coagulase-negative staphylococci, accounting for 37.7% of bloodstream infections in paediatric intensive care units reporting to the National Nosocomial Infections Surveillance System in the USA between 1992 and 1999 (National Nosocomial Infections Surveillance System 1999). Good hand hygiene before accessing or dressing central venous catheters, combined with aseptic technique during catheter manipulation, is essential in preventing infection (Healthcare Infection Control Practices Advisory Committee 2002, National Institute for Clinical Excellence 2003). Hands must be decontaminated either by washing with an antimicrobial liquid soap and water or by using an alcohol hand rub; in addition, hands that are visibly soiled or contaminated must be washed with soap and water before using an alcohol hand rub.

ALERT
Good hand hygiene before accessing or dressing central venous catheters, combined with aseptic technique during catheter manipulation, is essential in preventing infection.

Catheter site care

Following hand antisepsis, clean gloves and a no touch technique or sterile gloves should be used when changing the insertion site dressing. A sterile, transparent, semipermeable polyurethane dressing should be used to cover the catheter site, as it allows continuous visual inspection of the site, permits the child to bathe or shower without necessitating dressing change, and does not require changing as frequently as gauze dressings. Tegaderm or OpSite 3000 is recommended (Gillies et al 2003). However, if the insertion

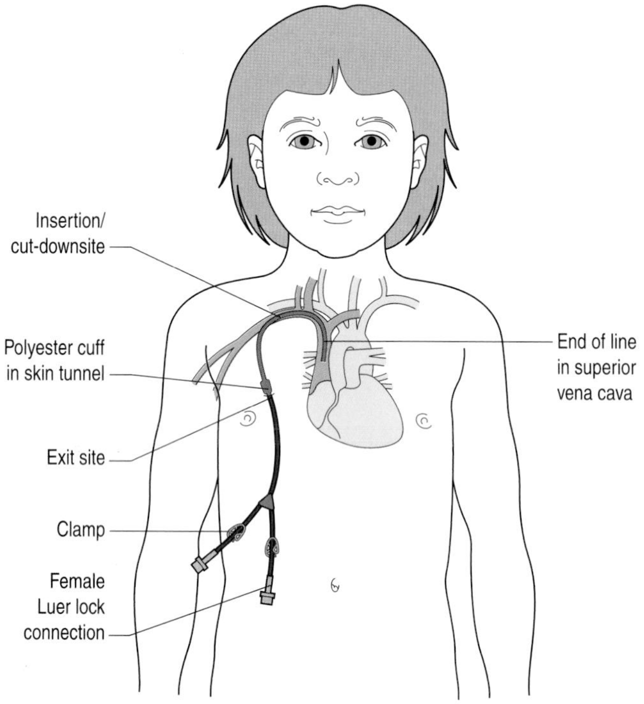

Fig. 26.1 • Position of central venous line. (After Trigg & Mohammed 2006, with permission.)

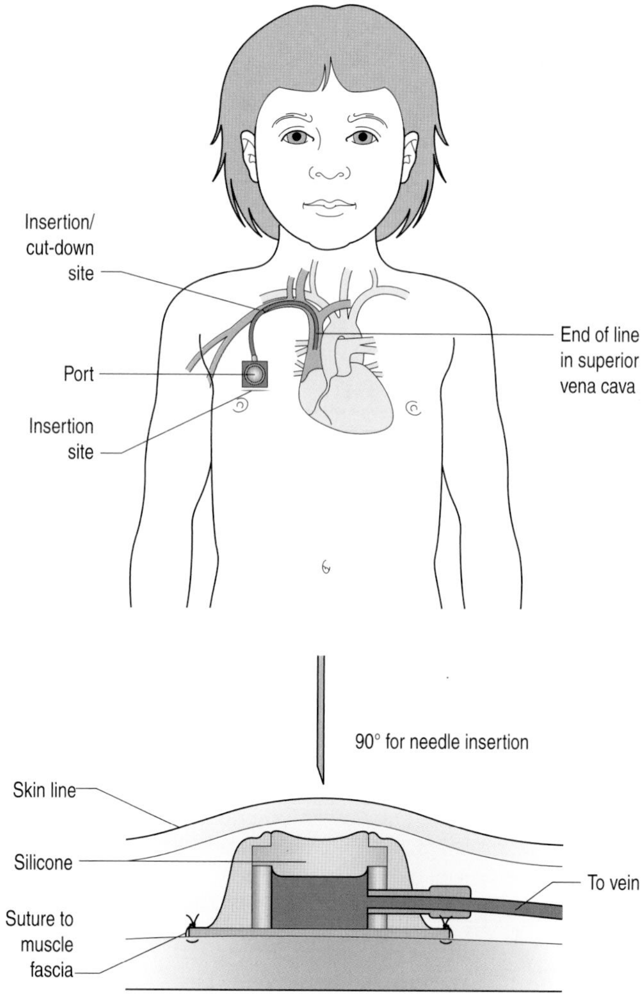

Fig. 26.2 • (**A**) Port in situ. (**B**) Cross-section of port. (After Trigg & Mohammed 2006, with permission.)

site is bleeding or oozing, a sterile gauze dressing is preferable; these dressings should be changed when they become damp, loosened or soiled and replaced at the earliest opportunity by a transparent dressing. Transparent dressings should be changed every 7 days, or sooner if they are no longer intact or if moisture collects under the dressing (National Institute for Clinical Excellence 2003). It is advisable to coil the catheter under the dressing to help prevent catheter dislodgement.

Chaiyakunapruk et al (2002) concluded that the use of chlorhexidine gluconate rather than povidone–iodine can reduce the risk for CRBSI by approximately 49% in hospitalised patients who require short-term catheterisation, therefore individual sachets of antiseptic solution or individual packages of an alcoholic chlorhexidine gluconate solution should be used to clean the catheter site during dressing changes and allowed to air dry. An aqueous solution of chlorhexidine gluconate should be used if the manufacturer's recommendations prohibit the use of alcohol with the product (National Institute for Clinical Excellence 2003). There is also evidence that aqueous chlorhexidine 2% is superior to either 10% povidone–iodine or 70% alcohol in lowering CRBSI rates when used for skin antisepsis prior to central venous catheter insertion (Healthcare Infection Control Practices Advisory Committee 2002). It should be noted that it is the responsibility of healthcare personnel to ensure that catheter site care is compatible with the catheter materials by checking the manufacturer's recommendations.

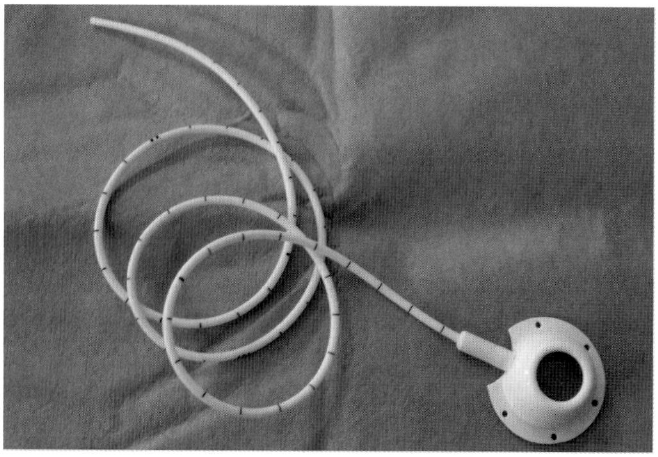

Fig. 26.3 • Port.

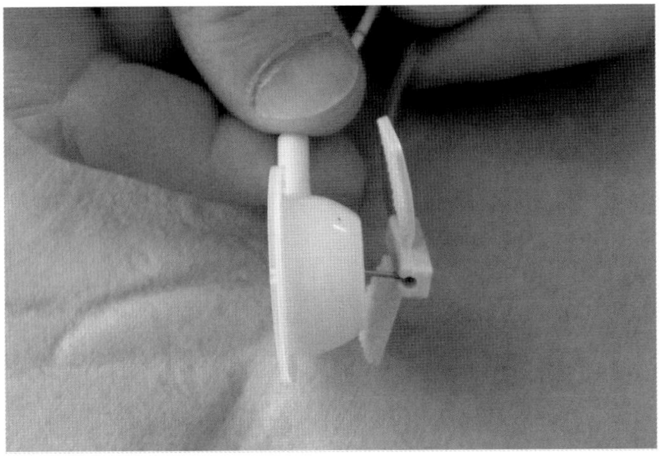

Fig. 26.4 • Port with winged needle.

Catheter management

As most modern catheter hubs, connections and ports are made from alcohol-resistant materials, they should be decontaminated using either alcohol or an alcoholic solution of chlorhexidine gluconate before and after they have been used to access the system (Healthcare Infection Control Practices Advisory Committee 2002).

In-line filters should not be used routinely for infection prevention, as there is no reliable evidence to support their preventing infections associated with intravascular catheters or infusions and they may become blocked, especially with solutions such as dextran, lipids and mannitol, which in turn increases the number of line manipulations (Healthcare Infection Control Practices Advisory Committee 2002).

The flushing and filling of the lumen of the catheter with antibiotics, although effective in neutropenic patients, should not be used routinely to prevent CRBSI, as it may lead to an increased number of antimicrobial-resistant micro-organisms. Neither should systemic antimicrobial prophylaxis be used routinely to prevent catheter colonisation or CRBSI, either before insertion or during the use of a central venous catheter (Healthcare Infection Control Practices Advisory Committee 2002).

When administering parenteral nutrition, single-lumen catheters should be used whenever possible. If a multilumen catheter is used, one port must be exclusively dedicated for total parenteral nutrition.

Systematic reviews by Randolph et al (1998), Goode et al (1991) and Peterson & Kirchoff (1991) of randomised controlled trials evaluating the effect of heparin on the duration of catheter patency and on the prevention of complications associated with the use of peripheral venous and arterial catheters concluded that heparin at doses of 10 U/mL for intermittent flushing is no more beneficial than flushing with normal saline 0.9% alone. Therefore a sterile 0.9% sodium chloride injection should be used to flush and lock catheter lumens. Anticoagulant flushes may be used providing that this is recommended by the manufacturer. However, systemic anticoagulants should not be used, as there are no data that demonstrate that warfarin reduces the incidence of CRBSI (Healthcare Infection Control Practices Advisory Committee 2002).

If needleless devices are used, to reduce the incidence of sharps injuries the manufacturer's recommendations for changing the needleless components should be followed and the access port decontaminated with either alcohol or an alcoholic solution of chlorhexidine gluconate before and after using it to access the system.

Gillies et al (2003) recommend that changing intravenous infusion sets that do not contain lipids, blood or blood products at intervals of <96 h does not affect infusate-related infections or CRBSIs; however, National Institute for Clinical Excellence (2003) guidelines suggest changing them no more frequently than at 72-h intervals unless they become disconnected or a catheter-related infection is suspected or documented. Administration sets for blood and blood components should be changed every 12 h or according to the manufacturer's recommendations, and administration sets used for total parenteral nutrition infusions should generally be changed every 24 h. However, if the solution contains only glucose and amino acids, administration sets in continuous use do not need to be replaced more frequently than every 72 h.

Line safety

Always keep the ends of the line pinned to a tape flap on the chest or securely pinned to the child's shirt; alternatively, 'wiggly' bags can be made for lines to sit in. This will prevent the line from getting caught on clothing or accidentally pulled. Parents of infants frequently use a one-piece undershirt that snaps between the legs and pin the C line to the shirt. A child with a central line is not allowed to participate in contact sports such as rugby, football or volleyball, as a direct blow to the chest can damage the line. Because of the risk of infection, swimming is not allowed.

ALERT

If the line becomes damaged then clamp the line above the break close to the exit site and report it immediately.

Table 26.1 summarises possible complications of central lines.

The basic equipment required for accessing central lines is similar for each procedure, with variations according to the required task:

- Trolley or medium-sized tray
- Sterile dressing pack
- Two sachets of cleaning fluid
- Needles (blue, 23 G, or green, 21 G)

Table 26.1. Complications of central lines

Complication	Causes	Management
Infection and potential CRBSI	• Poor aseptic technique • Poor hand-washing technique • Insufficient education and assessment of healthcare personnel • Inappropriate catheter and exit site care	• Blood cultures. • Exit site swabs. • Intravenous antibiotics. • In extreme cases, the line may have to be removed.
Occlusion	• Catheter kinking • Catheter integrity impaired by thrombus formation or blood or drug precipitate	• Visually check the external parts of the line and try altering the child's position. • If the line still appears blocked do a chest X-ray to exclude internal kinks. • Consider using an antifibrinolytic agent such as urokinase to dissolve the clot. • Consider regular heparinisation as a preventive measure. • Can occur if some solutions are not infused correctly; refer to experience personnel for removal.
Catheter misplacement	–	• There is evidence that ultrasound-guided placement of central lines reduces the complication rate associated with this procedure (Dunning 2003)
Accidental pulls to the central line	–	• Check the exit site; if there is any drainage on the dressing (clear or bloody), put pressure on the dressing and refer to experienced staff. • If the line appears to extend out from under the dressing farther than usual or if there is a large amount of bleeding report the incident immediately.
Damage to the central line	–	• Clamp the line above the break close to the exit site. Report the incident immediately as the break may be able to be repaired under aseptic conditions.
Air embolism	–	• Clamp the line close to the exit site. Turn the child so that he/she is lying on his/her heart side. Report incident immediately. If the child exhibits any shortness of breath, chest pain or bleeding report immediately.

- Orange needle (25 G) or filter needle
- Bare cannulae for tunnelled catheters
- Gripper needles of appropriate size and length for use with implanted ports
- 10-mL syringes
- 5 mL of Hepsal.
- 10-mL of normal saline 0.9%
- Appropriate blood bottles
- Prescription chart
- Sterile latex-free gloves
- Dressing
- Sharps container.

Procedures Box 26.1 Taking blood from a central venous line

Action
Explain the procedure to the child and carer.
Reason *Gains consent and cooperation.*

Action
Expose the end of the line.

Action
Decontaminate your hands either by washing with an antimicrobial liquid soap and water or by using an alcohol hand rub; hands that are visibly soiled or contaminated must be washed with soap and water before using an alcohol hand rub.

Procedures Box 26.1 Taking blood from a central venous line—cont'd

Reason *Avoids microbial contamination.*

Action
Ensure that appropriate blood bottles are available.

Action
Using aseptic technique, open a dressing pack and empty the equipment on to the pack.

Reason *Provides a clean field to work from.*

Action
Gel your hands.

Reason *Avoids microbial contamination.*

Actions
Check the expiry date and draw up normal saline 0.9% or Hepsal using a filter needle with glass ampoule, 10-mL syringe and expelling air bubbles.

Discard the needles.

Reasons *A filter needle reduces the risk of drawing up glass particles.*
The pressure of fluids through a central line must not exceed 40 p.s.i. (2068 mmHg), and using a syringe smaller than 10 mL may rupture the line.
Prevents injecting air.

Action
Put on sterile gloves.

Reason *Prevents microbial contamination and protects against contamination from the patient's blood.*

Action
Place a sterile towel on the lap with the line laid on it.

Reason *Maintains a clean surface for the procedure.*

Action
Wipe the bung with cleaning fluid and allow to dry.

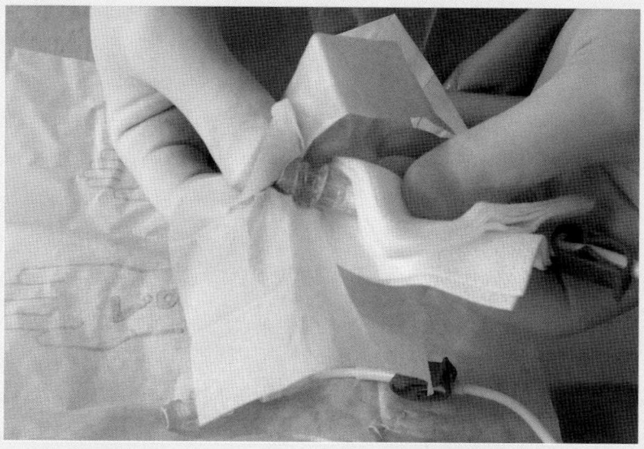

Reason *Prevents microbial contamination.*

Actions
Hold the bung with sterile gauze, unclamp the line and withdraw 4–5 mL of blood slowly.

Clamp the line.

Discard this blood unless it is required for blood cultures.

If clotting studies are required remove 10 mL of blood if the line has previously been heparin-locked.

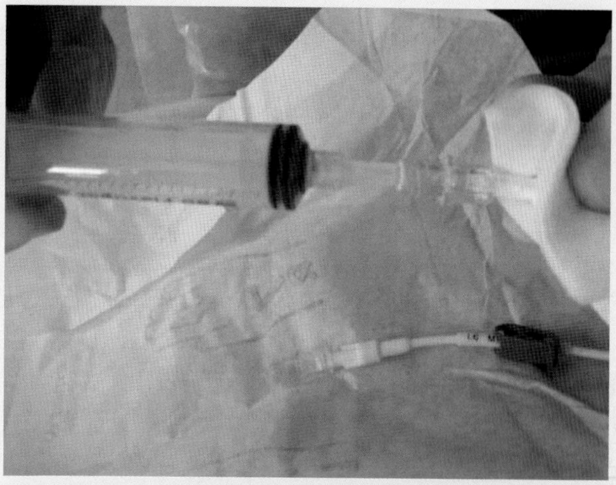

Reason *Removes blood that contains the previous flush.*

Actions
Insert a new syringe, unclamp the line and withdraw blood required for samples.

Clamp the line and place the syringe on a tray.

Reason *Obtains an uncontaminated blood sample.*

Actions
Insert the syringe containing normal saline 0.9% flush into the bung, unclamp the line and flush with normal saline 0.9%.

Clamp the line.

Reason *Flushes the line.*

Action
If Hepsal flush is being used, insert the syringe into the bung, unclamp the line, flush and clamp while pushing in the final 0.5 mL.

Reason *Heparin-locks the line and maintains positive pressure.*

Action
If accessing multiple lumens clean and flush each lumen in the same manner.

Reason *Ensures that all lumens are flushed.*

Action
Secure the line into the bag or fix it to the tag.

Reason *Prevents catheter misplacement.*

Action
Put blood in appropriate bottles following local policy for the order of draw and transfer of blood into specimen bottles.

Reason *Ensures safe and appropriate sample transfer.*

Action
Dispose of all sharps and equipment as per local policy.

Reason *Prevents injury to self and others.*

Action
Document the samples taken in the child's records.

Procedures Box 26.2 Administration of drugs

Action
Explain the procedure to the child and carer.

Reason *Gains consent and cooperation.*

Action
Expose the end of the line.

Action
Decontaminate your hands either by washing with an antimicrobial liquid soap and water or by using an alcohol hand rub; hands that are visibly soiled or contaminated must be washed with soap and water before using an alcohol hand rub.

Reason *Avoids microbial contamination.*

Action
Using aseptic technique, open a dressing pack and empty the equipment on to the pack.

Reason *Provides a clean field to work from.*

Action
Gel your hands.

Reason *Avoids microbial contamination.*

Actions
Check the expiry date and draw up medications and normal saline 0.9% or Hepsal using a filter needle with glass ampoule, 10-mL syringe and expelling air bubbles.

Discard the needles.

Reason *A filter needle reduces the risk of drawing up glass particles.*
The pressure of fluids through a central line must not exceed 40 p.s.i. (2068 mmHg), and using a syringe smaller than 10 mL may rupture the line.
Prevents injecting air.

Action
Put on sterile gloves.

Reason *Prevents microbial contamination and protects against contamination from the patient's blood.*

Action
Place a sterile towel on the lap with the line laid on it.

Reason *Maintains a clean surface for the procedure.*

Action
Wipe the bung with cleaning fluid and allow to dry.

Reason *Prevents microbial contamination.*

Action
Hold the bung with sterile gauze, unclamp the line, flush with 5 mL of normal saline 0.9%, clamp the line, discard the flush syringe, attach the syringe containing medication, unclamp the line and administer the medication according to the manufacturer's recommendations, then clamp the line.

Reason *Administers medication according to local policy and manufacturer's recommendations.*

Actions
Insert a syringe containing normal saline 0.9% flush into the bung, unclamp the line and flush with normal saline 0.9%.

Clamp the line.

Reason *Flushes the line.*

Action
If Hepsal flush is being used, insert the syringe into the bung, unclamp the line, flush and clamp while pushing in the final 0.5 mL.

Reason *Heparin-locks the line and maintains positive pressure.*

Action
If accessing multiple lumens clean and flush each lumen in the same manner.

Reason *Ensures that all lumens are flushed.*

Action
Secure the line into the bag or fix it to the tag.

Reason *Prevents catheter misplacement.*

Action
Dispose of all sharps and equipment as per local policy.

Reason *Prevents injury to self and others.*

Procedures Box 26.3 Connecting or changing an infusion set

Action
Explain the procedure to the child and carer.

Reason *Gains consent and cooperation.*

Action
Expose the end of the line.

Action
Decontaminate your hands either by washing with an antimicrobial liquid soap and water or by using an alcohol hand rub; hands that are visibly soiled or contaminated must be washed with soap and water before using an alcohol hand rub.

Reason *Avoids microbial contamination.*

Action
Check and prime the appropriate administration set with the prescribed intravenous fluid.

Reason *Ensures safe administration of intravenous fluid.*

Action
Using aseptic technique, open a dressing pack and empty the equipment on to the pack.

Reason *Provides a clean field to work from.*

Action
Gel your hands.

Reason *Avoids microbial contamination.*

Procedures Box 26.3 Connecting or changing an infusion set—cont'd

Action
Put on sterile gloves.

Reason *Prevents microbial contamination and protects against contamination from the patient's blood.*

Action
Place a sterile towel on the lap with the line laid on it.

Reason *Maintains a clean surface for the procedure.*

Action
Wipe the bung with cleaning fluid and allow to dry.

Reason *Prevents microbial contamination.*

Actions
Hold the bung with sterile gauze, unclamp the line, flush with 5 mL of normal saline 0.9%, clamp the line, discard the flush syringe and attach the intravenous administration set.

If the line is already attached to an infusion, clamp the line, clean the connection and allow to dry, remove and attach the new set.

Check that the whole system is complete and secure.

Open the clamp and set the infusion to the prescribed rate.

Action
Dispose of all sharps and equipment as per local policy.

Reason *Prevents injury to self and others.*

When accessing an implanted port for use the principles of asepsis remain the same, therefore the only differences are in how to access the device. Local anaesthetic cream should be applied at an appropriate time interval prior to accessing the port and removed prior to cleaning. After putting on sterile gloves the skin should be cleaned with chlorhexidine gluconate, working in a spiral from the raised centre outwards for at least 4 cm. Repeat this at least twice and allow to dry. Stabilise the port with the thumb and forefingers. Insert the gripper needle at an angle of 90% to the skin into the septum of the device until the needle contacts the base. Do not twist or rock the needle once inserted. Proceed with blood sampling, drug administration or connecting to intravenous infusion as required. When a port is in long-term use the needle must be changed every 2 weeks, or weekly if the child is neutropenic. While in use the port should be covered with an occlusive dressing, which is changed either when the needle is changed or when the dressing becomes soiled. To deaccess the port remove the dressing, put on sterile gloves, stabilise the device between the thumb and finger, and remove the needle by pulling straight up and out. Apply pressure to the site if there is any bleeding. When the port is no longer in use the skin's integrity is not broken, therefore a dressing is required only if the child requests it.

Now test your knowledge

- What type of dressings should be used on a central line site?
- What should you clean the catheter site with when changing the dressing?
- How often should you change the catheter site dressing?
- What advice would you give to a parent phoning the ward worried that the child's central venous line catheter has become dislodged?

References

Chaiyakunapruk N, Veenstra DL, Lipsky BA, Saint S (2002) Chlorhexidine compared with povidone–iodine solution for vascular catheter-site care: A meta-analysis. Annals of Internal Medicine 136(11):792–801

Dunning J, Williamson J (2003) Ultrasonic guidance and the complications of central line placement in the emergency department. Emergency Medicine Journal 20(6):551–552

Fridkin SK, Jarvis WR (1996) Epidemiology of nosocomial fungal infections. Clinical Microbiology Reviews 9(4):499–511

Gillies D, O'Riordan E, Carr D, O'Brien I, Frost J, Gunning R (2003) Central venous catheter dressings: a systematic review. Journal of Advanced Nursing 44(6):623–632

Goode CJ, Titler M, Rakel B et al (1991) A meta-analysis of effects of heparin flush and saline flush: quality and cost implications. Nursing Research 40:324–330

Healthcare Infection Control Practices Advisory Committee (2002) Guidelines for the prevention of intravascular catheter-related infections. Centers for Disease Control. Morbidity and Mortality Weekly Report 51(RR-10). Online. Available: http://www.cdc.gov/mmwr

National Institute for Clinical Excellence (2003) Infection control. Prevention of healthcare associated infection in primary and community care. Oaktree Press, London

National Nosocomial Infections Surveillance System (1999) Data summary from January 1990–May 1999, issued June 1999. American Journal of Infection Control 27:520–32.

O'Grady NP, Alexander M, Dellinger P et al (2002) Guidelines for the prevention of intravascular catheter-related infection [special report]. Infection Control and Hospital Epidemiology 23(12).

Peterson FY, Kirchoff KT (1991) Analysis of the research about heparinized versus nonheparinized intravascular lines. Heart and Lung 20:631–640

Randolph AG, Cook DJ, Gonzales CA, Andrew M (1998) Benefit of heparin in peripheral venous and arterial catheters: systematic review and meta-analysis of randomised controlled trials. British Medical Journal 316:969–975

Trigg E, Mohammed T (eds.) (2006) Guidelines for hospital and community, 2nd edn. Churchill Livingstone, London

27 Venepuncture

Sue Frost • Janet Kelsey

Children's nurses in a variety of settings are extending their practice to include venepuncture to enable care to be delivered in a less fragmented and more timely manner, thus meeting the demands of clinical areas and providing high-quality care. While undertaking this skill you should always adhere to the *Code of Professional Conduct* (Nursing and Midwifery Council 2004), *Guidelines for Records and Record-keeping* (Nursing and Midwifery Council 2005) and your trust's policies and procedures. Informed consent, verbal, written or implied, should be gained from the child or carer as appropriate.

In infants it may be necessary to use the veins in the head (Fig. 27.1), but venepuncture is usually performed on the veins of the upper arm or hands. The most widely used are the median cubital, the basilic and the median cephalic veins in the antecubital fossa (Fig. 27.2); however, these can be difficult to locate in well-nourished infants (Das & Sharma 2002). Therefore below the age of about 2 years the veins on the dorsum of the feet (Fig. 27.3) or hands (Fig. 27.4) may be easier to access. Goren et al (2001) found that transillumination of the palm of the hand with an otoscope can help in identifying suitable veins for venepuncture in young infants. In babies the scalp and feet may be used.

It should be noted that venepuncture is reported as being most painful in the hands and feet, with veins in the front (palm side) of a wrist being especially sore. If the child is likely to require peripheral venous cannulation then the smaller veins should be used to preserve larger veins for cannulation. Children with little or no sensation in their lower limbs may prefer their legs or feet to be used; however, care should be taken to inspect the site for tissue damage, as these children may not be able to detect any pain or swelling. The lower extremities are not routinely used for venepuncture, as there is an increased risk of deep vein thrombosis in some patients.

ALERT
Do not use sites that may interfere with the child's normal activity.

Classification of veins

Veins of the upper arm are both deep and superficial (Fig. 27.5). Deep veins are located deep within the arm and usually run parallel to their corresponding artery. They are also in close proximity to nerves. Superficial veins are located just below the skin and are often visible. The veins of the hand (Fig. 27.5) are much smaller than those of the arm; there are a greater number lying close to the skin and peripheral nerve receptors, therefore venepuncture here causes greater pain.

Superficial veins are:

- cephalics
- basilic
- median antecubital.

Deep veins are:

- radial
- ulnar
- brachial
- auxillary.

Veins of the hand are:

- dorsal metacarpal
- dorsal venous network or arch.

The venous anatomy of each child varies but the general structure is similar.

When performing venepuncture, care must be taken to avoid adjacent structures such as arteries and bony prominences. If a nerve is touched by a needle the child will experience pain and discomfort or altered sensation. The needle should be removed, the incident documented and the medial staff informed if it does not improve. If an artery is punctured there will be painful spasm and excessive bleeding. The needle should be removed, pressure applied for 5–10 min and the incident documented. Puncture of a bone also causes pain and discomfort; the needle should be removed and the incident documented and reported to the medical staff. Valves in a vein can sometimes be observed as bumps; puncturing a valve is noted by increased resistance and may damage the valve, so remove the needle and document the incident (Campbell et al 1999).

Factors influencing vein choice

See Box 27.1.

Choosing a vein

See Box 27.2.

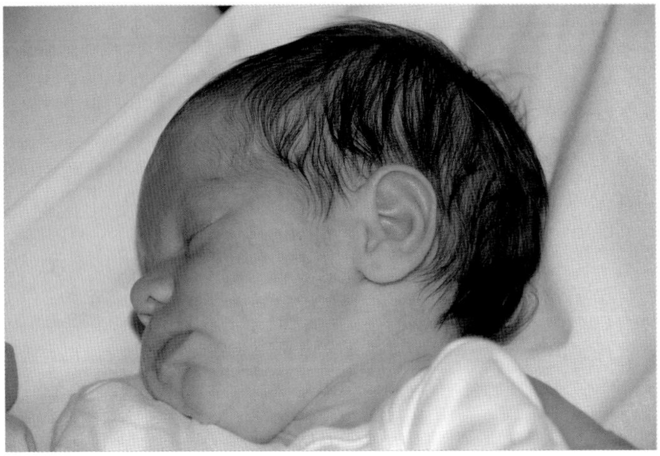

Fig. 27.1 • In infants it may be necessary to use the veins in the head.

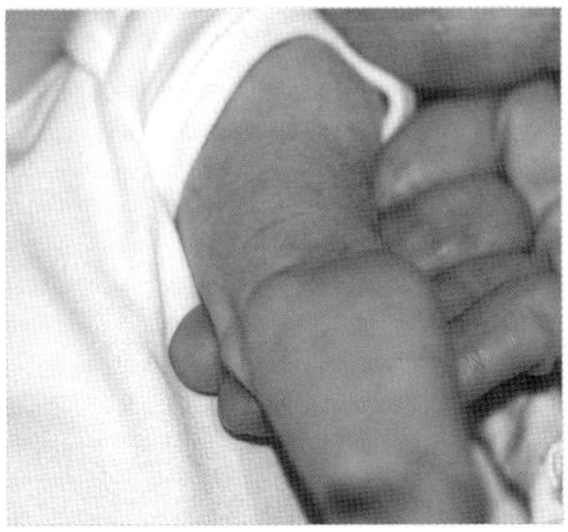

Fig. 27.2 • Veins in the antecubital fossa.

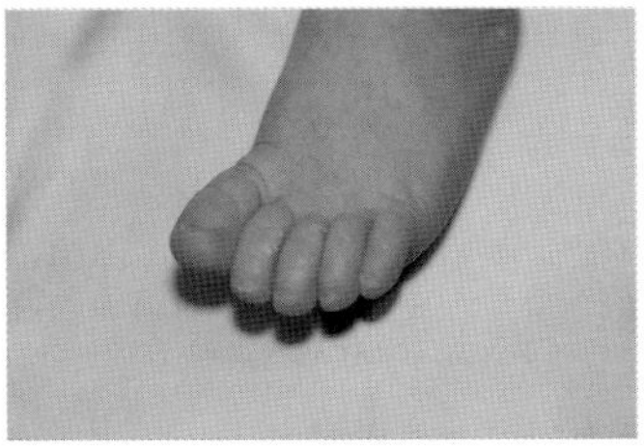

Fig. 27.3 • Veins of the dorsum of the foot.

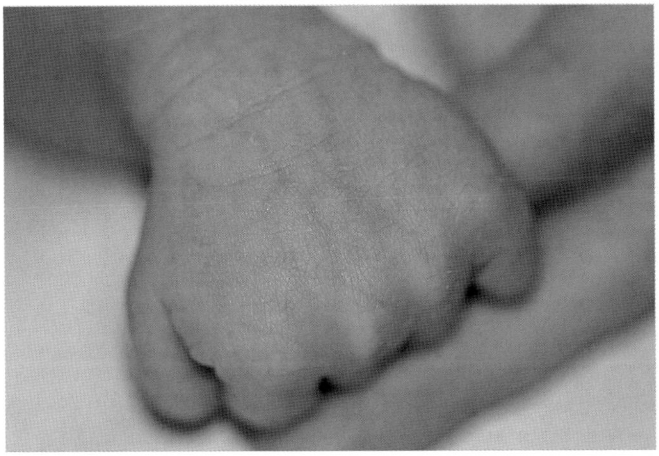

Fig. 27.4 • Veins of the dorsum of the hand.

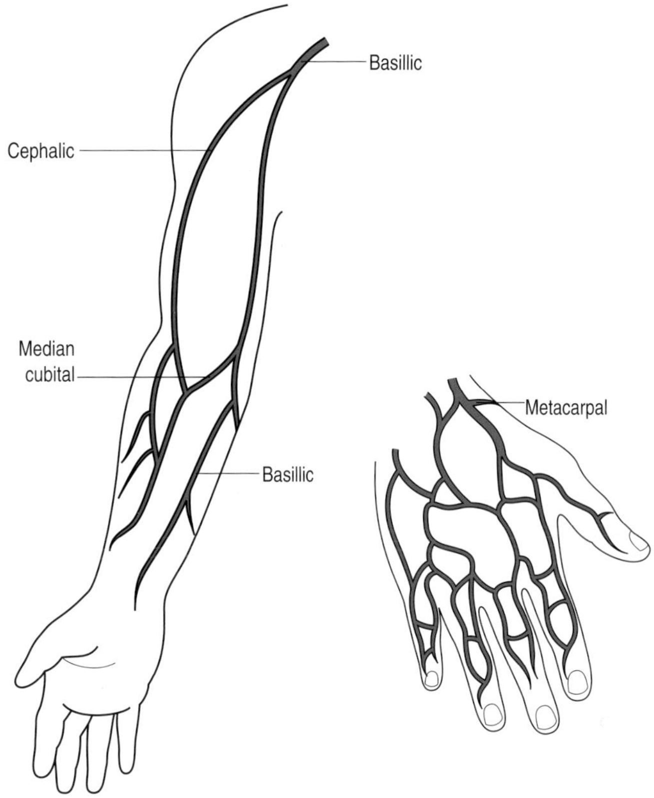

Fig. 27.5 • Anatomy and physiology of veins of the arm and hand.

Preparation

Circumstances such as anxiety, reduced body or environmental temperature, and mechanical or chemical irritation, which cause venous constriction, will make venepuncture more difficult. Children continue to see venepuncture as a frightening experience (Duff 2003); the child's memory and expectation of venepuncture as a traumatic experience can lead to venous constriction (Vessey et al 1994). It is therefore vital that children are psychologically prepared for venepuncture in order to reduce distress and enable successful venepuncture.

Box 27.1. Factors influencing vein choice

- Age of patient
- Previous use and condition of veins
- Weight (well nourished, obese, malnourished)
- Clinical status of child (e.g. dehydration, shock, fracture, phlebitis)
- Other clinical procedures required (e.g. cannulation)
- Child's preference
- Child's cooperation

Box 27.2. Choosing a vein

Veins to use

- Veins that are bouncy, soft and refill when depressed (Fig. 27.6)

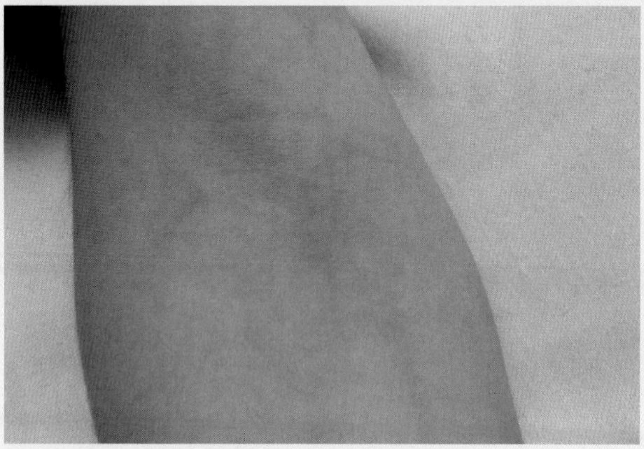

Fig. 27.6 • A suitable vein for venepuncture.

- Veins that are visible and easily palpable
- Veins on the non-dominant side
- Veins with a large enough lumen
- Veins that are well supported and straight

- **Veins to avoid**
- Veins that are thrombosed, sclerosed or fibrosed
- Veins that are inflamed, bruised or irritated from previous venepuncture or near to obvious valves
- Veins that are thin, fragile, mobile, small or superficial
- Veins near bony prominences, painful areas or sites of infection, oedema or phlebitis
- Veins that have undergone multiple punctures
- Veins in the lower extremities, except in exceptional circumstances
- Veins near arteries
- Veins on limbs affected by the clinical condition
- Veins near broken skin
- Veins in a limb with an intravenous infusion attached

Pain

Pain and distress caused by venepuncture can be reduced and eliminated by the use of appropriate analgesia, such as:

- eutectic lidocaine and prilocaine cream (eutectic mixture of local anaesthetics, EMLA)
- tetracaine gel (Ametop)
- ethyl chloride spray
- nitrous oxide and oxygen gas mixture (Entonox).

EMLA and Ametop act by causing a reversible block to conduction along nerve fibres; the numbing effect induced wears off a few hours after application. Both drugs are known to be effective for venepuncture (Arrowsmith & Campbell 2000). EMLA cream is indicated for use on normal, intact skin before minor skin procedures including venepuncture. It is contraindicated in premature infants and infants less than 1 month old because of the risk of methaemoglobinaemia, which is exacerbated if used in conjunction with sulphonamide antibiotics (Buckley & Benfield 1993), although Taddio et al (1997) showed it to be safe with most neonates. The manufacturers recommend that it is not used in infants less than 12 months of age. Accidental ingestion of EMLA may be toxic, and adverse reactions may occur if EMLA gets into contact with the eyes. Other adverse effects include transient paleness, redness and oedema. In addition, vasoconstriction has been reported, which may render venepuncture more difficult (Browne et al 1999). Prior to venepuncture the contents of the tube should be applied to one or two areas in a thick layer and covered with an occlusive dressing, sealed to ensure no leakage (Abraxis Pharmaceutical Products 2007) and left undisturbed. Immediately before the procedure (at least 60 min after application) the dressing and cream should be removed. Numbing of the skin should occur 1 h after application, reaching a maximum at 2–3 h (1 h for children less than 3 months old) and lasts for 1–2 h after removal of the cream. It must be removed with a gauze swab or tissue before venepuncture. It should be stored below 30°C. Ametop is recommended for use in children more than 1 month of age but not for premature infants. It is rapidly absorbed from mucous membranes and should not be applied to inflamed, traumatised or highly vascular surfaces. Adverse effects include hypersensitivity to tetracaine, also erythema, oedema, pruritus and blistering (rare). As with EMLA, the gel can be divided between two sites and sealed with an occlusive dressing. The gel and dressing are removed after 30 min for venepuncture and after 45 min for venous cannulation. Arrowsmith & Campbell (2000) report that EMLA produced more significant blanching and Ametop more erythema at the site of application owing to the different actions of the anaesthetic agents but the difference did not influence the number of attempts required to cannulate. The study confirmed that Ametop provided more effective analgesia for cannulation in a significantly higher proportion of children than EMLA did.

ALERT
The manufacturers of EMLA recommend that it is not used in infants less than 12 months of age. Ametop is recommended for use in children more than 1 month of age but not for premature infants.

Ethyl chloride is a surface anaesthetic spray. It is a volatile liquid; when sprayed on to the skin it rapidly evaporates and during evaporation it cools the skin down to below 10°C, preventing nerve impulses being generated. Ethyl chloride should be sprayed on to the skin for 5–10 s to achieve its anaesthetic effect. DeJong et al (1990) reported it as effective as EMLA for cannulation in children, and Cohen & Holubkov (1997) found that when combined with distraction vapocoolant spray significantly reduces immediate injection pain compared with distraction alone and is equally effective as, less expensive than, and faster acting than EMLA cream. The same study did not find vapocoolant spray suitable for intravenous cannulation. Inhalation of ethyl chloride should be avoided, as it may produce narcotic and general anaesthetic effects, deep anaesthesia or fatal coma with respiratory or cardiac arrest. Ethyl chloride is flammable and should never be used in the presence of an open flame or electrical cautery equipment.

Nitrous oxide is also effective for relieving pain (Beh et al 2002). A mixture of nitrous oxide and oxygen containing 50% of each gas (Entonox, Equanox) is used to produce analgesia without loss of consciousness. Self-administration using a demand valve may be used in children who are able to self-regulate their intake (usually those over 5 years of age). Side effects include over-sedation in 0.33% of children (Gall et al 2001), which is reduced if the child self-administers via a demand valve; euphoria; loss of inhibitions; dry mouth; disorientation; sensations of floating; hearing blurred voices; dizziness; nausea and vomiting (Bruce & Franck 2000). The child should not eat or drink for 1 h prior to nitrous oxide to reduce the risk of vomiting.

Sucrose has been found to decrease the response to noxious stimuli such as heel sticks and injections in neonates (Stevens et al 2001). Sucrose is safe and effective for reducing procedural pain from single painful events; however, an optimal dose to be used in preterm and/or term infants has not been identified (Stevens et al 2004). The effect seems to be strongest in the newborn infant and decreases gradually over the first 6 months of life (Blass & Hoffmeyer 1991, Stevens et al 2001). However, the use of sucrose in neonates who are of very low birth weight, unstable and/or ventilated also needs to be addressed (Stevens et al 2004).

The use of a pacifier alone or in conjunction with sucrose also has been shown to have analgesic effects in neonates undergoing routine venepuncture (Carbajal et al 2003). Skin-to-skin contact of an infant with his or her mother and breastfeeding during a procedure also decrease pain behaviours associated with painful stimuli (Gray et al 2000, 2002).

Supportive holding

Holding or immobilising children is a practice used to ensure success in carrying out therapeutic and diagnostic interventions.

LINK CHAPTER **6**

Equipment (Fig. 27.7)

Vacuum collection systems should be used whenever possible for the collection of blood. The use of partial fill systems may be beneficial in children, as these vials cause less vacuum and

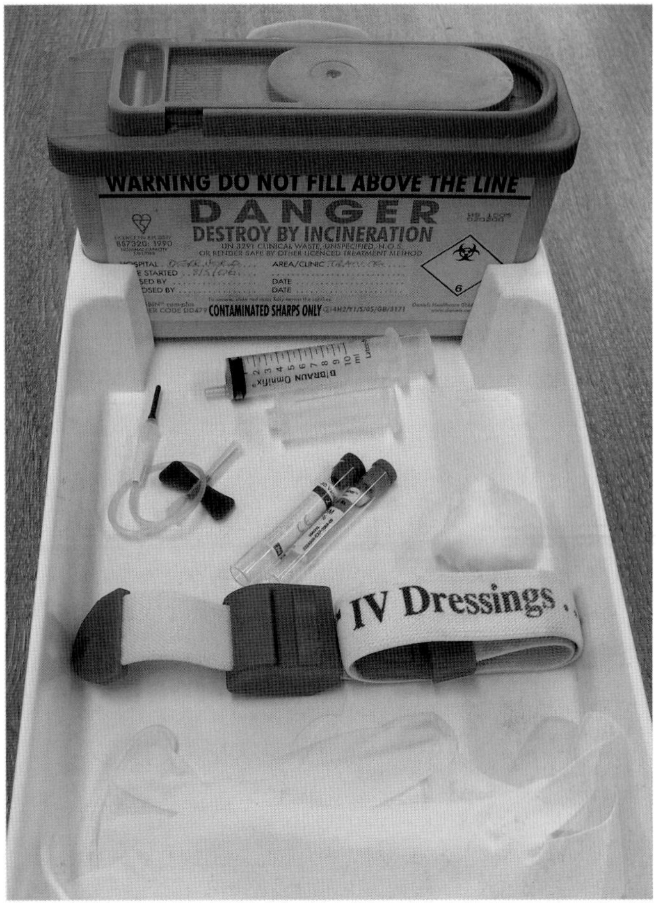

Fig. 27.7 • Venepuncture equipment.

less draw on the vein, helping to prevent vein collapse. When a vacuum system needs to be avoided due to small fragile veins, butterfly needles or single-wing needles may be used with a syringe. The required volume of blood should be transferred into the sample tubes with a blood transfer device to prevent inoculation injuries and the blood haemolysing as it is pushed through a second needle (Becton Dickinson Phlebotomy Education Programme 2004). Under no circumstances must a needle be inserted into the rubber stopper, as this creates an increased vacuum in the bottles, causing the potential for the lids to come off.

Tourniquets are used to encourage venous filling and can be used along with other techniques such as asking patients to open and close their fist, lowering the limb below heart level and applying warmth to the area. Tapping of the vein is not recommended, as this may hurt the patient, so gentle massage of the area is advised instead. Tourniquets must be clean and applied 8–10 cm above the site, tight enough to engorge the veins but a radial pulse must still be present; it should not be left in place for any longer than 2–3 min. It should be removed within 1 min when taking the sample, as some results can be affected if it is left on longer (Campbell et al 1999). Rubber gloves should not be used for a tourniquet, as these are uncomfortable for the patient and can cause tissue damage.

ALERT
Tourniquets should not be left in place for any longer than 2–3 min.

Blood volumes, order of draw and mixing guidelines

Although children have a smaller circulating blood volume than adults – approximately 80 mL/kg in infants (Davenport 1996) – it is important to collect sufficient blood to enable tests to be performed (Table 27.1). Blood should be drawn and mixed according to local policy guidelines.

Patients should be identified correctly before commencing the procedure and samples and forms labelled by the bedside to prevent misidentification of the samples.

Infection control

Hands should be cleaned and gloves always worn when taking blood, along with other appropriate universal precautions that may be required (e.g. goggles, aprons). Patients who are a high infection risk should have their samples clearly labelled as such. The use of a syringe as opposed to a closed system may increase the risk of inoculation injury (Higgins 2004).

Needlestick injury

Those undertaking venepuncture may be exposed to a variety of blood-borne viruses due to needlestick injuries, which can occur during and after the procedure. Sharps should be used safely and disposed of carefully. You should also familiarise yourself with local trust inoculation injury policy.

Table 27.1. Maximum amounts of blood to be drawn from patients under 14 years of age

Weight (kg)	Maximum volume at one time (mL)	Maximum amount during 1 month (mL)
2.7–3.5	2.5	23
3.6–4.5	3.5	30
4.6–6.9	5.0	40
7.0–13.9	10.0	60–90
14.0–18.5	10.0	100–130
18.6–27.0	20	140–200
27.1–19.9	25.0	200–400

(After Buckbee 1994, with permission.)

Blood spillage

Blood spillage should be dealt with according to local trust policy.

Complications

Bruising and haematoma can occur as a result of unskilled venepuncture technique or in patients who bleed easily. It can be prevented by correct insertion technique, less movement of the needle while in the vein, correct use of tourniquet and applying pressure following withdrawal of the needle for at least 2 min. Pain can be prevented by the use of appropriate pain relief and anaesthesia, allowing the skin to dry after cleaning with alcohol and avoiding nerves. Arterial puncture can be prevented by accurate assessment and choice of vein (Lavery & Ingram 2005).

Procedures Box 27.1 Venepuncture

Equipment
- Clinically clean tray containing prepared equipment
- Vacutainer needle or Safety-Lok winged infusion set, needle holder or syringe
- Appropriate vacuumed specimen tubes with order-of-draw card
- Sterile dressing or swab for puncture site
- Tourniquet
- Gloves, goggles, aprons as required for universal precaution measures
- Small sharps box to be taken to patient
- Specimen request form

Actions
Identify the patient and explain the procedure.
Check that informed consent is given.

Procedures Box 27.1 Venepuncture—cont'd

Reason *Ensures patient safety and informed consent.*

Action
Allow the patient time to ask questions and discuss previous problems with blood taking.

Reason *Involves the patient in treatment and helps the operator to understand the history, which may affect vein choice.*

Action
Assemble the equipment necessary for venepuncture (including appropriate size blood collection bottles) and check that the area has suitable lighting and privacy.

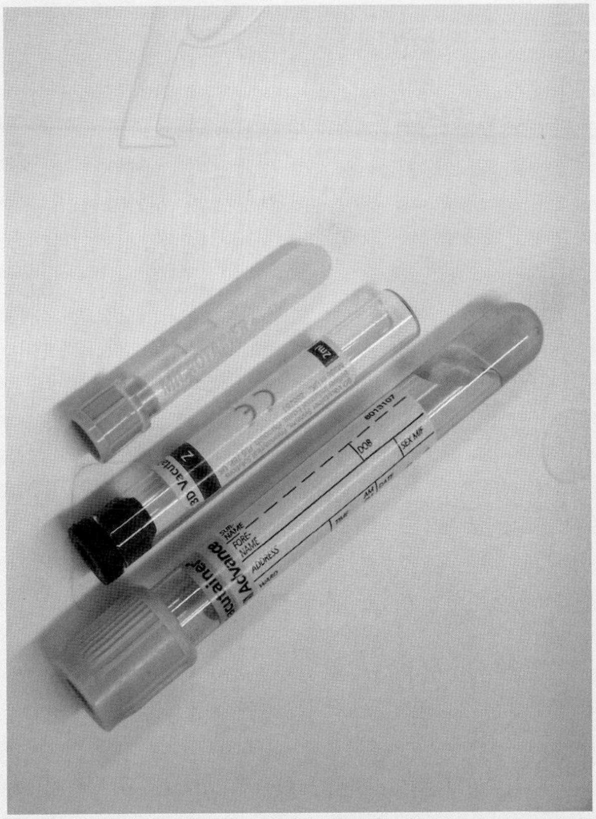

Reason *Reduces time and avoids interruptions.*

Action
Wash hands using soap and water and dry thoroughly, or use an alcohol gel according to infection control guidelines.

Reason *Minimises the risk of infection.*

Action
Check all packaging before opening and prepare the equipment on a clean receptacle.

Reason *Maintains asepsis.*

Actions
Choose which arm to use; avoid the same side where an infusion is present.

Support and/or hold the chosen limb.

Reason *Ensures that both the patient and the operator are comfortable.*

Actions
Apply the tourniquet 8–10 cm above the puncture site.

Ensure that arterial flow is not obstructed.

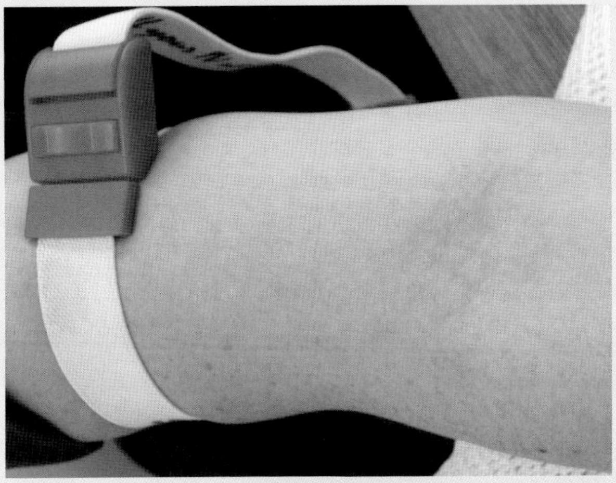

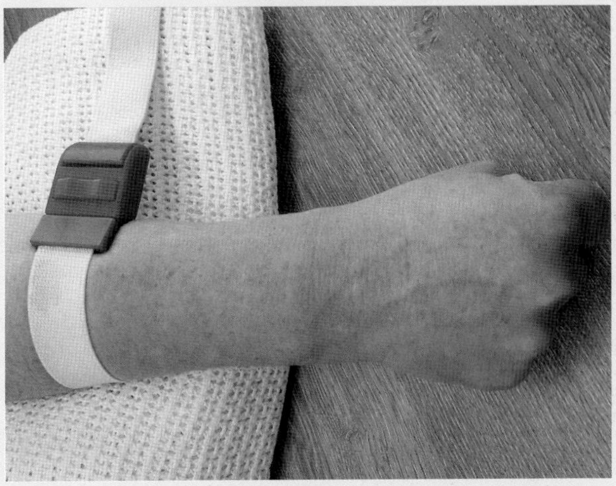

Reasons *Avoids possible contamination of the sample. Aids patient comfort.*

Action
If there is difficulty seeing a suitable vein you may do the following:

- Ask the patient to clench and unclench the fist
- Gently stroke the vein
- Apply warmth to the area.

Reason *Increases the prominence of veins.*

Action
Select a vein and remove the tourniquet until ready to proceed.

Reason *Prolonged application of tourniquet can cause tissue damage and altered blood results.*

Action
Select a suitable device based on vein size and site.

Reason *Reduces trauma.*

Procedures Box 27.1 Venepuncture—cont'd

Action
Gloves and other protective measures should be worn according to local trust policy.

Reasons *Minimises the risk of contamination.*
Fulfils universal precaution measures.

Action
Inspect the device carefully.

Reason *Detects faulty equipment; if present, discard.*

Action
Put on the tourniquet again.

Action
If the patient is immunologically compromised or you are taking blood for blood cultures then clean the skin with a 70% alcohol wipe and allow to dry.

Reason *Prevents infection and contamination of blood cultures.*

Action
Anchor the vein by applying manual traction on the skin below the proposed insertion site.

Reasons *Immobilises the vein.*
Provides counter-tension to facilitate smoother needle entry.

Action
Insert the needle smoothly at an angle of 30°, ensuring that the bevel of the needle is pointing up.

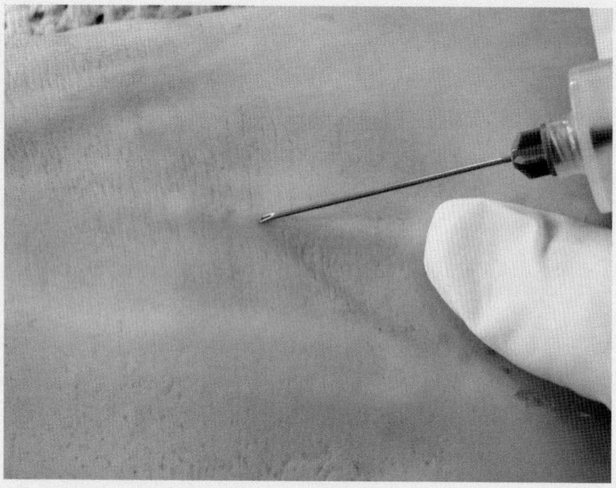

Reason *Facilitates successful venepuncture.*

Action
Do not exert any pressure on the needle.

Reason *Prevents through puncture occurring.*

Actions
Push the Vacutainer bottle on to the needle holder using firm but gentle pressure, ensuring that the needle remains still.

Bottles to be drawn in the order on the order-of-draw card.

Reasons *Avoids contamination of samples.*
Decreases the pressure within the vein.

Action
Release the tourniquet when blood has filled the first Vacutainer tube (i.e. within 1 min).

Reason *Prevents inaccurate results, as leaving the tourniquet in place for more than 1 min can alter certain levels in the blood.*

Action
Place a gauze swab over the puncture site.

Reason *Prevents blood spillage.*

Action
Remove the needle but do not apply pressure until the needle has been withdrawn.

Reason *Prevents pain on removal.*

Action
Dispose of the needle safely into the sharps box taken to the patient.

Reason *Ensures safe disposal of waste and reduces the risk of needlestick injury.*

Action
Apply digital pressure directly over the puncture site until bleeding has stopped – about 2 min, possibly longer with clotting disorders.

Reason *Stops leakage and haematoma formation.*

Actions
When a syringe has been used with a butterfly, transfer the blood to the appropriate specimen bottles as soon as possible, making sure that the correct quantity is placed in each container.

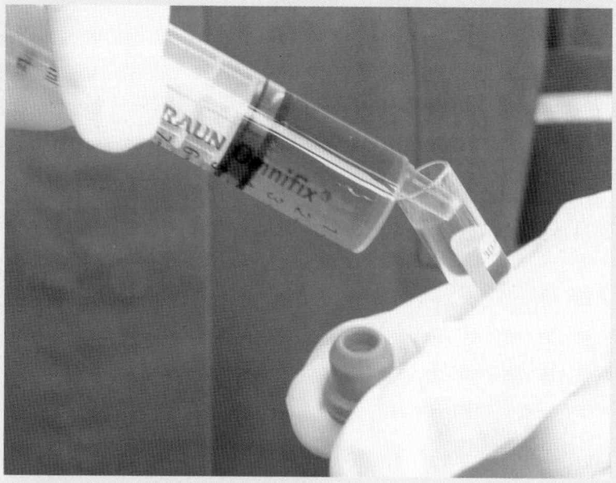

The transfer should be undertaken using a blood transfer device or by removing the tops off the bottles; do not use a needle to transfer.

Reasons *Ensures that an adequate amount is available for each test.*
Prevents inoculation injuries.

Action
Mix well, as directed by local order-of-draw card.

Reason *Ensures that the blood is correctly presented to the laboratory and the patient does not have to have the procedure repeated.*

Action
Label the bottles with relevant details while still at the patient's bedside and place with the form into the correct bag and seal correctly.

Procedures Box 27.1 Venepuncture—cont'd

Reason *Ensures the correct patient identification against each sample taken and aids the correct return of results.*

Action
Inspect the puncture site and apply dressing.

Reasons *Checks that puncture site has sealed.*
Covers the puncture site and prevents the introduction of bacteria.

Action
If adhesive dressing is to be used check if the patient is allergic to it.

Reason *Prevents allergic skin reaction.*

Action
Ensure that the child is comfortable.

Reason *Checks if any further action needs to be taken.*

Action
Discard of waste into appropriate containers.

Reason *Reduces the risk of cross-contamination.*

Action
Reassure and reward the child according to age and developmental stage.

Reason *Rewards the child's cooperation and promotes further cooperation.*

Action
Follow the trust procedure for collection and transport of specimens to the laboratory.

Reason *Ensures that specimens reach their intended destination.*

Action
Document actions in the patient's records.

Reasons *Maintains accurate records.*
Provides a reference in the event of queries and prevents duplication of treatment.

Action
Instigate postprocedural play if child is distressed.

Reason *Reduces the anxiety of patients displaying distress after the procedure.*

Now test your knowledge

- Find out where the order-of-draw information is kept within your place of work.
- How long should the tourniquet remain tightened for and why?
- What techniques could you use to prepare a 3-year-old to have venepuncture?
- What is the inoculation policy in your place of work?

References

Abraxis Pharmaceutical Products (2007) Online. Available: http://www.emla-us.com/

Arrowsmith J, Campbell C (2000) A comparison of local anaesthetics for venepuncture. Archives of Disease in Childhood 82:309–310

Becton Dickinson Phlebotomy Education Programme (2004) Use of the BD Vacutainer System. Serial no. UKv1.0062. Becton Dickinson, Franklin Lakes

Beh T, Splinter W, Kim J (2002) In children, nitrous oxide decreases pain on injection of propofol mixed with lidocaine. Canadian Journal of Anaesthesia 49(10):1061–1063

Blass EM, Hoffmeyer LB (1991) Sucrose as an analgesic for newborn infants. Pediatrics 87(2):215–218

Browne J, Awad I, Plant R, McAdoo J, Shorten G (1999) Topical amethocaine (Ametop™) is superior to EMLA for intravenous cannulation. Canadian Journal of Anaesthesiology 46(11):1014–1018

Bruce E, Franck L (2000) Self-administered nitrous oxide (Entonox®) for the management of procedural pain. Paediatric Nursing 12(7):15–19

Buckbee K (1994) Implementing a pediatric phlebotomy protocol. Medical Laboratory Observer 26(4):32–35

Buckley M, Benfield P (1993) Eutectic lidocaine/prilocaine cream. A review of the topical anaesthetic/analgesic efficacy of a eutectic mixture of local anaesthetics (EMLA®). Drugs 46(1):126–151

Campbell H, Carrington M, Limber C (1999) A practical guide to venepuncture and management of complications. British Journal of Nursing 8(7):426–431

Carbajal R, Veerapen S, Couderc S, Jugie M, Ville Y (2003) Analgesic effect of breast feeding in term neonates: randomized controlled trial. British Medical Journal 326(7379):13

Cohen E, Holubkov R (1997) Vapocoolant spray is equally effective as EMLA cream in reducing immunization pain in school-aged children. Pediatrics 100(6):5

Das B, Sharma A (2002) Acquired brachial arteriovenous fistula in an ex premature infant. Clinical Pediatrics 41(2):131–132

Davenport M (1996) Paediatric fluid balance. Care of the Critically Ill 12(1):26–31

DeJong P, Verburg MP, Lillieborg S (1990) EMLA® cream versus ethylchloride spray: a comparison of the analgesic efficacy in children. European Journal of Anaesthesiology 7(6):473–481

Duff AJA (2003) Incorporating psychological approaches into routine paediatric venepuncture. Archives of Disease in Childhood 88:931–937

Gall O, Annequin D, Benoit G, Van Glabeke F (2001) Adverse events of premixed nitrous oxide and oxygen for procedural sedation in children. Lancet 358(9292):1514–1515

Goren Laufer J, Yativ N, Kuint J et al (2001) Transillumination of the palm for venepuncture in infants. Pediatric Emergency Care 17(2):130–131

Gray L, Watt L, Blass EM (2000) Skin-to-skin contact is analgesic in healthy newborns. Pediatrics 105:e14

Gray L, Miller LW, Philipp BL (2002) Breastfeeding is analgesic in healthy newborns. Pediatrics 109:590–593

Higgins D (2004) Practical procedures – venepuncture. Nursing Times 100(39):30–31

Lavery I, Ingram P (2005) Venepuncture: best practice. Nursing Standard 19(49):55–65

Nursing and Midwifery Council (2004) The code of professional conduct. NMC London

Nursing and Midwifery Council (2005) Guidelines for records and eecord-keeping. NMC London

Stevens B, Yamada J, Ohlsson A (2001) Sucrose analgesia in newborn infants undergoing painful procedures (Cochrane review). Cochrane Library issue 3. Update Software, Oxford

Stevens B, Yamada J, Ohlsson A (2004) Sucrose for analgesia in newborn infants undergoing painful procedures. Cochrane Database of Systematic Reviews issue 3, article no. CD001069. DOI: 10.1002/14651858.CD001069.pub2

Taddio A, Stevens B, Craig K et al (1997) Efficacy and safety of lidocaine–prilocaine cream for pain during circumcision. New England Journal of Medicine 336(17):1197–1201

Vessey J, Carlson KL, McGill J (1994) Use of distraction with children during an acute pain experience. Nursing Research 43(6):369–372

28

Blood glucose monitoring

Philomena Morrow

This chapter aims to present a review of the principles of good technique when monitoring blood glucose levels in children and young people with diabetes mellitus. The main source of reference is the National Institute for Clinical Excellence clinical guidelines (2004), as they address the diagnosis and management of children and young people with type 1 diabetes from a rigorous evidence-based perspective.

Self-management of diabetes is the ultimate goal for all children and young people and their families (Morrow 2006). Self-monitoring of blood glucose allows for rapid and accurate measurement. All diabetic management regimens and self-management skills rely on frequent blood glucose monitoring. Blood glucose varies at different times of the day, as levels are affected by a variety of factors including time since last meal, the content of meals and exercise. Preprandial blood glucose monitoring is recommended in patients who alter their insulin dose according to their blood glucose level, because this is when the bolus insulin dose is given.

Children and young people with newly diagnosed type 1 diabetes should be offered a structured programme of education covering the aims of insulin therapy, the delivery of insulin, self-monitoring of blood glucose, the effects of diet, physical activity and illness affecting glycaemia content, and the detection and management of hypoglycaemia (Morrow 2006).

LINK CHAPTER **29**

Blood glucose testing lowers glycaemia haemoglobin (National Institute for Clinical Excellence 2004). There is a significant decrease in haemoglobin A1c (Hb_{A1c}) following training in blood glucose testing compared with urine glucose testing (National Institute for Clinical Excellence 2004).

Optimal glycaemia control can be assessed and maintained only by frequent and accurate blood glucose monitoring. Children and young people with type 1 diabetes and their families should be informed that the target for long-term glycaemia control is an Hb_{A1c} level of less than 7.5% without frequent disabling hypoglycaemia, and that their package of care should be designed to attempt to achieve this. They should be encouraged to use blood glucose measurements for short-term monitoring of glycaemic control, because this is associated with reduced levels of glycated haemoglobin. Optimal targets for short-term glycaemic control are a preprandial blood glucose level of 4–8 mmol/L and a postprandial blood glucose level of less than 10 mmol/L (National Institute for Clinical Excellence 2004).

The development of memory monitors has shown that patients with diabetes often make incomplete or incorrect recordings of blood glucose values in their diary records. A continuous monitor with a memory and further training in blood glucose testing may aid patients who make recording errors (National Institute for Clinical Excellence 2004). Severe haemolysis of blood samples may affect readings from some monitors, and the use of small sample volumes can lead to erroneously low readings with most models of monitors. Other technological influences and clinical conditions (e.g. low temperature) may sometimes affect results. These findings suggest that there is a need for formal training and updating skills in the use of monitors so that accurate results may be obtained (National Institute for Clinical Excellence 2004).

Frequency of self-monitoring of blood glucose testing

Self-monitoring of blood glucose provides information on glucose levels during the day, but marked glycaemia excursions can be missed in periods when no glucose level is taken. Hb_{A1c} was significantly lower when patients performed glucose testing four or more times a day compared with twice a day (National Institute for Clinical Excellence 2004).

Glycated haemoglobin testing

When there is a high amount of glucose in the blood some of it gets attached to the haemoglobin. At any particular time the amount that is attached shows the amount of glucose that has been in the blood over past 6–12 weeks.

The part with the glucose is called Hb_{A1c}, and this is what is measured with the aim to maintain the Hb_{A1c} level under 7.5%. (Tests for Hb_{A1c} should be carried out two to four times a year.) Children and young people with Hb_{A1c} over 9.5% should be offered extra help to improve glucose control.

To try to keep to targets, children and young people should be taught how to adjust their insulin and diet. How often someone should check his or her blood glucose depends on individual circumstances. Checking before meals and at bedtime is encouraged, and occasionally at night-time, and patients should adjust their insulin if they need to. If unwell they should check blood glucose more than four times a day.

Educational requirements in relation to blood glucose monitoring should be adopted to suit the needs of the child and family and provided at a rate that is in keeping with what suits them (McEvilly 2003). When being taught the practical skill they need to know the importance of the procedure and how to interpret the results (Denial 2006). It is vital that the principles of performing a capillary blood glucose measurement are followed both within the acute care setting and during patient and carer education (Denial 2006). Before meals, aim for blood glucose between 4 and 8 mmol/L, and blood glucose 2 h after meals less than 10 mmol/L.

Prior to undertaking blood glucose monitoring it is important to prepare the child and family for the procedure to help alleviate any distress that they may experience. All equipment necessary must be made available (Fig. 28.1). The monitor code and test strips must be the same, so it is vital that codes are checked for compatibility (Fig. 28.2). The manufacturer provides detailed step-by-step instructions on quality control checks, which must be strictly adhered to and carried out prior to undertaking monitoring. If a meter detects a malfunction it will display the error message and an appropriate symbol. Treatment decisions cannot be made based on an error message. A quality control check must be repeated as well as the procedure. It is important to realise that the blood glucose result may be extremely high and above the system's reading range. If this confirms how a child feels or appears then the doctor must be contacted immediately.

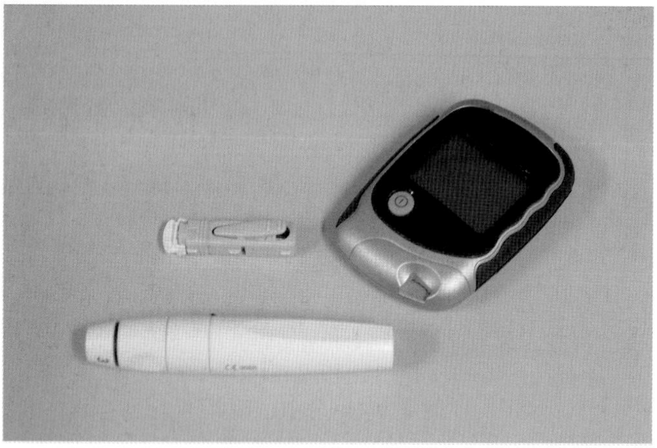

Fig. 28.1 • Equipment required for blood glucose monitoring.

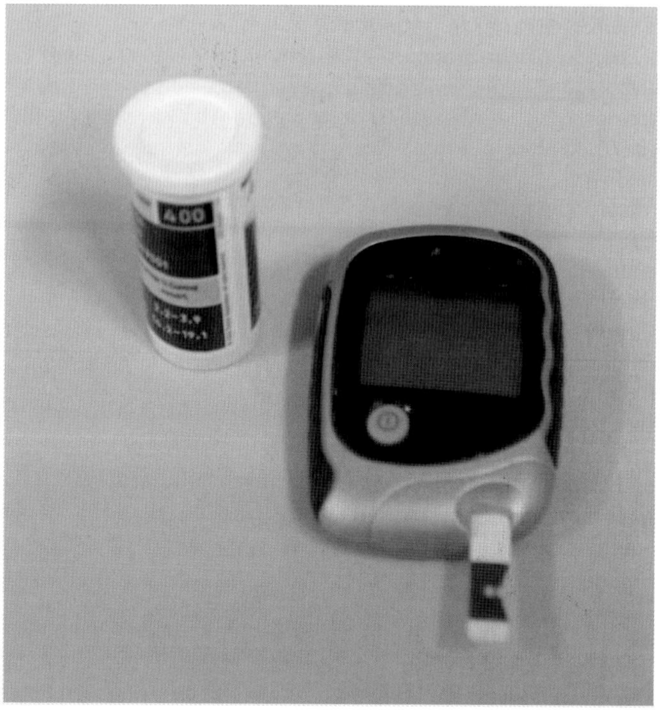

Fig. 28.2 • It is important to check the test strip code with the monitor code.

Procedures Box 28.1 Blood glucose monitoring

Action
Carry out a quality control check on the monitor according to the manufacturer's instructions.

Reason *Ensures the accuracy of the monitor in recording blood glucose levels.*

Action
Research is needed to investigate the clinical implications of alternative site monitoring, for example the arm as opposed to the finger (National Institute for Clinical Excellence 2004).

Reason *Repeated sampling of previous puncture sites should be avoided.*

Actions
The person taking the blood sample should wash her or his hands and wear gloves.

The child's hands should be thoroughly washed.

Reasons *Prevents cross-infection.*
May measure the sugar content of the child's last meal.

Action
Warm and shake the hands.

Reasons *Increases capillary blood flow, thus making it easier to obtain blood for testing from a warm, well-perused site. The aim is to obtain blood from capillaries located at the junction of the lower dermis and upper subcutaneous tissue.*

Action
With the hand in the downward position prick the fingertip with a lancet and squeeze a drop of blood out of the finger.

Procedures Box 28.1 Blood glucose monitoring—cont'd

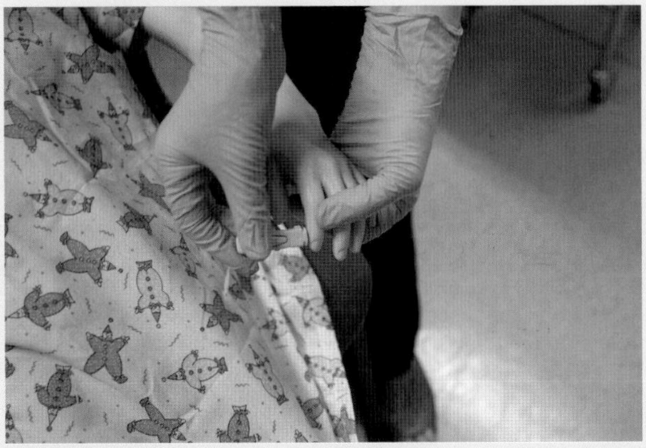

Reason *An incision device with a suitable lancet length should be used.*

Action

Apply gentle pressure.

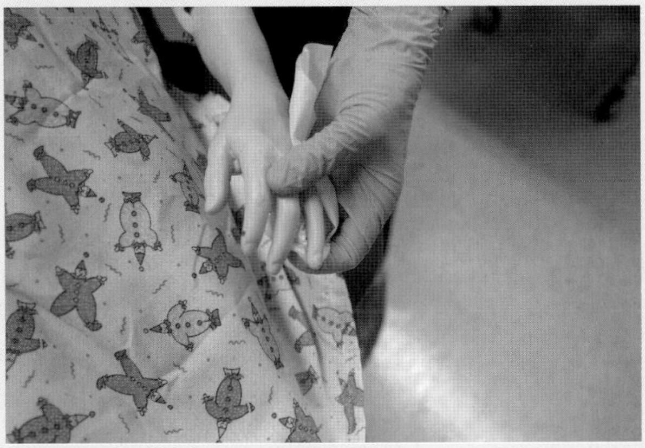

Reason *Encourages good blood flow.*

Actions

Press the finger against the diabetic testing strip; the strip may remain attached to the monitor at this stage – review the manufacturer's instructions.

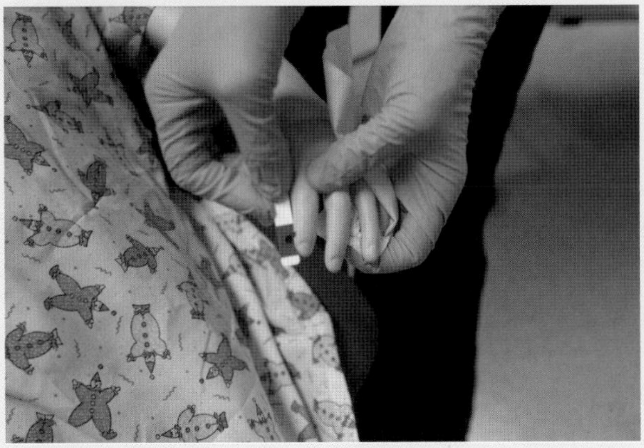

Reasons *Allows measurement of blood glucose with the blood glucose meter.*
When the strip has taken up sufficient blood the meter will bleep.

Actions

The sample should be analysed immediately.

Continue to observe the meter until the final blood result is indicated.

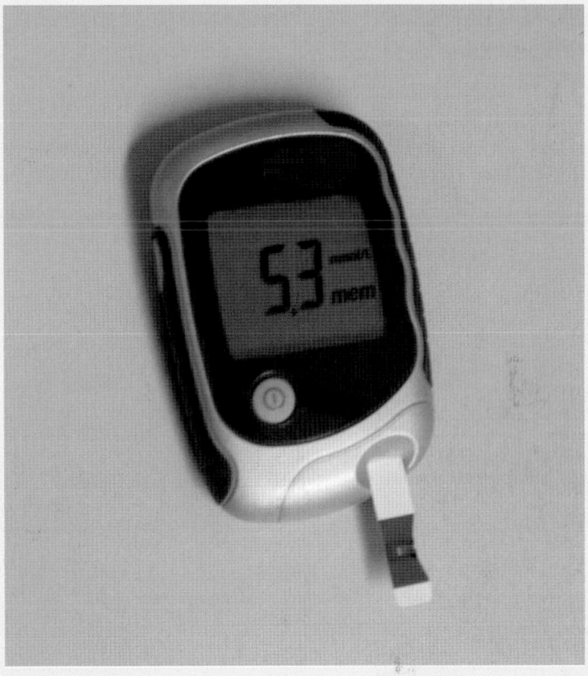

Reason *Avoids glycolysis.*

Action

When sampling is complete apply gentle pressure on the site with a cotton wool ball or swab.

Reason *Stops bleeding.*

Actions

Dispose of used sharps and other equipment appropriately.

Clean the monitor.

Wash your hands.

Reason *To adhere to health and safety regulations.*

Action

Record the level of blood glucose and time of monitoring.

Reasons *To identify the need for interventions.*
To monitor treatment regimens.
To adhere to Nursing and Midwifery Council (2005)guidelines for records and record keeping.

New advances in glucose monitoring

New methods for measuring blood glucose are currently being perfected and include non-invasive, semi-invasive and subcutaneous measuring. Non-invasive methods measure glucose without breaking the skin. Semi-invasive methods measure glucose with a minimal breech to the outer skin layer. Surgical methods measure glucose by means of an implanted device.

Blood glucose monitoring in infants

Clinical correlates of low blood glucose concentrations such as jitteriness, lethargy, pallor, apnoea and altered alertness or tone are non-specific and can occur with a variety of other pathologies (Deshpande & Taplin 2005). In order to assess the glycaemic status in infants accurate, precise and rapid measurements of blood glucose concentrations are needed. It is essential that nurses receive specialised training for this age group and are assessed in their competency to do so.

Now test your knowledge

John is a 12-year-old who has been diagnosed as having type 1 diabetes mellitus for the past 4 years. He enjoys been involved in many sporting activities and feels that his diet is satisfactory and he adheres to his insulin therapy regimen. However, he has been admitted to hospital for investigations for frequent episodes of hypoglycaemia. John has admitted that he monitors his blood glucose level only sometimes. Outline the support that John requires to enable him to recognise the importance of recording his blood glucose. Outline a step-by-step teaching programme to ensure that the procedure of blood glucose monitoring is carried out correctly.

References

Denial M (2006) Chapter 5. In Trigg E, Mohammed T (eds) Practices in children's nursing. Churchill Livingstone, London

Deshpande S, Taplin M (2005) Point of care analysis of blood glucose in infants. Advances in Practice 1(6):199–202

McEvilly A (2003) Chapter 12:6. In Barnes K (ed.) Paediatrics. A clinical guide for nurse practitioners. Butterworth Heinemann, London

Morrow P (2006) Chapter 34. In Glasper A, Richardson JA (eds) Textbook of children's and young people's nursing. Churchill Livingstone, London

National Institute for Clinical Excellence (2004) Type 1 diabetes: diagnosis and management of type 1 diabetes in children and young people. RCOG Press, London

Nursing and Midwifery Council (2005) Guidelines for records and record keeping. NMC, London

Further reading

British Society for Paediatric Endocrinology and Diabetes Online. Available: http://www.bsped.org.uk

Clinical Resource Efficiency Support Team Online. Available: http://www.crestni.org.uk

Department of Health Diabetes National Service Framework. Online. Available: http://www.doh.gov./nsf/diabetes

Diabetes UK Online. Available: http://www.diabetes.org.uk

Endocrine Society Online. Available: http://www.endo-society.org

Journal of Diabetes Nursing Online. Available: http://www.diabetesnursing.com

29

Insulin therapy

Philomena Morrow

This chapter aims to present a review of significant aspects of insulin therapy in the care of the child and young person with type 1 diabetes.

Diabetes mellitus is a chronic, severe metabolic condition. The majority of children in the UK with diabetes have type 1 (Diabetes UK 2005). However, the prevalence of type 2 is increasing in all ages and across races. Children who are obese and come from minority ethnic groups appear to be at higher risk of developing type 2 diabetes (Diabetes UK 2005).

Type 1 diabetes is caused by a cessation of insulin production, which is thought to be the result of an autoimmune response to an infection or some environmental trigger in a child who is born with a genetic risk to this diabetic state. The autoimmune response progressively destroys the beta cells of the islets of Langerhans in the pancreas, where insulin is produced (Morrow 2006). The insulin-producing capacity of the pancreas fails and there evidently is a loss of the body's ability to utilise glucose.

The management of type 1 diabetes mellitus requires a multidisciplinary, family-centred approach whereby the holistic, individual needs of the child and family are provided and supported. Therefore children and young people should receive high-quality specialist care within a service that encourages partnership in decision making, supports them in managing their diabetes and helps them to adopt a healthy lifestyle (Department of Health 2003). This should be evident in an agreed care plan that reflects the child's or young person's developmental needs (Diabetes UK 2005) and is written in an appropriate format and language and, when appropriate, parents should be fully engaged in this process (Department of Health 2003).

LINK CHAPTER **1**

The provision of high-quality information, education and psychological support that facilitates self-management is therefore essential in ensuring that children and young people with diabetes remain in the best possible health and have a good quality of life (National Institute for Clinical Excellence 2004). Improved diabetes control from diagnosis can reduce the incidence of microvascular complications and delay their progression (Diabetes UK 2005).

Insulin injections, blood glucose monitoring and dietary adjustment become part of the everyday management. The support and education provided must recognise difficulties that impact on all family members and empathise with them.

LINK CHAPTER **28**

Insulin therapy

Insulin plays a key role in the regulation of carbohydrate, fat and protein metabolism. It is a polypeptide hormone and is inactivated by gastrointestinal enzymes and therefore must be administered by injection, the dosage of which will vary according to age, weight, dietary intake, exercise and stress levels. During adolescence, insulin requirements increase due to insulin resistance (Morrow 2006). The higher doses are reduced at the end of growth and puberty. Insulin is a ready-to-use solution that is measured in units. The strength of insulin used is 100 U/mL.

LINK CHAPTER **1**

ALERT

Insulin has the potential to cause serious harm. Accuracy in interpreting the insulin prescription, understanding the information on the insulin label, selecting the correct syringe to measure insulin for administration and checking patient identity is essential. A second practitioner (one of whom is a registered nurse) should perform an independent second check of insulin doses. The second check must include all aspects of administration, irrespective of the route or method of administration; be conducted from preparation through to actual administration of the prepared dose to the correct patient and documentation of administration; and include the use of any infusion devices and calculations when applicable (Northern Ireland Medicines Governance Team 2005).

All staff involved in the administration of insulin should receive training in the use of the insulin syringe and in the dangers of using any other type of syringe to administer insulin.

All staff involved in administration of insulin should receive practical training in how to draw up a dose from a vial correctly using an insulin syringe and how to prepare a dose correctly using an injection device, for example a prefilled injection pen (Northern Ireland Medicines Governance Team 2005).

Administration is generally twice daily for the majority of children and young people and by subcutaneous injection with a 5- to 8-mm needle and syringe or pen injector. Mixtures of insulin preparations may be required, and appropriate combinations have to be determined for the individual child (British National Formulary 2006). The insulin regimen should therefore be tailored to achieve the best possible glycaemic control without disabling hypoglycaemia (Scottish Intercollegiate Guidelines Network 2001). Every nurse should know the onset, peak and duration of the insulin being administered (Table 29.1), as well as signs and symptoms of hypoglycaemia and hyperglycaemia (Craig 2005).

The insulin regimen may be a combination of short-acting soluble insulin with isophane intermediate insulin twice daily. A multiple-injection regimen of a soluble or rapid-acting insulin before meals and a long-acting insulin at bedtime may be suitable for some children and young people (*British National Formulary* 2006).

Table 29.1. The three main types of insulin preparation

Insulin type	Action	Examples of preparations
Short-acting	Rapid onset of action (10–60 min) with peak action between 2 and 4 h with subcutaneous injection. Intravenous administration onset of action is approximately 5 min with a 30-min duration.	Soluble insulin: • Hypurin • Actrapid • Velosulin • Humulin • Insuman • NovoRapid • Humalog
Immediate-acting	Onset of action with subcutaneous injection approximately 1–2 h, maximal effect 4–12 h, with duration of 16–35 h.	Isophane insulin: • Hypurin bovine isophane, porcine isophane • Pork Insulatard • Insulatard • Humulin 1 • Insuman-Basal Biphasic insulins (premixed preparations of short-acting and intermediate-acting insulin), for example: • Humalog Mix 25 • Humalog Mix 50 • Hypurin Porcine 30/70 Mix • Pork Mixtard 30 • Mixtard 10, 20, 30, 40, 50 • Humulin M3 • Insuman Comb 15, 25, 50
Long-acting	Onset and duration as for intermediate-acting insulins.	Insulin detemir: • Levemir Insulin glargine: • Lantus Insulin zinc suspension: • Hypurin Bovine Lente • Monotard Insulin zinc suspension (crystalline): • Ultratard Protamine zinc insulin: • Hypurin Bovine Protamine Zinc

(From *British National Formulary* 2006.)

Administration of insulin

Diabetes UK (2005) recommends that all children and young people have access to the correct insulin type and dose and access to appropriate meters.

Insulin is generally given by subcutaneous injection half an hour prior to a meal. Rapid-acting insulin should be given immediately before or after a meal.

Injection devices

Pens hold the insulin in a cartridge and a meter presets the required dose. This administration method is convenient to use and is now more popular than syringe and needle. However, not all insulin preparations are available in cartridge form, so for some U-100 (Fig. 29.1) or U-50 (Fig. 29.2) insulin syringes and needles have to be the route of administration.

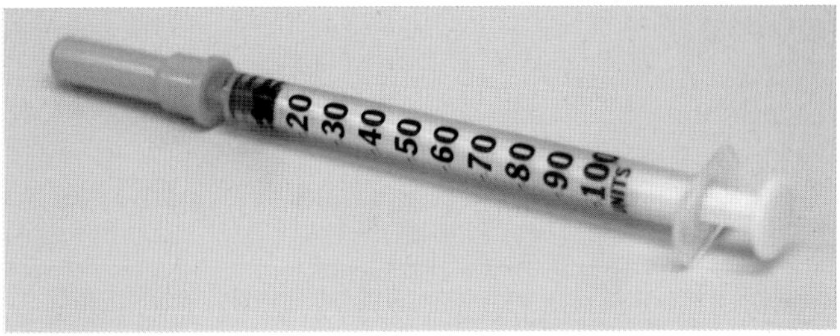

Fig. 29.1 • Standard U-100 insulin syringe.

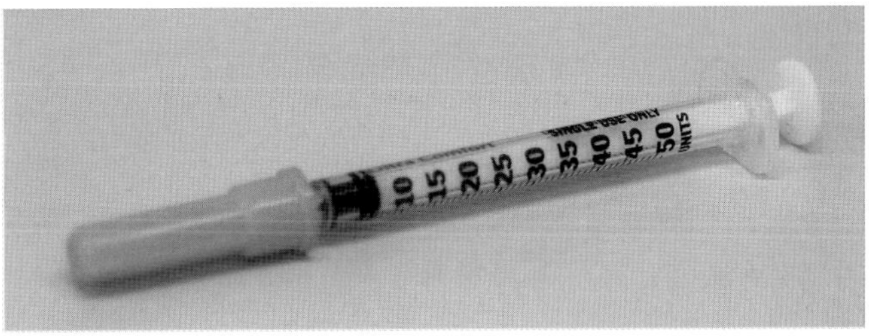

Fig. 29.2 • Lo-dose U-50 insulin syringe.

Procedures Box 29.1 Preparation for and management of the administration of insulin with a U-100 or U-50 syringe

Actions
Adhere to policy for safe administration of medicines (Department of Health, Social Services and Public Safety 2004, Nursing and Midwifery Council 2005).

Each stage of insulin preparation and administration must be checked by two nurses.

Reason *Ensures the safety of the child by adhering to standards for good practice.*

Action
Identify and prepare all equipment and the medical prescription and monitoring chart for insulin.

Reason *It is the nurse's responsibility to be familiar with the different types of insulin and to use a drug reference to prevent medication errors.*

Actions
Insulin type: carefully read the label and compare it to the drug order.

Check that it has not passed its expiry date.

Reasons *The insulin label includes the brand and generic names, supply dosage or concentration, storage instructions and expiration date; insulin action times and insulin species (e.g. human insulin) are drug label components.*
The following letters are important visual identifiers when selecting insulin type (Picker 2004):

- *R: rapid-acting (regular, lispro)*
- *L: intermediate-acting (Lente)*
- *N: neutral protamine Hagedorn*
- *U: long-acting (Ultralente insulin).*

Actions
Open vials of insulin are stored at room temperature, unopened vials stored in the refrigerator.

Once a vial is opened it should be used with in 30 days, and this is to be recorded on the label.

Reason *Insulin is a protein and tends to break down and become ineffective if wrongly stored.*

Action
Syringe: U-100 or U-50.

Reason *Insulin is given with an insulin syringe that requires no calculation; the number of units of insulin ordered by the physician equals the number of units that are displayed on the insulin syringe.*

Action
Needle: 5 or 8 mm.

Reason *A 5-mm needle reduces the risk of intramuscular injection in children with little subcutaneous fat.*

Action
Use a sharps disposal box.

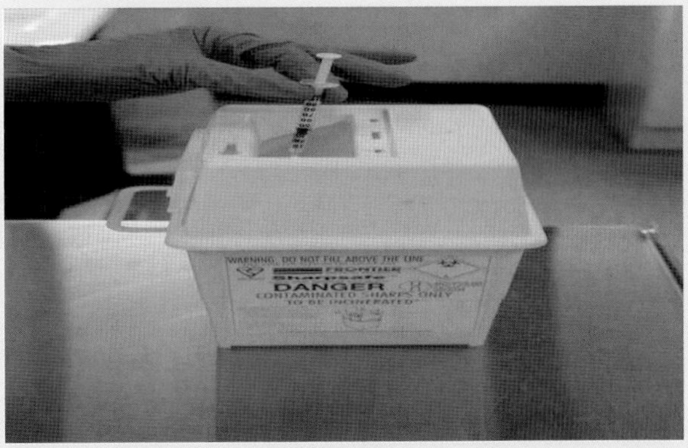

Reason *To adhere to health and safety regulations.*

Action
Gently roll the vial of insulin between the palms of the hands several times.

Procedures Box 29.1 Preparation for and management of the administration of insulin with a U-100 or U-50 syringe—cont'd

Reason *Mixes the insulin completely.*

Action
Wipe the top of the insulin vial with an alcohol wipe and allow to dry.

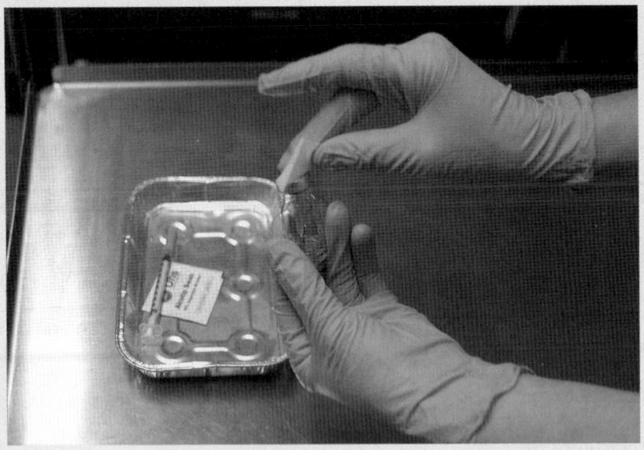

Reason *Reduces the risk of infection.*

Action
Remove the needle cover and, holding the vial, push the needle through so that the tip is not suspended in the solution.

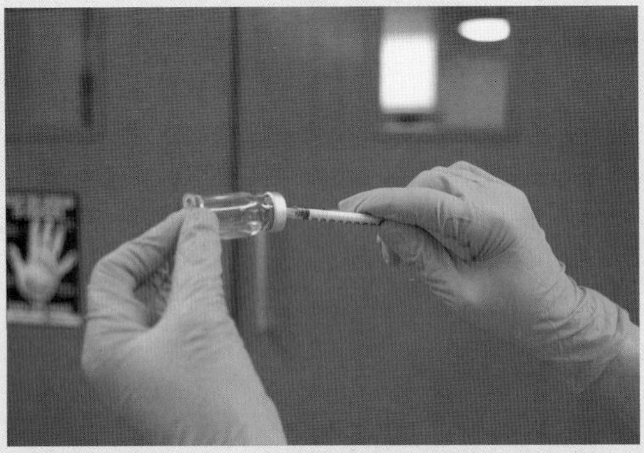

Action
Withdraw the piston of the syringe so that air in the vial is drawn up to equal the units that are going to be injected.

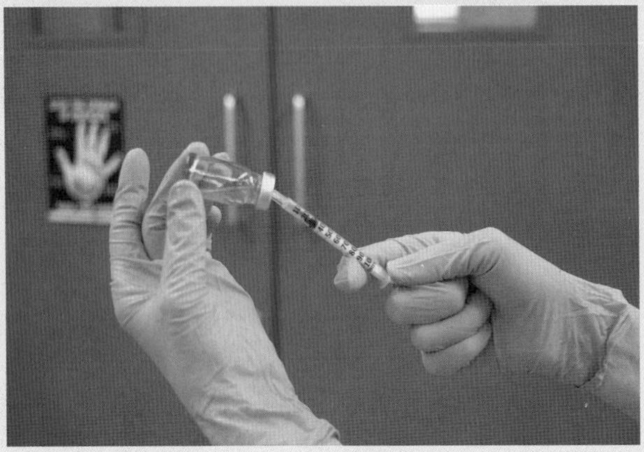

Reason *Draws air into the syringe that has not been exposed to the atmosphere, thus preventing the risk of contaminating the solution.*

Action
Without withdrawing the needle reinject the air back into the insulin vial.

Reason *Facilitates movement of solution from vial to syringe.*

Action
Turn the bottle up and position the needle within the solution, and pull back the piston gently until the required dose of insulin is measured.

Action
Remove air bubbles by tapping the syringe to allow them to rise to the top, thus they can be pushed back into the vial.

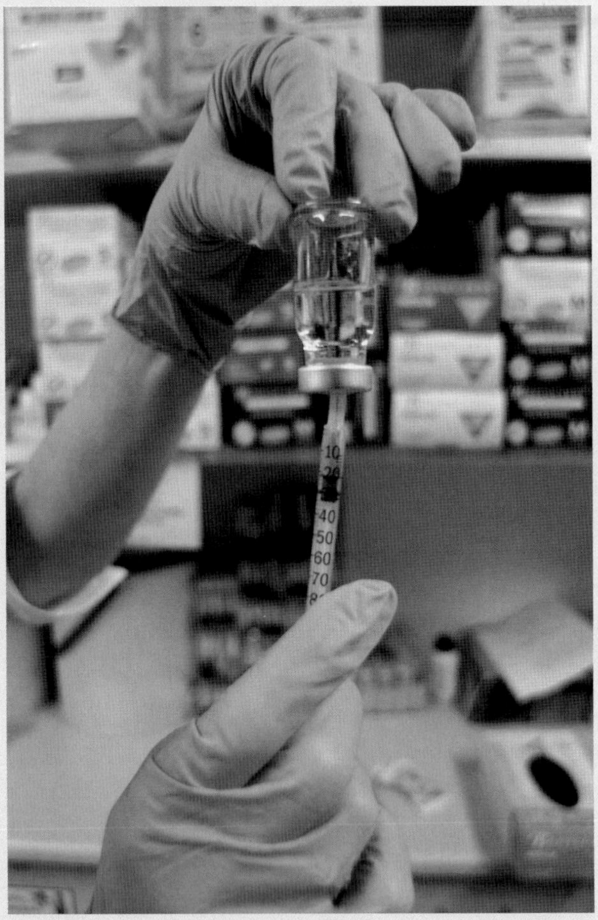

Reason *Air bubbles may increase pain and discomfort if injected into the site.*

Action
Recheck that the correct dose has been drawn up before removing the needle.

Action
When two insulins have to be mixed in the syringe it is important to draw up the regular insulin or rapid-acting analogue before the intermediate-acting insulin.

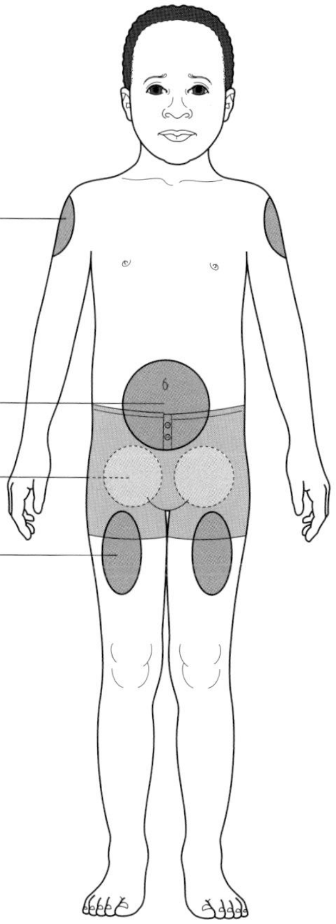

Fig. 29.3 • Main insulin injection sites.

Insulin injection technique

Significant research studies focusing on insulin injection technique have indicated that the correct technique may be as important for reliable insulin absorption and optimal glucose control as the type and dose of insulin delivered. Proper technique ensures that the injection is administered subcutaneously, and this requires individualisation (vertical or at an angle) in children, as there may be differences in subcutaneous thickness. Boys over 14 years old had statistically significantly thinner subcutaneous tissue at all injection sites than age-matched girls (Shin & Kim 2006).

To ensure the most reliable and consistent absorption of insulin, injections should therefore be made into subcutaneous adipose tissue. There is a difference in absorption rate and duration of different insulins when injected into subcutaneous fat and muscle. Intramuscular injection speeds up absorption and can lead to unexpected hypoglycaemia (King 2003, Strauss et al 2002). In some children intramuscular injections of insulin increases pain perceptions.

Insulin injection sites (Fig. 29.3)

Insulin is absorbed at different rates from different sites, so routine is required for consistent absorption. Insulin works faster when injected near the stomach and slower when injected into the thigh or buttocks. Injection into the arms or stomach is

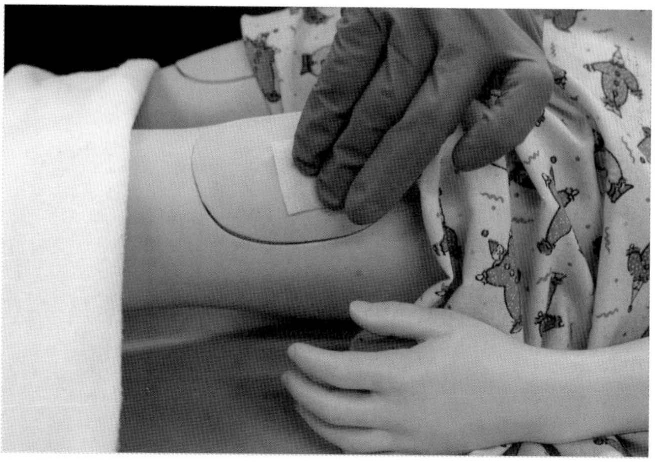

Fig. 29.4 • Cleaning the injection site with alcohol.

recommended in the morning and legs and buttocks in the evening (Barnes 2003).

It is advised to rotate sites to avoid damage to muscles and to prevent subcutaneous atrophy (Karch 2006). Absorption of insulin is impaired in lipohypertropic tissue, yielding a 25% lower plasma insulin (Johansson et al 2005).

If the skin is to be cleaned using alcohol (Fig. 29.4) and other disinfecting agents these must be allowed to evaporate before injection (Royal College of Paediatrics and Child Health 2002).

Injection technique

- Lift up the area of skin to ensure that this is a subcutaneous injection (Figs 29.5–29.6).
- Inject at a 90° or 45° angle as determined by subcutaneous thickness and depress the plunger of the syringe at a slow, steady rate (Fig. 29.7).
- When the plunger has been fully depressed wait 10 s before removing the needle and then release the lifted skin fold.

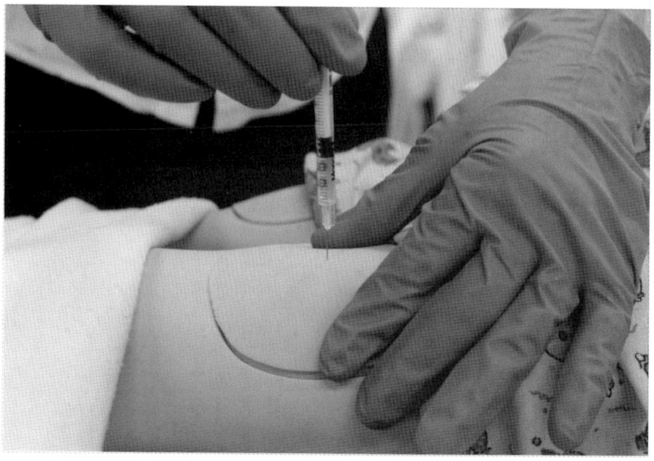

Fig. 29.5 • Preparing to inject the insulin.

- Dispose of sharps as advised and other equipment appropriately.
- Attend to hand hygiene.

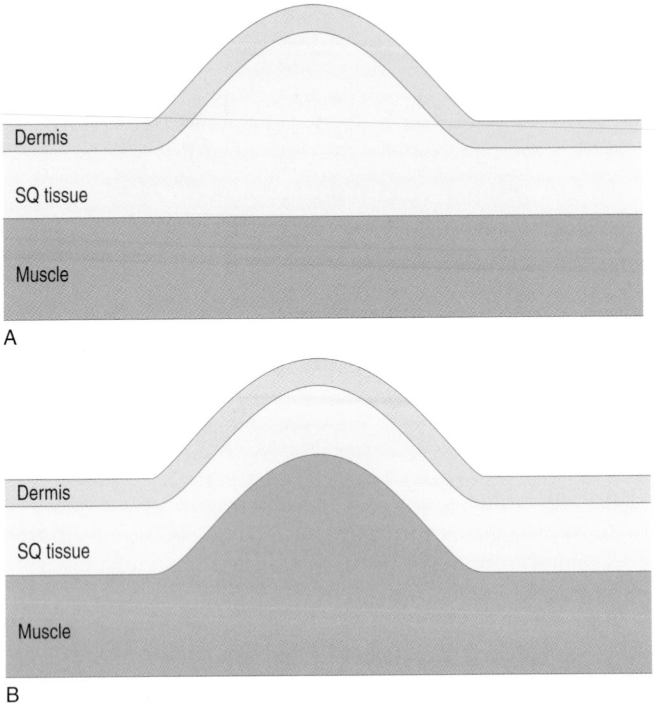

Fig. 29.6 • (**A**) Correct pinch. (**B**) Incorrect pinch.

Insulin pen injector

The insulin pen injector has at one end a small needle; on the other is a plunger that is pressed to deliver the insulin. A dial on the cartridge allows the desired dosage of insulin to be selected (Fig. 29.8).

Insulin pen with needle attached

Prior to administration of insulin via this method the same checking procedures are required as for administration by the U-100 or U-50 syringe and needle.

Intravenous administration

Children and young people with ketosis, hyperglycaemia, vomiting and dehydration require to be admitted to hospital, where their condition can be assessed and managed. Treatment with insulin is essential to return the blood sugar level to normal limits and prevent further lipolysis and ketogenesis. Insulin should be given intravenously while at the same time dehydration and electrolyte imbalances are corrected (Diabetes UK 2005). Guidelines for the management of diabetic ketoacidosis may be reviewed at the website of the British Society for Paediatric Endocrinology and Diabetes (2007).

Continuous subcutaneous infusion

Continuous subcutaneous infusion of short-acting insulin is recommended by the National Institute for Clinical Excellence

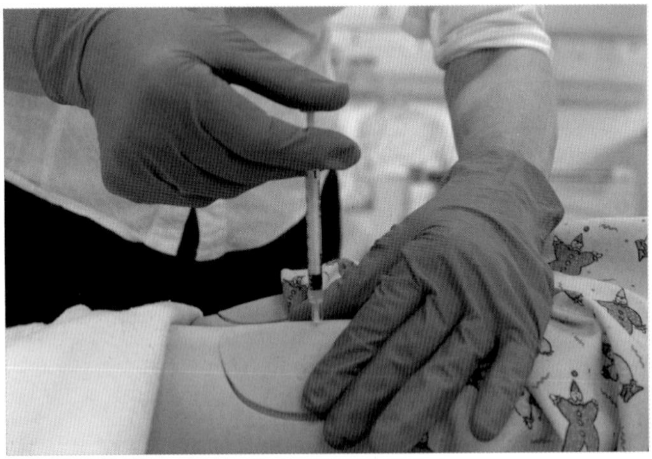

Fig. 29.7 • Inject the insulin at a slow, steady rate.

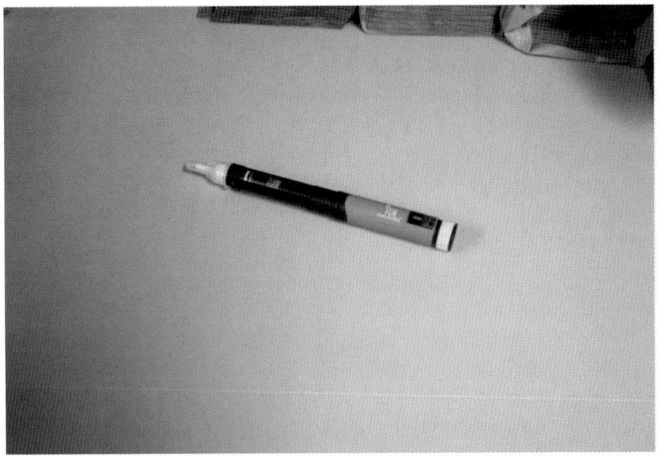

Fig. 29.8 • An insulin pen injector.

Procedures Box 29.2 Injection technique using a pen device

Actions
Remove the cap from the pen and ensure that the insulin it contains is adequately suspended.

Dial the required insulin dose by turning the dose selector until the dose arrow points to the required insulin dose.

Action
Attach a new needle to the pen and remove the protective cap.

Reason *To adhere to health and safety practices*

Procedures Box 29.2 Injection technique using a pen device—cont'd

Actions
Expel any air from the system.

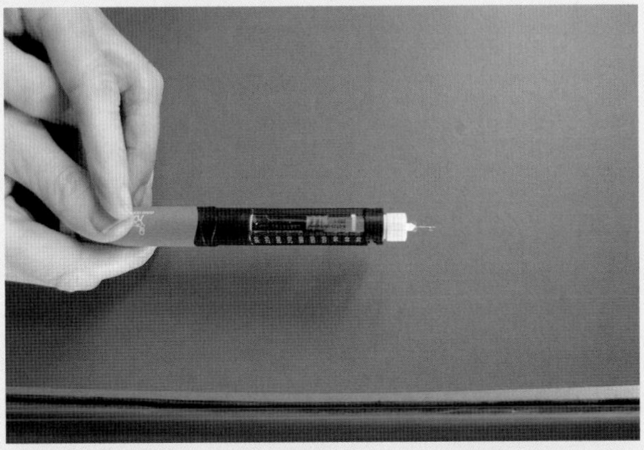

Press the injection button so that insulin is expelled through the needle tip.

Reason *Ensures that the pen and needle are working properly and are ready for use.*

Actions
Insert the needle using the recommended technique.

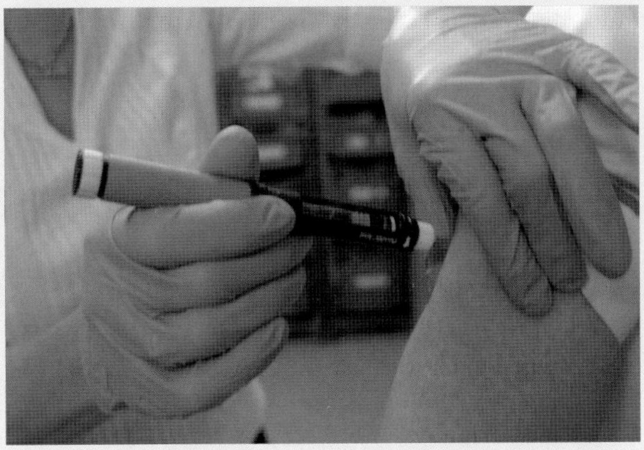

Inject the full dose by depressing the push button fully.

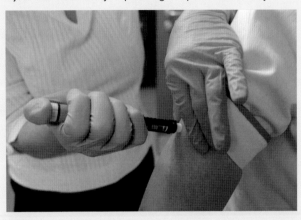

Action
Wait for at least 10 s before withdrawing the needle.

Reason *Ensures that the full dose of insulin has been injected.*

Action
Detach and discard the needle using the needle remover into the sharps box and replace the pen cap on to the pen.

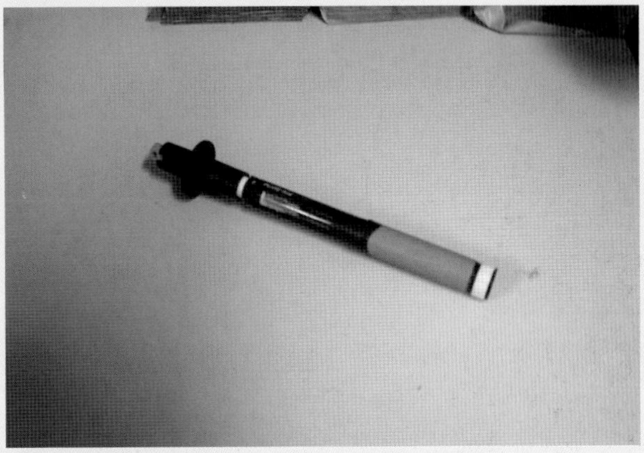

Reason *To adhere to health and safety practices and prevent contamination.*

(2004) for children who suffer repeated or unpredictable hypoglycaemia despite optimal multiple-injection regimens. Such intensified regimens need more intensive education and clinical support, both of which must be available if these treatment regimens are offered and to be effective (Diabetes UK 2005).

PUMP management

All administration devices and techniques require training, advice and supervision from an experienced healthcare team. PUMP is a network of multidisciplinary healthcare professionals with experience in pump use and can be contacted through their website (PUMP 2007).

Inhaled insulin

Inhaled insulin is a rapid-acting, dry powder human insulin. It is administered via the pulmonary route using a specifically designed handheld inhaler device. This allows insulin to be delivered to the alveoli in the lungs, from where it is absorbed into the bloodstream. Recommendations for its use are undergoing appraisal by the National Institute for Clinical Excellence.

Needle phobia

Children and young people who present with a needle phobia can have difficulty in adhering to treatment regimens. It is important that this condition is recognised and strategies implemented to reduce the discomfort associated with frequent subcutaneous injections. To help with needle phobia a simple device such as Pen Mate (Fig. 29.9) hides the needle from view (Morrow 2006).

The alternative methods of insulin delivery as mentioned above will be a major support to this treatment group. However, until such therapies are available play interventions should be undertaken by a play specialist or children's nurse who has attended a needle phobia workshop and has demonstrated competency in practical assessment. Stages of needle play may be viewed on the website of the National Association of Hospital Play Staff (2007).

LINK CHAPTER 3

Now test your knowledge

A 6-year-old girl has been diagnosed as having type 1 diabetes mellitus. Discuss the process necessary to educate the child and parents about insulin therapy.

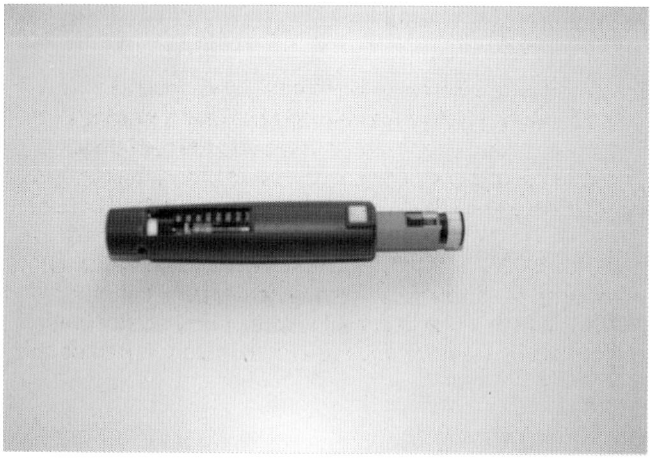

Fig. 29.9 • Pen Mate.

References

Barnes K (2003) Paediatrics. A clinical guide for nurse practitioners. Butterworth Heinemann, London

British National Formulary (2006) British National Formulary. BMJ Publishing Group, London

British Society for Paediatric Endocrinology and Diabetes (2007) Online. Available: http://www.bsped.org.uk/dka.htm

Craig GP (2005) Clinical calculations made easy, 3rd edn. Lippincott Williams & Wilkins, Philadelphia

Department of Health (2003) National Service Framework for Diabetes. Clinical care of children and young people with diabetes. Department of Health, London

Department of Health, Social Services and Public Safety (2004) Use and control of medicines, 2nd edn. DHSSPS, Belfast

Diabetes UK (2005) Resources to support the delivery of care for children and young people with diabetes. Diabetes UK, London

Johansson UB, Amsberg S, Wredling R, Arnqvist HJ, Lins PE (2005) Impaired absorption of insulin aspart from lipohypertrophic injection sites. Diabetes Care 28:2025–2027

Karch AM (2006) Focus on nursing pharmacology, 3rd edn. Lippincott Williams & Wilkins, Philadelphia

King L (2003) Subcutaneous insulin injection technique. Nursing Standard 17(34):45–51

Morrow P (2006) Chapter 34. In Glasper A, Richardson J (eds) A textbook of children's and young people's nursing. Churchill Livingstone, London

National Association of Hospital Play Staff (2007) Online. Available: http://www.nahps.org.uk/needle.htm

National Institute for Clinical Excellence (2004) Type 1 diabetes: diagnosis and management of type 1 diabetes in children and young people. RCOG Press, London

Northern Ireland Medicines Governance Team (2005) Recommendations to improve the safe use of insulin in secondary care in Northern Ireland. DHSSPS, Belfast

Nursing and Midwifery Council (2005) Guidelines for records and record keeping. NMC, London

Picker GD (2004) Dosage calculations, 7th edn. Thomson Delmar, Scarborough

PUMP (2007) Online. Available: http://www.insulin-pump

Royal College of Paediatrics and Child Health (2002) Position statement on injection technique. RCPCH, London

Scottish Intercollegiate Guidelines Network (2001) Management of diabetes. Section 2: children and young people with diabetes. Royal College of Physicians, Edinburgh

Shin H, Kim MJ (2006) Issues and innovations in nursing practice. Journal of Advanced Nursing 54(1):29–34

Strauss K, De Gols H, Hannet I, Partanen TM, Frid A (2002) Apan – European epidemiological study of insulin technique in patients with diabetes. Practical Diabetes International 19(3):71–76

Further reading

British Society for Paediatric Endocrinology and Diabetes Online. Available: http://www.bsped.org.uk

Clinical Resource Efficiency Support Team Online. Available: http://www.crestni.org.uk

Department of Health Diabetes National Service Framework. Online. Available: http://www.doh.gov./nsf/diabetes

Diabetes UK Online. Available: http://www.diabetes.org.uk

Endocrine Society Online. Available: http://www.endo-society.org

Journal of Diabetes Nursing Online. Available: http://www.diabetesnursing.com

30 Blood gas sampling and analysis

Zoe Wood

Arterial blood gas (ABG) analysis has become an integral part of the child health nurse's role when caring for the critically ill child. Close observation of blood pH from an ABG sample can alert the nurse to any disturbances in the pH level, which could result in abnormal respiratory and cardiac function, derangement in blood clotting and drug metabolism. It can give essential information about:

- A, oxygenation
- B, ventilation
- C, circulation (Cooper 2005).

With the appropriate training a nurse can learn the clinical skills required to obtain an ABG sample, use a gas analyser to obtain the results and finally interpret the results, recognising any abnormalities and taking corrective action (Ahern et al 1995).

Arterial cannula

There are two ways to obtain an ABG sample:

1. An aseptic direct arterial puncture (stab) with a heparinised syringe (heparinised to stop clotting), using local anaesthesia
2. An indwelling arterial cannula.

There are many benefits in using the arterial cannula rather than an arterial stab:

- It provides a continuous and accurate blood pressure
- It avoids recurrent puncture from an arterial needle
- You can obtain ABGs and other essential bloods regularly
- It reduces infection by lesser wounds sites
- It has less morbidity than single-puncture samples (Oh 1997).

There can be disadvantages:

- Accidental disconnection could result in hypovolaemia
- Inappropriate care could result in ischaemia and necrosis (Marieb 2001).

The most common arteries chosen for use are the radial, brachial and femoral. Driscoll (1997) notes a contradiction for using the femoral in children, as it can cause the risk of septic arthritis and nerve damage. Brachial is not recommended for long term, as there is the risk of catheter fracture (Adams & Osbourne 1997). The radial is the artery of preference (Dougherty & Lister 2004).

An indwelling cannula needs to be cared for by appropriate trained staff. Only saline should be used to flush; other solutions injected into the cannula could compromise circulation to the limb and result in ischaemia and necrosis (Marieb 2001) or loss of the limb. Heparin is the only other solution that may be used; this can help with the patency of the cannula. To avoid any mistakes with unprescribed infusions into the cannula it is always important to label the arterial line as such. There are red needleless devices available to help identify the cannula as an arterial cannula, as seen in Figure 30.1.

The nurse caring for an arterial cannula must be aware of local policies and procedures and take part in the training provided. Regular observations should be recorded – temperature, colour of the limb, comparing it with the body's opposite limb (Dougherty & Lister 2004); and capillary refill time – and when possible ask the child if there is any pain.

ALERT

If the limb is cold and discoloured and you are concerned that there is any circulation compromise then the cannula should be removed immediately. Remove it as you would a peripheral cannula, but you may need to apply pressure longer (remember to turn off the saline monitoring device). Apply gauze and pressure to the puncture site for about 5 min or until the wound stops bleeding. If there is any bleeding or swelling reapply pressure (Driscoll 1997), document and continue to observe that the circulation has been restored.

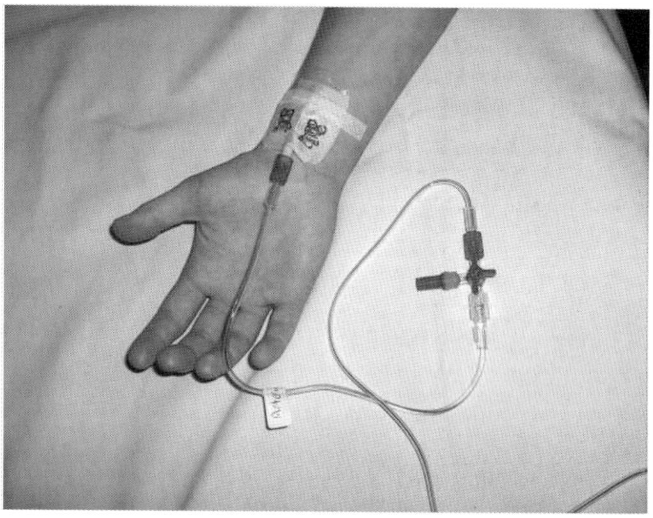

Fig. 30.1 • An arterial cannula.

Procedures Box 30.1 Obtaining an arterial blood sample from an indwelling arterial cannula

Action
Collect the required equipment:

- Sterile gloves
- Heparinised syringe
- 5-mL syringe
- Sterile wipe
- Sterile dressing cloth
- Sharps bin.

Action
If you do not have a gas analyser on the unit warn the laboratory that a sample is on its way.

Reason *Ensures that the sample gets analysed immediately; any delay will affect the results.*

Action
Wash and dry your hands and put on a plastic apron.

Reason *Prevents cross-infection.*

Action
Explain to the child and parent that you are going to access the cannula.

Reason *Promotes psychological support.*

Action
Ensure that the area where the cannula rests is on to a sterile dressing cloth.

Reason *Reduces the risk of infection.*

Action
Place the syringes and sterile wipe open on to the sterile dressing.

Reason *Ensure that you open the syringes and wipe without touching the cloth to help with clean technique.*

Action
Switch off the saline device, which is keeping the cannula patent.

Reason *Stops saline entering the sample.*

Actions
Wash and dry your hands and put on sterile gloves.

Use the sterile wipe to thoroughly clean the three-way tap.

Reason *Reduces the risk of infection.*

Action
Attach the 5-mL syringe to the three-way tap; turn the tap off from the monitoring equipment.

Action
Pull the syringe and open the three-way tap to the syringe and withdraw approximately 5 mL of blood.

Reason *This blood may have saline in it and will not be an appropriate sample.*

ALERT
It is important to withdraw the sample slowly to allow artery refill and to prevent backflow.

Action
Observe the fingers and limb throughout the procedure

Reason *Ensures that there is no circulation compromise.*

Action
Turn off the tap and discard the sample into the sharps bin.

Reason *Ensures safe disposal of blood.*

Actions
Place the arterial syringe on to the three-way tap and fill the syringe slowly until the required amount is collected.

Open the three-way tap to the monitoring equipment.

Clean the three-way tap and port site.

Use the saline device to flush the cannula.

If the cannula is attached to a pressure bag you can slowly advance saline to flush the cannula; however, if this is not available an extra syringe of saline needs to be ready to flush the cannula.

ALERT
Only saline can be flushed into arterial cannulae; anything else could result in the loss of the child's limb.

Action
Expel any air bubbles from the blood gas syringe.

Action
Seal the syringe.

Reason *If this is not done it allows carbon dioxide and oxygen to diffuse out, thus altering their concentration and producing inaccurate results.*

Action
Ensure that the monitoring equipment is recording.

Action
Observe and record the circulation of the fingers and limb.

Reason *Ensures that there has been no circulation compromise and that this has been documented.*

Action
Label the sample with the patient's details and that it is an arterial sample.

Reason *So the laboratory processes the sample correctly.*

Actions
Dispose of the equipment and remove your gloves.

Record in the patient's notes that a sample has been taken.

Sample analysis

Today many critical care units caring for children provide their own gas analysis device that can analyse an ABG sample without sending the sample to the laboratory. For those hospitals that do not have these on their units the biochemistry department will process the sample. Whatever the method of analysis it is important that the sample is analysed as soon as possible. Any delay in analysis will lead to an inaccurate result; gaseous exchange and metabolism continue in the blood even when it is removed from the body (Beaumont 1997, Woodrow 2004). Transporting the sample on ice can help if you anticipate a delay in analysis, slowing any metabolic activity. It is recommended to avoid vigorous shaking, as this may cause haemolysis (Woodrow 2004).

Interpretation of ABG results

The blood's potential hydrogen (pH) is between 7.35 and 7.45; any disruption from these limits indicates an acid–base imbalance or disorder, inhibiting normal enzyme activity.

The varying hydrogen ion (H^+) levels can affect the pH of the blood. When the child is unwell the H^+ concentration can increase and the pH can fall below 7.35 (acidosis occurs, also referred to as acidaemia), or the H^+ concentration can fall during illness and the pH rises (alkalosis occurs, or alkalaemia).

The H^+ is present in the body in huge numbers, but it is presented in small numbers in the pH scale to make the concentration figures more manageable (Driscoll 1997, Woodrow 2004).

ALERT

It is important to remember when interpreting the results that the smallest changes in pH can have a significant effect on the body functions. A pH below 6.9 or above 7.8 is often incompatible with life.

Step 1

The gas result given to you by the laboratory or your own gas analyser gives you the readings below. (Note that each blood gas machine may vary with its reference range, but only slightly.) There will be other results available, but when beginning to learn how to interpret ABG results it is recommended to look at the readings below. These results are normal; can you see why?

- pH: 7.36 (reference range, 7.35–7.45)
- P_aCO_2: 5.0 (reference range, 4.0–6.0)
- Sodium bicarbonate (HCO_3): 23 (reference range, 22–26)

Note: in this chapter the blood results will be measured in kilopascals (kPa). However, some blood analysis machines record results in millimetres of mercury (mmHg). To convert the mmHg results into kPa divide by 7.5. For example:

***PCO*$_2$ = 40 mmHg ÷ 7.5 = 5.3 kPa**

When interpreting ABG results it may help to take it in steps; first distinguish if the child has an acidosis or an alkalosis:

- <7.35 = acidosis
- >7.45 = alkalosis.

Now test your knowledge

Question 1

What is pH 7.30 – acidosis or alkalosis?

Question 2

What is pH 7.50 – acidosis or alkalosis?

Step 2

Once you have established acidosis or alkalosis the next step is to decide if the cause of the acidosis or alkalosis is *respiratory* or *metabolic*.

To help with this, look at the carbon dioxide levels in the arterial blood (P_aCO_2) and the HCO_3:

- The P_aCO_2 normal reference is between 4.0 and 6.0. Any deviation from this range indicates respiratory involvement.
- The HCO_3 normal reference is between 22 and 26. Any deviation from this range indicates metabolic involvement.

Respiratory acidosis

The body excretes 13 000 000 000 nmol of H^+ a day through the lungs. If there is respiratory compromise the body is left with many excess H^+ ions; these ions then accumulate in the blood (Driscoll 1997), presenting an increase P_aCO_2 levels in the ABG. This increase in H^+ makes the pH fall below 7.35 and the P_aCO_2 level rises above 6.0, causing a *respiratory acidosis*. Conditions that can cause respiratory comprise leading to respiratory acidosis are pneumonia and asthma.

An example of respiratory acidosis is:

- pH <7.35 (*acidosis*)
- $P_aCO_2 > 6.0$ (*respiratory involvement*)
- HCO_3 normal (*normal value, no metabolic involvement*).

Remember to look at patient's diagnosis to confirm the results.

Metabolic acidosis

The daily metabolism uses 1 570 000 000 nmol of H^+, which is excreted safely mainly by urine (Driscoll 1997). The body produces a buffer to absorb the H^+; HCO_3 produced by the kidneys is the body's biggest buffer. However, when there has been a compromise in production of HCO_3 then there will be an excess of H^+ in the blood, causing an acidosis, but this time a *metabolic acidosis*. Conditions that can cause metabolic acidosis are diabetic ketoacidosis, diarrhoea and starvation.

An example of metabolic acidosis is:

- pH <7.35 (*acidosis*)
- P_aCO_2 normal (*normal value, no respiratory involvement*)
- $HCO_3 <22$ (*metabolic involvement*).

Respiratory alkalosis

If the child is unwell and there is a rapid increase in breathing this can produce an excess removal of carbon dioxide out of the lungs. This will cause a rise in the pH (decrease in H^+), therefore if the pH rises above 7.45 and the cause is low carbon dioxide this is *respiratory alkalosis*. Causes of respiratory alkalosis are over-ventilation of an artificial ventilator and hyperventilation.

An example of respiratory alkalosis is:

- pH >7.45 (*alkalosis*)
- $P_aCO_2 <4.0$ (*respiratory involvement*)
- HCO_3 normal (*no metabolic involvement*).

Metabolic alkalosis

Metabolic alkalosis is when the body either loses acid or gains a base. Prolonged vomiting, gastric aspiration and renal loss after diuretics treatment are conditions that can cause it (Driscoll 1997). The pH rises above 7.45, along with the bicarbonate in the blood.

An example of metabolic alkalosis is:

- pH >7.45 (*alkalosis*)
- P_aCO_2 normal (*no respiratory involvement*)
- HCO_3 >26 (*metabolic involvement*).

You can use a table to help you to remember (Table 30.1).

Now test your knowledge

(Use the table below to help.) Interpret the ABG results and identify the acid–base disorder (answers in the *Answers to Questions* appendix).

Question 3

A child has presented with asthma and ABG results of:

- pH: 7.23
- P_aCO_2: 9.2
- HCO_3: 23.

Question 4

A known diabetic patient arrives unwell and presents with ABG results of:

- pH: 7.29
- P_aCO_2: 5.0
- HCO_3: 12.

Question 5

A child who has been vomiting for 3 days presents with ABG results of:

- pH: 7.49
- P_aCO_2: 4.0
- HCO_3: 30.

Table 30.1. Respiratory and metabolic acidosis and alkalosis

Acid–base disorder	pH	$PaCO_2$	HCO_3
Reference range	7.35–7.45	4.0–6.0	22–26
Respiratory acidosis	↓	↑	Normal
Metabolic acidosis	↓	Normal	↓
Respiratory alkalosis	↑	↓	Normal
Metabolic alkalosis	↑	Normal	↑

Compensation

If your blood gas results do not fit the results in Table 30.1 then you need to consider other acid–base disorders (Table 30.2). The respiratory–metabolic link ensures that if the lungs or the kidneys become overwhelmed then they will compensate for each other (Cooper 2005). The body will attempt to normalise the pH. For example, if there is a metabolic imbalance causing a disturbance in the pH then the respiratory system will attempt to compensate to try and normalise the pH. When interpreting compensation imbalances, remember that generally the acid–base disorder is in the system that is furthest from its normal range (Driscoll 1997). Remember the child's illness history; this can also help indicate where compensation is happening.

Now test your knowledge

(Use the table to help.) Interpret the ABG results and identify the acid–base disorder.

Question 6

A known child with diabetes presents with increased respirations, a central refill time of 3 s and ABG results of:

- pH: 7.33
- P_aCO_2: 3.0
- HCO_3: 15.

Question 7

A febrile child with a persistent cough for 3 weeks in respiratory distress, with central refill time of 3 s and ABG results of:

Table 30.2. Acid–base disorders with renal and respiratory compensation

Acid–base disorder	pH	$PaCO_2$	HCO_3
Reference range	7.35–7.45	4.0–6.0	22–26
Respiratory acidosis with renal compensation	↓	↑	↑
Metabolic acidosis with respiratory compensation	↓	↓	↓
Respiratory alkalosis with renal compensation	↑	↓	↓
Metabolic alkalosis with respiratory compensation	↑	↑	↑

- pH: 7.35
- P_aCO_2: 9.8
- HCO_3: 28.

Question 8

A child with prolonged vomiting, low oxygen saturations and ABG results of:

- pH: 7.43
- P_aCO_2: 7
- HCO_3: 30.

Note how in question 7 the child's body has normalised his acidosis.

Mixed acidosis or alkalosis

The critically ill child may also be unlucky enough to have a mixture of respiratory and metabolic acid–base disorders (Table 30.3).

Table 30.3. Summary of acid–base disorders

Acid–base disorder	pH	$PaCO_2$	HCO_3
Reference range	7.35–7.45	4.0–6.0	22–26
Respiratory acidosis	↓	↑	Normal
Metabolic acidosis	↓	Normal	↓
Respiratory alkalosis	↑	↓	Normal
Metabolic alkalosis	↑	Normal	↑
Respiratory acidosis with renal compensation	↓	↑	↑
Metabolic acidosis with respiratory compensation	↓	↓	↓
Respiratory alkalosis with renal compensation	↑	↓	↓
Metabolic alkalosis with respiratory compensation	↑	↑	↑
Mixed metabolic acidosis and respiratory acidosis	↓	↑	↓
Mixed metabolic and respiratory alkalosis	↑	↓	↑

Now test your knowledge

(Use the table to help.) Interpret the results and identify the acid–base disorder.

Question 9

A hyperventilating child with renal impairment and ABG results of:

- pH: 7.56
- P_aCO_2: 2.0
- HCO_3: 28.

Question 10

A child presents with pneumonia and dehydration and has ABG results of:

- pH: 6.9
- P_aCO_2: 9.0
- HCO_3: 13.

Use Table 30.3 to help answer the following questions. Until you become proficient at interpreting blood gas results carry a table with you or ensure that you have access to one.

Question 11

Respiratory arrest leading to a cardiac arrest in a previously well child with ABG results of:

- pH: 6.9
- P_aCO_2: 11
- HCO_3: 9.

Question 12

A child with acute asthma, recent dehydration and vomiting and with ABG results of:

- pH: 7.46
- PCO_2: 2
- HCO_3: 21.

Remember that these results are only one part of the picture; you must always look at the child's ABC observations as well as other continuous monitoring in situ.

References

Adams S, Osbourne S (1997) Critical care nursing: science and practice. Oxford University Press, Oxford

Ahern J, Filder S, Peters R (1995) A guide to blood gases. Nursing Standard 9(94):50–52

Beaumont T (1997) How to guides: arterial blood gas sampling. Care of the Critically Ill 13:1

Cooper N (2005) Acute care: arterial blood gases. Student BMJ. http://student.bmj.com/issues/04/03education/105.php

Dougherty L, Lister S (2004) The Royal Marsden Hospital manual of clinical nursing procedures, 6th edn. Blackwell Publishing, Oxford

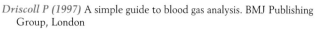

Driscoll P (1997) A simple guide to blood gas analysis. BMJ Publishing Group, London

Marieb E (2001) Human anatomy and physiology, 5th edn. Benjamin Cummings, San Francisco

Oh T (1997) Intensive care manual, 4th edn. Butterworth, Sydney

Woodrow P (2004) Arterial blood gas analysis. Nursing Standard 18(21):45–52,54–55

31 Specimen collection

Emma V.P. Jasper

Children and young people are admitted to hospital to undergo investigations to determine the cause of an acute onset of illness or as part of treatment regimens, enabling diagnosis and treatment. The collection of specimens is frequently the responsibility of the nursing staff, therefore it is important that the nurse has an understanding about the correct technique to collect the specimen and the importance of this collection to obtain reliable results.

To enable successful diagnosis, specimens must be:

- collected at the right time
- collected using the correct technique
- sent to the laboratories as soon as possible.

The greater the amount of specimen that is collected, the greater the chance that an organism will be isolated and, therefore, diagnosis and treatment decisions can be made (Dougherty & Lister 2004).

Principles of specimen collection

Contamination

Care must be taken when collecting specimens to avoid contamination. Contamination leads to misleading results. Collection pots and swabs should not be opened until the specimen is ready for collection, and the equipment used for the collection is sterile. As with any exposure to body fluids, protective clothing, gloves and masks should always be worn in accordance with local trust policy.

Consent

Informed consent should be obtained from patients and their family. The gaining of informed consent also ensures that the sample is collected correctly. Dignity and privacy should be maintained at all times.

Types of specimen

The majority of specimens collected in practice are either bacterial or viral:

- Bacterial specimens: the specimen is cultured in the laboratory for 24–48 h; this allows bacteria to be isolated and *sensitivities* to be identified, which enables the correct antibiotic treatment to be commenced.
- Viral specimens: viruses do not survive outside the human body for very long, therefore a transport medium is required to store the sample for its transport to the laboratory.

Documentation

To ensure correct analysis, diagnosis and treatment the specimen must be labelled correctly in accordance with local trust policy. This includes the:

- patient's name
- ward or department or patient's address
- hospital number
- date the specimen was collected
- time the specimen was collected
- diagnosis
- relevant signs and symptoms
- relevant history
- any ongoing microbial drugs
- type of specimen
- consultant's name
- name of requesting doctor (Dougherty & Lister 2004).

Any specimen that is incorrectly labelled may be discarded by the laboratory staff and the specimen will need to be repeated (Health Services Advisory Committee 1991 cited in Dougherty & Lister 2004). The specimen collection should be documented in the child's nursing or medical notes.

Specimen collection

Nasopharyngeal aspirate

Nasopharyngeal aspirate is a method of collecting secretions from the nasopharyngeal area of the upper airway using suction and a 'sputum trap' to collect the sample (Fig. 31.1).

Nasopharyngeal aspirates are taken from children of all ages, but they are most commonly performed in paediatric practice during the winter months to diagnose the cause of respiratory infections such as bronchiolitis. The nasopharyngeal aspirate is obtained with the use of suction; to prevent trauma to the nasopharyngeal area correct suction pressures should be used, as indicated in Table 31.1.

The collection of nasopharyngeal aspirates can be upsetting for parents to watch; after the explanation of how the procedure is performed they should be given the option of whether

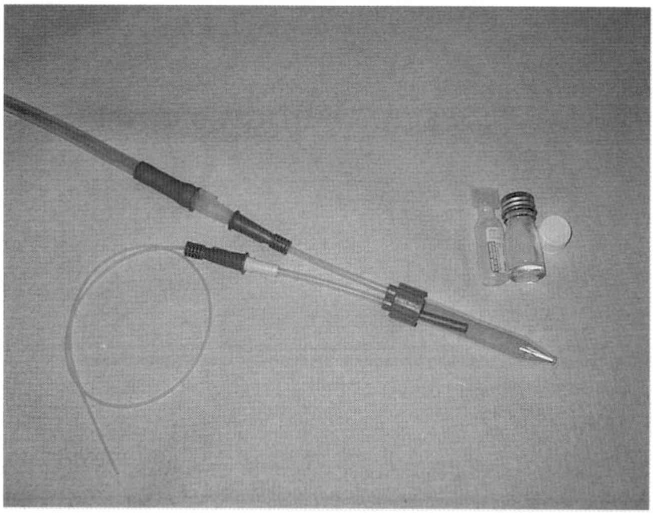

Fig. 31.1 • Nasopharyngeal specimen collection: vacuum-assisted nasal aspirate method.

Table 31.1. Suction pressures

Patient age	Catheter size (French)	Suction pressure (mmHg)
Premature infant	6	80–100
Infant	8	80–100
Toddler or preschool	10	100–120
School age	12	100–120
Adolescent or adult	14	120–150

(From Dougherty & Lister 2004, with permission.)

they wish to be present with their child or not, and their decision and wishes should be respected.

Babies or young children may also need to be supportively held for the procedure to ensure their safety and to allow the sample to be collected as quickly as possible, to prevent distress for the child and family. This should be performed by another member of staff.

Throughout the procedure the baby or child needs to be closely observed due to the suction catheter entering the airway for any signs of respiratory distress, for example changes in breathing pattern or cyanosis (blueness) around the lips and nose, in which case the sample collection must be stopped and the catheter removed.

Procedures Box 31.1 Nasopharyngeal aspirate collection

Action
Explain to the child and family why the specimen is required and the method to be used to collect the specimen.

Reasons *Ensures that informed consent is obtained. Ensures parental and child's understanding.*

Action
Consult local trust policy regarding the collection of nasopharyngeal aspirates.

Reason *To adhere to policy and procedure.*

Action
Decontaminate your hands either by washing with an antimicrobial liquid soap and water or by using an alcohol hand rub; hands that are visibly soiled or contaminated must be washed with soap and water before using an alcohol hand rub.

Reason *Avoids microbial contamination.*

Action
Prepare the equipment to be used, including the correct suction catheter size and suction pressure.

Reasons *Obtains the sample as quickly and safely as possible. Reduces the anxiety of the child and family. Prevents trauma to the nasopharyngeal area.*

Action
Adhere to local universal precautions before obtaining the sample.

Reason *Prevents cross-infection.*

Action
The child's or baby's head may need to be supportively held by a trained colleague.

Reason *Ensures the safety of the patient when obtaining the sample.*

Action
Once the equipment is prepared turn on the suction unit.

Action
Insert the catheter into the nostril (do not apply suction at this stage) and gently push the catheter upwards and backwards towards the posterior pharynx.

Reasons *Prevents trauma of the area during catheter insertion. The sample needs to be obtained from the pharynx area; if it is not far enough then the sample will not be adequate.*

Action
Remember to always observe the baby or child throughout the procedure; if there are any changes in her or his condition, stop collection and remove the catheter immediately.

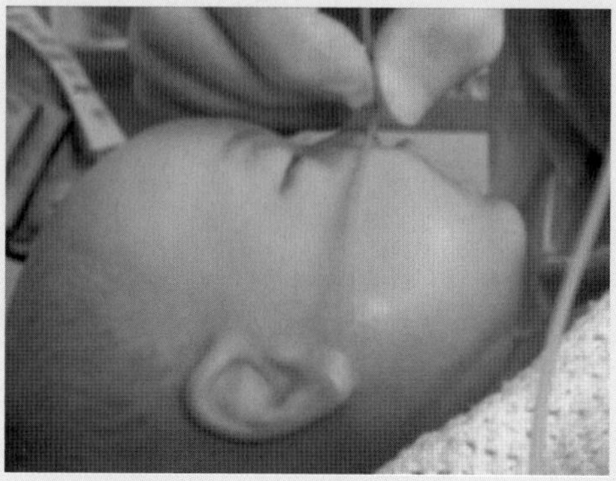

Procedures Box 31.1 Nasopharyngeal aspirate collection—cont'd

Action
Apply suction and gently remove the catheter from the nostril.
Reason *Obtains the sample.*

Action
The sputum trap should be kept upright during the procedure.
Reason *Prevents loss of specimen into the suction tubing.*

Action
The catheter may need to be cleared with the use of viral medium or 0.9% sodium chloride (according to local policy); there should be visible secretions in the collection media.
Reasons *Allows secretions in the suction catheter to be transferred into the sputum trap.*
Allows the sample to be tested.

Action
Turn off suction, disconnect the catheter from the suction unit and secure the lid on the sputum trap.
Reason *Prevents spillage.*

Action
Dispose of equipment adhering to universal precautions and replace with new.
Reason *Prevents contamination.*

Stool samples

Stool samples allow the identification of bacteria and viruses that cause gastrointestinal illness. A good amount of faecal matter should be obtained as soon as the symptoms develop, thus allowing for the causative organisms to be identified as soon as possible and treatment to be commenced. Stool samples are collected in stool collection pots, which contain a small spoon attached to the lid to enable the sample to be collected without contamination; however, there are other forms of stool samples that require different methods of collection, for example faecal occult blood.

Procedures Box 31.2 Stool collection

Action
Explain to the child and family how and why the sample requires collection and the method to be used.
Reason *Ensures their understanding and obtains consent to perform the procedure.*

Action
Consult local trust policies regarding stool sample collection.
Reason *To adhere to trust policies and procedures.*

Action
Use universal precautions to collect the sample in accordance with local policy.
Reason *Prevents cross-infection.*

Action
Provide facilities and collection equipment for the child or young person to provide a stool sample.
Reasons *Ensures privacy.*
Allows the sample to be collected.

Actions
Once the baby, child or young person has passed the stool for collection, using the spoon provided in the stool collection pot transfer faecal matter into the pot (the greater the amount, the greater the chance of isolating organisms) and secure the lid.
Ensure that there is no faecal matter on the outside of the pot.
Reasons *Obtains the sample for testing.*
Ensures that none of the sample is wasted.
Prevents contamination and cross-infection.

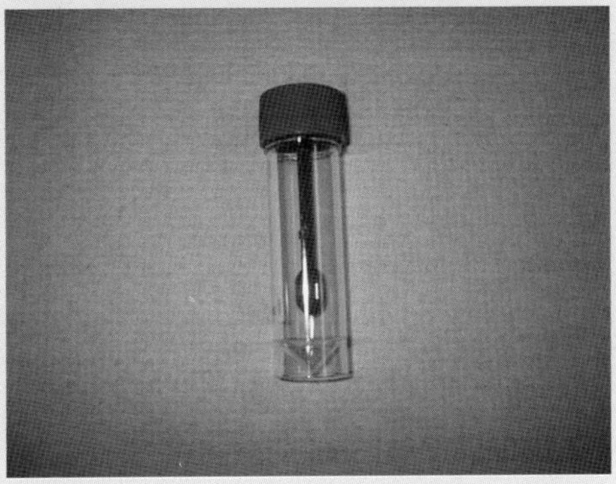

Action
Remove your gloves and wash your hands.
Reason *Prevents cross-infection.*

Action
Label the sample correctly and transport it to the laboratory for testing.
Reason *Allows a diagnosis to be obtained as soon as possible.*

Action
Results may take 24–48 h to return; the family should be informed of this.

Action
Document in the child's or young person's medical or nursing notes.
Reason *Indicates that the sample has been collected and sent for analysis.*

Faecal occult blood collection

Faecal occult blood identifies blood in the stool sample, which indicates bleeding somewhere in the gastrointestinal tract; however, the sample should not be collected if there is visible blood noticed in the stool. The test requires samples of faecal matter that have been collected from stools passed over a 3-day period, one sample per day. The test is performed with the use of faecal occult blood cards obtained from the laboratory. The instructions inside the packet should always be followed to allow the correct method of collection. The completed pack should be returned to the laboratory within 48 h of finishing the collection to allow the best results to be obtained (Beckman Coulter 2006).

Swabs

Swabs are used in practice to collect organisms from wounds, the throat, the nose and other parts of the body (Fig. 31.2). Swabs should be collected before any antimicrobial or antiviral treatment is commenced, and there should be a sufficient amount of exudate collected on the swab. Bacterial swabs are stored at room temperature in sterile packaging. The packaging should not be opened until the specimen is ready to be collected; the sample is then taken and the swab transferred into the charcoal medium carrier provided. Viral swabs require the use of an antibiotic containing viral medium for transport to the laboratory (Gould & Brooker 2000). The swabs and the medium are refrigerated and have a use-by date that should be checked before obtaining the sample. The swab should be transported to the laboratory as soon as possible after it has been collected; if there is any delay then the sample should be refrigerated. Viruses are small, therefore a good amount of any exudate should be collected to enable analysis to be performed (Gould & Brooker 2000).

Urine collection

One of the most common specimens collected in paediatric practice is urine. Urine is collected to identify causes of unexplained pyrexia, the presence of a urinary tract infection (especially when no other source of infection can be found on physical examination), pregnancy in young females of child-bearing age or the cause of abdominal pain in surgical patients; it is also collected for other tests, for example protein:creatinine ratios. The sample should be as fresh as possible and sent for analysis as soon as possible once collected.

Once the sample has been collected (adhering to local policy), the sample needs to be transferred to a receptacle appropriate for the test requested by the medical staff. If there are any concerns about what collection pot to put the sample in, then the laboratory should be contacted to avoid using the incorrect pot, for example some urine tests for biochemical testing cannot be tested if in a microbiological boric acid pot. Local trust policies should be read and adhered to in relation to urine collection.

Types of collection equipment

Collection methods (Fig. 31.3) are:

- urine collection pads
- urine collection bags
- clean catch or midstream
- suprapubic aspiration
- catheter sampling.

Midstream urine collection is the most reliable urine collection method due to the low contamination rate (Alam et al 2005); however, it is also time-consuming and difficult in the younger child. Before the specimen is collected the young person should be given information about how to collect the sample and the importance of this for the ongoing investigation or treatment.

When handling body fluids local universal precautions should be followed and local policy regarding urine testing should be adhered to.

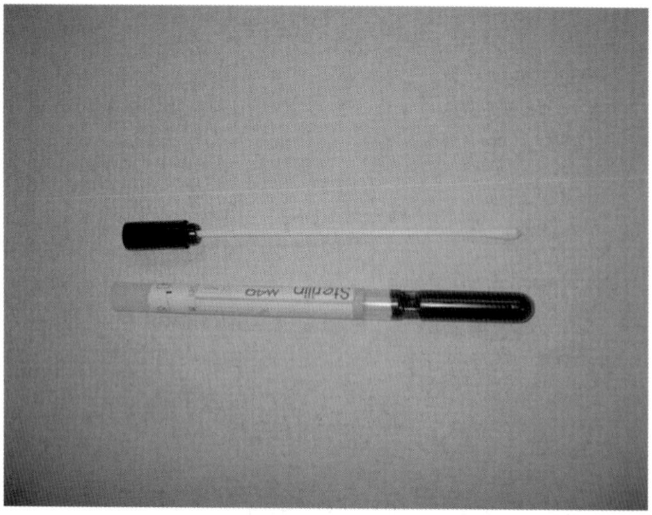

Fig. 31.2 • A swab.

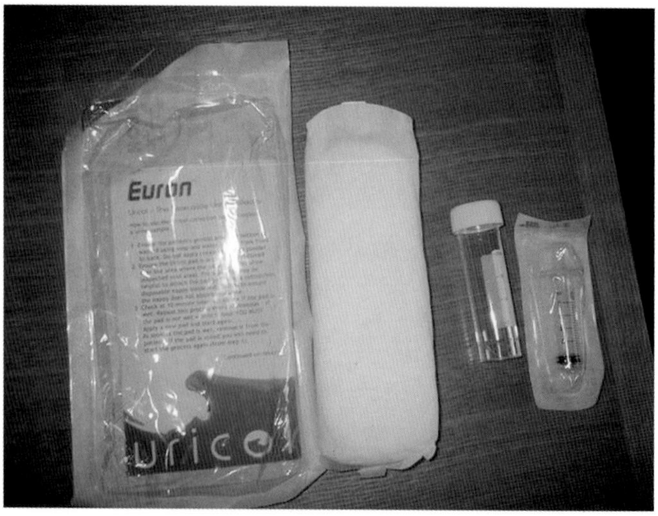

Fig. 31.3 • Urine collection methods.

Procedures Box 31.3 Midstream urine collection

Action
Explain to the child or young person and parents or carers the reason for needing the sample collection.

Reason *Ensures their understanding, has implications for care and gains informed consent to obtain a specimen.*

Action
Consult local trust policy regarding the collection of midstream urine samples.

Reason *To adhere to local policy or procedures.*

Action
Provide the child or young person with a sterile container.

Reasons *Used to collect the urine sample.*
Prevents contamination.

Action
Provide the child or young person with facilities to collect the sample.

Reason *Ensures dignity and privacy.*

Action
The patient must wash his or her genitalia with water and ensure that the area is dry.

Reason *Prevents contamination.*

Action
The child or young person needs to pass a small amount of urine as normal.

Reason *Eliminates bacteria from the perurethral area.*

Actions
Place a sterile container under the genitalia and collect the urine sample; the patient must not fully empty her or his bladder.

Remove the container, and the patient can pass urine normally.

Reason *Ensures a midstream sample.*

Action
Using local trust policy for universal precautions, transfer the urine into an appropriate specimen pot.

Reason *Avoids unnecessary exposure to body fluids and adheres to local policy or procedure.*

Action
Label the specimen correctly.

Reason *Ensures that the urine can be analysed correctly and facilitates transport to the correct laboratory.*

Action
Transfer the sample to the laboratory.

Reason *Ensures that the sample can be analysed by laboratory staff correctly.*

Action
Document in the child's or young person's medical or nursing notes.

Reason *Indicates that the sample has been collected and sent for analysis.*

Urine collection pads

Urine collection pads are commonly used in paediatric practice for babies and younger children who are still in nappies. They are easy to use and non-invasive and have been shown to have low contamination rates if used correctly, making them reliable for the identification of urinary tract infections (Feasey 1999).

The most important factor when using the urine collection pad is the length of time that the pad is left in situ. The longer the pad is left unchecked, the greater the risk of it becoming contaminated due to contact with skin flora. The pad should be checked every 10 min and replaced with a new pad if no urine has been obtained within 30 min (Liaw et al 2000). The pad will need to be replaced if soiled with faeces.

Procedures Box 31.4 Collecting urine with a urine collection pad

Action
Explain to the family the reason for the collection of the urine sample using the urine collection pad.

Reason *Ensures their understanding, has implications for care and gains their informed consent.*

Actions
Using local universal precautions wash the baby's genitalia with water only; do not use baby wipes or apply any creams afterwards.

Parents or carers may wish to do this for their child; their preferences should be discussed.

Reasons *Prevents contamination.*
Prevents unnecessary exposure to body fluids.
Allows parental participation in the child's care.

Action
Turn a clean nappy inside out.

Reason *Prevents the nappy soaking up the urine.*

Action
Remove the urine collection pad from the sterile packet; be sure not to touch the pad.

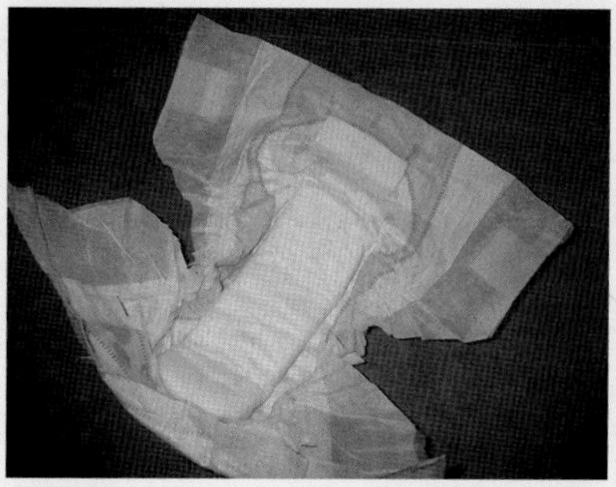

Procedures Box 31.4 Collecting urine with a urine collection pad—cont'd

Reasons *Allows the urine collection pad to collect urine. Prevents contamination.*

Action
Place the pad in the nappy and secure the nappy in place.

Reason *Prevents dislodgement of the pad.*

Action
Check the pad at 10-min intervals.

Reason *To obtain a sample as soon as possible and prevent unnecessary exposure to skin flora and possible contamination.*

Action
If the baby has not passed urine after 30 min, the pad must be replaced.

Reason *Prevents contamination from exposure to skin flora.*

Actions
When the baby has passed urine remove the pad.

Using a sterile 5-mL syringe, aspirate the urine and transfer it to the correct specimen pot.

Reason *Collects the sample.*

Action
Note that 0.5 mL is adequate for analysis (Rao et al 2004).

Reason *For correct analysis by laboratory staff.*

Action
Label the specimen and transport it to the laboratory.

Reason *Enables clear identification of the source of the specimen.*

Action
Document the collection in the patient's medical or nursing notes.

Reason *Indicates that the sample has been collected and sent for analysis.*

Adhesive urine bags

These are another option for the younger patient; however, there have been many identified problems with their use and therefore they may not be commonly used in practice. Identified problems include:

- high contamination rates
- difficulty in application
- discomfort for the patient, especially if they have to be reapplied
- leakage
- expense (Feasey 1999, Poole 2002).

Procedures Box 31.5 Urine collection with adhesive urine bags

Action
Inform the parent or carer of the need for urine collection using the adhesive bag.

Reason *Ensures their understanding, has implications for care and gains informed consent.*

Action
In accordance with local trust universal precautions, wash your hands and apply gloves.

Reasons *Prevents exposure to body fluids. Prevents cross-infection.*

Action
Wash the baby's genitalia with water and dry.

Reason *Reduces the risk of contamination from skin flora.*

Action
Do not use baby wipes or apply any creams.

Reason *Prevents displacement of the adhesive bag.*

Action
Remember that parents or carers may wish to undertake this procedure.

Reason *Allows parental participation in the child's care.*

Action
Apply the adhesive bag (suitable for the sex of the baby or child), ensuring that it is securely in position.

Reasons *Prevents displacement. Obtains the sample.*

Action
Check the bag at regular intervals.

Reason *Obtains the sample as soon as possible and prevents prolonged attachment to the skin.*

Action
When urine has been passed into the bag, carefully remove the bag from the skin.

Reasons *Prevents discomfort to the child. Obtains the sample.*

Action
Transfer the sample from the bag to the specimen pot with a sterile syringe.

Reasons *Avoids contamination. Avoids wastage of urine collected.*

Action
Label the specimen and send it to the laboratory.

Reason *Enables clear identification of the source of the specimen.*

Action
Document in the patient's notes.

Reason *Indicates that the sample has been taken.*

Catheter sampling

A sample can be obtained from an existing catheter, or the child may need to be catheterised to obtain the sample and then the catheter removed. Catheterisation is performed only by health professionals trained and assessed in the procedure. This is a reliable method of collecting a urine sample, but it is not commonly used due to it being invasive and uncomfortable for the child (Feasey 1999). Samples are taken straight from the catheter tubing via a sampling port, requiring a needle and syringe to obtain the sample, therefore care is needed to avoid needlestick injury. Because of this risk, manufacturers have produced catheters that have a needleless sampling port, in which a syringe can be inserted into the port but no needle is required. Samples of urine should be taken from the sampling port and not the collection bag on the end, as the sample is fresher and less contaminated.

Procedures Box 31.6 Catheter sampling

Action
Explain to the child or young person and parent or carer what the procedure involves and the way the sample will be collected.
Reason *Ensures their understanding, has implications for care and gains their informed consent.*

Action
Ensure privacy and dignity.

Action
Adhere to local trust universal precautions; wash your hands and apply gloves.
Reason *Prevents cross-infection.*

Action
Clamp the catheter using clamp-on tubing and ensure that urine collects in the tubing.
Reason *To gain an adequate sample.*

Action
Clean the access port on the tubing with an alcohol swab and allow to dry.
Reason *Reduces the risk of cross-infection and contamination.*

Needle ports

Action
Using a sterile needle and syringe, insert the needle into the access port at a 45° angle and gently aspirate the urine, withdraw the needle and dispose of it in the sharps bin (do not resheath the needle before disposal).
Reasons *The degree of angle reduces the risk of the needle perforating the tubing. Safe disposal prevents needlestick injury.*

Action
Note that some children may have needle phobia, therefore explanation is needed and the procedure may need to be performed with minimal exposure to the child.

Needleless ports

Action
Using a syringe insert into the port, turn into place and aspirate urine.
Reason *Prevents needlestick injury.*

Action
Reclean the port with an alcohol swab.
Reason *Reduces contamination.*

Action
Transfer urine from the syringe into the specimen pot.
Reason *Reduces contamination if transferred as soon as the sample is taken.*

Action
Unclamp the tubing.
Reason *Allows patient comfort and urine drainage.*

Action
Label the specimen and send it to the laboratory.
Reason *Enables clear identification of the source of the specimen.*

Action
Document in patient's notes.
Reason *Indicates that the sample has been sent.*

Suprapubic aspiration

Suprapubic aspiration, as with catheterisation, is not routinely used in paediatric practice due to its invasiveness and discomfort for the child (Feasey 1999). It involves a needle being inserted from the outside of the abdomen into the bladder and a sterile sample being taken. This is possibly the most reliable method of obtaining a sample and is often used for children who have had recurrent positive microbiological urine cultures from clean catch or midstream urine tests. This procedure should always be performed by medical staff.

There are two common types of urine specimen pots available in practice for routine specimens: a clear top universal pot and a red-topped boric acid pot. Boric acid is a preserving agent, allowing the sample to be preserved, especially if it is going to a take a while for it to reach the laboratory, for example from a community general practitioner surgery, via a courier service, to the local main hospital laboratory. There is an indication line on the pot that shows the amount of urine needed in relation to the amount of boric acid. If there is not enough urine to reach this line the pot should not be used, as the boric acid:urine concentration ratio is incorrect. Boric acid pots are used for samples requiring microscopy, culture and sensitivity testing; they should not be used for samples requiring other biochemical testing, for example protein:creatinine ratio – these should be sent in a universal pot (if in any doubt contact the laboratory).

Samples that will reach the laboratory within a short space of time, for example from the ward to the laboratory via a vacuum transport system, can be sent in a clear top universal pot, as they will be collected by the staff and dealt with and stored quickly. Urine samples can be kept in a specimen fridge if they are not required to be sent urgently. Because of their content, boric acid pots should be kept out of the reach of children, and if parents are discharged with one they should be advised of this.

This chapter has covered the principles of specimen collection. It should always be remembered that individual hospital and community trusts have their own policies and procedures in place regarding the collection of specimens and their transportation to the laboratories. If in doubt the relevant laboratory should be contacted and advice obtained. Policies, procedures and professional advice should always be followed, and student nurses should be aware of these before undertaking any procedure, especially one they have not performed before. This will ensure the safety of the student, the trained colleague accountable for supervising the student, the laboratory staff and most importantly the child and their family.

Now test your knowledge

Ellie is a 6-month-old baby and has been admitted to the ward due to pyrexia and vomiting. No other cause for the temperature has been identified on clinical examination. The doctors have asked for a urine sample to be collected to exclude a urinary tract infection:

- Discuss the method most appropriate for the collection of the specimen for this baby and its subsequent transportation to the laboratory.

David is a 12-year-old boy and has been complaining of a sore throat for a few days. The doctor has examined David and has made the diagnosis of tonsillitis, with visible exudate, that will require antibiotic treatment. The doctor has asked you to collect both viral and bacterial swabs and send them to the laboratories for analysis. However, David is admitted in the early hours of the morning and the laboratory is closed until 9 a.m:

- Discuss the most appropriate way to collect the swabs from David and how they should be safely transported to the laboratory for analysis.

References

Alam MT, Coulter JBS, Pacheco J (2005) Comparison of urine contamination rates using three different methods of collection: clean catch, cotton wool pad and urine bag. Annals of Tropical Paediatrics 25:29–34

Beckman Coulter (2006) Hemoccult. Beckman Coulter, Fullerton

Dougherty L, Lister S (eds) (2004) The Royal Marsden Hospital manual of clinical nursing procedures, 6th edn. Blackwell Publishing, Oxford

Feasey S (1999) Are Newcastle urine collection pads suitable as a means of collecting specimens from infants? Paediatric Nursing 11(9):17–21

Gould D, Brooker C (2000) Applied microbiology for nurses. Macmillan Press, London

Liaw LCT, Mayar DM, Pedlar SJ, Coulthard MG (2000) Home collection of urine for culture from infants by three methods: survey of parents' preferences and bacterial contamination rates British Medical Journal 13(320):1312–1313

Poole C (2002) Diagnosis and management of urinary tract infection in children. Nursing Standard 16(38):47–52

Rao S, Bhatt J, Houghton C, Macfarlane P (2004) An improved urine collection pad method: a randomised clinical trial. Archives of Disease in Childhood 89:773–775

32 Collection and assessment of urine specimens and urinary catheterisation

Caroline Sanders • Lucy Bray • Sarah Doyle

Urine is produced by the kidneys and is a waste product of the body; it is normally pale yellow, amber or clear depending on fluid intake and diet (Fig. 32.1). The volume of urine produced will be dependent on the fluid intake; it is common for urine to be darker first thing in the morning due to reduced fluid intake and the body concentrating urine while asleep (antidiuretic hormone production). The colour of the urine can be associated with the by-products of recently eaten foods and insufficient water intake. In illness the volume and composition of urine can change, and analysis of the urine can reveal pathological links to metabolism, renal function, fluid balance and infection.

Urine can indicate:

- infection
- systemic illness (increased frequency, dysuria, renal problems)
- metabolic disorders
- pregnancy
- use of alcohol or drugs
- diet (changes in colour after eating certain foods or colourings or taking certain medication, or a change in odour after eating a specific food, such as asparagus).

In both male and female infants the expected bladder capacity can be calculated using the formula suggested by Holmdahl et al (1996):

bladder capacity (mL) = 38 + (2.5 × age in months)

Other formulae exist for older children (Hjalmas 1976, Koff 1983):

bladder capacity (mL) = (age × 30) + 30

Inspection of urine

The colour, nature and odour of urine have been considered as indicators for disease. Sometimes children or their parents will use the colour of the child's urine as an indicator that the child is unwell and will report if they have noticed a change in the colour of the child's urine, often noting haematuria or very concentrated urine:

- Dark, scanty and strong-smelling urine or cloudy urine: infection in the bladder or lower urinary tract; however, caution needs to be used as clear urine (pale yellow with no apparent cloudy appearance) cannot completely eliminate a urinary tract infection (UTI; Bulloch et al 2000)
- Bloody urine (haematuria; Fig. 32.2): infection or renal stones
- Red-stained urine can be due to blood in the urine (haematuria)
- Yellowish urine with bilirubin in the urine: liver disorder, jaundice, cirrhosis, etc.
- Frothy urine: caused by jaundice and is due to the presence of bile salts of albumin in the urine
- Fragments can be noted in the urine if the family has been asked to sieve the urine following treatment for renal stones. In some cases a stone can be passed, but this is very uncommon
- An injury to the bladder or lower urinary tract can result in clots forming in the bladder and being passed as thick dark red debris
- Parasites in the urine: the parasite that is the more frequently seen in urine is *Trichomonas*; however, other parasites can be seen in the urine sediment (but this is rare and is usually seen in exposed populations).

Dietary factors affecting the colour of urine include the following:

- Vitamin B supplements can turn urine bright yellow.
- Reddish brown urine may be caused by blackberries, beetroot or rhubarb in the diet.
- Excessive intake of carotene can make the urine appear more orange.

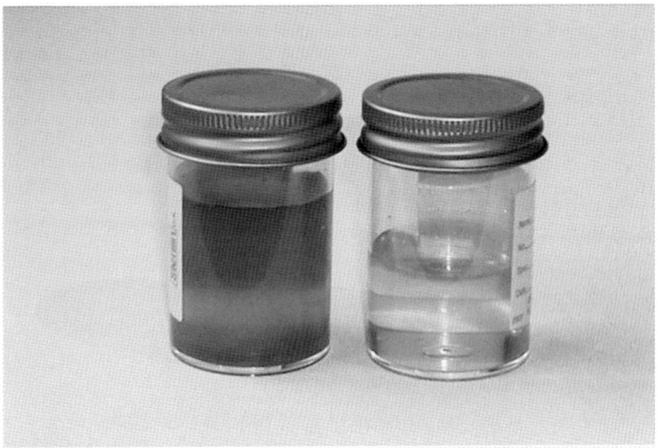

Fig. 32.1 • The urine on the right is the normal appearance of urine; the sample on the left is darker and more concentrated.

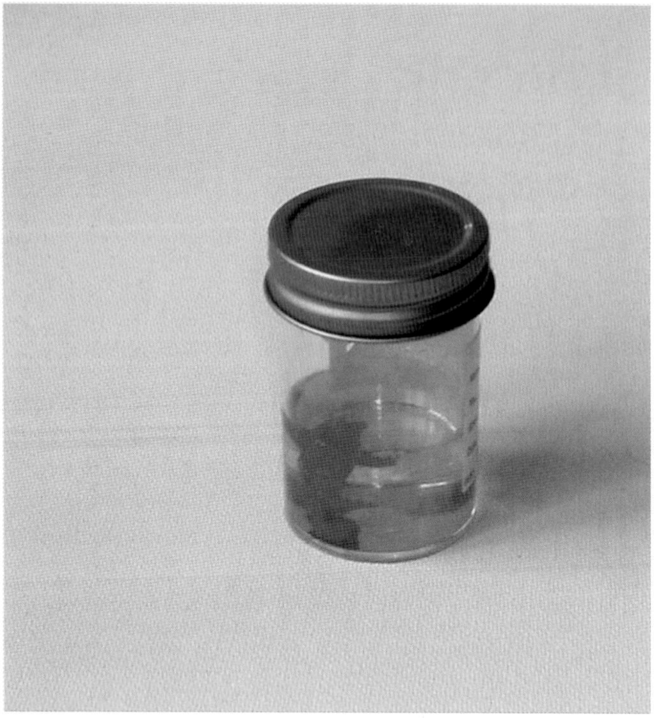

Fig. 32.2 • An example of frank (visible) haematuria; normally blood in the urine is not as obvious as this and can just look darker in nature.

Additional factors for consideration

- Burning urination, difficulty in urination and painful urination: infection and obstruction (dysuria).
- Reduced volume (oliguria): infection, obstruction, renal stones, kidney failure, etc.
- Increased volume of urine (polyuria): hypertension, diabetes, nephrotic syndrome, intake of beer or other alcohol or drugs, endocrinal disorders.
- Absence of urine (anuria): obstruction, kidney failure or stenosis.

Odour of urine

Odorous (strong-smelling) urine is usually caused by a high alkaline condition, which is frequently associated with bacteria in the urine. Other odours are reported in the urine, such as the following:

- Sweet or sugary, which is associated possibly with glucose in the urine and therefore suggestive of diabetes or kidney damage.
- A pleasant smell of maple syrup, suggestive of maple syrup urine disease (an inherited disease of amino acid metabolism).
- Offensive urine or proteins in the urine (proteinuria): diabetes, kidney damage due to drugs, toxins, etc.
- Diet can affect the odour of urine, for example asparagus can give urine a sulphurous odour.

Urinalysis

Urinalysis is 'the analysis of urine using physical, chemical and microscopical tests to determine the proportions of normal and abnormal constitutes' (Martin 2003). It is a valuable screening and diagnostic tool and is relatively simple and cost-effective; it can also aid a practitioner in the assessment, planning, implementation and evaluation of appropriate patient care. It can be effective in screening for certain conditions, such as diabetes mellitus or renal conditions such as nephrotic syndrome and glomerular nephritis. It is also used to identify and exclude the presence of UTIs.

Once a urine sample is collected it should be tested within 1 h (Cook 1996). If this is not appropriate then the sample must be refrigerated, but only for a maximum of 48 h, and then the specimen should return to room temperature prior to testing. A minimum of 10–20 mL is required for a microscopy, culture and sensitivity (Simerville et al 2005), although at some hospital trusts a smaller volume can be negotiated with the local laboratory.

Initially urine should be visually inspected for colour, consistency, obvious debris and visible blood.

Urine samples can be dip-tested with a variety of urinalysis reagent strips (Fig. 32.3). Urinalysis strips have absorbable pads that respond and react to the urine constitutes to provide a degree of positive or negative result:

- *Glucose* should not normally be present in urine. When there is an excess of glucose in the blood plasma it then leaks into the urine. The most common cause of this is diabetes mellitus or excessive glucose intake, but it can also be present due to renal tubular disorders or at times of severe stress, such as following a grand mal seizure. In the

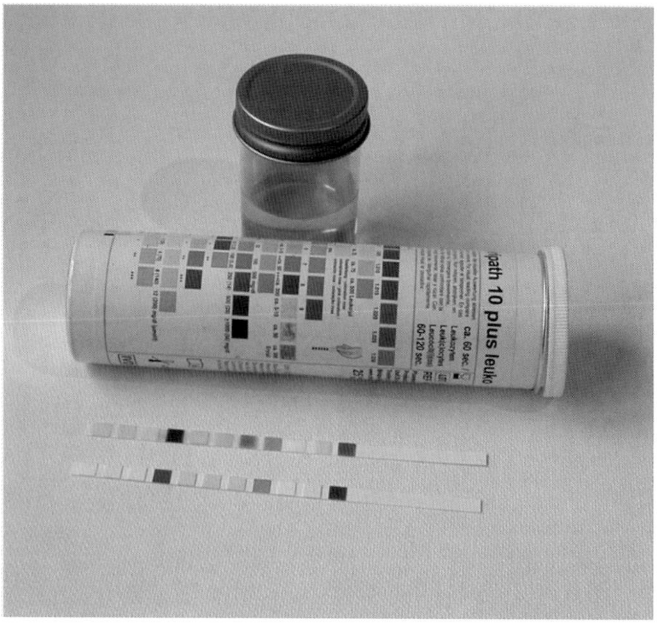

Fig. 32.3 • An example of urinalysis sticks with the reactive boxes displayed.

neonatal period the presence of glucose could relate to the inherited disorder of galactosaemia (Jefferson 1990). The urine of neonates and children on total parenteral nutrition should be regularly tested for glucose to detect glycosuria and its consequent risk of osmotic diuresis and dehydration. Also, certain medications such as salicylates can influence this result, therefore it is advisable to test urine prior to these medications being taken. If glucose is detected this should be reported to senior nursing staff or medical staff.

- *Ketones* are produced during fat metabolism, therefore ketone presence indicates that there has been some breakdown of the body fat stores. This is not uncommon during periods of fasting such as pre- or post surgery or during occasions of vomiting. In the patient with uncontrolled diabetes it can be an indication of diabetic ketoacidosis, which has the potential to be life threatening and should be taken seriously and promptly treated.
- *pH* demonstrates the acidity or alkalinity of urine and consequently the pH of body fluids. Normal pH for urine is 4.0–8.0 (Fillingham & Douglas 2004). Acidic urine can be prone to calculi and present during fasting and diabetic ketoacidosis. Alkaline urine can be an indication of UTI due to the ammonia produced from certain organisms, but not all organisms can produce ammonia and this tends to be due to *Proteus mirabilis* and other Gram-negative organisms. The pH of urine can be greatly influenced by the diet of the patient, and this should be taken into consideration when interpreting results. For accurate assessment pH measurement should be performed on fresh urine.
- *Specific gravity* is the concentration of urine and demonstrates hydration level. When specific gravity is low (less than 1.010) this indicates high levels of hydration such as when there is a high volume of fluid consumption or in specific conditions that increase diuresis, such as diabetes insipidus. High specific gravity (greater than 1.020) is an indication of increasing dehydration (Liao & Churchill 2001). Normal specific gravity should be between 1.003 and 1.030 (Simerville et al 2005).
- *Protein* is normally excreted in urine in microscopic amounts that are normally undetectable by urinalysis. Urine strips are particularly sensitive to albumin, which is a large protein molecule. If protein is detected in urine this can indicate one of two pathologies: protein can be present during a UTI but also can be present when there is increased permeability of the glomerular basement membrane and may indicate a renal disorder such as glomerular nephritis or nephrotic syndrome. Nephrotic syndrome increases the risk of hypovolaemia and susceptibility to infection. Children with this syndrome may present with an acute abdomen, and all these children should have their urine checked for protein and glucose. A low level of benign proteinuria may also be present during an acute febrile illness (Jefferson 1990).
- *Blood* present in urine can be highly specific; it can indicate UTI, calculi, trauma, bleeding disorders, renal disorders and even some cancers. It must be taken into context that urine strips are particularly sensitive to blood. Personal history must be taken into account, and any female menstruating or any person self-catheterising may have urine positive to blood. Therefore a positive result (Fig. 32.4) must be interpreted as a small part of a larger plan of care, but it is always taken seriously.
- *Bilirubin and urobilinogen* should not be present in a urine sample and may indicate a liver or gall bladder disorder. Urinalysis is essential if jaundice is in any way atypical in infants. Jaundice associated with bile in the urine indicates a significant liver or biliary tract disease. The results can be influenced by how recent the sample has been obtained, and therefore prompt testing is important.
- *Nitrites* are produced when Gram-negative bacilli such as *Proteus mirabilis*, *Pseudomonas*, *Escherichia coli* and *Klebsiella* convert nitrate into nitrites when there is a UTI present. Not all organisms are able to convert the nitrate, and therefore nitrites indicate a UTI but a negative result for nitrites does not exclude a UTI.
- *Leucocyte esterase* is an enzyme present within white cells, therefore a positive test for leucocytes confirms the presence of white cells in an inflammatory response. This is quite likely to be a UTI but it is not definitive, as it is a generalised white cell inflammatory response (Trigg & Mohammed 2006). The presence of leucocytes and nitrites together are more reliable as a result indicative of a UTI.

Urine testing strips are valuable tools for analysing urine. Any urine sample tested that produces a positive result for glucose, protein, blood (without cause), bilirubin, urobilinogen, nitrites and leucocytes with dip strip testing should be sent to the laboratory for further investigation.

A common investigation carried out in the laboratory is urine microscopy; this specifically counts the cellular levels in urine. A white cell count of greater than 100×10^6 is an indication

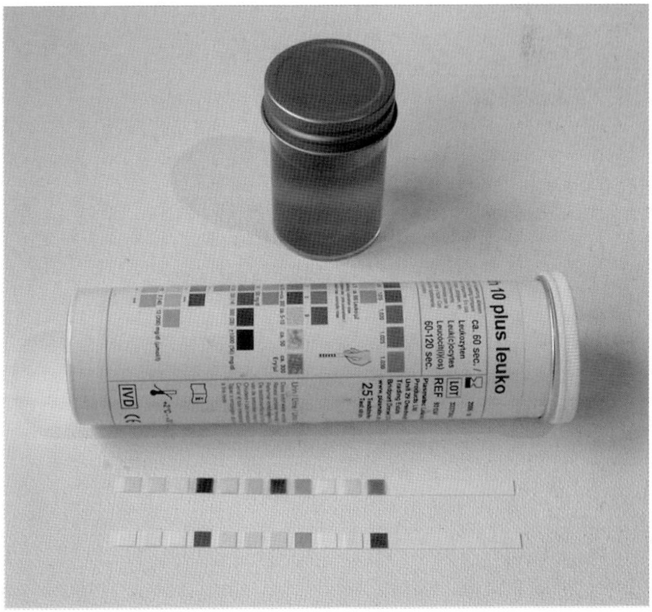

Fig. 32.4 • An example of a positive test for blood on a urinalysis strip, with the dark green indicator on the dipstick.

of a positive UTI, but a culture must be attained to confirm this and sensitivity to drugs can be performed to ensure that the correct antibiotic is prescribed. Urine can be cultured to detect a specific pathogen and then sensitivities to particular antibiotics can be ascertained. A mixed growth sample must be repeated to exclude contamination and ensure correct treatment. Children who perform intermittent self-catheterisation over a long period may be colonised with a specific pathogen; for these children antibiotic treatment is used only when the child is symptomatic (Simpson 2001).

Twenty-four–hour urine collection can be obtained to determine the levels of clearance the kidneys provide for certain substances such as creatinine, which is used to determine kidney function.

Urine sample collection

The accuracy of urine collection can have a significant impact on the quality of the urine sample obtained. Contamination of a urine sample can have a negative effect on patient care, as it can mislead diagnosis, involving unnecessary treatment or a repeated sample, which have implications on patient care and cost-effectiveness (Lewis 1998).

Suprapubic aspiration and clean intermittent catheterisation are considered the gold standard for urine sample collection but have many implications (Rao et al 2004). Both are considered invasive procedures and require the practitioner to have a certain degree of knowledge, skill and competence to perform. The most preferred non-invasive method is a midstream urine sample, or in non-toilet-trained children a urine collection pad.

LINK CHAPTER **31**

Suprapubic aspiration

Obtaining an uncontaminated urine sample from a sick neonate or infant can be problematic (Austin et al 1999). Suprapubic aspiration has been reported as the optimal method for obtaining urine samples for culture from infants (Barkemeyer 1993). This procedure is performed by an experienced doctor in children under 2 years. However, it may be unrealistic to expect this practice to be widely accepted, as the procedure is anxiety-provoking for parents and doctors and does have risks involved (Ross 2000). For sick infants with a high probability of a UTI suprapubic aspiration, although invasive, is a recognised method to obtain a sample of urine. Organisations will have local policy to guide clinical practice, and issues of consent must be discussed with the parents as suprapubic aspiration can carry a risk, although complications are very rare (Barkemeyer 1993).

Minor risks are:

- local bleeding from the puncture site
- transient haematuria.

More serious complications (very rare) are:

- gross haemorrhage
- haematoma
- bowel perforation
- peritonitis
- abdominal wall abscess
- bacteraemia.

Contraindications to suprapubic aspiration reported in the literature have included:

- cellulitis
- absence of a palpable bladder
- large inguinal hernia
- abdominal distension
- massive organomegaly.

Procedure

If a decision has been made to perform a suprapubic aspiration this should be undertaken before carrying out the rest of the infection screening in the sick child, as he or she may void during other upsetting procedures. Evidence exists in the literature to support suprapubic aspiration using ultrasound, as this will inform the doctor of where there is likely to be urine present. Local policy should be in place, but generally the following equipment and support will be required:

- Topical or local anaesthetic can be applied to the area (unless the sample is required urgently from a critically unwell infant).
- Analgesia or pain relief needs to be administered (Rosenblum et al 2006).
- Equipment: an assistant to hold the baby, a urine collection bottle, a sterile 23-G needle (25 G for premature babies), a sterile 2- or 5-mL syringe, a portable scanner if one is available, an alcohol swab, sterile gloves and a cotton swab.

If a scanner is available undo the nappy and scan the bladder to establish if urine is in the bladder; ALWAYS keep the sample bottle nearby, as the baby may well void at this stage. If no scanner is available establish if the nappy is wet or dry, and if there is a dry nappy and a history of no void in the past 30 min this may increase the chance of a successful suprapubic aspiration. If possible give the baby fluids, as a hydrated baby will be making more urine. Also, if the bladder is dull to percussion (indicating the presence of urine) there is a greater chance of a successful aspiration.

A video is available online that clearly demonstrates the procedure (Royal Children's Hospital Melbourne 2007):

1. Ask parents or carers if they wish to stay.
2. Ask a nurse to hold the infant supine with the legs extended.
3. Make sure that someone is ready with the sample bottle to catch the urine if the baby voids.
4. Wipe the skin with an alcohol swab (allow to dry) and fix the needle to the syringe.

5. Using sterile procedure to collect the sample, identify the insertion point (midline, lower abdominal crease; use a scan picture if available).
6. Insert the needle at right angles to the skin, aspirating gently as the needle advances.
7. If you have no success, withdraw the needle to just under the skin and insert it again at an angle aimed slightly away from the pelvis, again gently aspirating.
8. If this fails then stop the procedure; however, if urine is obtained place it in the sample bottle.

Following the procedure apply a small dressing or plaster and advise the family that there may be a small amount of local bleeding and that the urine may be tinged pink when they next change the nappy.

Urinary catheterisation

Rationale for catheterisation

Urinary catheterisation is the insertion of a tube into the bladder, using aseptic technique, for the purpose of evacuating or instilling fluid (Mallett & Dougherty 2000). The procedure can be required for a variety of reasons, from urinary retention and investigations (e.g. urodynamics, micturating cystourethrogram) to during acute illness or pre- or postoperatively to measure urine output and/or promote healing (Macauley 1997). It is acknowledged that indwelling urethral catheters should be used only after reviewing other possible management strategies, and when necessary the catheter should be removed as soon as possible (Department of Health 2001). Alternatives to indwelling urethral catheterisation include intermittent catheterisation, medication, voiding programmes, incontinent pads and suprapubic catheterisation (Simpson 1999). UTIs are one of the most commonly acquired hospital infections, the majority of which (80%) are associated with urinary catheters (Niel-Weise & van den Broek 2005, Parkin & Keeley 2003). The risk of developing catheter-acquired infections increases with the period of catheterisation, with the highest risk factor associated with catheterisation lasting longer than 6 days, which increases the risk by nearly sevenfold (Gentry & Cope 2005). Practice regarding catheterisation can often be ritualistic rather than evidence-based; it is important that nurses carrying out this procedure have received specific training and are competent practitioners.

LINK CHAPTER **1**

Selection of an appropriate catheter

Some clinical areas do not stock paediatric catheters, and feeding tubes are sometimes used to catheterise paediatric patients; this can result in harm to the patient and is not recommended (Smith 2003). Appropriate and licensed catheter materials available include polytetrafluoroethylene, hydromer polymer, hydrogel, silicone elastomer and 100% silicone (Fig. 32.5).

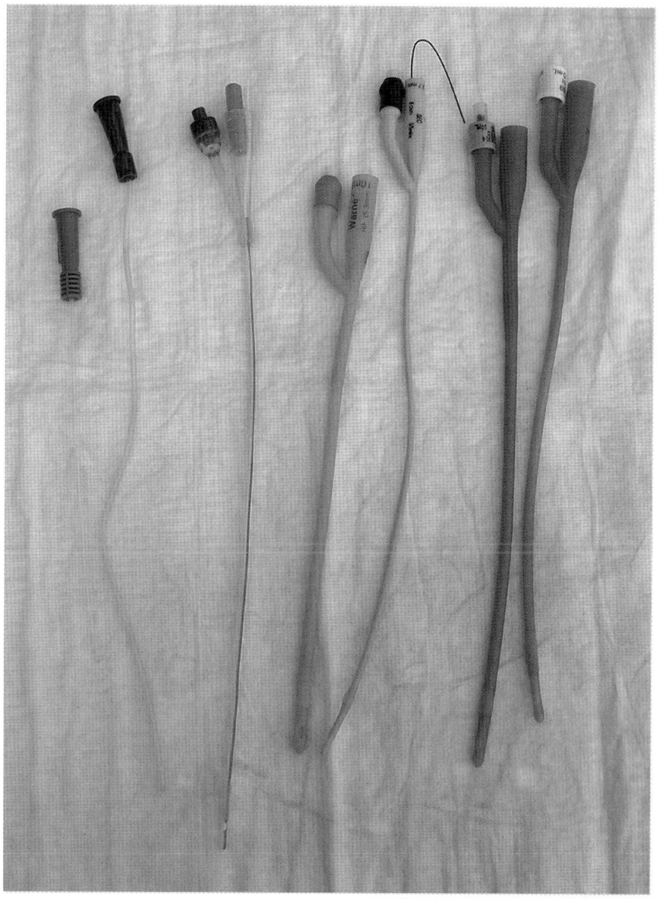

Fig. 32.5 • A range of catheters.

There is little research evidence on the most appropriate catheter material for use in paediatric patients (Smith 2003). Hydrogel-coated and 100% silicone catheters are commonly used in practice (Bray & Sanders 2006). Latex-coated or latex catheters should not be used in patients who are at risk of latex allergy; this includes children with chronic illness, especially those with neural tube defects and other urogenital abnormalities (Sapan et al 2002).

There are four available catheter lengths: paediatric (30 cm), male (40–44 cm), female (23–26 cm) and female (15 cm). If an inappropriate length is used this can result in trauma to the patient. There is a range of different diameter sizes (Charriere, Ch) available; in paediatric practice sizes 6–12 Ch are appropriate for use. The smallest diameter catheters should be used that will effectively empty the bladder (Pellowe et al 2001).

Selection of appropriate lubrication

The use of lubrication during catheterisation is necessary to protect the urethra from trauma. National Institute for Clinical Excellence guidelines (2003) advise that an 'appropriate lubricant from a single-use container should be used during catheterisation to minimise trauma and infection'.

LINK CHAPTER 1

Increasingly, anaesthetic gels (Instillagel, Fig. 32.6, and lidocaine gels) are being used for lubrication; this serves to make the procedure as pain-free as possible and can reduce the incidence of infection due to such preparations being in sterile ready-to-use packs (Gentry & Cope 2005). If using lidocaine gel it is necessary to identify any patients who may be at risk of possible systemic effects; these can include patients with liver disease, hypotension, cardiac problems, pregnancy and epilepsy, and children (Addison & Mould 2000).

There is little evidence to strongly support the use of antibiotics during indwelling urinary catheterisation to prevent urinary-related infections (Rao 1998), although limited evidence does suggest that prophylactic antibiotics can reduce the rate of bacteriuria in adult catheterised patients (Niel-Weise & Van den Broek 2005). A standardised approach to the use of antibiotics in urinary catheter management would be of benefit to patients and staff (Fraczyk & Godfrey 2004), but as these currently do not exist it is recommended that the use of antibiotics is decided in line with local policy and procedures.

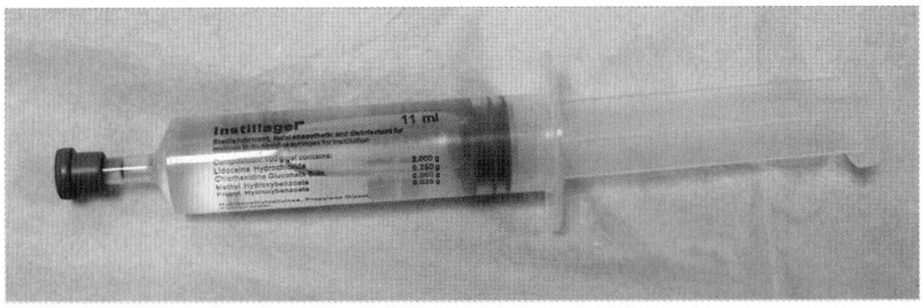

Fig. 32.6 • Instillagel.

Procedures Box 32.1 Passing a urethral catheter on a child

Action
Ensure the child's consent and adequate preparation and procedures for distraction.

LINK CHAPTER 1

Reason *Catheterisation is a sensitive procedure that requires preparation and negotiation to prevent anxiety and emotional upset.*

Action
Ensure that adequate pain relief is discussed with the child and family.

Reason *Enables a positive experience of the procedure and negotiation of analgesia options.*

Action
Collect the required equipment:

- Selected catheter
- Sterile gauze
- Sterile saline
- Sterile water
- Lubrication gel
- 5- to 10-mL syringe
- Sterile pack with gloves
- Plastic apron
- Catheter drainage bag
- Tape to secure.

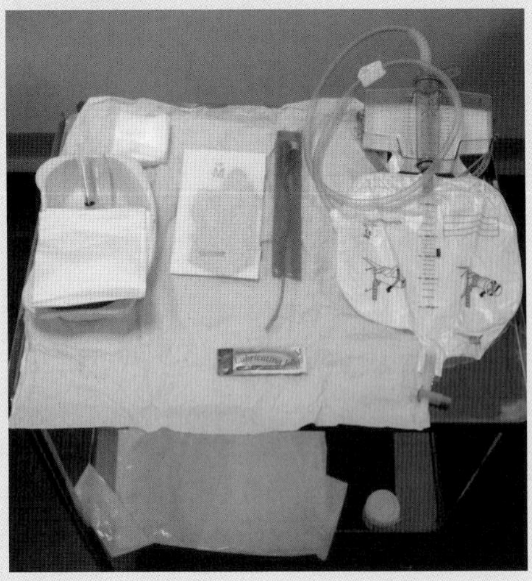

A cleaned trolley with the equipment required for catheterisation is shown.

Action
Prepare a private setting.

Reason *Enables privacy and dignity.*

Action
Arrange the presence of appropriate staff and family members.

Reason *The presence of appropriate family support mechanisms is well documented as improving the outcome for a child.*

Action
Wash and dry your hands and put on a plastic apron.

Reason *Prevents cross-infection.*

Action
Apply gloves, and using sterile saline on gauze clean the urethral meatus.

Reason *There is no evidence to support cleansing the urethral meatus as a sterile procedure; it is recommended to use sterile saline on gauze (Bray & Sanders 2006).*

Action
Clean the trolley and lay out the sterile field or pack with equipment for catheterisation.

Reason *Catheterisation is a sterile procedure and should be undertaken using a strict aseptic technique (National Institute for Clinical Excellence 2003).*

Action
Wash and dry your hands and put on sterile gloves.

Reason *Prevents cross-infection and bacterial contamination of the catheter.*

Action
Apply the chosen sterile lubrication to the tip of the catheter, ensuring even coverage.

Procedures Box 32.1 Passing a urethral catheter on a child—cont'd

Reason *Prevents urethral trauma and maintains sterile procedure.*

Action
Leave most of catheter within the sterile internal packaging.

Reason *Reduces the chance of infection and allows urine (when inserted) to drain into an enclosed container.*

Action
Locate the urethral meatus and insert the catheter slowly.

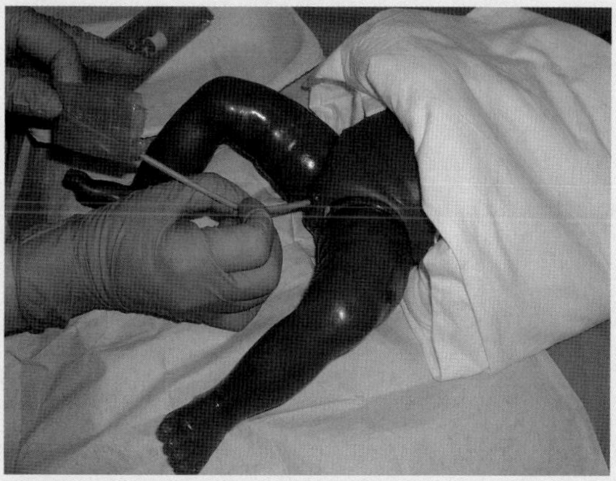

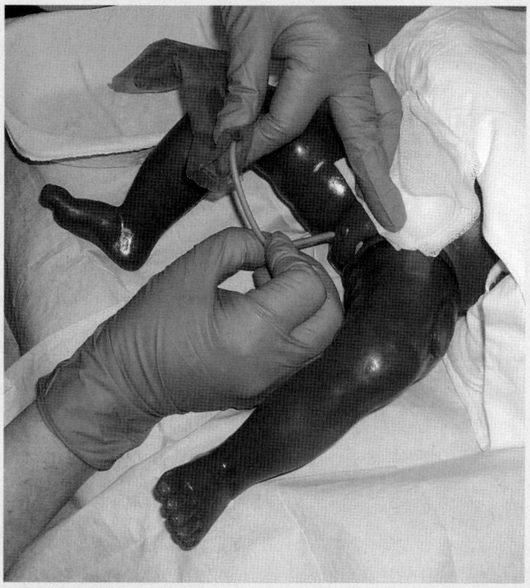

Reason *Prevents urethral trauma and possible mislocation.*

Action
If catheterising a boy, support the penis in a semierect position; pressure or resistance might be felt while bypassing the urethral sphincter.

In this example of catheterisation of a boy, the catheter is in place as urine has drained from the catheter hub, and the syringe to inflate the balloon is attached.

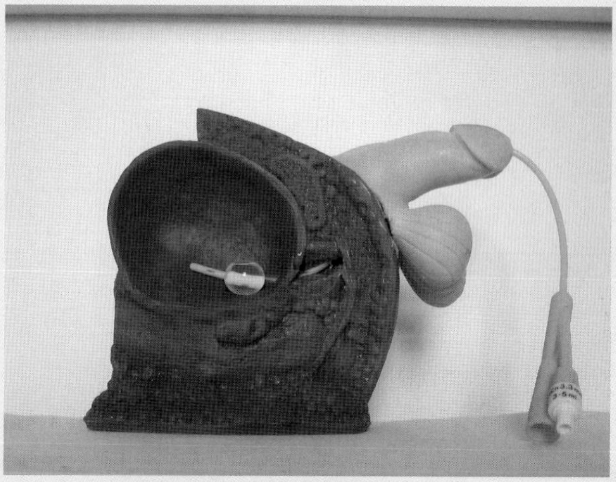

Reason *It is important to gently apply pressure to bypass this and enter the bladder; knowledge of anatomy is important to ensure safe practice.*

Action
Continue to insert the catheter until urine drains.

Reason *Ensures correct placement of the catheter.*

Action
If catheterising girls and urine is not present, leave the catheter in situ and begin the procedure with a new sterile catheter; practitioners need to check that two tubes are not inserted into the urethra.

Reason *The catheter left in situ helps locate the incorrect opening (most commonly the vagina); a new catheter must be used to prevent contamination, as the urinary system is sterile.*

Action
If any further difficulty is experienced the procedure should be stopped and appropriate senior staff contacted.

Reason *To prevent trauma, both physical and emotional, to the child.*

LINK CHAPTER **1**

Action
When urine drains from the hub insert the catheter at least a further 2 cm.

Reason *Prevents possible inflation of the balloon in the urethra and ensures correct placement (Bray & Sanders 2006).*

Action
Attach the syringe filled with sterile water to the inflation channel hub on the catheter.

Reason *Sterile water prevents contamination; saline must not be used as it can crystallise and cause harm to the patient on removal of the catheter.*

Action
The balloon should be slowly inflated with the recommended amount on the catheter.

Reason *The guidance from the manufacturers on inflation must be adhered to, as over- or under-inflation can cause uneven inflation, causing the catheter tip to lie against the bladder wall, resulting in irritation (Getliffe 2003).*

Procedures Box 32.1 Passing a urethral catheter on a child—cont'd

LINK CHAPTER 1

Action
If any resistance is felt during balloon inflation, stop the procedure and reposition the catheter.

Reason *Prevents inflation of the balloon when not correctly in the bladder.*

Action
Attach a sterile drainage bag.

Reason *Prevents contamination and allows drainage.*

Action
Gently pull back on the catheter to ensure that it is secure.

Reason *Checks the location and prevents trauma.*

Action
Apply hydrocolloid dressing to the child's leg.

Reason *Protects the skin against strong adhesive tapes.*

Action
Secure the catheter using appropriate tape, checking for any possible allergies.

Reason *The catheter must be secure to prevent possible trauma.*

Action
Document the make, type and batch number of the catheter used along with the water inserted and the time and place of catheter insertion.

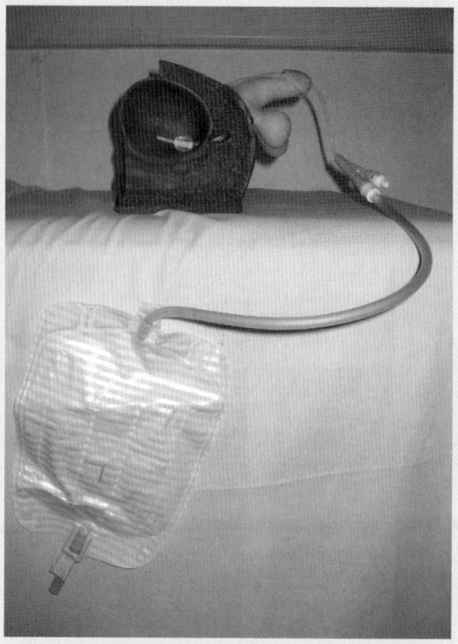

A model demonstrating a catheter inserted with the balloon inflated in the bladder and a sterile drainage bag attached is shown.

Reason *Allows identification of risk and infection sources and possible product issues.*

Suprapubic catheters

Suprapubic catheterisation is increasingly being used as an alternative to urethral catheterisation (Addison & Mould 2000) and involves the insertion of a catheter directly into the bladder via an incision in the abdominal wall (Shah & Shah 1998). It is associated with many advantages, including no risk of urethral trauma, no risk of urethral necrosis or urethritis, more comfort for wheelchair users and evidence of reduced infection (Robinson 2005). Initial suprapubic catheterisation in children is done under general anaesthetic and is a surgical procedure undertaken by a qualified clinical practitioner trained to undertake the procedure (Robinson 2003). Not all indwelling catheters are licensed for use as suprapubic catheters (Medical Devices Agency 2001); it is therefore important for practitioners to check the necessary licensing, which can be done by either contacting the manufacturers or checking inside the National Health Service Catalogue available on all wards and to community staff (Robinson 2005).

Commonly, a suprapubic catheter is sized between 12 and 16 Ch with a 10- to 20-mL balloon volume; the female length catheter can be used successfully depending on body shape, dexterity and the drainage system that will be used (Robinson 2005). Previously the use of 100% silicone catheters was advised for suprapubic catheterisation (Doherty & Winder 2000); however, the Medical Devices Agency (2001) have since highlighted concern about the use of 100% silicone catheters due to cuffing of the balloon following deflation and possible pain caused to patients during removal. As this is observed to a lesser extent in latex products (Parkin et al 2002), when no latex allergy occurs it is recommended that these catheters are used as an alternative to silicone-based products. It has been suggested by manufacturers that following balloon deflation the catheter should be left in place for 5 min to allow the balloon to return to its original shape, although the influence of this on practice has been questioned (Evans et al 2001). It is recommended to gently rotate the catheter while removing it suprapubically; often a little force is required (Robinson 2005). Some manufacturers now produce a catheter for suprapubic use with an integral balloon that does not increase in diameter on inflation and does not misshape on deflation (Robinson 2005).

Emptying of a catheter

As soon as a catheter is inserted and attached to a sterile catheter bag this then forms a closed drainage system. There are a variety of different urine collection bags that can be attached to the catheter; they include bags that can be strapped to the leg to allow the child to be mobile, and there are some that have additional measuring reservoirs in which the urine can be held in the system to enable accurate measurement of urine produced over a planned time period of time (Fig. 32.7).

Emptying a catheter bag must be a clean procedure, as the closed system is utilised to try to maintain a sterile environment (Winn 1996). In emptying a catheter bag the closed system is broken, and this therefore increases the risk of introducing

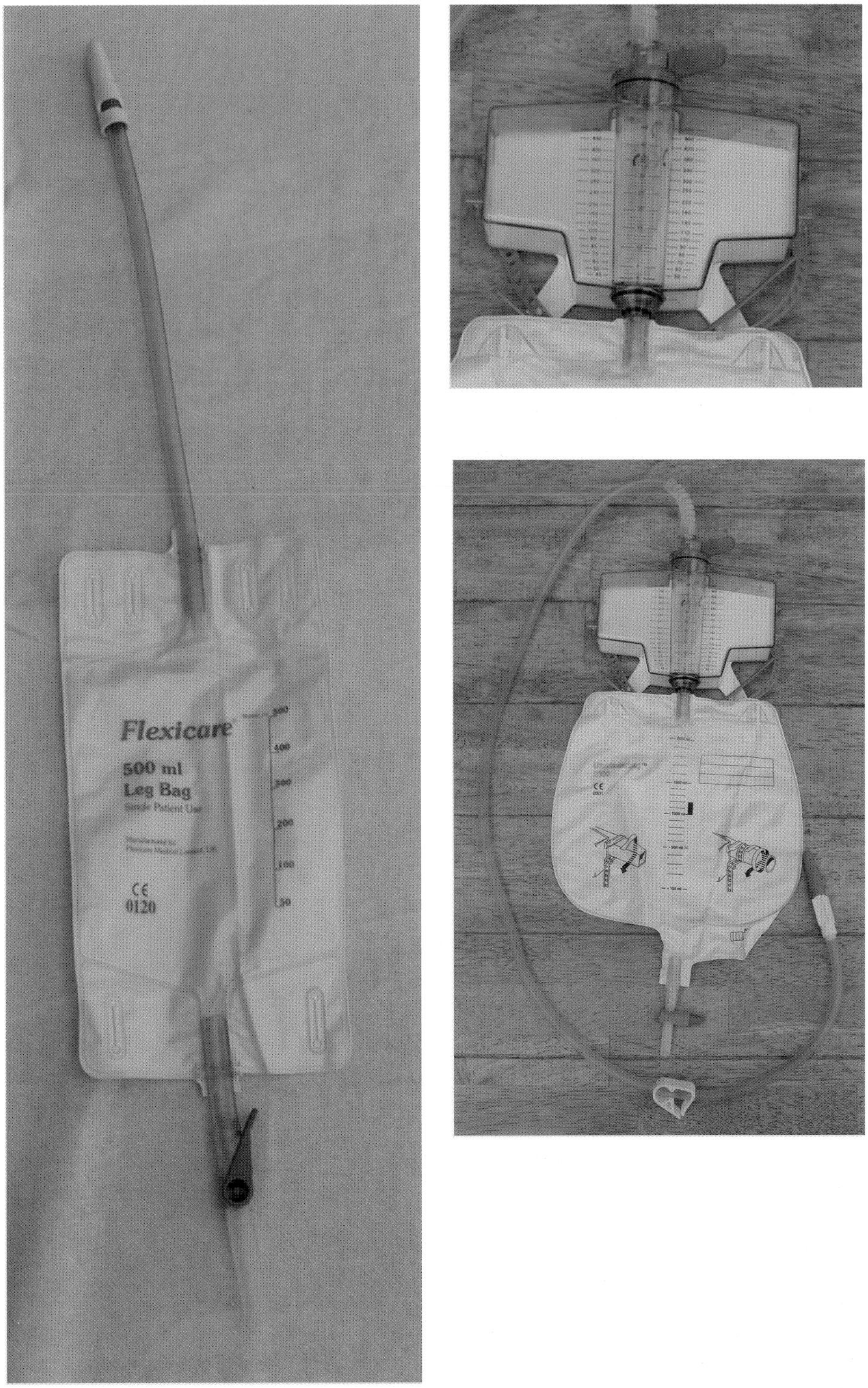

Fig. 32.7 • Urine collection bags.

pathogens. Unnecessary sampling of urine from a catheter closed drainage system should be avoided, and a catheter should be emptied only when clinically required (Department of Health 2001, 2003). If the utmost care is taken and effective infection control measures are undertaken then this can limit the potential for pathogen introduction but not eliminate it, as merely having a urinary catheter in situ introduces a risk of infection (Simpson 2001). The longer a catheter is in situ, the higher the risk of UTI (Curran 2001). Being vigilant in maintaining the closed system can limit the risk of UTI (Langley et al 2001). Nurses have a key role to play in maintaining the closed urinary drainage system (Winn 1996).

Procedures Box 32.2 Emptying a catheter bag

Action
Collect the equipment needed:

- Swabs soaked with 70% isopropyl alcohol
- A clean jug or container
- Disposable gloves.

Action
Explain and discuss the procedure with the child and her or his carer.

Reason *Ensures that the child and carer understand the procedure and that the carer and child (dependent on age and developmental stage) give valid consent.*

Action
Wash your hands using antibacterial soap and water and put on disposable gloves.

Reason *Avoids cross-infection.*

Action
Clean the outlet valve with a swab soaked with 70% isopropyl alcohol.

Reason *Reduces the risk of infection and removes pathogens.*

Action
Allow the urine to drain into the jug or container without the outlet valve contacting the jug.

Reason *Empties the drainage bag and accurately measures the volume of the contents as required.*

Action
Close the outlet valve and clean it again with a new alcohol-soaked swab.

Reason *Reduces the risk of cross-infection and removes residual urine droplets.*

Action
Cover the jug and dispose of the contents appropriately, having noted the amount of urine for fluid balance records.

Reason *Reduces the risk of environmental contamination and maintains Nursing and Midwifery Council guidelines for accurate documentation.*

Action
Wash your hands with antibacterial soap and water.

Reason *Reduces the risk of infection.*

LINK CHAPTER **31**

Removal of a urinary catheter

While there is extensive literature on the type, maintenance and techniques for insertion of urinary catheters, limited attention has been given to the policies and procedures for their removal (Griffiths & Fernandez 2005). Evidence suggests that the timing of catheter removal is a balance between avoiding infection (by early removal) and circumventing voiding dysfunction (by later removal) (Griffiths & Fernandez 2005). Catheter-associated bacteriuria is common and increases by 5–8% each day during the period of catheterisation (Getliffe 1996). There is evidence to suggest that early rather than delayed catheter removal influences shorter hospital stay (Griffiths & Fernandez 2005).

No evidence exists to suggest that clamping prior to removal of the catheter compared with free drainage has any beneficial effects, or that there are any benefits of between midnight and early morning catheter removal (Griffiths & Fernandez 2005). These findings are based on an adult population.

Before catheter removal the water in the catheter balloon has to be drained; this balloon will have expanded and stretched at inflation (Robinson 2003). At deflation the balloon membrane collapses and deforms, resulting in surface changes to the deflated balloon; these changes can form the shape of creases, ridges or cuffing, and all these can cause discomfort to the patient on catheter removal and possible trauma of the urethra (Robinson 2003).

Manual syringe aspiration is the most common method used to deflate catheter balloons, in which a syringe is attached to the deflation valve and pulled back until no more water is emitted. Some authors have suggested that following deflation of the balloon 0.5 mL should be reinserted to reduce ridges and creases before removal of the catheter (Semijonow et al 1995). This is not based on research evidence, and it can take up to 4 mL to fully remove any disruptions to the balloon surface; additionally, catheters are manufactured for single inflation and deflation (Robinson 2003). Previous practice may have involved deflation by cutting the inflation valves; this has been found to still involve the formation of creases and ridges (Robinson 2003) and is not recommended by manufacturers. Self-syringe aspiration has been discussed as a possible alternative to manual aspiration, as it has been shown to leave a small volume of water behind in the balloon that may act as a cushion and prevent misshape following deflation (Robinson 2003), although this is currently not recommended as there is no supportive evidence.

Procedures Box 32.3 Removing a urethral catheter

Action
Ensure the child's consent and adequate preparation and procedures for distraction.

Reason *This involves a procedure that may cause anxiety and distress.*

Action
Ensure that adequate pain relief is discussed with the child and family.

Reason *Enables a positive experience of the procedure and negotiation of analgesia options.*

Action
Prepare a private setting and arrange the presence of appropriate staff and family members.

Reason *The presence of appropriate family support mechanisms is well documented as improving the outcome for a child.*

Procedures Box 32.3 Removing a urethral catheter—cont'd

Action
Collect the required equipment:

- Sterile gauze
- Sterile saline
- 5- to 10-mL syringe
- Sterile pack with gloves
- Plastic apron.

Action
Clean the trolley and lay out the sterile field or pack with equipment for catheter removal.

Reason *Prevents cross-infection.*

Action
Wash and dry your hands and put on sterile gloves.

Reason *Prevents cross-infection.*

Action
Attach an appropriate size syringe to the inflation and deflation hub and gently draw back on the syringe.

Reason *Deflates the balloon and reduces cuffing.*

Action
The full quantity of original water inserted may not be present.

Reason *Osmosis causes the water in the balloon to decrease in volume over time.*

Action
When all the water has been withdrawn, gently apply pressure to the catheter and pull in a smooth action away from the body.

Reason *Prevents urethral trauma and discomfort for the child.*

Action
If any resistance is felt, reattach the syringe to the inflation and deflation valve and repeat the withdrawal technique.

Reason *Omits any residual water in the balloon.*

Action
If any further difficulty is experienced the procedure should be stopped and appropriate senior staff contacted.

Reason *To prevent trauma, physical and emotional, to the child.*

Action
When the catheter is removed, ensure that the child drinks adequate fluids and that adequate pain relief is provided to aid the first urethral passing of urine.

Reason *Encourages normal micturition to resume.*

Now test your knowledge

- A 1-year-old child is presented at the walk-in centre with a day's history of temperature and being off her food, with her parents anxious about a 'pink' nappy that she has just had. How might you collect and store and test a sample of urine and what might you observe for?
- Critically evaluate how you would prepare a 4-year-old child (a boy) for the insertion of a urethral catheter prior to an investigation for vesicoureteric reflux. What support and guidance would be required to prepare the parent to assist you in this procedure?
- A 2½-year-old child attends the clinic with his mother; she is worried that he has restarted wetting again after being dry for the past 3 months. She reports that he has been more tired than usual over the past week and drinking more fluids. What could a urine sample detect?
- What considerations should be given to a child who has an indwelling catheter in place? Can you assess the areas of risk?

References

Addison R, Mould C (2000) Risk assessment in suprapubic catheterisation. Nursing Standard 14(36):43–46

Austin BJ, Bollard C, Gunn TR (1999) Is urethral catheterisation a successful alternative to suprapubic aspiration in neonates? Journal of Paediatrics and Child Health 35(1):34–36

Barkemeyer BM (1993) Suprapubic aspiration of urine in very low birth weight infants. Pediatrics 92(3):45

Bray L, Sanders C (2006) Nursing management of paediatric urethral catheterization. Nursing Standard 20(24):51–60

Bulloch B, Bausher J, Pomerantz W, Connors JM, Mahabee-Gittens M, Dowd MD (2000) Can urine clarity exclude the diagnosis of urinary tract infection? Pediatrics 106:60–64

Cook R (1996) Urinalysis: ensuring accurate urine testing. Nursing Standard 10(46):49–52

Curran E (2001) Reducing the risk of healthcare-acquired infection. Nursing Standard 16(1):45–52

Department of Health (2001) Guidelines for preventing infections associated with the insertion and maintenance of short-term indwelling urethral catheters in acute care. Journal of Hospital Infection 47(suppl.):S39–S46

Department of Health (2003) Winning ways: working together to reduce healthcare associated infection in England. Stationery Office, London

Doherty W, Winder A (2000) Indwelling catheters: practical guidelines for catheter blockage. British Journal of Nursing 9(18):2006–2014

Evans A, Godfrey H, Fraczyk L (2001) An audit of problems associated with urinary catheter withdrawal. British Journal of Community Nursing 6(10):511–519

Fillingham S, Douglas J (2004) Urological nursing. Baillière Tindall, London

Fraczyk L, Godfrey L (2004) Current practice of antibiotic prophylaxis for catheter procedures. British Journal of Nursing 13(10):610–617

Gentry H, Cope S (2005) Using silver to reduce catheter-associated urinary tract infections. Nursing Standard 19(50):51–54

Getliffe K (1996) Care of urinary catheters. Nursing Standard 11(11):47–50

Getliffe K (2003) Catheters and catheterization. In Getliffe K, Dolman M (eds) Promoting continence: a clinical and research resource. Baillière Tindall, London

Griffiths R, Fernandez R (2005) Policies for the removal of short-term indwelling urethral catheters. Cochrane Database of Systematic Reviews, issue 1, article no. CD004011.pub2

Hjalmas K (1976) Micturition in infants and children with normal lower urinary tract: a urodynamic study. Scandinavian Journal Urology and Nephrology 37:9–17

Holmdahl G, Hanson E, Hansom M et al (1996) Four-hour voiding observation in healthy infants. Journal of Urology 156:1809–1812

Jefferson I (1990) Urine analysis in paediatrics. In Newall R, Howell R (eds) Clinical urinalysis. Miles, Buckinghamshire

Koff SA (1983) Estimating bladder capacity in children. Urology 21:248

Langley JM, Hanakowski M, Leblanc J (2001) Unique epidemiology of nosocomial urinary tract infection in children. American Journal of Infection Control 29(2):94–98

Lewis J (1998) Clean-catch versus urine collection pads: a prospective trial. Paediatrics Nursing 10(1):15–16

Liao J, Churchill B (2001) Peadiatric urine testing. Paediatric Clinics of North America 48(6):1425–1434

Macauley M (1997) Urinary drainage systems. In Fillingham S, Douglas J (eds) Urological nursing, 2nd edn. Baillière Tindall, London

Mallett S, Dougherty L (2000) The Royal Marsden Hospital manual of clinical nursing, 5th edn. Blackwell Science, Oxford

Martin E (2003) Concise medical dictionary. Oxford University Press, Oxford

Medical Devices Agency (2001) Problems removing urinary catheters. MDA, London

National Institute for Clinical Excellence (2003) Infection control: prevention of healthcare associated infection in primary and community care. NICE, London

Niel-Weise B, van den Broek P (2005) Antibiotic policies for short term catheter bladder drainage in adults. Cochrane Database of Systematic Reviews, issue 3, CD005428

Parkin J, Keeley F (2003) Indwelling catheter-associated urinary tract infections. British Journal of Community Nursing 8(4):166–170

Parkin J, Scanlan J, Woolley M, Grover D, Evans A, Feneley R (2002) Urinary catheter deflation cuff formation: clinical audit and quantitative in vitro analysis. BJU International 90(7): 666–671

Pellowe C, Loveday H, Harper P, Robinson N, Pratt R (2001) Preventing infections from short term indwelling catheters. Nursing Times 87(37):67–68

Rao G (1998) Risk factors for the spread of antibiotic-resistant bacteria. Drugs 55:323–330

Rao G, Bhatt J, Houghton C, Macfarlane P (2004) An improved urine collection pad method: a randomised clinical trial. Archives of Disease in Childhood 89:773–775

Robinson J (2003) Deflation of a Foley catheter balloon. Nursing Standard 17(27):33–38

Robinson J (2005) Suprapubic catheterization: challenges in changing catheters. British Journal of Community Nursing 10(10):461–463

Rosenblum A, Goldman M, Lavi G, Goldman D, Kozer E (2006) Pain in infants and younger than 2 months of age during suprapubic aspiration and transurethral bladder catheterisation – a single blind randomised controlled study. Journal of Emergency Medicine 30(2):238–238

Ross JH (2000) Urinary tract infections: 2000 update. American Family Physician 62(8):1777

Royal Children's Hospital Melbourne (2007) Suprapubic aspiration procedure. Online. Available: http://www.rch.org.au/clinicalguide/forms/SPAvideo_procedure.cfm

Sapan N, Nacarkucuk E, Canitez Y, Saglam H (2002) Evaluation of the need for routine pre-operative latex allergy tests in children. Pediatrics International 44:157–162

Semijonow A, Roth S, Hertle L (1995) Reducing trauma whilst removing long term indwelling balloon catheters. BJU International 75(2):241

Shah J, Shah N (1998) Percutaneous suprapubic catheterisation. Urology News 2(5):11–12

Simerville JA, Maxted WC, Pahira JJ (2005) Urinalysis: a comprehensive review. American Family Physician 71(6):1153–1162

Simpson L (1999) Improving community catheter management. Professional Nurse 14(12):831–834

Simpson L (2001) Indwelling urethral catheters. Nursing Standard 15(46):47–53

Smith L (2003) Which catheter? Criteria for selection of urinary catheters for children. Paediatric Nursing 15(3):14–18

Trigg E, Mohammed T (eds) (2006) Practices in children's nursing: guidelines for hospital and community. Elsevier, Edinburgh

Winn C (1996) Basing catheter care on research principles. Nursing Standard 10(18):38–40

33 Assessment and management of wounds in children

Lesley E. Wayne

The skills involved in assessing and managing wounds in children far exceed those normally needed to deal with adult wounds and require all the specialist knowledge inherent in the care of paediatric patients.

Many children and their carers will be anxious and afraid (Williams 1995), and gaining the child's cooperation and compliance can difficult. For many children sustaining a wound through injury will be a new and traumatic experience incurring all the natural fears and anxieties.

Commonly, children have been physically restrained while undergoing treatment for wounds, so increasing their anxiety and distress. This practice is not only distressing for all concerned but also largely unnecessary.

The psychological and emotional welfare of the child and carer is integral to paediatric wound assessment and management. Not only can children be apprehensive about the impending procedure and fearful of pain, but they may also be concerned about the end result (e.g. fearing loss of function or scarring). The child's cognitive developmental stage is crucial in directing the practitioner in devising the treatment and management plan.

Pictures or diagrams are useful to support verbal explanations.

The child's expert is their main carer, so consult and include her or him when preparing the child for the forthcoming procedure.

Definition of a wound

A wound is 'any injury caused by physical means that results in disruption of normal continuity of tissues and structures' (*Dorland's Illustrated Medical Dictionary* 1988, cited by Foster 2007).

Wounds can be categorised as:

- contusion (bruise)
- abrasion (graze)
- laceration (tear)
- incision (with a sharp implement)
- puncture (stab)
- burn (from dry heat) or scald (from wet heat) (Dougherty & Lister 2004a).

Wound assessment and examination

The assessment and examination of patients presenting with wounds is complex.

Procedures Box 33.1 Assessment and examination of acute wounds

Take a detailed history, including the following:

Action
The time elapsed since the injury occurred.

Reason *This is important for deciding on whether to primarily close the wound and the need for tetanus prophylaxis (wounds not cleaned for 24 h are considered to be tetanus-prone).*

Action
The history should also ascertain the mechanism of injury.

Reason *The mechanism will indicate whether there is likely to be damage to underlying structures or the presence of a foreign body.*

Action
Check tetanus status and any known allergies.

Reason *Tetanus infection can gain entry through an open wound, particularly a wound sustained in a dirty environment.*

Action
Specify the anatomical location of the wound.

Reason *The location of the wound will affect healing rates and choice of treatment.*

Action
Specify the dominant hand in an upper limb injury.

Reason *Injuries to a dominant hand require especial care when assessing and managing the injury.*

Action
Specify:

- type of wound (e.g. flap, laceration, cut, puncture wound, amputation, crush injury)
- wound measurements (length, depth, breadth)
- direction and shape of the wound (e.g. transverse, oblique, longitudinal, L-shaped, stellate); is it a straight incision or ragged and is there any skin loss?

Reasons *Ensures the accuracy and clarity of the wound assessment.*
Aids review of the wound by other professionals (see Reynolds & Cole 2006).

Procedures Box 33.1 Assessment and examination of acute wounds—cont'd

Action
Specify whether the tissue is:
- viable (i.e. healthy undamaged tissue)
- non-viable (i.e. damaged and contused, without adequate blood supply).

Reason *Healthy tissue is conducive to optimal healing, whereas non-viable tissue is unlikely to survive and needs removal to ensure optimal healing.*

Action
Note any associated bruising, haematoma, swelling, erythema and circulatory or sensory deficit.

Reasons *A haematoma will need evacuation before wound closure.*
Sensory deficit may indicate nerve damage and will require further assessment.
Circulatory deficit will need to be addressed in order to preserve and restore healthy tissue.

Action
Determine if the wound is clean, dirty or contaminated.

Reason *Dirty, contaminated wounds are likely to become infected, preventing wound healing.*

Action
Control local bleeding.

Reason *Haemostasis is necessary to prevent the possible development of a haematoma and to promote wound healing.*

Action
Expose patients who have sustained trauma, as appropriate.

Reason *Further wounds or injuries may be missed if a full examination is not undertaken.*

Action
Evaluate distal neurovascular function.

Reason *If there is a deficit in the neurovascular function further assessment will be required and action taken to restore function.*

Action
Exclude involvement of underlying structures (e.g. tendons and nerves distal to the wound, joints and fractures).

Reason *Damage to underling structures could result in loss of function.*

Action
Assess motor function.

Reason *Ascertains whether the patient has full motor function; a deficit may indicate an underlying injury.*

Action
Consider the use of X-rays.

Reason *Excludes the presence of a radiopaque foreign body or bony injury.*

(Guly 1996, Wayne & Bunn 2007.)

Wound management

The objectives of wound management are not only to promote healing but also to ensure the child's psychological well-being. It is perfectly possible to give quite young children (4–5 years) choices about their treatment and involve them in carrying out the techniques. Teaching and involving children in cleansing their own wound not only teaches them about wound care and management but also gains their consent, gives them control of the situation and acts as a distraction technique.

Wound management should include the following:

- 'Written and/or verbal consent as appropriate
- Age appropriate explanations
- Local/topical anaesthetic/analgesia as required
- Thorough cleansing and exploration of wound, ensuring that the base of wound is visualised and the extent of the wound is determined; use retractors and magnifying lights if necessary
- Removal of slough, contaminants and damaged tissue
- Occasionally a tourniquet may be required to aid haemostasis when examining digits; remember to remove it! (Wayne & Bunn 2007).

The prime objectives of wound management are:

- to preserve viable tissue
- to avoid infection
- to restore tissue continuity and function
- to minimise scar formation.

Preservation of tissue: handling

Preservation of viable tissue is essential. Damaged tissue should therefore be handled as gently as possible in order to preserve the blood supply, maximise healing and prevent further damage.

Devitalised tissue should be debrided (National Institute for Clinical Excellence 2001), for although the body can remove devitalised and damaged tissue by autolysis, if large amounts remain healing can be impeded and it may be a source of infection. Various dressings are available to enhance autolysis by providing a moist environment (Dougherty & Lister 2004b); however, surgical debridement is usually considered to be the most effective method of removing necrotic material (Tissue Viability Nurses Association 2005).

Prevention of infection: cleansing agents and techniques

Infected wounds take longer to heal and scar formation may be increased. Infection can persist if necrotic or foreign material is left in the wound (Dulecki & Pieper 2005, National Institute for Clinical Excellence 2001). Thorough wound cleansing is essential in the management of traumatic wounds.

Cleansing techniques

Cleansing techniques commonly employed include high-pressure irrigation, swabbing, low-pressure irrigation, showering, bathing and washing the affected area under a running solution (Moore 2005).

Swabbing

Swabs are often used for applying the cleansing agent but may leave fibres in the wound, so prolonging the inflammatory response and thereby increasing the risk of infection (Blunt 2001).

Irrigation

Utilising the force of an irrigation solution to assist in the removal of debris is frequently advocated as the method of choice. Beware, however: too low a pressure may result in inadequate cleansing of the wound, while using too high a pressure may cause further trauma to the tissues (Blunt 2001, Fernandez et al 2004, McKirdy 2001).

Scrubbing

Adhered grit and gravel may be removed from the wound bed by gently scrubbing with a stiff brush after anaesthetising the wound with local anaesthetic. Abrading the wound in this manner is effective in preventing tattooing and infection, although care must be taken to avoid causing further trauma to the wound and delaying healing (Moore 2005).

The various methods employed to cleanse wounds have therefore advantages and disadvantages, and the choice of method must be a clinical decision made by the practitioner based on the assessment of the wound, the patient involved and the situation.

Cleansing agents

Tap water it is suggested is as effective in preventing bacterial infection as sterile normal saline solution for simple wounds (Griffiths 2001, Valente et al 2003). The use of antiseptics and disinfectants are no longer recommended as routine cleansing agents, indeed their use may prove to be systemically toxic and actually impair healing (Blunt 2001). Solutions should be used at body temperature in order to ensure that the macrophages can work effectively (Young 1995, cited in McKirdy 2001). A decrease in temperature can also have an adverse effect on the availability of oxygen within the wound (Thomas 1990, cited in McKirdy 2001).

Restoration of tissue continuity and function: minimise scar formation

Wound management in children can present the practitioner with particular challenges. Previous experiences, fears and anxieties will impinge on the child's coping strategies. Many children are frightened by the thought of needles, and closure of the wound by suturing may be a terrifying prospect for the child. It is therefore essential that the child's cognitive developmental stage and emotional status are considered when deciding on the most appropriate management procedure. First, consider whether wound closure is appropriate. Some wounds should not be closed, for example those heavily contaminated and at high risk of infection, such as human or animal bites. Other wounds, due to the nature of the trauma, cannot be closed, for example those with excessive skin loss. These wounds should be left to heal by secondary intent and dressed with a suitable dressing.

Wounds that may require closure include:

- lacerations
- incisions
- penetrating injuries.

ALERT
Care must be taken to explore these wounds thoroughly to exclude damage to underlying structures or the presence of a foreign body.

Crush injuries

ALERT
Wounds of this type may have a significant amount of skin loss, rendering them unsuitable for suturing. Closure with adhesive skin closure strips should be considered (Reynolds & Cole 2006).

Wound closure

There are several methods of wound closure available, for example:

- adhesive strips
- tissue adhesive
- suturing
- staples.

The method selected will depend on various factors. The child's developmental stage, psychological status and leisure activities, and the site and type of wound and its dimensions will all influence the practitioner's choice of method. The two former methods, however, are likely to cause the least distress in their application and therefore whenever possible should be the methods of choice.

Adhesive strips and tissue adhesive

Perforated flexible adhesive tape that allows 'spot welding' with tissue adhesive is now available for use when closing wounds over joints.

Method of application of adhesive strips

Strips should be applied on clean, dry skin at even intervals, leaving a small gap between each adhesive strip to prevent the skin becoming macerated and impairing healing (Fig. 33.1).

Tissue adhesive

Tissue adhesive can be used for superficial or deep dermal wounds when haemostasis has been achieved. It should not be used on friable skin or when good skin apposition is not

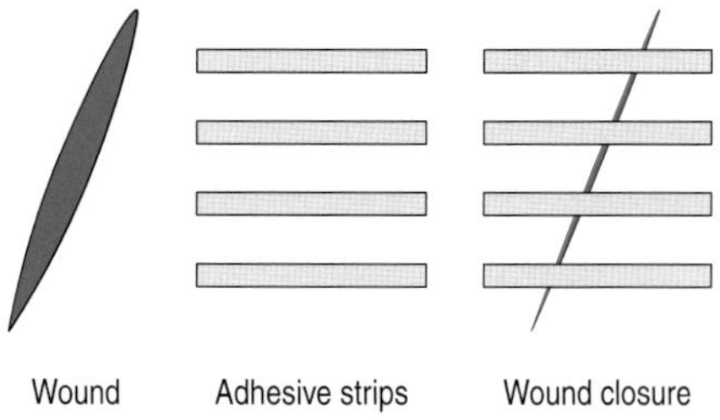

Fig. 33.1 • The application of adhesive strips.

achievable. It should not be used on infected tissue. It is advisable to refer to the manufacturer's instructions when applying tissue adhesive, as there may be some slight variation in their suitability of application and preferred method. When using adhesive on the face it is necessary to protect the eyes to prevent adhesive running into them. While adhesive will not damage the eyes it is nevertheless a very unpleasant experience and may result in the lids sticking together. Lying the patient down during application and covering the eyes with a damp gauze pad can avoid this (Reynolds & Cole 2006).

Generally, less is more when applying adhesive, i.e. the adhesive should be applied as a thin layer; a second layer can be applied if necessary. Application in thick layers will lessen its efficacy and may result in the wound dehiscing. Tissue adhesive can be used in conjunction with adhesive strips. This technique is useful to assist in drawing the skin edges together and holding them while the adhesive is applied. The adhesive is applied along the wound edges either in one continuous line or by using a spot welding method. The wound edges should be held together for approximately 30s to 1 min. Ensure that good closure has been achieved. The patient is advised that the adhesive will be absorbed in approximately 5 days. If adhesive strips have also been used the patient should be advised to leave them in situ until the wound is healed.

Sutures

It may be necessary to close certain wounds, such as large or jagged wounds and wounds under tension or over joints, with sutures. Closure of wounds by this method is normally undertaken in wounds that are less than 6h old. Lack of careful preparation may lead to infection and cause the wound to dehisce. After initial cleansing of the surrounding skin, the wound edges are infiltrated with a local anaesthetic. The wound can then be cleansed and prepared as appropriate, taking care to remove all foreign debris and excise any devascularised tissue. A clean incised laceration will require no excision, although skin edges may require trimming if they are ragged. The base of the wound should be visualised and explored to check that there is no injury to underlying structures. Wounds over joints should be thoroughly explored to ensure that there is no breach to the joint capsule and possible subsequent infection. Remember to assess traumatic wounds for underlying fractures.

Procedures Box 33.2 Using adhesive strips and tissue adhesive

Action
The wound should be thoroughly cleansed.

Reason *Avoids infection.*

Action
Haemostasis must be achieved; it may therefore be necessary to apply pressure to the wound for several minutes and when appropriate elevate the limb.

Reason *If the wound is still bleeding the adhesive strips will not adhere and tissue adhesive will not form a strong bond.*

Action
The surrounding skin needs to be dry.

Reasons *If not dry, adhesive strips will fail to stick.*
Application of adhesive to a moist area will produce a thermal reaction and cause pain.

Action
The skin edges should be apposed and not inverted (curled under).

Reason *Inverted edges impede healing and the resulting scarring is increased.*

Action
There should not be too much tension on the wound.

Reason *If there is too much tension it will not be possible to appose the skin edges, resulting in greater scarring.*

Actions
You will need a certain amount of compliance by the child; whenever appropriate, encourage the child to participate in the wound preparation and closure.

You will find that quite young children are quite good at this and are quite keen to apply their own adhesive strips (under supervision!).

Reasons *Compliance is required to achieve the best attainable results.*
Participation also ensures the child's consent; it is a good distraction technique and teaches the child how to care for a wound.

Suture materials

Needles

Atraumatic sutures are most commonly used. A variety of modern suture materials are now available for use in skin closure, and selection is largely a matter of personal preference. Non-absorbable materials such as monofilament nylon are most commonly used for skin closure, as they are less irritating to the tissues. Silk is now less commonly used, as it has been shown to be more prone to causing irritation and subsequent infection. Absorbable suture materials are used when deeper structures are involved. Choice of suture size is dictated by the extent, tension and site of the wound; when there is tension over the wound it may be necessary to select the stronger suture material (Table 33.1).

Equipment

See Box 33.1.

Suture technique

Obtain informed consent from the patient and/or parent or guardian.

Simple interrupted sutures

Traumatic wounds to the skin are usually closed by simple interrupted sutures. Knots should be positioned away from the skin edge and tied with just enough tension to bring the wound edges into apposition and slightly everted. Sutures should be placed at regular intervals along the wound, with an even tension. Knots should all be tied on the same side of the wound.

Table 33.1. Site of wound and suture gauge

Wound site	Suture gauge	Time left in situ (days)
Face	5.0 or 6.0	4–5
Head	4.0 or 3.0	7
Torso	4.0 or 3.0	7–10
Limbs	4.0	7 up to 10
Over joints	4.0	14

Box 33.1. Suture equipment

- 5-mL syringe
- Orange needle, long (gauge 25)
- Green needle for drawing up (gauge 21)
- Pair of scissors
- Needle holder
- Pair of non-toothed forceps
- Pair of toothed forceps
- Galipot
- Waterproof paper drapes (two)
- Paper hand towel
- Rubbish bag
- Personal protection: eye goggles, apron, gloves

Figure 33.2 is a diagrammatic representation of a simple interrupted suture technique.

Vertical mattress sutures

A vertical mattress suture consists of a double stitch that is inserted perpendicular to the wound edges (Fig. 33.3). Mattress sutures are used to evert the skin edges when the wound is under tension and/or the skin edges are inverting (Zuber 2002). Because scars eventually retract, eversion of the wound edges lessens scarring (Zuber 2002).

Staples

Inserting staples can be painful, and I would generally not recommend their use on young children. They are, however, sometimes used to close scalp wounds and are quick and easy to insert. The method used is similar to that when using a paper stapler (see manufacturers' instructions, as techniques vary slightly depending on the stapler used and the depth of the wound). The skin edges should be pushed up to evert them slightly to ensure good apposition. After inserting the staple release the handle completely, lift it away from the skin and check the staple insertion. Remove any that are not correctly implanted.

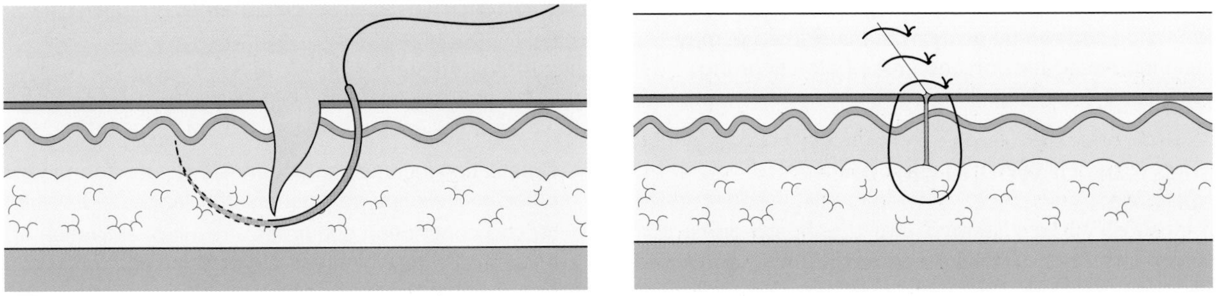

Fig. 33.2 • Simple suture. **(A)** The initial bite depends on the location of the wound and the needle gauge used. Ensure that the needle size is appropriate for the wound. **(B)** Ensure that the skin edges are everted and apposed. Bites should be adequate and equal on both sides.

Procedures Box 33.3 Staple removal

Action
Remember to give the patient a staple remover if you are referring her or him elsewhere for their removal.

Reason *Other healthcare facilities may not have the appropriate equipment.*

Action
Check that staples are in situ and are not rotated.

Reason *Rotated staples will need readjustment before removal.*

Action
Hold the staple remover with the lower jaw underneath.

Reason *The tips of the staple remover need to be inserted beneath the staple.*

Action
Lift the staple slightly and squeeze the handles together.

Reason *Facilitates removal.*

Action
Lift the staple away from the skin and discard.

Reason *Removes the staple.*

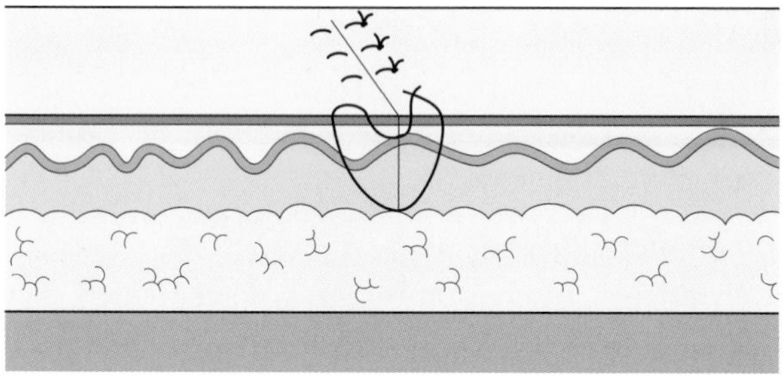

Fig. 33.3 • Vertical mattress suture. This is used when the skin edges are inverting. Initial bites are full thickness on both sides; complete the suture with bites through superficial layers. The suture is completed on the same side as the entry site.

ALERT

- **It is essential before closing any wound that you check for the presence of foreign bodies and remove them.**
- **Ensure that there is no tendon injury and that the nerve and vascular supply is intact.**
- **Overlapping or inverted skin edges will not allow optimal healing and will give a poor cosmetic result.**
- **Sutures tied too tight may tear the skin and devitalise the tissue, resulting in scarring.**
- **Sutures tied too loose will not hold the skin edges in opposition, delaying healing and increasing the risk of scarring.**
- **Sutures placed too near the wound edges may tear the skin.**
- **Sutures placed too far away from the skin edge may cause increased tension and cross-hatch scarring (Reynolds & Cole 2006).**

Classification of wound closure

Wound closure can be classified into three categories: primary, secondary and delayed primary closure (sometimes referred to as tertiary). Primary closure, as the term suggests, involves closing a wound within hours of its occurring. Secondary healing allows the wound to close spontaneously by contraction and re-epithelialisation. Delayed primary or tertiary wound closure involves initial cleansing and debridement of the wound. It is subsequently left open under a moist dressing for an extended period of time (several days). Finally, if there is no sign of infection, the wound is formally closed by suturing or by another mechanism. Wounds caused by animal bites or those that are very contaminated are usually treated by delayed primary closure (Rosenberg & de la Torre 2006).

Phases of wound healing

Normal wound healing is complex and comprises three different phases. Each phase needs to take place for healing to occur.

First phase: the inflammatory phase

The inflammatory phase takes place from the time of injury to between 2 and 5 days. Its characteristics include inflammation and haemostasis. Vasoconstriction occurs within seconds of the injury occurring in order to stem the bleeding. Clotting factors are activated and platelet aggregation takes place. The body's defences, i.e. white blood cells, are employed to protect against bacterial infection. Prostaglandins and histamine are released, instigating vasodilation of the injured area, which facilitates the removal of debris and delivery of nutrients to injured tissue.

Second phase: the proliferative phase

The proliferative phase takes place from day 2 to 3 weeks or until healing has taken place. During this phase the following occur: granulation, contraction and epithelialisation:

- Granulation includes angiogenesis, i.e. the formation of new blood vessels and collagen synthesis.
- Wound contraction occurs as a result of activation of myofibroblasts, which secrete proteins and form collagen or elastic fibres between cells.
- Epithelialisation: epithelial cells migrate to resurface the area.

Third phase: maturation

Maturation begins at about 3 weeks and can take up to 2 years. During this time there is reduced vascularisation. Collagen is synthesised, so increasing the tensile strength of the wound.

Scar remodelling and contraction take place. The final appearance of a scar may not be known for a considerable length of time. It is worth informing the patient that the appearance of scar tissue can be helped by gentle massage with a non-perfumed moisturising cream (Dougherty & Lister 2004c, Foster 2007, Stuart 2006).

Factors affecting wound healing

These can be divided into two categories: intrinsic factors and extrinsic factors.

Intrinsic factors (i.e. those pertaining to the patient) include:

- wound location (e.g. wounds to the shin do not have as good a blood supply as those to other areas)
- blood supply (if compromised tissues become ischaemic, leading to further tissue injury)
- pH of the wound (related to the degree of oxygenation)
- age (wounds heal more rapidly in children, as cell division is more rapid)
- infections (local or systemic)
- the health status of the patient (underlying disease such as diabetes, renal disease, respiratory disorders and cancers)
- dehydration
- nutritional status of the patient (anorexia or obesity will delay healing, as a good nutritional status is vital for healing to occur).

Extrinsic factors (i.e. those factors external to the patient) include:

- wound surface temperature (wounds heal more rapidly if the temperature is maintained at normal body temperature)
- moisture or humidity at the wound surface (wound healing is optimal in a moist environment, which promotes epithelialisation)
- inappropriate wound management (such as incorrect dressings, poor surgical technique, poor or rough handling of the tissues)
- suture materials
- infection
- drugs (e.g. steroid therapy, non-steroidal anti-inflammatory drugs, cytotoxic drugs, alcohol)
- chemicals (all antiseptics are cytotoxic; MacLellan 2000)
- radiation treatments
- retained foreign bodies
- smoking (oxygenation and contraction of the wound are impaired)
- adverse psychosocial factors (Alexander et al 2000).

Reviewing old wounds

In addition to assessing the tissue status of healing wounds and chronic wounds it is vital to measure the progress of the wound. There are a variety of wound site measurement techniques.

The following methods are among those most commonly used (Fette 2006):

- Simple measurements of the wound can be made using a tape measure. Measurements can, however, be difficult to calculate if the wound has an irregular shape.
- Wound tracing using a grid. The outline of the wound is traced directly on to sterile transparent film marked with a measured grid. Tracings can be kept in the patient's notes and subsequent tracings can be easily compared with the others, giving an immediate indication of the progress of the wound. Reliability and accuracy can be affected by inaccuracies in tracing the wound boundary.
- Scaled photographs. This method of assessment uses a photographic film that incorporates a scaled ruler at the edge of the photograph. The ruler is used to calculate the wound dimensions. Photographs also enable comparisons to be made, but these can be inaccurate due to magnification error.
- Moulds. 'A three-dimensional mould of the wound can be created by taking a cast of the wound cavity using a saline or alginate filling' (Fette 2006).

Procedures Box 33.4 Assessing the progress of healing wounds and chronic wounds

Actions
Ascertain if the dressings are intact and in situ.

Ascertain if they are clean or dirty, contaminated, dry or wet.

Reason *The status of the dressings will indicate patient compliance and the likely condition of the wound.*

Action
Ascertain if there is any exudate, and if so, how much and what it looks like.

Reasons *Provides information about the wound status and healing, for example a small amount of serous fluid may be normal while a large amount may indicate damage to the tissues, as in a burn or underlying pathology.*

- *Blood: is it old or new? The latter possibly indicates that haemostasis has not been achieved or that the wound has sustained further trauma.*
- *Pus: green may indicate a* Pseudomonas *infection, yellow and purulent may indicate* Staphylococcus *infection.*
- *Exudate due to wound dressing breakdown occurs with hydrocolloids.*

Action
Check for other signs, such as swelling, erythema, heat and 'tracking'.

Reason *May indicate localised infection.*

Procedures Box 33.4 Assessing the progress of healing wounds and chronic wounds—cont'd

Action
Measure the extent of the erythema and draw around it.

Reason *At a subsequent review it will then be obvious whether the infection is settling or increasing.*

Action
Check odour:

- Does the wound smell?
- What does it smell of?

Reason *A fruity smell suggests Staphylococcus organisms, whereas foul smells are indicative of Gram-negative bacteria.*

Action
Check tissue appearance.

- Red?
- Pink?
- Cream or yellow, adhering to the wound surface?
- Black?

Reason

- *Red indicates healthy granulation tissue.*
- *Pink indicates epithelialising tissue.*
- *Cream or yellow, adhering to wound surface, is slough (i.e. dead tissue, which will impede healing).*
- *Black tissue is necrotic (i.e. non-viable tissue due to reduced blood supply).*

Actions
What percentage of the wound appears to be slough or necrotic tissue?

Where is the dead tissue?

Reason *The amount and location will dictate how debridement should be undertaken.*

Action
Remember to draw an accurate diagram of the wound and label it.

Reason *This will indicate the progress of the wound on future assessment.*

(Freedline & Fishman 1995, Stuart 2006.)

Wound dressings

Dressing selection will depend on a variety of factors:

- The age of the patient
- Patient activities and lifestyle
- Comfort and cosmetic appearance
- The type and size of the wound
- The position of the wound
- The ease of application and removal
- The desired frequency of dressing change
- Cost.

The ideal dressing should, however:

- keep the wound moist but not cause maceration
- protect against infection and prevent excessive sloughing
- remove exudates and toxic substances
- be free of toxic chemicals, particles or fibres
- keep the wound at an optimum temperature for healing to take place
- keep the wound at the optimum pH value
- allow gaseous exchange
- be absorbent
- be left undisturbed by the need for frequent changes
- allow for change without trauma
- protect the wound from further injury
- provide an environment for optimal healing to take place (Dougherty & Lister 2004c, Plymouth Area Joint Formulary 2004).

When selecting which dressing to use, all the factors affecting wound healing and compliance need to be considered in order to select a dressing that will not only provide the optimal healing environment but will also be comfortable and acceptable to the patient. It is important to refer to the research literature to ensure that your practice is current.

A brief review of the management aims is given in Table 33.2; for a more comprehensive list of wound dressings and their properties please refer to Dougherty & Lister 2004c.

Dressing fixation

The fixation of the dressing is largely a matter of practicality and individual preference, for example bandages such as boxing gloves are practical for small children and flexible tapes are useful when there is movement. Note that it is never necessary to tape the bandage on to skin. Stockinette may be placed over the bandage to maintain its position, and the tape can then be applied over the stockinette. Flexible tape can easily be removed using plaster remover wiped over the tape.

On completing your assessment and treatment remember to reward the child with stickers, colouring books, etc. A number of puzzle books and colouring books are available free from various agencies such as health promotion organisations and the fire service.

Documentation

Finally, do not forget to document your findings and treatment. Accurate documentation is essential.

Documentation of the wound:

- records the patient history
- is a record of your patient assessment, treatment and management

Table 33.2. Selection of dressings

Management plans/aims	By colour	By tissue type	General principle(s)	Dressings and preparations
Remove the cause Rehydrate tissue Address systemic influences Treat topically	Black	Necrotic ↓	Rehydrate tissue to facilitate autolysis, and maintain moist environment; this may not be appropriate in patients with peripheral vascular disease	Hydrocolloids, hydrogels, honey, debriding enzymes, capillary action
	Yellow	Sloughy ↓	Rehydrate tissue, absorb excess exudates	Alginates, hydrocolloids, hydrogels, foams, polysaccharide beads or paste, honey, debriding enzymes
	Green	Infected ↓	Symptom control including absorption, odour control	Alginates, silver sulfadiazine (not suitable for children under 1 year), povidone–iodine (not suitable for children under 2 years), polysaccharide beads or paste, honey
	Red	Granulating ↓	Maintain moist environment, protect delicate tissues	Soft silicone wound contact material, semipermeable membranes
	Pink	Epithelialising ↓, complete healing	Maintain moist environment, protect delicate tissues	Soft silicone wound contact material, semipermeable membranes
		Clean acute wounds	Maintain moist environment and temperature, protect tissues	Soft silicone wound contact material, semipermeable membranes (abrasions, minor burns), hydrocolloids
		Contaminated acute wounds	Prevent infection	Inadine (not suitable for use in children under 2 years), silver sulfadiazine (not suitable for use in neonates)

(After Dougherty & Lister 2004c, National Institute for Clinical Excellence 2001 and Plymouth Area Joint Formulary 2004.)

- reminds or informs practitioners about previous consultations and findings when the patient is reviewed
- provides a baseline for future comparison and monitoring of progress
- is a legal record; notes made by the practitioner at the time of consultation are assumed in law (unless proved otherwise) to be an accurate record of what took place and findings
- communicates information to other health professionals
- can provide evidence for research and audit (Guly 1996, Templeton 2004).

To conclude, wound assessment and management in children can be challenging and may require a lot of patience and ingenuity on behalf of the practitioner. It is, however, immensely rewarding to see a child (and his or her carer), who has been apprehensive, tearful and afraid, happy and smiling when you have completed your task. The sense of achievement is enormous.

References

Alexander M, Fawcett JN, Runciman PJ (2000) Nursing practice: hospital and home – the adult, 2nd edn. Churchill Livingstone, Oxford, p 742

Blunt (2001) Wound cleansing: ritualistic or research-based practice? Nursing Standard 16(1):33–36

Dougherty L, Lister S (2004a) Wound management. In Dougherty L, Lister S (eds) The Royal Marsden Hospital manual of clinical nursing procedures, 6th edn. Blackwell Publishing, Oxford, p 789

Dougherty L, Lister S (2004b) Wound management. In Dougherty L, Lister S (eds) The Royal Marsden Hospital manual of clinical nursing procedures, 6th edn. Blackwell Publishing, Oxford, p 802

Dougherty L, Lister S (2004c) Wound management. In Dougherty L, Lister S (eds) The Royal Marsden Hospital manual of clinical nursing procedures, 6th edn. Blackwell Publishing, Oxford, p 808–809

Dulecki M, Pieper B (2005) Irrigating simple acute traumatic wounds: a review of the current literature. Journal of Emergency Nursing 31(2):156–160

Fernandez R, Griffiths R, Ussia C (2004) Effectiveness of solutions, techniques and pressure in wound cleansing. Joanne Briggs Institute Reports 2(7):231–270

Fette AM (2006) A clinimetric analysis of wound measurement tools. Online. Available: http://www.worldwidewounds.com/2006/january/Fette/Clinimetric-Analysis-Wound-Measurement-Tools.html April 2006

Foster EM (2007) Wound care principles and products: the short course. American Pediatric Surgical Nurses Association. Online. Available: http://www.apsna.org/mc/page.do?sitePageId=24267 3 Apr 2006

Freedline A, Fishman TD (1995) Ulcer documentation. Wound Care Information Network. Online. Available: http://www.medicaledu.com/ 1 Apr 2006

Griffiths RD (2001) Is tap water a safe alternative to normal saline for wound irrigation in the community setting? Journal of Wound Care 10(10):407

Guly H (1996) History taking, examination and record keeping in emergency medicine (Oxford Handbooks in Emergency Medicine). Oxford University Press, Oxford, p 47

McKirdy L (2001) Wound management: burn cleansing. Journal of Clinical Nursing 15(5). Online. Available: http://www.jcn.co.uk/journal.asp

MacLellan DG (2000) Chronic wound management. Australian Prescriber 23:6–9 Online. Available: http://www.australianprescriber.com/magazine/23/1/6/9/16.05.2006

Moore Z (2005) The assessment and management of traumatic wounds. Practice Nurse 30(4):54,56,58

National Institute for Clinical Excellence (2001) Guidance on the use of debriding agents for difficult to heal surgical wounds. NICE, London

Plymouth Area Joint Formulary (2004) Wound management. In Plymouth Area Joint Formulary. Plymouth Hospitals NHS Trust, Plymouth

Reynolds T, Cole E (2006) Techniques for acute wound closure. Nursing Standard 20(21):55–64

Rosenberg LZ, de la Torre J (2006) Wound healing, growth factors. eMedicine. Online. Available: http://www.emedicine.com/plastic/topic457.htm

Stuart S (2006) ABC of wound healing: wound assessment. Student BMJ 14(89):132. Online. Available: http://www.studentbmj.com/issues/06/03/education/98.php 1 Apr 2006

Templeton S (2004) Nursing documentation and legal considerations in wound management. Online. Available: http://www.wound.sa.edu.au/newsletters/2004/sawma_documentation_and_legalities_wound_management.pps 23 Mar 2006

Tissue Viability Nurses Association (2005) Conservative sharp debridement: procedure, competencies and training. Online. Available: http://www.tvna.org/generic_forms/sharp_debridement_revise.pdf 8 May2006

Valente JH, Forti RJ, Freundlich LF, Zandieh SO, Crain EF (2003) Wound irrigation in children: saline solution or tap water? Annals of Emergency Medicine 41:609–616

Wayne L, Bunn L (2007) Treatment of children with minor injuries. In Cleaver K, Webb J (eds) Accident and emergency nursing. Blackwell Publishing, Oxford

Williams C (1995) Children's understanding of treatments in the A/E department. British Journal of Nursing 4(7):385–387

Zuber TJ (2002) The mattress sutures: vertical, horizontal, and corner stitch. American Family Physician 66(12). Online. Available: http://www.aafp.org/afp/20021215/2231.html 9 Jun 2006

34 Occlusive treatments for childhood eczema and other skin conditions

Stephen Gill

Various forms of wound coverings and dressings have historically been used for all manner of skin conditions and wounds, and while many practices are commonly used, very few treatments for eczema have a foundation of evidence-based practice (BMJ Knowledge 2007). However, significant anecdotal and non-randomised evidence strongly supports the use of moisturisers and bandaging techniques (BMJ Knowledge 2007). Some of these occlusive bandaging techniques have been applied to children with eczema to good effect, as described by Atherton (1994), Goodyear et al (1991), and Turnbull & Atherton (1994) for use in the acute and chronic phases of the condition and employed both in hospital and in the home. These have been made easier to do since the production of tubular bandages and bandage suits. However, bandaging regimens are usually regarded as second-line treatments due to their cost and time-consuming nature, etc. (BMJ Knowledge 2007), and, moreover, bandaging should not be regarded as a replacement but as an add-on therapy to standard treatment for eczema. This chapter therefore includes a background to childhood eczema as well as an overview of treatments that should be tried before bandaging. Three of the commonest occlusive treatments for childhood will be discussed in this chapter, and these are:

1. dry occlusive bandaging
2. wet wraps
3. paste bandages.

There are some variations on these themes and some discussion will take place regarding them.

Bandages are used in eczema for two main reasons:

1. To *cover* and protect the skin and reduce its sensitivity by forming a close-fitting layer over the skin
2. To *hold* an appropriate amount of steroid and generous amounts of emollient on the skin in order to rehydrate it over an extended period of time.

Eczema is a condition that can have a profound effect on the quality of life (Lewis-Jones & Finlay 1995), being an inflammatory skin disorder that is intensely pruritic with excoriations and dry skin as the major visible signs. There are various forms of eczema seen in children; the commonest and arguably most troublesome is atopic eczema, affecting 12–13% of all school age children (Emerson et al 1998), which has furthermore been described as the 'commonest skin disease in the western world' (University of Dundee 2006). This same article's genetic research report strongly links different forms of eczema to a deficiency in the gene that produces filaggrin, a protein essential for maintaining skin barrier function. Indeed, many of the aspects of eczema seem to be related to the dysfunctional epidermal barrier, although whether the defective skin provides the environment or the bacterial growth creates the environment is less clear.

When the skin barrier is compromised, skin that is sore, weeping, encrusted and breaking down is likely to have some form of infection alongside the inflammation. Eczematous skin is more spongy and characterised by microfissuring. This provides an ideal environment for pathogenic microbial growth, and these microbes can be bacterial, fungal or viral. The site of the affected skin and the history can sometimes give clues to likely offending organisms. For instance if the flexures of the skin are involved then fungal growth, i.e. candidiasis, is likely to occur in these damper areas. It is usually considered unhelpful to use wet occlusive bandaging techniques on infected skin, as pathogenic organisms may proliferate under wet dressings, so recognition of infection is an important nursing observation.

Atopic eczema is often regarded as essentially a disorder of the body's immune response to certain stimuli (Ring et al 2004) and is one of the atopic triad of asthma, eczema and hay fever. Triggering of eczema by exposure to environmental substances has given rise to the so-called hygiene hypothesis, in which a cleaner environment and fewer life-threatening diseases have left the body's immunity looking for something to defend against (Ring et al 2004). While the exact mechanism producing eczema remains the province of research and mystery, a major trigger is thought to be the bacterium *Staphylococcus aureus*. When the microbe is attacked by the body's immune system it releases powerful exotoxins that in turn trigger off a superantigenic response. This is signified by T-lymphocyte activation, mast cell degranulation and cytokine release (McFadden et al 1993, Skov et al 1995).

While *S. aureus* is a pathogenic organism that grows well on eczematous skin (Goodyear 1993), it is more of a danger to the patient with eczema than to others. It is a bacteria often linked with wound infections but it is also a common commensal found in the nose, axillae and perineum of otherwise healthy individuals. As such, some degree of balance is required in the treatment of the individual with eczema when considering his or her positioning on the ward. Most children with intact skin are unlikely to be harmed by coming into contact with a child with eczema unless they have some form of immunocompromisation or the organism is identified as methicillin-resistant *S. aureus*, and the psychological problems of skin disease and isolation of the child with eczema need to be considered (Gill 2006, Papadopoulos & Bor 1999).

Staphylococcus aureus is an opportunistic organism that can be present in both viral and fungal infections and usually reveals itself by having a yellow encrustation on the skin. A less common but nonetheless important organism that infects the skin and worsens eczema is streptococci. Both are likely to be identified by the result of a skin swab for bacteriology and treated with appropriate antibiotics.

Again, the broken skin barrier can allow viral organisms to occupy the affected site as well, and an example of this is a herpetic infection on eczematous skin known as eczema herpeticum. This is usually regarded as a medical emergency requiring urgent treatment. Eczema herpeticum usually occurs quickly, perhaps overnight, and parents will often say that the rash is different to the usual eczema – this is often a trustworthy parental observation. It usually affects a smaller area of skin than the rest of the eczema, and the lesions start as pustules similar to chickenpox. These pustules are itchy and delicate and often scratched open before admission to hospital. They are also monomorphic, which means that they all look the same at the beginning and all go through a similar uniform progression from pustule to open crater-like appearance to raw pink resolving patches. This is in comparison with chickenpox lesions, which tend to 'crop' with healing lesions and more pustules present at the same time. It is likely to be quite harmful to wet wrap skin infected with eczema herpeticum, so nurses should familiarise themselves with the appearance of this condition before deciding to wet wrap.

Typical regimens and basic techniques employed for treating childhood eczema

A typical regimen for eczema will usually include the following basic elements (Gill 2006):

- A moisturiser (emollient) to be applied liberally and frequently throughout the day and at night as required.
- A soap substitute for washing the skin (this may be an emollient that contains a gentle antiseptic). Soap substitutes are often applied to the skin before bathing.
- A bath oil. This sometimes contains a gentle antiseptic.
- A topical steroid. This may be a plain steroid or contain a mixture of steroid–antiseptic, steroid–antifungal or steroid–antiseptic–antifungal.
- Avoidance of any known triggers for an individual's eczema (Tan et al 1996), including soaps, shampoos and bubble bath products.
- A bedtime sedative, usually an antihistamine.

Topical treatment regimens for eczema are often adjusted in accordance with the visible presenting features, which are characterised by three main physical elements:

1. dry skin
2. inflamed areas of the skin
3. infection.

Thus:

- if the skin is dry the moisturiser needs applying more frequently or a greasier one chosen as an alternative
- if the skin is inflamed and sore then a topical steroid is used as an anti-inflammatory treatment
- if the skin is weepy and encrusted then antimicrobial agents may be required.

It should be borne in mind that unless a child is septicaemic, even quite severe eczematous infections can permit a normal body temperature due to the peripheral vasodilatation of blood vessels near the skin's surface and subsequent heat loss through the skin (Buxton 1998). Because basic observations are poor indicators of severity or improvement it is more important to observe the child's general demeanour and skin condition. If the skin appears weepy and encrusted (impetiginised) and the general demeanour of the child is a picture of misery then the eczema is likely to be infected and require appropriate antimicrobial treatment. Lesser colonisations are often treated with antibacterial regimens, including antiseptic bath oils and emollients and antiseptic–steroid combination therapies.

Basic techniques for applying treatments to delicate skin are:

- applying emollients
- using shampoos
- applying topical steroids.

Applying emollients

The skin that is affected by eczema is very sensitive, and as any form of friction is likely to stimulate the itch–scratch–itch cycle, this should be strenuously avoided. This includes the application of emollients, so they should be first softened in the hands prior to application. This will also warm up the treatment as you use it to avoid a cold shock to the skin. Apply moisturisers by gently stroking them on in the same direction as hair growth or with the 'grain' of the skin. If using a cream as the main emollient, as either a leave-on treatment or as a soap substitute to be washed off in the bathing process, the cream should be left looking a little white on the skin. Rubbing till the white appearance of the cream has gone will often irritate the skin through friction. When the skin is extremely sensitive the emollients can be picked up in the hands to be gently warmed before simply 'laying' the grease-coated hands on to the patient. As a general guide, the more sensitive and sore the skin is the greater likelihood of requiring the simpler structure of ointments rather than creams.

Safety warnings

Emollients make most surfaces very slippery, and extreme care must be taken to ensure the safety of the child in the bath. Even older children may have difficulty sitting up or standing in the bath, and so they should not be left unattended. A small towel placed in the bottom of the bath may help give some grip, and it may be necessary to use a flannel or small towel to hold the child safely. Flannel gloves are a useful aid to give extra grip.

Greasy treatments are messy and slippery, so protection for surfaces and floors is required. Any emollients that fall on the floor should be cleaned up and disposed of as soon as it is practical to do so in order to avoid slipping hazards.

Using shampoos

Most shampoos (even medicated and prescribed shampoos) have a significant detergent effect on the skin. Therefore treatments to the hair that include any form of detergent shampoo should be performed separately to the bathing process, as the detergent will dry up the skin even more if it runs into the bath and comes into contact with the skin. As a general guide, this precaution should be taken with any form of hair treatment that bubbles and lathers. When a medicated shampoo is prescribed it is often necessary to use emollient on the scalp as well.

Using topical steroids

Topical steroids are prescribed medications. Therefore the type of steroid, where to apply it and the required frequency should be clearly stated on the prescription and should be adhered to as with any other prescribed drug. However, the application of steroids is not so clearly understood as the use of medicines or tablets and requires some discussion, as it is often an issue of confusion. Therefore the following guidelines may be used:

- Steroids go only on to areas of skin where it is inflamed and sore. Dry skin just needs moisturisers.
- Most steroids should not be used more than twice a day, and some are licensed as only once-daily drugs.
- Steroids are best applied to rehydrated skin, otherwise much larger amounts may be required if the epidermis is very dry. After a bath with soap substitute and bath oil the skin is usually more translucent and the inflamed areas are more easily visible for treating with topical steroids. Appropriate times are therefore just after a greasy bath or half an hour after emollients. If the intention is to apply dry or wet bandages then the best time to apply steroid is after the bath, just before applying copious amounts of emollients.
- The amount used should be visible on the skin. Some descriptions say that the steroid should glisten or be shiny when the correct amount is applied (Atherton 1994). Further information on the fingertip unit of measurement for topical steroids can be found in Long et al (1992).
- Generally speaking, ointments are preferential to creams due to their simpler construction, and preservatives in creams can be a source of skin irritation. However, the role of creams lies in their ability to stick to wet infected skin where ointments will not.

Bandaging techniques: general principles

The general rationale for using bandages is that they cover and protect sensitive skin and can also be used as a vehicle to hold a treatment next to the damaged skin. A good principle for choosing an appropriate bandaging strategy for eczema is to use the simplest method first and progress to more complex methods as required. Therefore the methods described here are presented in the order of the simplest strategy first, progressing to the more complex.

Bandaging regimens for eczema are usually carried out after preparatory emollient bathing has soothed and made the skin more comfortable. Bathing a child is an intimate procedure, and therefore the number of carers should be minimised and one of the parents involved in the care as often as possible, both to reassure the child and for parental education and involvement. The time spent bathing the child also presents an opportunity for the nurse to get to know the child and perform psychological assessment, in the knowledge that many children with skin conditions suffer from low self-esteem and psychological dysfunction (Dennis 2003, Papadopoulos & Bor 1999) and may require psychological referral.

The process of treating very sore and pruritic skin can be prolonged, painful and unpleasant, and so it demands the highest skills a children's trained nurse can muster to ease the situation and make the experience more pleasant. The skin is very delicate after bathing, and rubbing should be avoided. Instead the skin can be gently patted dry using soft towels or cuddly sheets. Bath time play is a useful strategy to distract the child and help the child to normalise the process, and bathing a special friend or dolly may help encourage a child to mentally work out his or her experiences.

A child may chill if the environment of the bathroom is too cold or if the child has to wait while bandages are cut to size. Minimal waiting time is therefore facilitated by having all equipment ready prior to starting and having all bandages cut to size before bathing starts. A single or double layer of tubular bandage is made into a suit by use of different sizes being cut to fit parts of the child's body (a double layer will hold more grease and therefore moisturise the skin for longer). There are presently four companies making these tubular bandages, the original being Tubifast and recent additions being Coverflex, Actifast and Comfifast. These bandages are non-elasticated but have high conformity to the body due to the weave of the material. They all stretch width-wise but there is very little stretch in the length. A more recent addition to these products is the ready-made bandage suits made by Comfifast and Tubifast. All these bandages are on prescription and permit the continuation of these treatments in the home.

The order of applications is as follows:

1. The areas of eczematous skin that require the application of topical steroid are treated according to the prescription.
2. Then copious amounts of greasy emollient are applied to the skin without disturbing the steroid underneath.
As a general guide the emollient should be thick enough to draw in if it is the correct amount. Only one part of the body is greased at a time prior to bandaging.
3. Grease then bandage the trunk first then grease and bandage the limbs. In this way the limb bandages can be secured to the vest in sequence.

Two ties are used to secure each limb bandage to the vest. These are made from 2.5-cm strips of the limb-sized bandage. If limb-bandages are not secured at all they will tend to become displaced, roll down and form an undesirable garter effect. Furthermore, if only a single tie is used the bandages will tend to be uncomfortable, as the bandage will tend to pull into the groin or armpit.

Dry occlusive bandaging

Indications

Dry and pruritic (itchy) and excoriated skin.

Method

Measuring and cutting the bandages to size for a single layer.

Measuring the bandages is not a specific science, as the wider a child is in a limb or the trunk dimension the more bandage length will reduce, as it will stretch only in the width. Another varying factor is the size of the child to be bandaged, therefore the following measurements are intended to be only approximate guidelines. When the best fit is achieved the old bandages can be removed and used as a template to cut future suits.

The vest is cut to length after measuring from the top of the ear to the hip, and a small straight cut of 1–2 cm is made approximately 10 cm down from the top of the bandage (Fig. 34.1). These cuts are for the arms to go through. Avoid over-cutting of the armhole, as the intention is to make the body suit as close-fitting as possible.

The arm bandages are measured from the top of the shoulder to the tip of the fingers and an extra adult hand span (15–20 cm) in length (Fig. 34.2). If the fingers are to be free then the end of the bandage is folded back by approximately 10 cm and a nick is made on both sides of the bandage (Fig. 34.3) to allow the finger and thumb to be used to secure the bandage at the lower end (Figs 34.4 and 34.5). These cuts are not necessary if the fingers are enclosed to make mittens. The bandage is then tied to the vest (Fig. 34.6). Figure 34.7 shows how to make a hole in the bandage for the child's thumb.

The leg bandages are measured from the top of the hip bone to the heel, along the heel and an extra 15–20 cm (a hand's span) for folding back to form a sock.

A balaclava can be used to rehydrate the face, neck and forehead either by 'buttering' it with grease before applying to the child or by fitting it over already greased skin. Balaclavas can either be bought ready made or be constructed using medium size tubular bandages. They are useful, if tolerated, but are inappropriate for a small child or an unattended one who may dislodge the bandage and choke, therefore this is reserved for older children who can easily protect their own airway by removing the balaclava themselves.

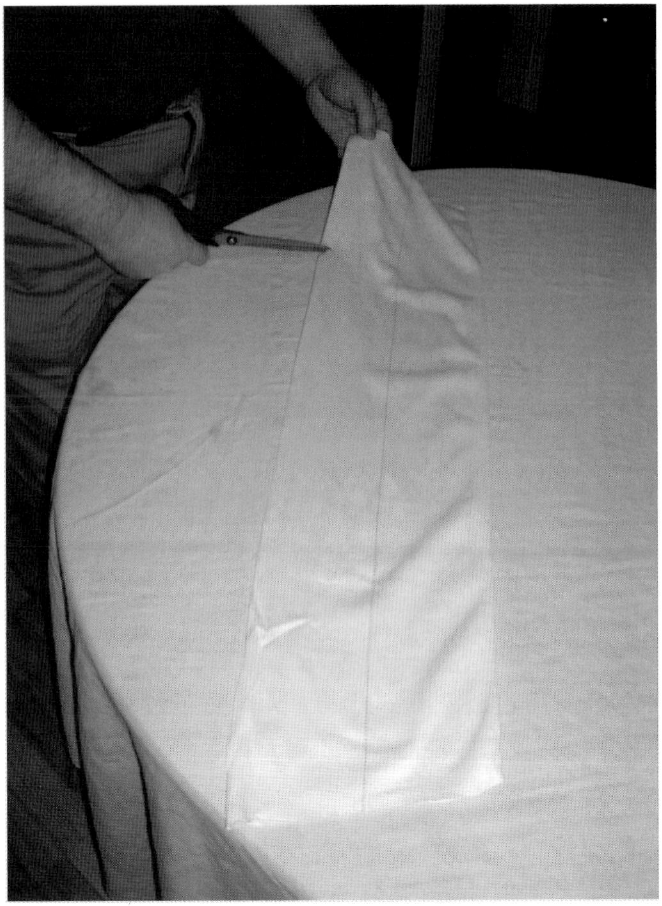

Fig. 34.1 • Cutting the bandage.

Two-layered dry occlusive bandaging

Indications

Dry and pruritic (itchy) and excoriated skin.

Method

An extra layer of bandage can be used to hold more emollient and an extra coating of greasy emollient can be applied in between the inner and outer bandage layer. It also gives an extra thickness of bandage to afford greater protection of sore skin.

Two vests are cut to length as described above. The limb bandages are measured as above and doubled in length so that two layers can be made from the longer length.

Wet wrapping

Indications

Dry and pruritic (itchy) and excoriated skin.

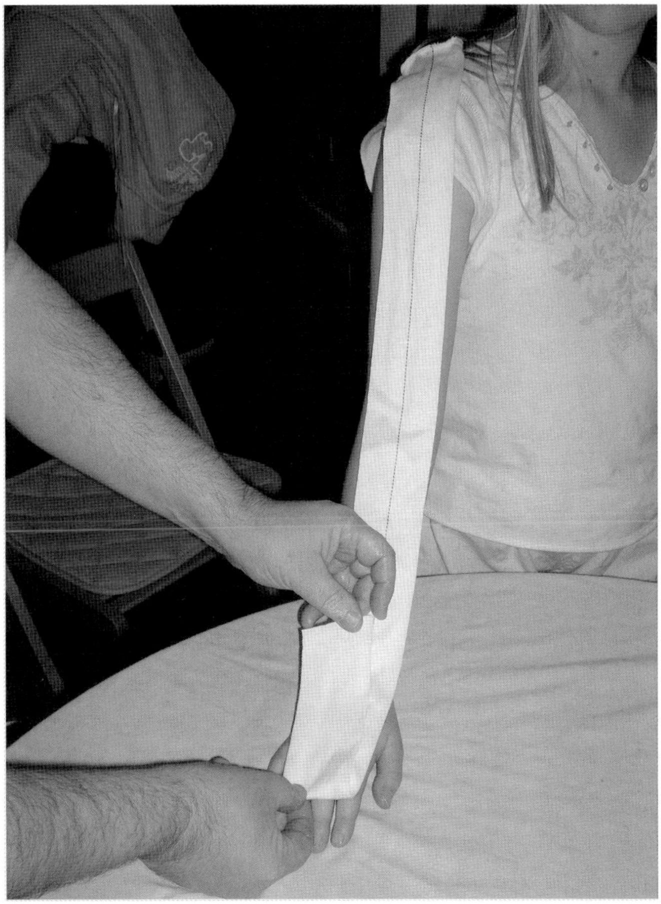

Fig. 34.2 • Measuring an arm bandage.

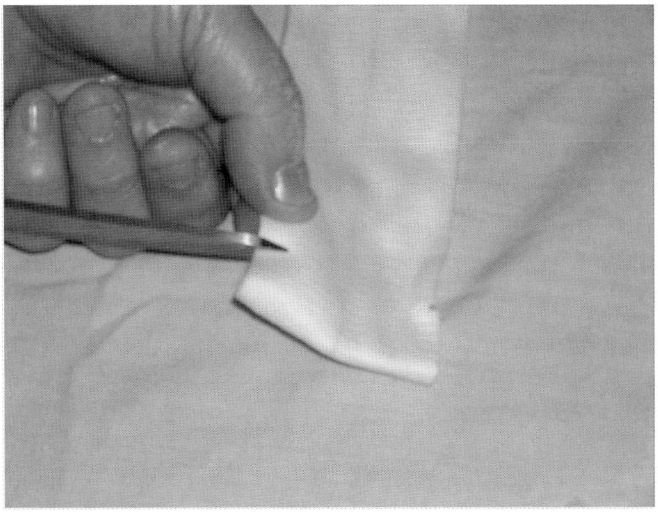

Fig. 34.3 • Cutting a nick in the bandage to allow the finger and thumb to be used.

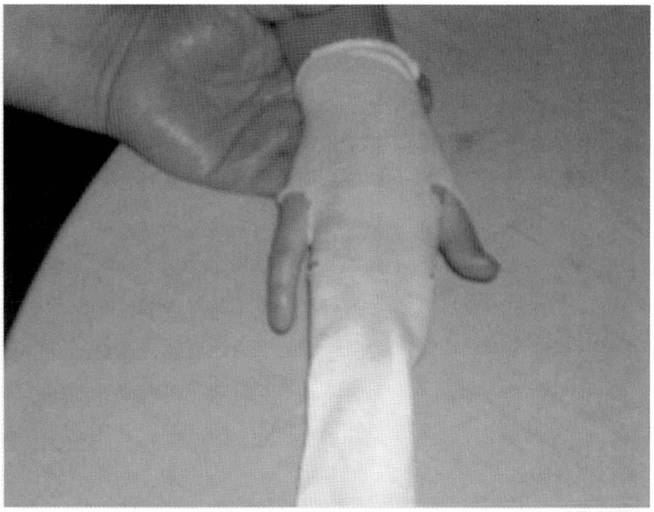

Fig. 34.4 • The child's finger and thumb secure the bandage.

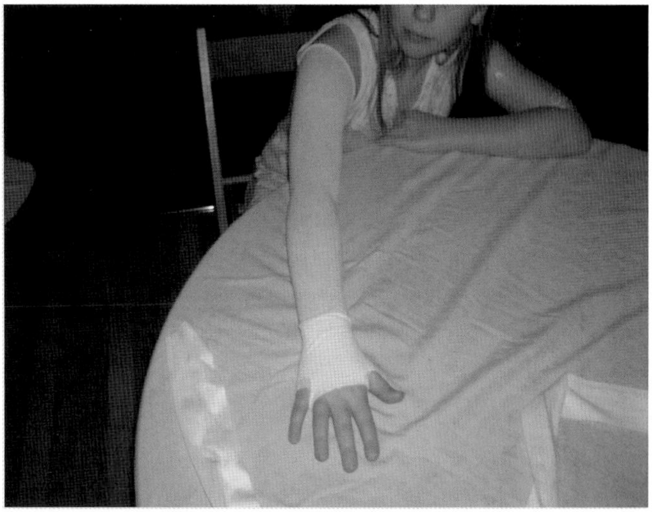

Fig. 34.5 • The completed bandage.

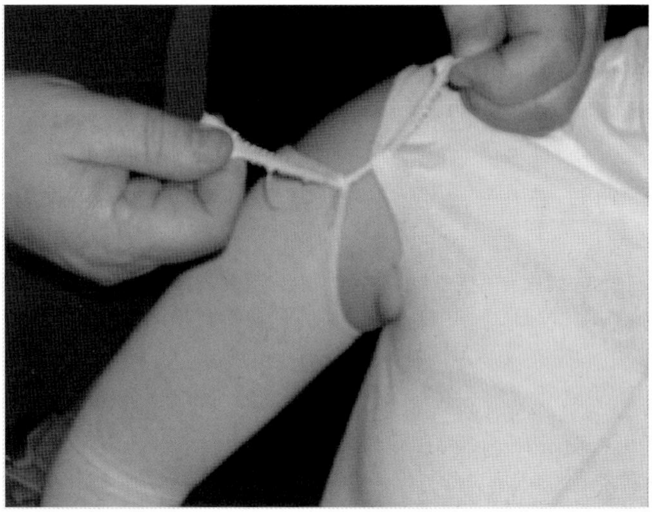

Fig. 34.6 • Tying the bandage to the vest.

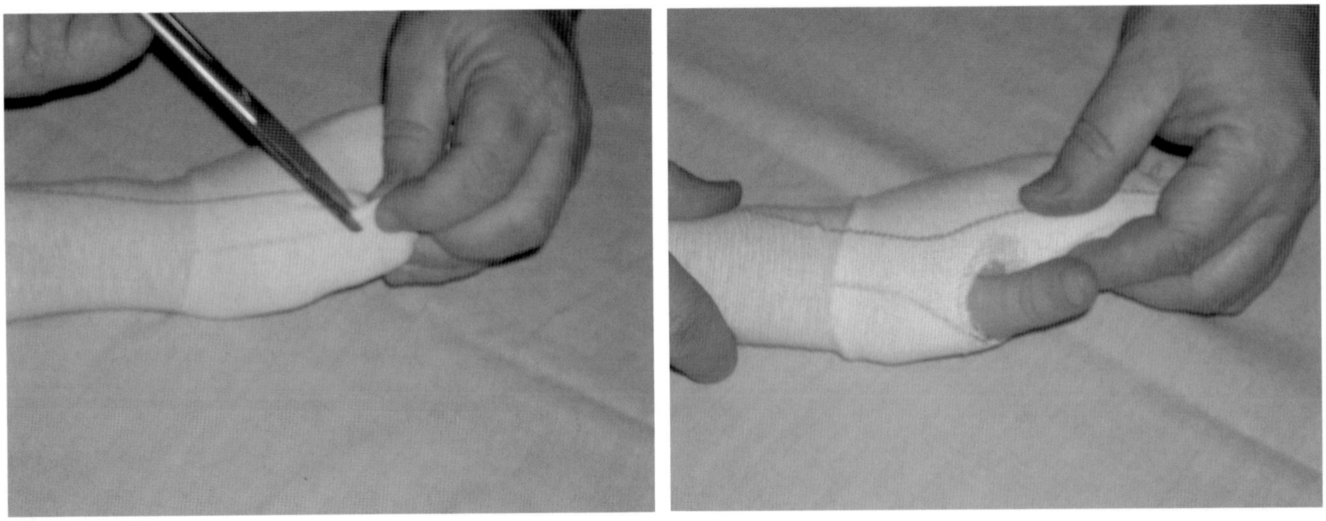

Fig. 34.7 • Making a hole in the bandage for the child's thumb.

The rationale of this technique is similar to that for other bandaging techniques in that it covers and protects the skin and also is a vehicle for holding an appropriate treatment, in this case an appropriate amount of steroid and liberal amounts of grease. The difference with wet wraps is that controlled evaporation of water is also used to cool the skin and thereby reduce extreme itching. Wet wrapping bandages are constructed in the same way as the two-layered dry occlusive suit described above, and the same method is employed by using appropriate topical steroid followed by a liberal coating of greasy emollient.

Method

The inner bandage is wet with warm tap water (hand hot) and gently squeezed so that excess water runs into the sink or bowl. The bandage is then applied immediately before it cools down. The outer layer is applied to cover the wet inner layer. Sequentially grease and bandage the child, securing the bandages as described above, and then put on day clothes or pyjamas to cover. The normal clothing helps to reduce the speed at which the water evaporates. If the bandages dry out they can be rewet if required by using a wet flannel or previously unused household plant spray. Remoisturise any uncovered skin as required.

Variations on the dry occlusive and wet wrapping themes

Selected areas of skin can be bandaged using shorter lengths, for example for the wrists or ankles when these are the worst affected areas rather than a whole body suit. This is sometimes described as patch wrapping.

The emollient used can be varied, but the greasier the better is a good general principle. Examples of emollients used in common practice are 50/50 liquid paraffin in white soft paraffin BP, emulsifying ointment BP*, oily cream BP (also known as hydrous ointment BP), Epaderm*, Hydromol ointment* and aqueous cream BP*. Preparations marked with an asterisk are water-soluble and are more appropriate for use with washable garments.

Topical steroids blended into an emollient were used in the original form of wet wrapping in this country, and a mixture of Cetomacrogol BP and Propaderm was used. These seem to be less favourable now due to difficulties in mixing and stabilising the mix. Also, this method is indiscriminate in its steroid application and treats non-active areas of skin with steroid as well as eczematous. However, it still has its devotees.

Sticky paste bandages

Indications

Paste bandages can be used for badly affected limbs that need the extra protection from thicker layers of bandage for deeply excoriated skin or with ulceration. Eczema that has a nodular appearance responds particularly well to this method.

The paste in the bandages is also therapeutic, and ichthammol and zinc paste are the usual constituents in paste bandages. Proprietary names include Viscopaste, Ichthopaste, Ichthaband and Steripaste.

Method

Topical steroid is applied to affected skin prior to bandaging in the appropriate amount, and they can be left in place overnight or for up to 72h. As the bandages can shrink or become stiff when they dry out a special technique is used to apply them. The aim of this technique is to avoid creating a restrictive bandage that impairs the circulation, and it involves folding the

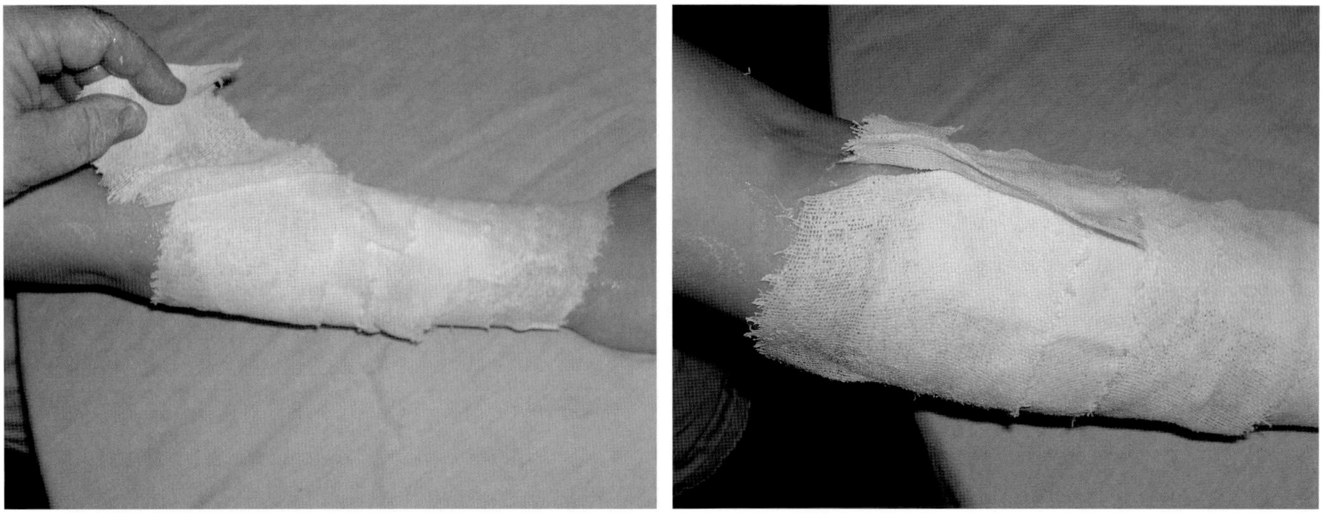

Fig. 34.8 • Applying sticky paste bandages.

bandage back on itself, creating a pleat in the bandage or using strips to cover the affected areas (Fig. 34.8). In this way a tight band around the limb is avoided.

These sticky paste bandages require a secondary covering, therefore a tubular, a conforming or an elasticated bandage such as Coban can be used. The advantages of using elasticised bandages such as Coban is that they are self-adherent and difficult for children to remove, and they are also quite resistant to being scratched through. However, caution should be used when elasticised bandages such as Coban are used: first, to ensure that no pre-existing latex allergy is present; and second, to ensure that only sufficient tension to retain the bandage is used, as too much tension can easily create a tourniquet effect on local circulation, with devastating results. A reasonable rule would therefore appear to be to refrain from using elasticised bandages on a child who is too young to tell the carer that the circulation is being cut off by the bandage.

Procedures Box 34.1 Bathing and bandaging procedure

Actions

Instruct the patient and family of the procedure, informing them of what you plan to do.

If they are new to the concept of bandaging for eczematous conditions they can be informed that bandaging is a method of protecting the skin and of intensifying the moisturising of sore skin.

Reasons *Informing the patient of the procedure will prepare him or her for the experience.*
This should aim to reduce any anxiety and uncertainty for both the patient and the family.

Action

Collect all the equipment required for the procedure:

- Bath oil
- Soap substitute and other emollients
- Shampoo or hair treatment, as prescribed
- Topical steroid, as prescribed
- Bandages (suit as selected according to age or tubular bandages measured and cut to size)
- 2.5-cm strips of bandage to use as ties to secure the bandages (a minimum of eight should be cut)
- Towels to dry off the child.

Reasons *Ensures that the child does not get cold while waiting around.*

Ensures that the child does not have to be left in order to get more equipment or treatment.

Actions

Run the bath and ensure that the ambient environment is comfortable but not too hot (a high temperature will worsen the eczema).

Test the water with your elbow or as per hospital policy; also ensure that the surfaces of the bath and surrounding area are clean.

Reason *Ensures the comfort and safety of the child.*

Action

Examine the skin to assess the level of eczema, signs of infection and the discomfort of the child; record your findings later.

Action

Apply emollient used as soap substitute before the child gets into the bath.

Reason *Reduces stinging of the skin by the bathwater or, as in the case of antiseptic soap substitutes, allows time for the bactericidal action.*

Action

Help and support the child to get into the bath safely.

Reason *Ensures the safety of the child, as the emollients make the child and bath very slippery.*

Procedures Box 34.1 Bathing and bandaging procedure—cont'd

Action
Allow the child to play in the bath; perhaps use a dolly or a friend to share the bathing experience.

Reason *Play reduces anxiety in what is often a painful experience.*

Action
Permit one of the parents or carers to participate in the procedure as much as possible.

Reason *Maintains continuity of care with a trusted carer and provides an opportunity to assess and augment parental skills.*

Action
All shampooing should be done quickly either at the end of bathing to limit detergent exposure or after bathing as a separate treatment.

Reason *Most shampoo has a detergent effect on the skin and will tend to dry the skin out if it is allowed to enter the bathwater.*

Action
Bathing should last no more than 10–15 min; if the skin on the fingertips looks shrivelled the child has been in for too long.

Reason *Optimises the skin treatment benefits.*

Action
Help the child out of the bath.

Reason *Ensures the continued safety of the child in a greasy and slippery environment.*

Action
Gently pat the skin dry.

Reason *Avoids damaging the skin when it is wet and more delicate.*

Actions
Apply the prescribed topical steroid on to the areas of active eczema to create a thin and shiny layer.

Note that gloves can be worn by the carer to do this, but in practice the steroid can easily be washed off before proceeding.

Reason *Treats the skin according to recommended dosing procedure.*

Actions
Apply liberal amounts of emollient all over without disturbing the topical steroid and prior to putting on the tubular bandages.

Paste bandages are impregnated with emollient already and therefore little or no extra emollient is required.

Some emollient scalp treatments, such as Cocois or emulsifying ointment in coconut oil 25%, can be used at this point.

Reason *Ensures rehydration of the skin and appropriate treatment of the condition.*

Action
Assess the child after bathing and reapply emollients to unbandaged areas as appropriate.

Reason *Assesses the need for further emollients in order to optimise skin care.*

Action
Clean the bath using appropriate bath cleanser to remove grease.

Reasons *Maintains a hygienic environment.*
Reduces the potential for infection and slipping hazards from the grease.

Actions
Assess the child's bandages throughout the day to ensure that they remain greasy and comfortably in place.

Tubular bandages can have the outer layer removed and dry bandages can be regreased.

Paste bandages can stay in place for a minimum of 24 h and a maximum of 72 h.

Reason *Ensures the continued comfort of the child.*

Action
Document your findings in the patient's records.

Reason *For safe and accurate record keeping.*

Now test your knowledge

- What advice would you give to the parent of a 3-year-old child when using emollients in the bath?
- What are the basic elements of a care regimen for a child with eczema?

References

Atherton D (1994) Eczema in childhood, the facts. Oxford University Press, Oxford

BMJ Knowledge (2007) Best treatments. Clinical evidence for patients from the BMJ. Online. Available: http:/www.besttreatments.co.uk/btuk/conditions/12803.html Oct 2006

Buxton P (1998) ABC of dermatology, 3rd edn. BMJ Publishing Group, London

Dennis H (2003) The relationship between parental attributions for the causes of childhood eczema and child psychological adjustment to atopic eczema. Unpublished doctorate, University of Birmingham

Emerson RM, Williams HC, Allen BR (1998) Severity distribution of atopic dermatitis in the community and its relationship to secondary referral. British Journal of Dermatology 139(1):73–76

Gill S (2006) An overview of atopic eczema in children: a significant disease. British Journal of Nursing 15(9):494–499

Goodyear H, Spowart K, Harper J (1991) Wet-wrap dressings for the treatment of atopic eczema in children. British Journal of Dermatology 125(6):604

Goodyear HM, Watson PJ, Egan SA, Price EH, Kenny PA, Harper JI (1993) Skin microflora of atopic eczema in first time hospital attenders. Clinical and Experimental Dermatology 18(4):300–304

Lewis-Jones MS, Finlay AY (1995) The Children's Dermatology Life Quality Index (CDLQI): initial validation and practical use. British Journal of Dermatology 132(6):942–949

Long C, Finlay A, Averill R (1992) The rule of hand: 4 hand areas = 2 FTU = 1 g. Archive of Dermatology 128:1129–1130

McFadden J, Noble W, Camp R (1993) Superantigenic exotoxin-secreting potential of staphylococci isolated from atopic eczematous skin. British Journal of Dermatology 128(6):631–632

Papadopoulos L, Bor R (1999) Psychological approaches to dermatology. British Psychological Society, Leicester

Ring J, Kramer U, Berhendt H (2004) A critical approach to the hygiene hypothesis. Clinical and Experimental Allergy Reviews 4(2):40–44

Skov L, Strange P, Baadsgaard O (1995) The potential role of *Staphylococcus aureus* superantigens in atopic eczema. Journal of the Academy of Dermatology and Venereology 5(suppl. 1):185

Tan BB, Weald D, Strickland I, Friedmann PS (1996) Double-blind controlled trial of effect of housedust-mite allergen avoidance on atopic dermatitis. Lancet 347(8993):15–18

Turnbull R, Atherton D (1994) Use of wet wrap dressings in atopic eczema. Paediatric Nursing March 6(2):22–32

University of Dundee (2006) External relations report on genetic research. Online. Available: http://www.dundee.ac.uk/pressreleases/2006/prsept06/eczemagene.html Oct 2006

35 Stoma care

Imelda T. Coyne

Stoma is the Greek word for mouth or opening. A stoma is simply a surgically created opening of the bowel or urinary system on the abdomen. It acts as an outlet for the elimination of body waste. A stoma is generally formed as a temporary measure in the surgical correction of congenital abnormalities that include Hirschsprung's disease, imperforate anus, necrotising entercolitis, cloacal exstrophy, Crohn's disease, ulcerative colitis, bladder tumour and familial polyposis coli. In some cases the stoma may be permanent, particularly with chronic inflammatory bowel conditions, tumours and trauma. Children with severe perineal burns or trauma often require a temporary colostomy to allow the injured area to heal (Minkes et al 2006). Stomas are usually known by the part of the bowel or urinary system that is used. The most common intestinal stomas are colostomies (formed from a piece of colon), ileostomies (formed from a piece of ileum) and urostomies (formed in the urinary tract using a section of ileum) (Collett 2002). Urinary diversions are known as urinary stomas, which include vesicostomies, ureterostomies and ileal conduits.

The most common type of stoma for children is a colostomy performed for anorectal malformations and Hirschsprung's disease. A colostomy can be placed in different areas of the colon, i.e. the sigmoid colon, descending colon, transverse colon and ascending colon (Black 2000a). It is normally sited in the left iliac fossa.

Despite improved surgical techniques, innovations in management and understanding, complications of colostomy remain substantially high (Cigdem et al 2006). The problems that can occur with either bowel or urinary stomas include stoma retraction, excoriation, prolapse, stomal obstruction or stenosis, peristomal hernia, and bleeding flatus or odour (Burch 2004, Chandramouli et al 2004, Collett 2002, Patwardhan et al 2001). Stoma prolapse is common in children, possibly because of decreased fascial development or inadequate fixing of the stoma to the abdominal wall during surgery. Generally, minor prolapses can be reduced easily but some prolapses require reduction under general anaesthetic. Stoma retraction may result from increased tension on the bowel caused by insufficient stomal length or poor stoma placement. Stenosis may occur as a result of inadequate suturing of the fascial layer or mucocutaneous separation (Boyd-Carson et al 2004). Bleeding may occur because of inadequate hemostasis preoperatively or mechanical trauma at the stoma site. Surgical revision is indicated in instances of vascular compromise such as ischaemia, obstruction and chronic bleeding. The most common complications are skin irritation and infection, which are frequently due to improper location of the stoma and/or poor stoma care (Minkes et al 2006). Contact dermatitis is usually caused by faecal contact with peristomal skin. Allergic dermatitis may occur due to sensitivity to appliances, topical creams or other ostomy supplies. When allergic reactions occur alternative appliances should be used. Fortunately most paediatric stomas are temporary diversions that are eventually closed with re-establishment of intestinal continuity. Hence many of the complications listed above are eliminated once the stoma is closed. However, persistent problems usually require surgical revision.

Preparing children for stoma formation

Although the stoma is generally a temporary measure for many children, it can result in physiological, psychological and emotional problems for the child and family. There is limited literature and research on children's experiences of coping with a stoma, which means extrapolation from research studies with adults (Bray & Sanders 2006). The research from adults' perspectives reports that many patients feel overwhelmed and frightened following surgery and in the long term they can experience stigmatisation, degradation and isolation (Black 2000b, Boyd-Carson et al 2004). Stoma formation causes profound changes because of physical damage, disfigurement, loss of bodily function and change in personal hygiene. Most patients adjust to the appearance of a stoma but experience difficulty managing the stoma in relation to fixing and removal of appliances, emptying bags, viscosity of stool, leakage and discontinuation of products. Many adults feel very anxious about possible leakage due to improperly fixed appliances or ballooning of bags and bad odour (Karadag et al 2003). Infants may not have similar anxieties due to their cognitive immaturity and lack of understanding. However, older children and parents may experience similar concerns about stoma formation. The range of anxieties indicates the need for adequate preparation of the child and family prior to surgery and in the aftercare of the stoma.

Most hospitals employ a specialist paediatric stoma nurse, and he or she should be involved in the preparation of the child and family for stoma formation. Because most stomas are formed in the neonatal period as an emergency measure it is often not possible to adequately prepare the family. However, older children may have concerns about altered body image, therefore adequate preoperative preparation is essential. Along with the stoma nurse, the play therapist and clinical psychologist can help with the preparation of the child and family. Preparation programmes may include leaflets, booklets, demonstration or role play with equipment, photograph albums and the use of toys as props (Bray & Sanders 2006). Research indicates that the early promotion of stoma management skills may significantly enhance the psychological adjustment to stoma formation (O'Connor 2005). Therefore children and parents will require ongoing patient education and support to ensure safe management of the stoma and prevention of problems (Borkowski 1998).

Stoma siting

Choosing a suitable site for a stoma is essential, as a poorly sited stoma may result in poor adherence of the appliance, odour, leakage of stool and subsequent skin excoriation. Rutledge et al (2003) state that stoma siting is the most important part of preoperative preparation, as the stoma site has a direct effect on the patient's quality of life and ability to manage the stoma. The intended stoma site should be marked preoperatively to avoid bony prominences, scars, wound sites and skin folds. The site should be marked with the child in both the supine and the sitting position (Rutledge et al 2003). It is important that the site is chosen carefully to ensure that appliances will be easy to apply and will stay fixed in position. There should be enough flat surface for the appliance to adhere to. Children who use wheelchairs, callipers or braces will have special requirements. Therefore they should be measured for the stoma siting while using the appliances. The child should be able to see the stoma while lying down, sitting and standing up. It is important that the child is able to see the stoma so that he or she can be self-caring in the future.

Stoma care appliances

There are a large range of colostomy appliances available and the variety continues to expand (Burch & Sica 2004, White & Berg 2005). Closed colostomy devices can be either one or two piece.

A one-piece appliance has an adhesive flange with a pouch bonded on to it (Fig 35.1). A two-piece appliance (Fig 35.2) allows the flange base plate to be left in place for several days, and only the bag is replaced when the stoma is active. Two-piece appliances can help reduce skin irritation or discomfort from frequent changes (Black 2000a). Both appliances can have a closed end or an open drainable end. Closed end pouches are used when stools are formed, while drainable pouches are used for loose stools. Children with stomas that produce formed stools can also use a colostomy plug. A face plate is attached to the skin and a plug is inserted into the stoma. The cap on the end of the plug is then clipped on to the face plate. The plug must be removed at least 12-hourly and a bag attached to the

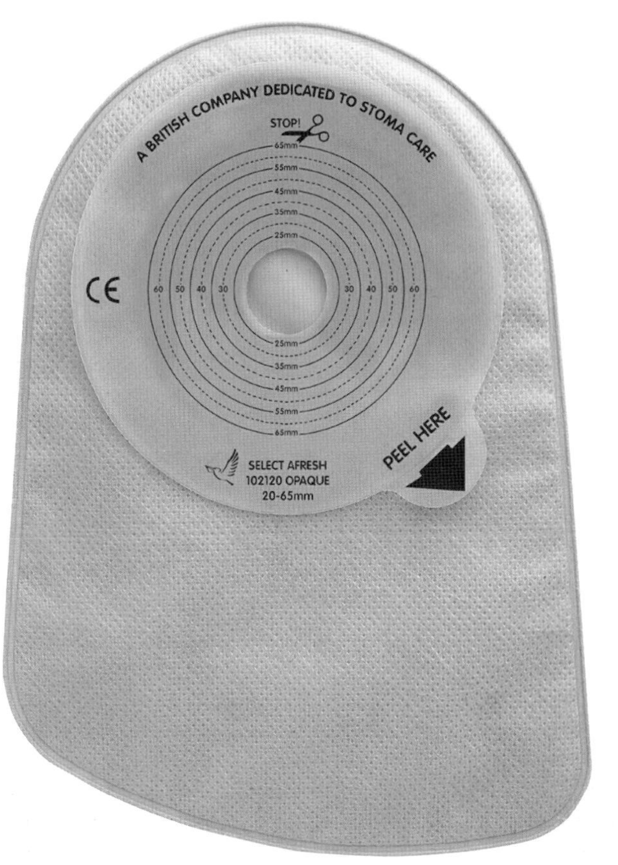

Fig. 35.1 • A one-piece colostomy appliance.

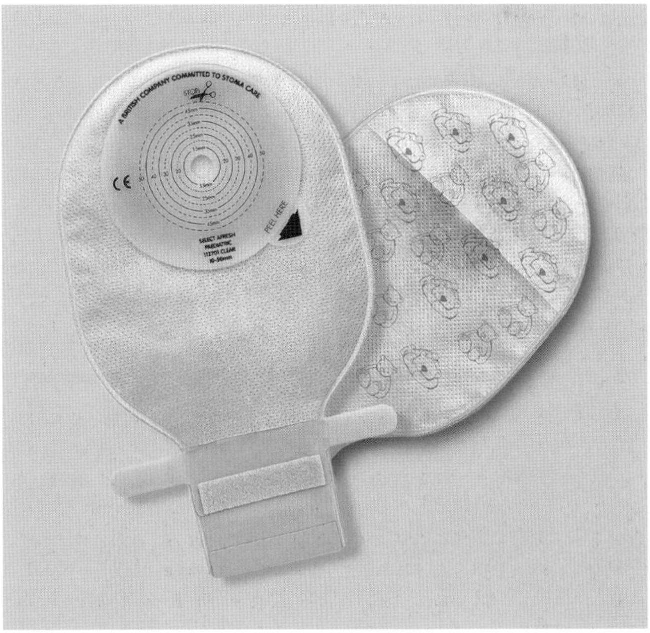

Fig. 35.2 • A two-piece colostomy appliance.

face plate to allow drainage of stool. Filter devices can be used to reduce ballooning of the pouch and neutralise the odour (White & Berg 2005). The child's and parents' views and their dexterity with different products should be a consideration in the selection of appliances. Using an inappropriate appliance is time-consuming and can cause unnecessary discomfort for the child (Chamberlain 1998).

Caring for a stoma

In the early postoperative period a clear transparent drainable pouch is used so that the stoma can be observed easily and can be drained rather than changed frequently (Burch 2005). Generally a one-piece drainable appliance is used in the early preoperative period, as stools will be loose and applying a two piece can be painful. Flatus filters are not used in the early postoperative period, as it is important to observe that the bowel function has returned by the presence of trapped flatus. Bowel function usually returns within 3–4 days. When a stoma is formed it is important to observe the colour of a newly fashioned stoma because of the complication of stenosis or retraction. The stoma is oval-shaped and red–pink in colour, and because it does not have a nerve supply it is not painful. It is essential that the skin area surrounding the stoma is cleansed properly, because excoriation is the most common complication (Burch 2004). Sore skin in the peristomal area results from the adhesion of the appliance, and further leakage of effluent will exacerbate the broken skin. The area around the stoma should be cleaned in the same way as after a normal bowel evacuation. The excess faecal matters should be removed with gauze squares or ordinary toilet paper (only for older children). The skin is washed with warm water, rinsed and then dried with a gauze or towel prior to a new appliance being put on (Black 2000a). All stomas will be oedematous in the early postoperative period, therefore the stoma will change in shape and size. At 6 weeks the stoma should have shrunk to its actual size, therefore parents should be advised wait the 6 weeks before organising precut appliances or ordering precut flanges from suppliers. It is essential that the appliance should fit around the stoma snugly with no peristomal skin exposed.

The advantage of the two-piece appliance is that the pouch may be changed frequently while the adhesive flange is left in situ, therefore the two-piece appliance is particularly suitable for children with sensitive skin or with skin that has become irritated. Constant changing of the appliance can cause abrasion to the peristomal skin and cause discomfort for the child. Sometimes it may not be possible to use a two-piece appliance if the stoma has been sited in an awkward position. In such cases the one-piece appliance can be more suitable due to its flexibility.

Older children with more formed stools may be able to manage their colostomy by irrigation rather than a pouch appliance. The colostomy is irrigated by the instillation of warmed water via a cone and irrigation equipment. Once the bowel contents are evacuated and the returned fluid is clear, the stoma can be closed with a small stoma cap. Alternatively a soft foam plug can be inserted into the stoma after irrigation. The disadvantages of irrigation are that it is time-consuming (approximately 1 h) and has to be performed daily. According to Burch (2005), less than 5% of colostomates in the UK chose irrigation as a form of colostomy maintenance.

Stoma output should always be observed and recorded, as loose or watery stools can indicate gastric upset or gastroenteritis. Some foods, such as spicy products, may cause loose stools. Loose stools should be taken seriously, as dehydration can occur very quickly in infants and children with ileostomies, and electrolyte replacement therapy may be necessary. Generally children are advised to eat a range of foods, thus ensuring adequate nutritional intake, and to avoid a particular food only if it causes digestion difficulties or loose or constipated stools. Children should be encouraged to combine a normal diet with adequate fluid and exercise to ensure satisfactory gastrointestinal functioning.

Procedures Box 35.1 Changing the stoma appliance

1

Action
Collect the required equipment:

- Disposable gloves
- Warm water
- Gauze squares
- Scissors
- Stoma bag
- Stoma flange
- Receptacle to empty the pouch into or bag to dispose of the used pouch and cleansing materials.

2

Action
Wash and dry your hands and put on a plastic apron.

Reason *To adhere to universal precautions.*

3

Action
Explain to the child and parent that you are going to change the stoma appliance.

Reason *Promotes understanding and preparedness.*

4

Action
Place the baby lying down; older children can be offered the choice of lying down or standing.

Reason *It is difficult to apply the appliance when a child is sitting up, because of skin creases.*

Procedures Box 35.1 Changing the stoma appliance—cont'd

5

Action
Ensure that the room is warm and free of draughts.

Reason *Babies, when exposed, lose heat quickly.*

6

Action
Assess the colour of the stoma.

Reason *A healthy stoma is red–pink in colour.*

7

Action
If the stoma appears darker in colour seek medical advice - surgery may be required.

Reasons *A slightly darker colour than normal may indicate stenosis.*
A darker colour such as purple or black indicates a compromised blood supply, which will lead to bowel necrosis.

8

Action
If the stoma has prolapsed seek nursing or medical advice; some minor prolapses can be reduced easily, but some prolapses require reduction under general anaesthetic.

Reason *If the prolapsed portion is darker in colour or tense to touch, this may indicate a compromised blood supply, which will lead to bowel necrosis.*

9

Actions
If the stoma is retracted use a pouch with a convex adhesive flange.

If the stoma remains retracted seek nursing or medical advice, because this may result in leakage of contents, a non-adhered appliance and excoriation.

Reasons *Retracted stomas can be managed by using a pouch with a convex adhesive flange, which will push out the stoma. If the stoma remains retracted it will need surgical refashioning.*

10

Actions
Put on disposable gloves to empty the drainable pouch.

The stoma may require measuring, therefore the pouch contents will be emptied into a jug, the amount recorded and then the contents emptied into a toilet.

Reason *To adhere to universal precautions.*
In the early postoperative period the output may need measuring, as dehydration can occur very quickly.

11

Action
Remove the old pouch by slowly peeling it off from top to bottom with one hand while supporting the skin with the other hand.

Reason *Prevents the skin from tearing and makes the procedure less painful for the baby or child.*

12

Action
Dispose of the appliance in a clinical waste bag.

Reason *To adhere to waste disposal policy.*

13

Action
Clean the peristomal skin with warm water and gauze squares.

Reason *Using water close to body temperature will be less intrusive for the baby or child.*

14

Action
Dry the perisotomal skin with a dry piece of gauze and ensure that the skin is dried thoroughly.

Reason *Wet skin will prevent the appliance from adhering.*

15

Action
Do not use cotton wool to dry the peristomal area.

Reason *Strands may adhere to the stoma and interfere with blood flow or prevent the appliance from adhering properly.*

16

Action
The pouch needs to be cut to fit around the stoma snugly with no peristomal skin exposed; a template or measuring device can assist in the trimming of the flange to the correct size.

Reason *Exposed skin will become excoriated with stool content.*

17

Action
Apply the new pouch.

18

Action
If a one-piece appliance is being used fold the paper adhesive backwards in half, placing the pouch on the underside of the stoma first, and then remove the remaining adhesive on the upper part and secure it carefully.

Reason *It is easier to apply the flange securely in stages than in one action.*

19

Actions
If a two-piece appliance is being used secure the flange first by placing on the underside of the stoma first and then the upper part, then attach the pouch.

Check that the pouch is attached securely.

Reason *Two-piece pouches will leak if the pouch has not been attached properly to the flange.*

20

Action
If a drainable appliance is being used ensure that the clip is secured correctly.

Reason *If the clip is not secure the stool contents will leak.*

Discharging children home with a stoma

A discharge plan should be prepared and agreed for each child and family prior to discharge in order to facilitate a smooth transition from care in hospital to care in the community. In order to ensure that sufficient time is allowed for arrangements to be made, a predicted date of discharge should be identified and agreed with the child and family.

The discharge planning process must include an assessment of the child's continuing health and social care needs and involve such essentials as the following:

- Date and time for discharge
- Referral to the multiprofessional team
- On discharge the children and family should be given 1–2 weeks' supply of the type of pouch the child is using and provided with written details of order numbers and manufacturers' names (Fig 35.3)
- Transport
- Arrangements for services after discharge.

It is likely that only some of the information provided at the hospital will be remembered, and follow-up visits by the healthcare team should be continued into the community. The first few weeks of having to cope at home can be difficult for the child and family, so this continuing support from the stoma team or community nurse is invaluable. The community children's nurse can liaise with other members of the healthcare team, such as the health visitor, general practitioner and school nurse, as well as ensure that the child has access to appropriate facilities at school to ensure privacy and assistance provided as required.

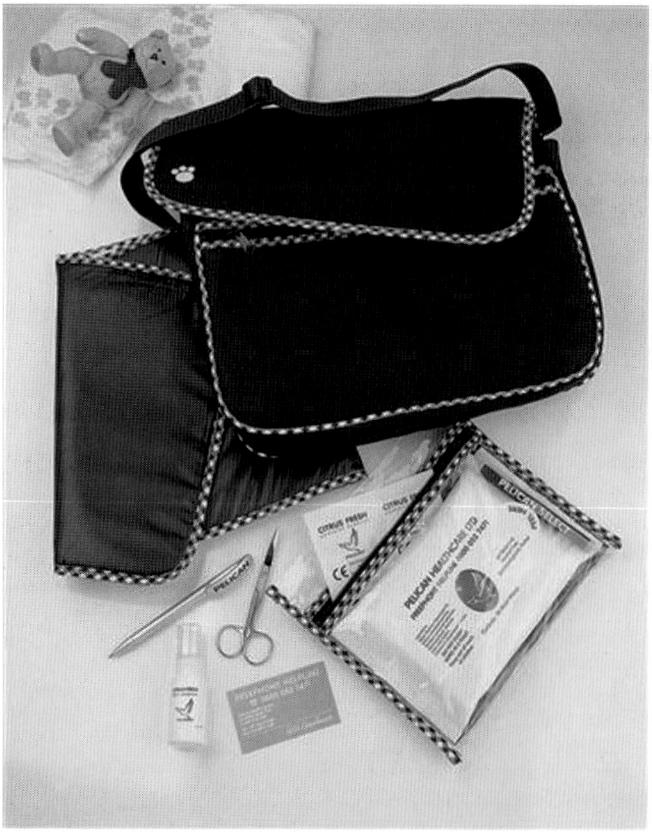

Fig. 35.3 • Supplies for stoma care. (Pelican Healthcare, with permission.)

Now test your knowledge

- Critically evaluate how you would prepare a 5-year-old child for changing of the stoma appliance. What support and guidance would be required to prepare the parent to assist you in this procedure?
- Describe the different types of stoma and understand the reason for their formation.
- Identify the stoma complications that will require urgent medical attention.

References

Black P (2000a) Practical stoma care. Nursing Standard 14(41):47–53

Black PK (2000b) Holistic stoma care. Ballière Tindall, London

Borkowski S (1998) Pediatric stomas, tubes and appliances. Pediatric Clinics of North America 45(6):1419–1435

Boyd-Carson W, Thompson MJ, Boyd K (2004) Mucocutaneous separation: clinical protocols for stoma care. Nursing Standard 18(17):41–43

Bray L, Sanders C (2006) Preparing children and young people for stoma surgery. Paediatric Nursing 18(4):33–37

Burch J (2004) The management and care of people with stoma complications. British Journal of Nursing 13(6):307–318

Burch J (2005) The pre and postoperative nursing care for people with a stoma. British Journal of Nursing 14(6):310–316

Burch J, Sica J (2004) Colostomy products: an update on recent developments. British Journal of Community Nursing 9(9):373–378

Chamberlain J (1998) Choosing the right product for the patient. WCET Journal 18(20):26–28

Chandramouli B, Srinivasan K, Jagdish S (2004) Morbidity and mortality of colostomy and its closure in children. Journal of Pediatric Surgery 38:596–599

Cigdem MK, Onen A, Duran H, Ozturk H, Otcu S (2006) The mechanical complications of colostomy in infants and children: analysis of 473 cases of a single centre. Pediatric Surgery International 22:671–676

Collett K (2002) Practical aspects of stoma management. Nursing Standard 17(8):45–55

Karadag A, Mentes BB, Uner A, Irkörücü O, Ayaz S, Ozkan S (2003) Impact of stoma therapy on quality of life in patients with permanent colostomies or ileostomies. International Journal of Colorectal Disease 18(3):234–238

Minkes RK, McLean SE, Mazziotti MV, Langer JC (2006) Stomas of the small and large intestine. Online. Available: http://www.emedicine.com/ped/topic2994.htm 15 Dec 2006

O'Connor G (2005) Teaching stoma management skills: the importance of self-care. British Journal of Nursing 14(6):320–324

Patwardhan N, Kiely EM, Drake DP, Spitz L, Pierro A (2001) Colostomy for anorectal anomalies: high incidence of complications. Journal of Paediatric Surgery 36(5):795–798

Rutledge M, Thompson MJ, Boyd-Carson W (2003) Effective stoma siting. Nursing Standard 18(12):43–44

White M, Berg K (2005) A new flangeless adhesive coupling system for colostomy and ileostomy. British Journal of Nursing 14(6):325–328

36 Neonatal jaundice and phototherapy

Sharon Nurse

Hyperbilirubinaemia is common in newborn babies because most will develop higher than normal unconjugated serum bilirubin (SBR) levels in the first week of life (Hansen 2002). It is vital that nurses caring for the jaundiced baby have a sound knowledge of the physiological processes that result in hyperbiliribinaemia and the rationale behind the care they provide.

Phototherapy is the most common mode of treatment used, which results in the bilirubin being excreted without the need for conjugation (Watson 2006).

Physiology of bilirubin production and excretion

Newborn babies have high levels of red blood cells containing haemoglobin, which are destroyed in significant numbers in the first week of life. The globin part of the cell is recycled as protein and the haem part becomes biliverdin and eventually bilirubin. Unconjugated or fat-soluble bilirubin cannot be excreted, so it travels to the liver attached to plasma proteins or albumin. In the liver the unconjugated bilirubin is acted on by the enzymes glucuronyl transferase and glucuronic acid. It is vital that oxygen and glucose are present for effective conjugation. Once treated the bilirubin becomes conjugated or water-soluble. It travels to the kidneys and gut as urobilinogen and stercobilinogen, respectively, and is excreted.

Pathophysiology of jaundice

Neonatal jaundice results from two processes occurring simultaneously:

1. Bilirubin production is elevated due to red blood cell destruction
2. Hepatic function is inadequate in the newborn to conjugate effectively.

These factors lead to physiological jaundice, which is the most common form in the newborn and usually occurs between the third and fifth day after birth.

Other causes of jaundice in the neonate

Physiological jaundice appears as a naturally occurring condition in newborn babies, but there are many other reasons why a baby may appear jaundiced.

Bilirubin levels

Visual assessment of jaundice varies with the experience and confidence of the practitioner (Yeo 1998). Most neonatal units will commence treatment in a term baby at SBR levels of 320 μmol/L, preterm babies (< 28 weeks) at levels of 150–180 μmol/L, and preterm babies (34 weeks) at levels of 200–240 μmol/L (Sweet 1999).

Each neonatal unit must have protocols for instigating treatment and should use graphs to plot the rate and rise of SBR levels, repeating blood tests when necessary.

Phototherapy

This treatment uses light to act on the unconjugated bilirubin under the skin, changing it to photobilirubin and lumirubin, after which it is transported to the liver for the final stages of conjugation before being excreted.

Phototherapy can help to lower bilirubin levels (Hansen 2002). Lamps emitting between 400 and 500 nm are specifically used for phototherapy because bilirubin absorbs this wavelength. The light is visible white, blue or green. Green light is more effective in absorbing bilirubin due to the power and range of the wavelengths (Vecchi et al 1983).

Types of phototherapy unit

Overhead lamps

These units have fluorescent tubes that can be a combination of white, blue and green. The lamps should be positioned at least 25–30 cm away from the infant, and the protective Plexiglass covering the tubes must be intact to protect the baby from excessive heat (Fig. 36.1). Bulbs may degenerate with time and so should be tested periodically to ensure maximum effectiveness.

Light sources are:

- fluorescent lamps
- quartz halogen lamps
- light-emitting diodes (LEDs).

Light sources can be used to deliver additional phototherapy from above or from the side of the baby (Fig. 36.2). Most manufacturers recommend keeping spotlights at least 52 cm away from the baby due to their heat emission.

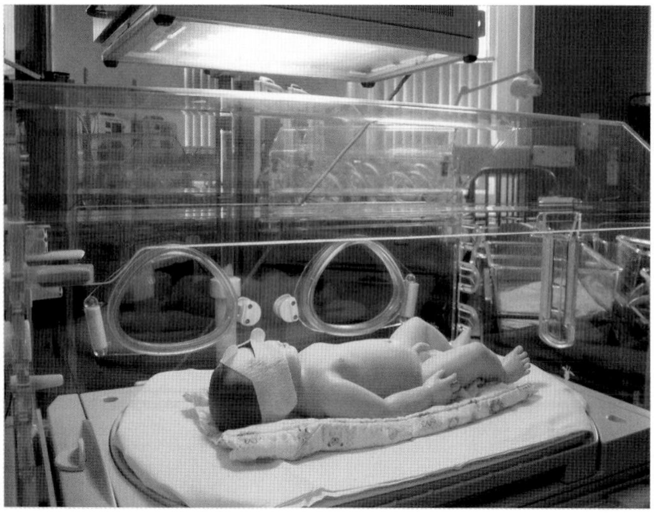

Fig. 36.1 • A phototherapy unit.

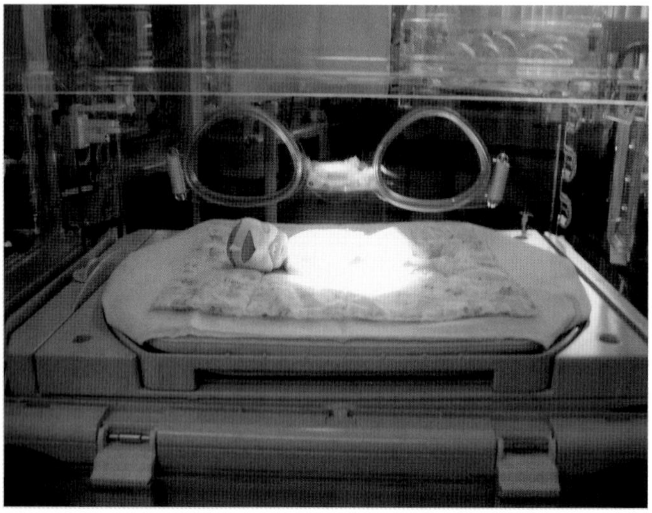

Fig. 36.2 • Light sources can deliver additional phototherapy.

Wentworth (2005) compiled a comprehensive survey of the range of equipment available, providing descriptions, considering the safety aspects and comparing them to identified effective criteria.

Biliblanket

A halogen bulb is directed into a fibre-optic mattress, the filter removing the ultraviolet rays, providing a blue–green colour (Fig. 36.3).

The baby lies on the mattress or blanket. This device can be useful as an additional source if overhead phototherapy is in place (double phototherapy). These blankets are suitable only for babies of > 28 weeks' gestation. Fibre-optic phototherapy is less effective than conventional treatment in lowering SBR levels (Mills & Tudehope 2000, Sarici et al 2001).

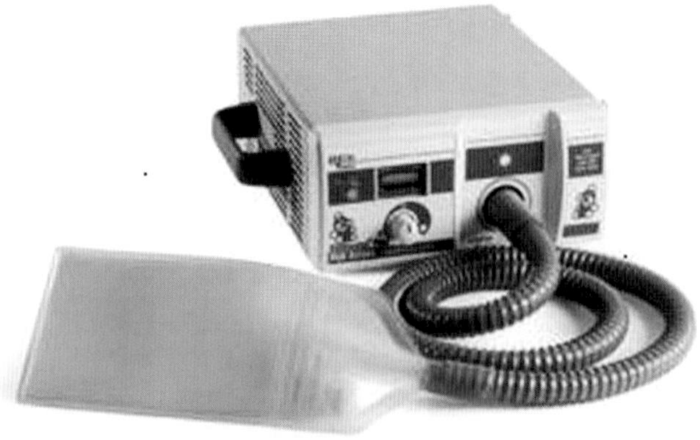

Fig. 36.3 • A Biliblanket.

Bilibed and babygro

A blue fluorescent tube is fitted into a plastic base and the top is formed like a Babygro. The baby lies on the base but fits the arms into a suit and so does not require eye covers (Fig. 36.4). This form of phototherapy is not suitable for high SBR levels.

There are many factors that can affect the efficacy of phototherapy, and these are listed in Box 36.1.

Care of the baby having phototherapy

The baby having phototherapy is clinically unstable and the treatment is not without side effects, so a comprehensive nursing plan is required. Parents need explanations about the treatment, and when possible, the baby should be nursed beside her or his mother in the ward. Nursing staff should be educated as to the care of the jaundiced baby and use of the equipment.

Like all treatments, phototherapy is not without its problems, and all nurses should be fully aware of potential problems and the importance of close monitoring of the baby while undergoing treatment. The possible side effects of phototherapy are listed in Box 36.2.

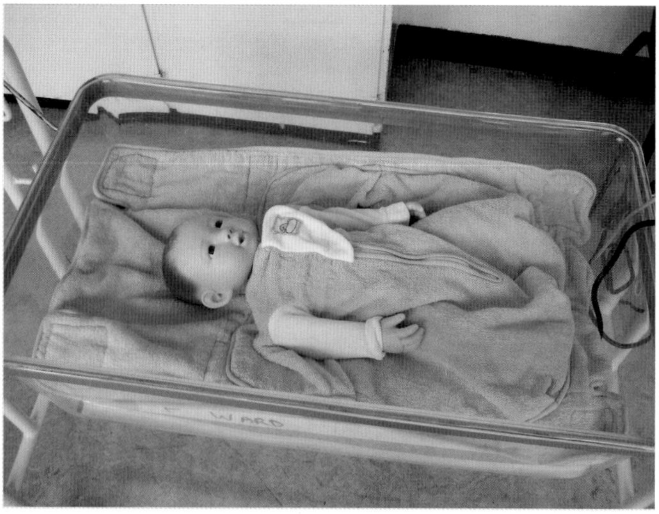

Fig. 36.4 • A Bilibed.

Box 36.1. Factors affecting the dose and efficacy of phototherapy

- Plexiglass may be stained or broken: it should always be checked prior to use; this glass emits ultraviolet rays and prevents burns.
- Fluorescent tubes have a limited lifespan: they must be tested or replaced after every 1000 h of use and serviced every 6 months.
- The photometer should be used to test the light output of each phototherapy unit.
- Distance of the unit from the baby: halving the distance doubles the amount of light to the baby (Hey 1995).
- Surface area of the baby exposed to light: the baby should be naked.
- Using reflective material inside the cot or incubator to reflect light to the baby.
- Using a curtain around the incubator and unit can multiply delivery several-fold.
- It is vital that the manufacturer's recommendations are closely adhered to when using their product.

Box 36.2. Possible side effects of phototherapy treatment in neonates

- Temperature instability leading to hypothermia or hyperthermia.
- Excessive fluid loss through transepidermal water loss, leading to dehydration and electrolyte imbalance.
- Eye damage from excessive bright light (Noell et al 1966).
- Risk of eye infections from the use of eye pads (Fok et al 1995).
- Skin rashes can be aggravated by the light.
- Skin may turn a grey–green colour if phototherapy is used for high conjugated bilirubin levels – this is called bronze baby syndrome.
- Sore, excoriated buttocks may result from loose stools containing bile salts.
- DNA damage induced in human cells exposed to phototherapy (Rosenstein & Ducore 1984).
- Chromatic radiance damage linked to sterility and genetic damage of sperm when the gonads were exposed to lights for long periods (Edwards 1995, Schwoebal & Sakraida 1997).
- Parental separation and potential interference in the bonding process.
- Nursing staff have complained of headaches when exposed to blue lights for long periods.
- Possibility of missing cyanosis in a baby nursed under blue lights.

Procedures Box 36.1 Care of the baby receiving phototherapy

1 Observations

Action
Daily weighing is required.

Reason *To accurately assess fluid requirements.*

Action
Routine observations such as heart rate, respiratory rate and blood pressure can be recorded as prescribed.

Reason *Tachypnoea and tachycardia could be signs of overheating.*

Action
A pulse oximeter should be used to record oxygen saturations.

Reason *Blue lamps can make it difficult to detect cyanosis.*

Action
Monitor change in colour.

Reason *To record the change in condition in resolving or deepening jaundice.*

2 Positionng

Action
Change the baby's position occasionally.

Reasons *There is very little evidence to support the frequent changing of position during treatment, but it is important to change position occasionally to ensure the comfort of the baby. Shinwell et al (2002) investigated the response of SBR level decline to position change and found that the supine position produced better results.*

Action
If spotlights are being used on small babies, it is important to have the light directly on the chest or trunk area.

3 Skin care

Action
Maximum exposure of skin is important, so babies are usually nursed naked without nappies.

Reason *Ensures maximum exposure of the skin to light (Dent 2000).*

Action
Keep the skin clean and dry, and clean only with water.

Reason *Prevents infection.*

Action
Skin can be protected with a clear topical ointment.

Reason *Protects the skin from transepidermal water loss (Dani et al 2001, Wananukul & Pralsuwanna 2002).*

Actions
Oil-based creams should not be applied to skin that is directly exposed to lamps.

Increased excretion of bilirubin causes excoriation of buttocks and can be treated by cleansing and leaving the skin exposed to air.

If a nappy is worn, small amounts of protective cream can be applied to the area.

Action
Male infants should have gonad protection.

Reason *Sperm DNA can be damaged by prolonged exposure to phototherapy lamps.*

Procedures Box 36.1 Care of the baby receiving phototherapy—cont'd

3 Continued

Action
Rashes should be left untreated but monitored.

4

Eye care

Action
The newborn baby's eyes should always be covered while undergoing phototherapy treatment (Behrman 1974).

Reasons *The newborn baby's eyes are extremely sensitive to light. Phototherapy lamps can cause retinal damage if the eyes are exposed for long periods unprotected.*

Action
Eye pads can be used effectively but should be changed at least 4-hourly.

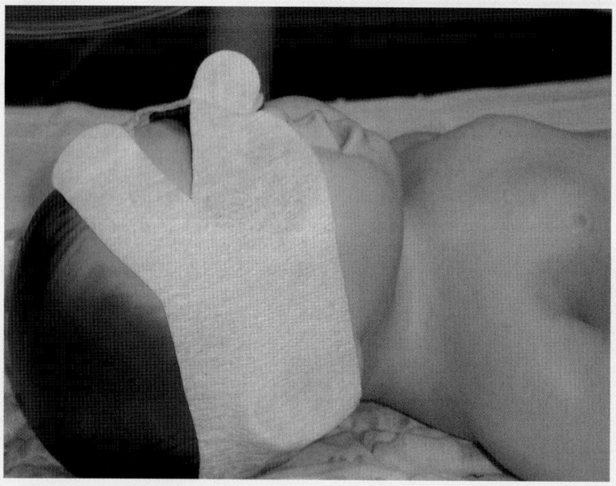

Reason *Prevents infection.*

Action
Avoid using tape to secure eye pads.

Reason *This causes epidermal stripping.*

Action
Avoid using tight bands.

Reason *This can impede blood flow to the brain.*

Action
The infant requires constant observation.

Reason *There is always the danger of the eye pads slipping down and covering the baby's nose and mouth, occluding the airways.*

Action
Clean the eyes every 4 h.

Reason *Prevents infection and lubricates the area.*

Action
Ensure that the eyes are closed when applying new pads.

Reason *Prevents corneal damage.*

Action
Plexiglass eye shields can be used to protect the eyes and do not require eye pads; however, careful positioning of baby is essential to avoid the baby sliding from under the shield (Fok et al 1997).

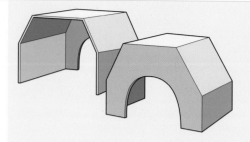

5

Thermoregulation

Actions
Axilla temperature should be checked at least 4-hourly.

A skin probe in the incubator could give a constant read-out of temperature when used in the 'air' mode.

Reasons *Although babies are nursed naked under phototherapy lamps, the bulbs can increase the environmental temperature, leading to temperature instability.*
Monitoring the incubator temperature is vital, as phototherapy may increase the ambient temperature (Dollberg et al 1995).

Action
Observe the baby.

Reasons *A red colour, extended posture and tachypnoea could all indicate an overheated baby.*
There can be significant increases in temperature when using overhead units (Pezzati et al 2002).

6

Fluid requirements

Actions
There can be up to a 20% increase in transepidermal water loss during halogen spotlight therapy, despite relative humidity (Grunhagen et al 2000); however, increasing fluid requirements during phototherapy remains controversial (Cloherty 1991).

To counteract excessive losses some authors advise increases of 10–20%/kg per 24 h.

Merenstein & Gardner (1998) suggested not increasing fluids routinely but using the specific gravity of the urine as an indicator of the need for extra fluid.

7

General guidelines for fluid assessment

Actions
All fluids should be calculated according to unit protocols.

Intake and output should be recorded accurately.

Action
Urinalysis and specific gravity should be checked 6- to 8-hourly.

Procedures Box 36.1 Care of the baby receiving phototherapy—cont'd

7 Continued

Reason *Ensures that fluid requirements are adequate and that renal function is maintained.*

Action

Observe and record losses via stools.

8

Fluid requirements for term infants

Actions

Give 3-hourly bottle or tube feeds.

Breastfed babies demand feed (assess mother's supply).

Give complementary feeds of expressed breast milk or formula by tube, cup or bottle.

Reasons *A good intake of protein is required to aid transport of bilirubin to the liver.*
Adequate glucose is needed to aid conjugation.

9

Fluid requirements for preterm infants

Action

Increases up to 20%/kg per day may be necessary.

Reason *Transepidermal fluid loss is greater.*

Action

Monitor urea and electrolyte results and compare with the specific gravity of the urine.

10

Rest and sleep

Action

Ensure good positioning using soft bedding and rolls and using pacifiers.

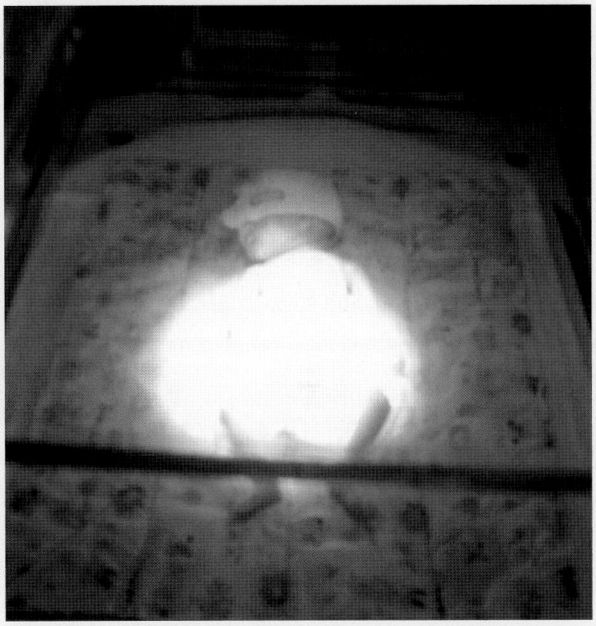

Reasons *Phototherapy can affect cardiorespiratory activity during active sleep, causing an increased heart rate and a reduced respiratory effort in response to apnoea (Bader et al 2006).*
Babies can also be more agitated under phototherapy.
Good positioning can facilitate developmental care while reducing agitation and promoting rest.

11

Involvement of parents

Actions

Kangaroo care using a fibre-optic blanket could be used for 1 h/day and does not appear to lessen the effectiveness of treatment (Ludington-Hoe & Swinth 2001).

Encouragement to continue breastfeeding is essential.

Physical contact should not be an issue during treatment.

Promoting parent–child relationships is vital at all times; parental contact should always be encouraged to promote bonding.

When possible, nurse the baby with his or her mother.

Reasons *It can be very distressing for parents to see their baby being nursed naked in an incubator with his or her eyes covered and requiring repeated blood sampling.*
There is added anxiety of the possibility of transfer to the neonatal unit.
Parents are not able to hold their baby for long periods due to the treatment, which may affect bonding.

Action

Provide parents with explanations and updates on their baby's condition and treatment.

Reasons *Parents may believe their baby to be in discomfort and may experience feelings of anxiety and sadness (Campos & Leitao 2005).*
Information and reassurance are essential to empower parents to assist in the care of their baby.

Now test your knowledge

Question 1

Why can unconjugated bilirubin not be excreted from the body in this form?

Question 2

Name the two processes that result in neonatal jaundice.

Question 3

When does physiological jaundice in the newborn usually appear?

Question 4

What is phototherapy?

Question 5

Name three types of phototherapy.

Question 6

Name three factors that can affect the efficacy of the phototherapy.

Question 7

Why is the use of an oxygen saturation monitor sometimes required when using blue lamps?

Question 8

Why do the baby's buttocks sometimes become excoriated?

Question 9

How often should eye pads be changed and why?

Question 10

How would you recognise overheating in a baby?

Question 11

How much extra fluid should a baby having phototherapy receive?

Question 12

How often should bottle- or tube-fed babies be fed?

Question 13

What is transepidermal water loss and how does it affect the baby under phototherapy?

Question 14

List five side effects of phototherapy.

References

Bader D, Kugelman A, Blum D, Riskin A, Tirosh E (2006) Effect of phototherapy on cardiorespiratory activity during sleep in neonates with physiologic jaundice. Israeli Medical Association 8(1):12–16

Behrman RE (1974) Preliminary report of the committee on phototherapy in the newborn infant. Journal of Paediatrics 84:135–147

Campos A, Leitao G (2005) Beliefs and feelings experienced by mothers of children under phototherapy. Revista gaúcha de enfermagem 26(1):50–56

Cloherty J (1991) Neonatal hyperbilirubinaemia. In Cloherty J, Sterk A (eds) Manual of neonatal care, 3rd edn. Little, Brown, Boston

Dani C, Martelli E, Reali M, Bertini G, Panin G, Rubaltelli F (2001) Fibreoptic and conventional phototherapy on the skin of premature infants. Journal of Pediatrics 138(3):438–440

Dent J (2000) Haematological problems. In Boxwell G (ed.) Neonatal intensive care nursing. Routledge Press, London

Dollberg S, Atherton HD, Hoath SB (1995) Effect of different phototherapy lights on incubator characteristics and dynamics under three modes of servo-control. American Journal of Perinatology 12(1):55–60

Edwards S (1995) Phototherapy and the neonate: providing safe and effective nursing care for jaundiced infants. Journal of Neonatal Nursing October (suppl.):9–12

Fok TF, Wong W, Cheung AF (1995) Use of eye patches in phototherapy: effects on conjunctival bacterial pathogens and conjunctivitis. Pediatric Infections Disease Journal 14(12):1991–1994

Fok TF, Wong W, Cheung AF (1997) Eye protection for newborns under phototherapy: comparison between a modified headbox and the conventional eyepatches. Annals of Tropical Paediatrics 17(4):349–354

Grünhagen D, Boer M, Beaufort A, Walther F (2002) Transepidermal water loss during halogen spotlight phototherapy in preterm infants. Pediatric Research 51:402–405

Hansen T (2002) Neonatal jaundice. Online. Available: http://www.eMedicine.com/

Hey EN (1995) Neonatal jaundice – how much do we really know? MIDIRS Midwifery Digest 5(1):4–8

Ludington-Hoe S, Swinth JY (2001) Kangaroo mother care during phototherapy: effect on bilirubin profile. Neonatal Network 20(5):41–48

Merenstein G, Gardner S (eds) (1998) Handbook of neonatal intensive care, 4th edn. Mosby, St Louis

Mills JF, Tudehope D (2000) Fibreoptic phototherapy for neonatal jaundice. Cochrane Library Issue 2. John Wiley, Chichester

Noell W, Walker V, Kang BS, Behrman S (1966) Retinal damage by bright light in rats. Investigative Ophthalmology 5:450–473

Pezzati M, Fusi F, Dani C (2002) Changes in skin temperature of hyperbilirubinaemic newborns under phototherapy: conventional versus fibreoptic devices. American Journal of Perinatology 19(8):439–443

Rosenstein B, Ducore J (1984) Enhancement by bilirubin of DNA damage, induced in human cells exposed to phototherapy light. Pediatric Research 18:3–6

Sarici SU, Alpay F, Dundaroz MR, Ozcan O, Gokcay E (2001) Fibreoptic phototherapy versus conventional daylight phototherapy for term newborns. Turkish Journal of Paediatrics 43(4):280–285

Schwoebal A, Sakraida S (1997) Hyperbilirubinaemia – new approaches to an old problem. Journal of Perinatal and Neonatal Nursing 11(3):78–97

Shinwell ES, Scialey Y, Karplus M (2002) Effect of position changing on bilirubin levels during phototherapy. Journal of Perinatology 22(3):226–229

Sweet B (1999) Neonatal jaundice. In Sweet B (ed.) Mayes' midwifery: a textbook for midwives. Baillière Tindall, London

Vecchi C, Donzelli G, Migliorini M, Sbrana G (1983) Green light in phototherapy. Pediatric Research 17:461–463

Wananukul S, Pralsuwanna P (2002) Clear topical ointment decreases transepidermal water loss in jaundiced preterm infants receiving phototherapy. Journal of Medical Associates, Thailand 85(1):102–106

Watson J (2006) Neonatal hyperbilirubinaemia. In Glasper A, McEwing G, Richardson J (eds) 2006 Oxford handbook of children's and young people's nursing. Oxford University Press, Oxford

Wentworth S (2005) Neonatal phototherapy – to-day's lights, lamps and devices. Infant 1(1)14–19

Yeo H (1998) The jaundiced baby. In Yeo H (ed.) Nursing the neonate. Blackwell Science, Oxford, p 221–241

37 Developmentally supportive positioning and handling of neonates

Joyce Robertson

Careful handling and positioning on a neonatal intensive care unit (NICU) is crucial to the baby's current well-being and future development. The quality of handling on the NICU affects the baby's vital signs and very survival. In addition to this, recent research has shown that the development of the baby's brain is shaped by the environment (Schore 2003a: 14, 2003b: 23). Therefore the infant's experience during handling and interactions on the NICU has the potential to influence future emotional and motor development. Evidence indicates that sensitive empathic handling and positioning probably has immediate, short-term and long-term benefits (Als et al 2004, Symington & Pinelli 2003).

Although basic guidelines about handling and positioning can be given, it is important to note that the quality of the baby's experience in the NICU depends on empathic responses from the nurse and a moment-by-moment reading of the baby's cues. It is not so many years ago that operations on NICUs were performed without anaesthetic, as it was thought that these babies did not experience pain. This is fortunately no longer the case, and steps are now taken to ensure that discomfort and pain are addressed by the use of drugs or other strategies such as non-nutritive sucking. Given the daily invasive and distressing procedures undergone by infants on NICUs, having a personal involvement with these babies and treating them as sentient human beings can be a painful experience for the nurse. He or she should ideally have access to support or supervision in order to have the opportunity to process his or her own feelings.

During all procedures the nurse should 'hold in mind' (Winnicott 1960) the experience of the baby. By 'holding in mind' Winnicott meant the often semiautomatic sense that the mother has for what her infant is experiencing at each moment. The control of noise, including if, when and how the nurse speaks in the vicinity of the infant; the monitoring of light around the incubator (very preterm babies do not have the motor skills to avert their eyes from bright lights); and how the nurse approaches and moves the baby will then flow naturally from this premise.

Neurobiological background

The biological structures of the brain are maturing during the growth spurt that starts during the last trimester of pregnancy (Dobbing & Sands 1973), hence the importance of providing the best possible environment for this. It is now recognised that the environment affects not only the memories and habits but the actual differentiation of brain structure (Cicchetti & Tucker 1994), so that a different brain is formed according to the environment. Figure 37.1 shows the concentration of a father (using his brain) as he attempts to attune to his baby's experience (the baby's brain) and provide what the baby's brain needs at this stage. Note the offering of his finger for the baby to grasp in an attempt to help the baby feel connected and more secure.

Peters (1998) describes how '(T)he continual activation of the hypothalamic–pituitary–adrenal (HPA) axis and production of cortisol' causes maladaptive changes in the sensitive endocrine system of the neonate. Stress in early infancy resulting in high cortisol levels can result in cell death, as 'the pruning and maintenance of synaptic connections is environmentally driven' (Schore 2003a). Perry et al (1995), talking about mental and physical responses to trauma, including physiological hyperarousal, describes how 'adaptive states, when they persist, can become maladaptive traits'. This applies to both emotional and motor development. Schore (2003a) says that stress causing high levels of cortisol can result in disturbances in the regulation of emotions in later life.

The interaction of the various bodily systems and functions

Dynamic systems theory (Lewis & Douglas 1998) explains how all the different systems in the body interact with each other and how stress in one system, such as the autonomic system, can affect the function of another system, such as the motor system. In the NICU, any handling may affect the various systems in the body, such as the sleep state, heart rate, circulation, respiration and muscle tone. Infants on the NICU who arch back stiffly in response to physiological hyperarousal, perhaps caused by environmental influences such as noise or by nursing intervention such as suctioning, often persist with this activity well into the first few months of life (Robertson 2005), hence the importance of hands-on support (see below).

Heidi Als from the USA, a psychologist by background, has pioneered a way of caring for babies on the NICU that is responsive to their cues and replicates as much as possible the intrauterine environment. This method of developmental care is called the Newborn Individualised Developmental Care and Assessment Programme (NIDCAP). Some of the cues that may show that the infant is getting stressed are change of colour,

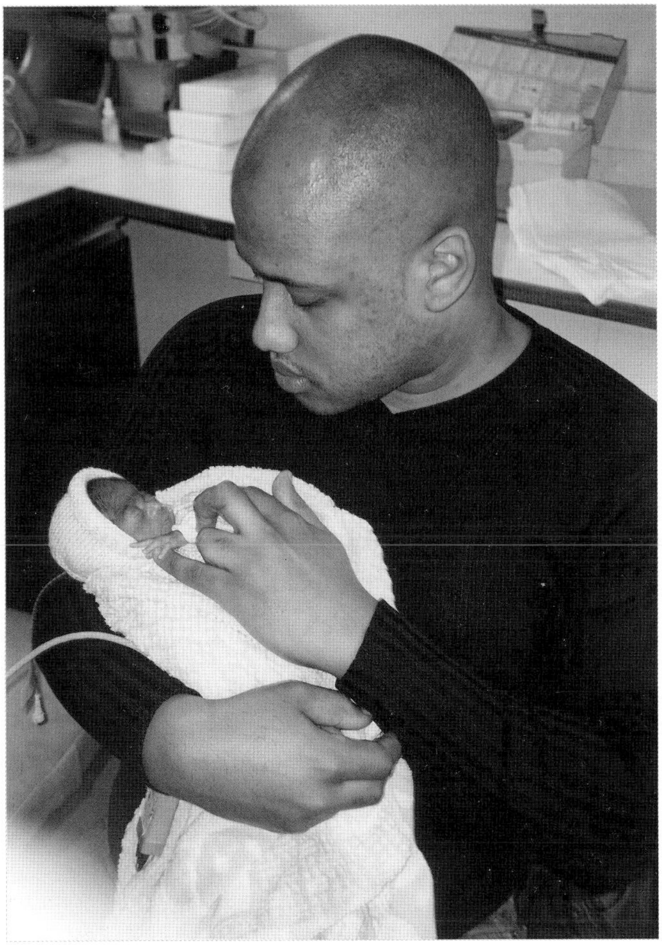

Fig. 37.1 • 'The infant's brain develops in the context of a relationship with another self, another brain.' (Schore 2003b: 23).

respiration or heart rate; hiccupping; yawning; looking away; and stiffening of limbs; as well as the arching back mentioned above.

Cues that indicate more stability are a stable colour, regular heart rate and respiration, a flexed posture, hand to mouth, relaxed muscle tone, and clear sleep and awake states. Sometimes babies use coping strategies that enable them to withstand potentially stressful situations such as over-stimulation by noise or handling. Some of these coping strategies are bracing limbs (e.g. against the side of the cot), going into a light sleep state, sucking, putting a hand on the face or head, or clasping the hands or feet together.

Full information on reading infant cues is not within the scope of this chapter, but more information can be found in the NIDCAP literature and on the NIDCAP website (NIDCAP Federation International 2007) and also in Warren (2000). Research by Als et al (2004) shows that babies cared for by the NIDCAP method show improved brain development compared with those cared for in the traditional way.

The NIDCAP literature also gives more information and guidelines about the use of kangaroo care. This is when a baby is nursed in skin-to-skin contact with the mother. This close contact provides conditions similar to those in utero (such as the sound of the mother's voice, breathing and heartbeat) and often helps the baby to be more settled, adopt a better posture and be more responsive (Fig. 37.2).

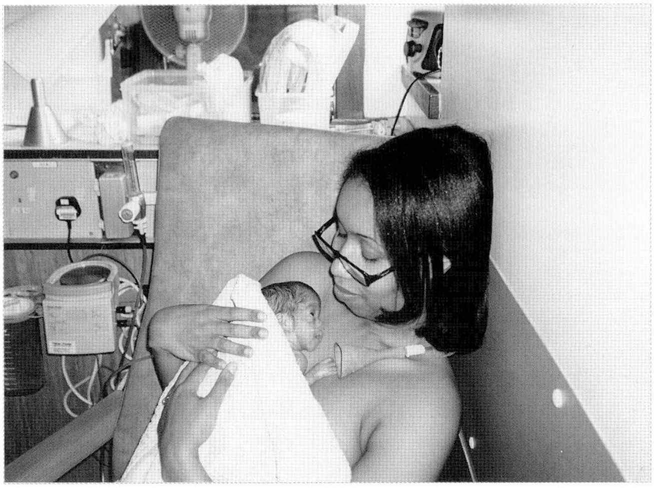

Fig. 37.2 • Kangaroo care: a baby at 32 weeks' gestation.

How position may affect future movement

Given the early neuroplasticity of the brain, it is important to consider the best ways of positioning and handling to promote optimal movement patterns. First of all, a percentage of preterm babies may develop cerebral palsy, but during their early days in the NICU it may not be clear which babies these are. The Prechtl assessment of infant movement is a useful tool for screening at-risk babies (Prechtl et al 1997). For those who will develop cerebral palsy, early positioning is of the utmost importance. For those babies who have an undamaged neurological system, thoughtful early positioning and handling are still important for the reasons outlined above.

The muscle tone in preterm babies is lower than in full-term babies. Therefore the preterm baby tends to adopt a flattened posture, as the limbs and body take up the position of the flat surface. When babies are nursed in the supine position without supports around the body, gravity causes the arms and legs to fall outwards into a frog-like position as the baby takes up the supporting surface (Fig. 37.3).

The place of sensory feedback and feed-forward is an important aspect in the neurological planning of movement (Ehrsson et al 2000). If a baby lies in the supine position without support, with abducted limbs and retracted shoulder girdle, the sensory feedback that will be registered is of this position as a starting position for movement. However, this is not the optimal position from which to move. The danger is that the baby may develop some adverse postural habits that persist after discharge. These are typically retraction of the shoulder girdle, abduction and outward rotation of the arms and legs, and even some associated muscle and ligamentous shortening. This can delay the development of motor skills.

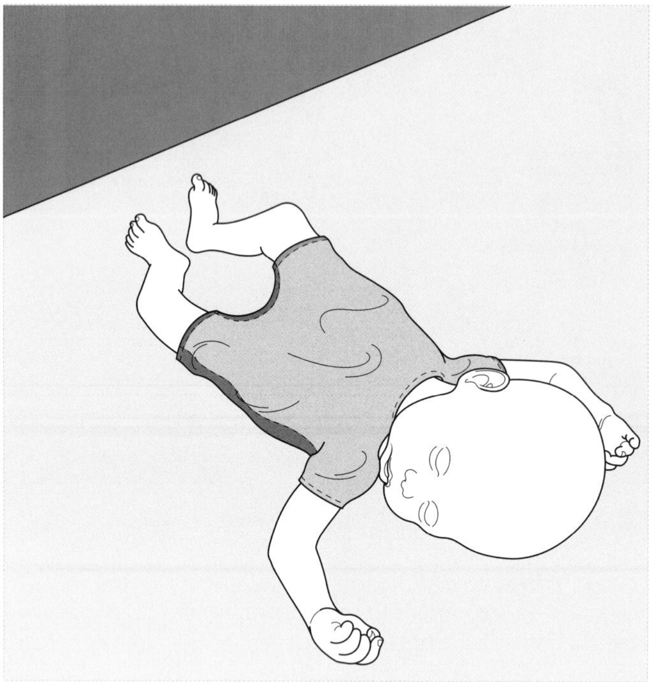

Fig. 37.3 • Posture without the use of supports.

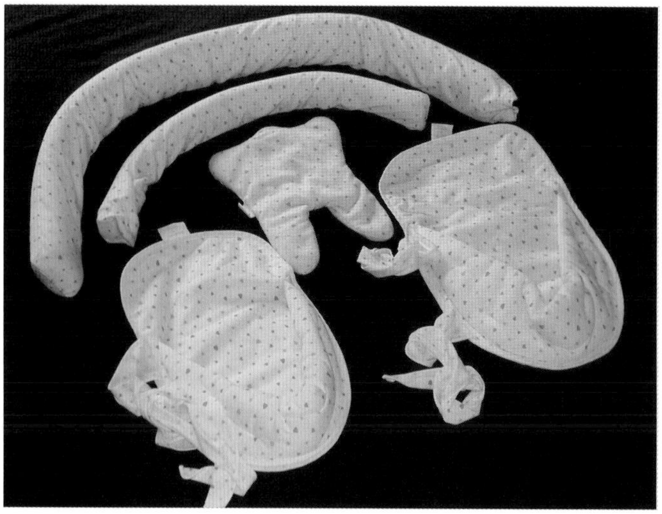

Fig. 37.4 • Positioning equipment. Above are large and small bendy bumpers. Below are large and small nests. In the centre is Freddie the frog.

The central nervous system is task-dependent in its organisation (Bower et al 1996). Therefore positions that allow the possibility of functional movement, such as sucking the thumb, will be the most useful. In addition, it is difficult for a baby in the supine position to make eye contact with any part of his or her own body due to the effort needed to bring the arms forward into the line of vision. It is important to position the baby so that the sensorimotor experiences are of a high quality, so that when movements are repeated the optimal neuronal pathways are reinforced.

Position

Various commercially produced positioning aids are available, but these are not essential as rolled towels, sheets and blankets can be used. In Figure 37.4 some commercially made supports are shown. Several different companies make such supports, but the ones illustrated are made by Children's Medical Ventures. The best position for a preterm baby is one that as far as possible replicates the position in utero, i.e. with a flexed trunk and limbs, as well as fulfilling the criteria mentioned above. The baby should have firm, deep boundaries to give physical containment and resistance to straightening the limbs. These boundaries can be created by using a commercially made nest and other positioning aids or by rolled towels and blankets. It is important that the nest is deep enough to give good containment of the limbs (Fig. 37.5) and provide a firm surface for the baby to push against as in utero (Fig. 37.6). Because of the interaction between the different systems, as explained in dynamic systems theory, this physical containment appears to 'contain' (Bion 1962) or settle the baby emotionally.

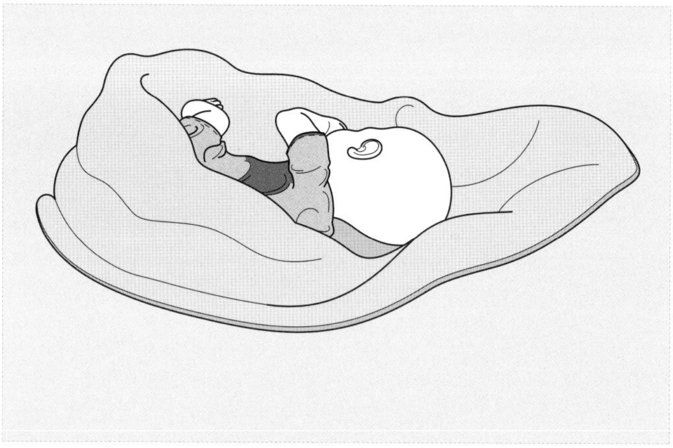

Fig. 37.5 • A deep nest to provide complete containment.

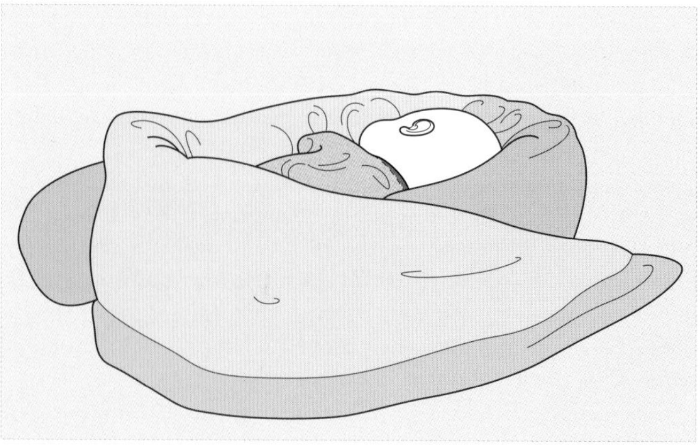

Fig. 37.6 • A firm boundary.

As well as containment, attention should also be paid to the alignment of each part of the body. In the supine position, the toes and knees should point upwards so that the legs are not too outwardly rotated. The head should be supported in midline, and an extended posture of the head and neck should be avoided. This alignment of the limbs and head also applies in side lying, and again, in this position the toes should point in the same direction as the eyes and the head should be well aligned on the trunk and not extended.

The position should ideally provide the baby with the possibility of seeing his or her own body and enable the baby to self-comfort, for example get the hand to face or mouth. Preterm infants often have relatively low muscle tone, and so their limbs take up the posture of the supporting surface. Therefore, as mentioned above, if placed in a supine position without supports to bring the shoulder girdle forwards, it is hard for the infant to bring the hands forwards into the line of vision or to the mouth for self-comfort. Visual and oral experience is helpful for motor development. The position should not expose the baby to stressful stimuli, for example bright lights.

In the prone position there is always some asymmetry, as the head is necessarily turned to one side. Ideally, the side to which the head is turned should be alternated. However, the limbs can still be well aligned, avoiding excess outward rotation of the arms and legs and encouraging protraction of the shoulder girdle. This can be achieved by using a blanket folded lengthways to a width slightly less than the width of the baby's body and placing this underneath the baby from above the head and down as far as the umbilicus (Fig. 37.7). This allows for some protraction of the shoulders and flexion or adduction of the arms. The legs should be flexed at the hips and knees and excess outward rotation prevented by using positioning aids or blankets under the sheet. A firm boundary also needs to be provided, for example by using the bendy bumper (Fig. 37.8).

If it is essential to keep a peripheral intravenous line in view, the baby can be nested as above, but the limb with the intravenous line can be lifted out of the nest (Fig. 37.9). After further boundaries are added, this limb can then be supported to prevent it flailing around by using a strap from the nest or a thick strip of bandage (Fig. 37.10).

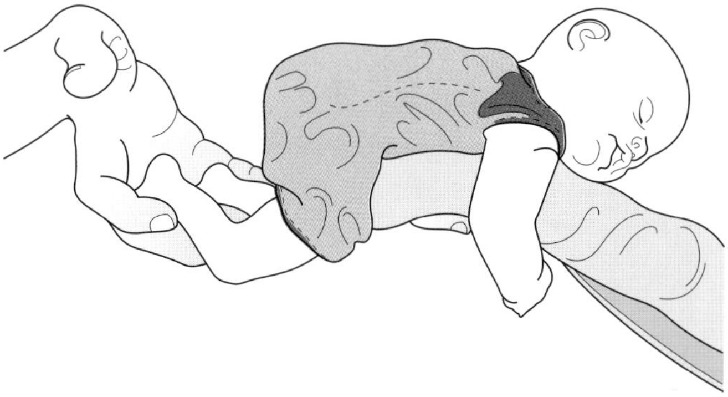

Fig. 37.7 • Prone position: the position of a folded blanket under the baby.

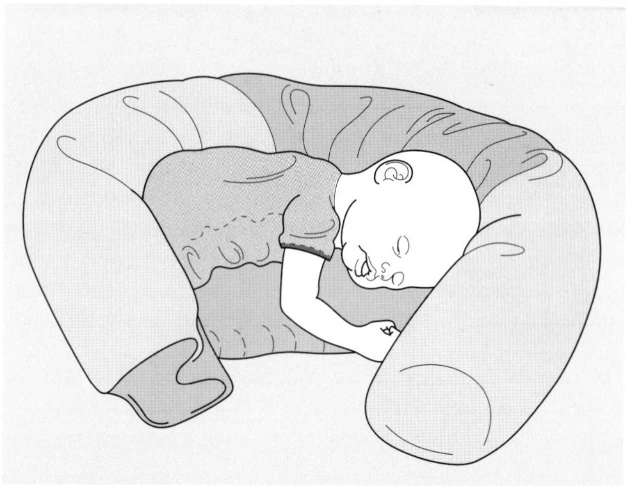

Fig. 37.8 • Prone position: a firm boundary is provided.

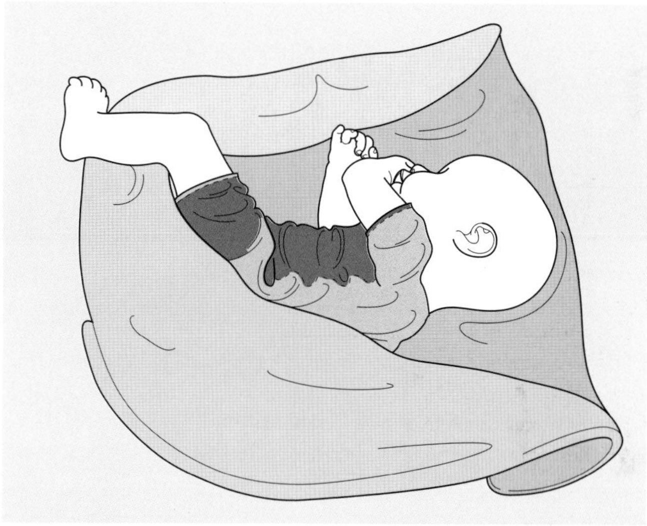

Fig. 37.9 • Leg out to view the intravenous line.

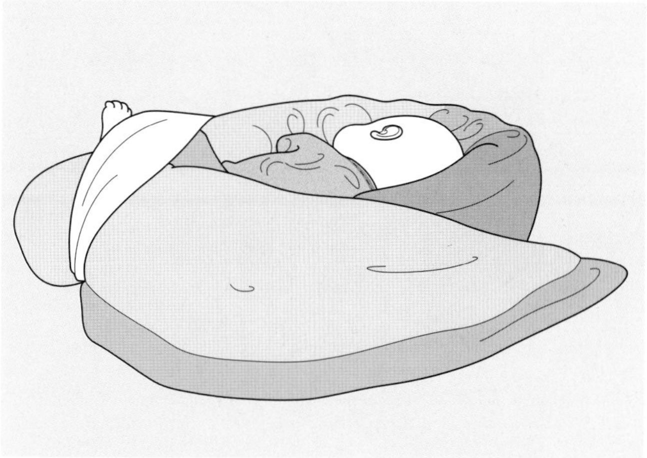

Fig. 37.10 • A strap supporting a limb outside the nest.

It is sometimes necessary to nurse preterm babies in a supine position, for example if they have just had abdominal surgery. Again, the baby should be placed well down into the nest, ensuring that the legs are well aligned (i.e. not in an outwardly rotated position) and that the knees and hips are flexed. Figure 37.11 shows the supine position using a gel cushion under the head and shoulders and a Freddie the frog to keep the shoulders slightly protracted, so that the baby can move his or her hands forwards to touch the face. A bendy bumper or towels under the sheet will then keep these supports in place and provide good containment and boundaries to push against (Fig. 37.12).

When preterm babies are extremely ill it is still helpful to provide support and containment, as when they are more comfortable their vital signs are likely to be better. Also, if the time of critical illness is extended, contractures of soft tissue can occur. Sometimes the supports may need to be modified to allow observation of lines and tubes, for example chest drains. In Figure 37.13 two Freddie Frogs and a gel cushion have been used to provide support but also allow full visual inspection of wound sites and lines.

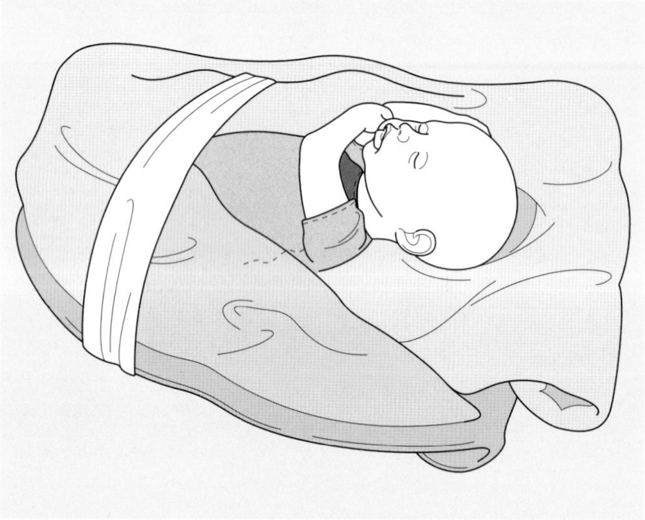

Fig. 37.11 • Supine position: shoulder protraction.

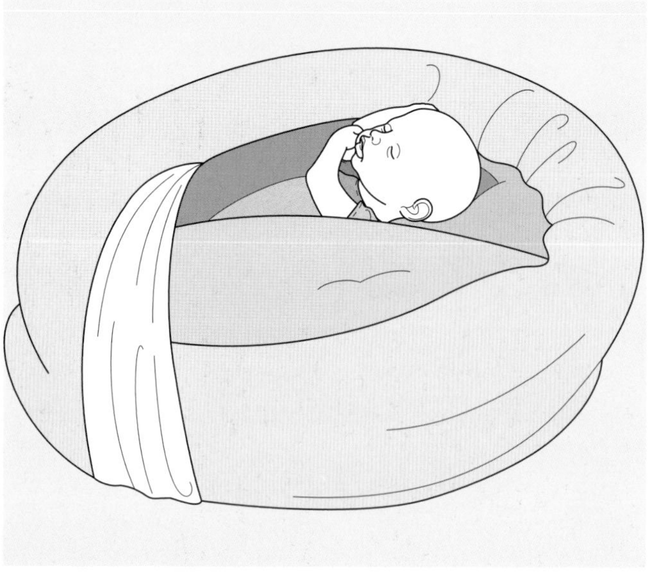

Fig. 37.12 • Supine position: firm boundaries.

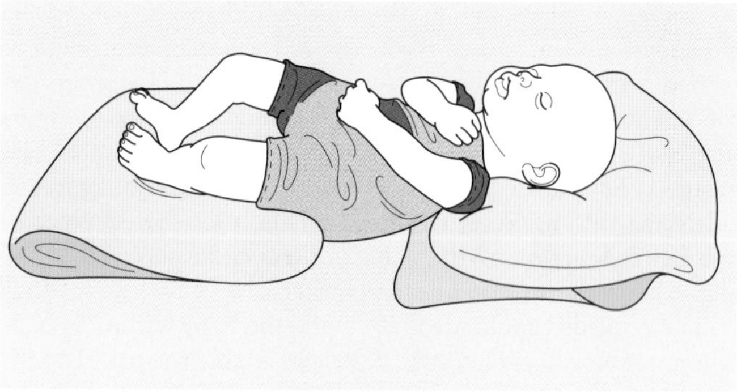

Fig. 37.13 • Support that allows visibility.

Sick babies in the NICU who are not preterm may also be happier when nested, as it seems to provide a feeling of security and it will also prevent contractures developing. Once the baby is at home, it is important for parents to follow the advice given to prevent cot death, i.e. by positioning in the supine position when asleep and allowing adequate air circulation around the baby's head to avoid overheating.

During uncomfortable or frightening interventions

These are best performed with the baby in side lying when possible. A containment hold may be provided by the nurse's hands enclosing the baby gently in a flexed position so that he or she does not startle and extend when the intervention (e.g. suction) is carried out (Fig. 37.14). When no other person is available and the procedure uses both the nurse's hands for some of the time,

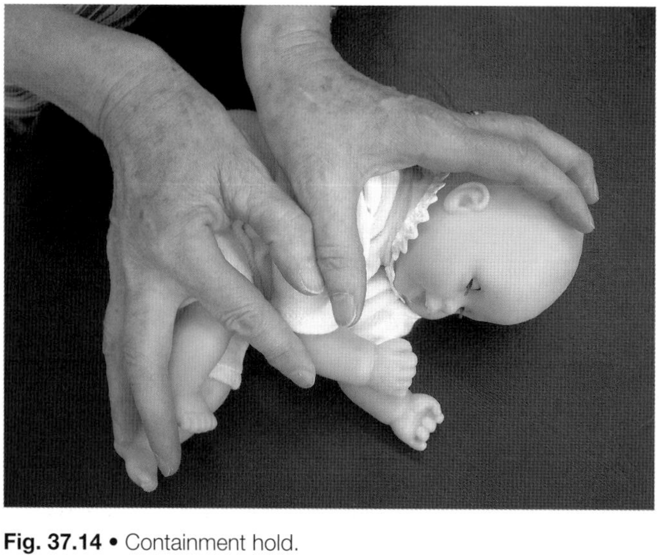

Fig. 37.14 • Containment hold.

the infant may be swaddled in a blanket, which has a similar effect. Alternatively, this may be a good opportunity to involve parents with their baby's care and to show them how to do the containment hold while the nurse carries out the intervention.

Other strategies during uncomfortable or potentially stressful procedures are for the baby to be offered a finger to grasp. Having something to grasp or brace against often settles an anxious baby. Non-nutritive sucking is another good way of calming a baby and preventing extension patterns of movement that occur during distress. Some NICUs use sucrose on the dummy during painful interventions such as heel pricks. Interventions should be paced to the baby's cues.

Moving the baby

Although babies obviously do not understand speech, Norman (2001) describes infants' understanding of the emotions expressed in the non-lexical aspect of language. Therefore, as when approaching any patient you are going to move, it is helpful to speak softly (so that the baby knows you are there) and then place your hands on the baby for a few seconds explaining that you are going to turn him or her. The baby will then get used to this routine and be prepared for the move and so start to gain some control over his or her body during the movement. Observe the baby closely during the move and pause as necessary. The speed of movement should be slow, and limbs should be contained by tucking them in or swaddling. If the baby is being taken out of the incubator, the nest can be used to contain the limbs.

Criteria for selecting the position

Criteria for selecting the position are:

- age-appropriate (e.g. well flexed with boundaries to push against at preterm age)
- ability to see own body
- mechanical implications of the position (limb position and ability to move)
- medical considerations (e.g. abdominal operation)
- physiological stability
- life support equipment, intravenous lines, drains, etc.
- need to facilitate efficient respiration and improve oxygen saturations
- reflux (research shows that elevated prone is the best position for nursing babies with gastro-oesophageal reflux and the second best position is elevated left side lying [Ewer et al 1999]; in practice these two positions are often alternated depending on what works best for the individual baby)
- the infant's tolerance of the position and ability to self-quiet and control states.

Advantages and disadvantages of the various positions

Side lying

Side lying (Fig. 37.15) is the position of choice, as it is easier to obtain a flexed, tucked posture and to promote symmetry. It discourages abduction deformities of limbs and scapula retraction, and also assists the infant's self-calming strategies. The baby can more easily have contact with his or her own body, such as hand to hand, foot to foot and hand to mouth. The infant also has a better possibility of seeing his or her own body. It is easier to avoid disturbance by bright lights than in the supine position. Some NICUs implementing developmental care are recommending that washing and cares are done in a side-lying position when possible, as the infant is usually calmer in this position.

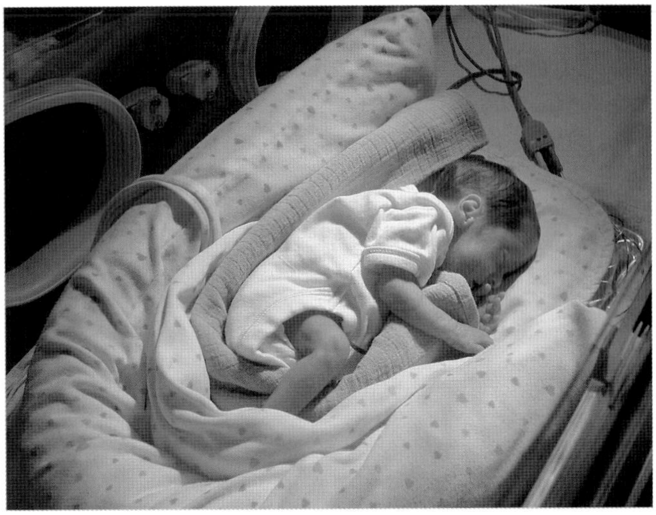

Fig. 37.15 • Side-lying position. (Courtesy of Katy Thompson.)

Prone

The prone position (Fig. 37.16) improves ventilation by improving the stability of the chest wall. This decreases the work of breathing and may conserve energy and result in lower oxygen consumption and so a decreased respiration rate. There is some evidence that the prone position also promotes sounder sleep (Bhat et al 2003, Sahni et al 2005). However, the prone position encourages asymmetry, as the head is turned to one side,

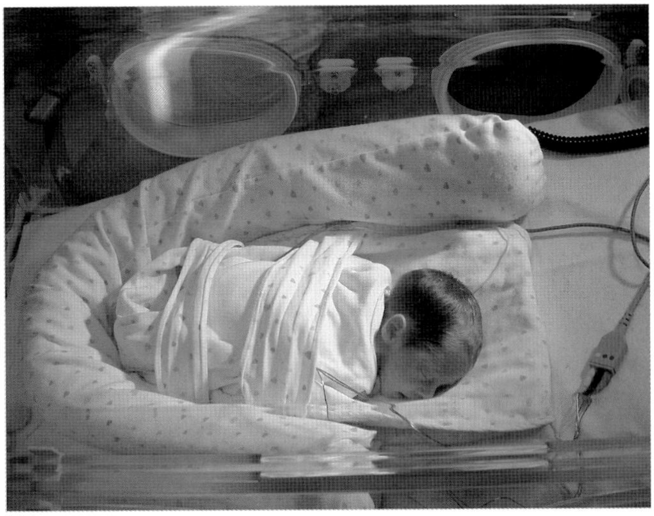

Fig. 37.16 • Prone position. (Courtesy of Katy Thompson.)

and it also encourages an abducted and retracted 'frog' posture unless the baby is very well positioned. There is less possibility for the baby to visually explore his or her body, and less possibility for self-regulation, although hand to face may be possible. Although less effective at preventing reflux (Ewer et al 1999), the prone position is sometimes used as an alternative to side lying when a baby with reflux needs for some reason to have an alternative to left side lying.

Supine

The supine position (Figs 37.17 and 37.18) may be necessary for medical reasons, for example after abdominal surgery, but if left unsupported the baby will adopt an extended position with abduction and outward rotation of the limbs. In an unsupported supine position it is harder for the baby to initiate and control movements due to the effect of gravity, and therefore it is more difficult for the infant to make eye contact with the rest of the body, to touch the body (e.g. hand to hand) and to self-comfort (e.g. by bringing the hand to the mouth). It is difficult for the baby to avoid bright lights. The work of breathing is increased and reflux is more likely.

If the infant has to be in a supine position it is important to create a flexed, tucked posture to replicate the in utero position and also create the possibility of the infant seeing the rest of his or her body. Ensure that the shoulder girdle and arms are brought forwards to prevent retraction of the scapulae. This makes it easier for the baby to move the arms forwards and to bring the hands towards the face and mouth. The legs can be flexed by a roll under the knees, and rolled towels or other supports such as wedges may be used to prevent excessive outward rotation of the legs. Ensure that the baby is in a deep nest so that there is a firm boundary to push against, and position the infant so that the feet do not hang over the edge of the nest.

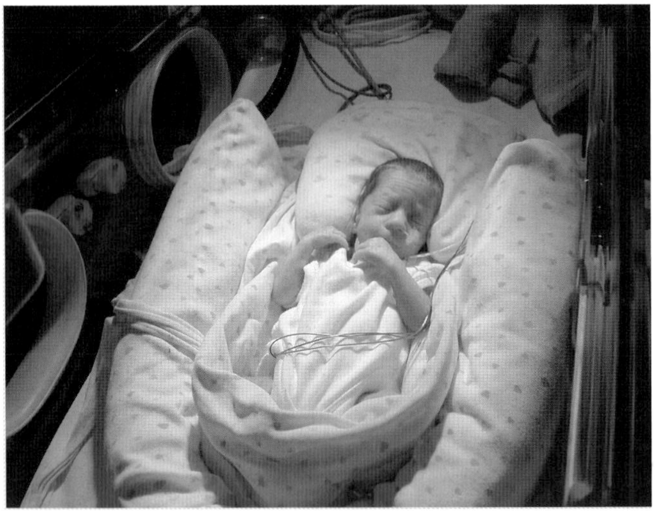

Fig. 37.17 • Supine position. (Courtesy of Katy Thompson.)

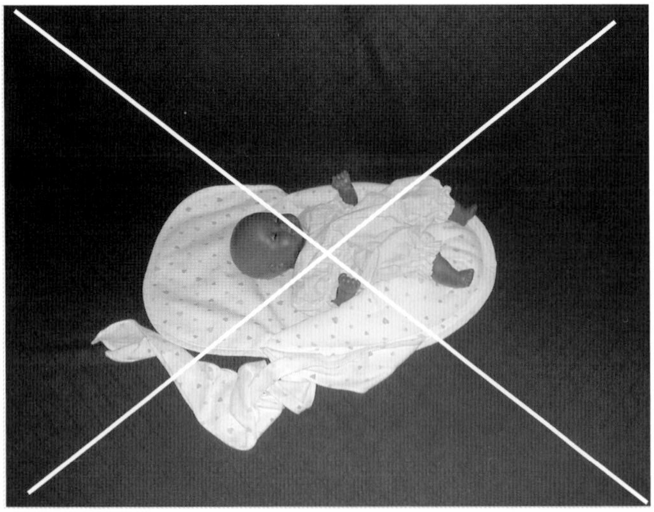

Fig. 37.18 • Incorrect supine position.

Position for feeding

Thoughtful handling of the baby should continue when oral feeding commences, often at around 33 or 34 weeks' gestation in the healthy preterm infant. Advice for breastfeeding is now more readily available, but there is generally less understanding of the importance of establishing good positions for bottle feeding. For those babies who are developing neurological problems, learning a safe position for feeding is crucial. Once a baby and mother have established the habit of a poor position it is hard to change. Sometimes the baby also tends to start feeding with the head slightly extended, and this then becomes the habitual preferred position, although it carries the danger of aspiration of feeds. Nurses anxious about the baby aspirating often feed the baby with the infant facing them at the end of their lap with one hand behind the baby's head. This does not give good support to enable efficient sucking and swallowing and it should not be used. If the baby needs to be held upright and facing the carer, give good support to the head and trunk by using a Vcushion or pillows on the nurse's lap. If the chair is high it may be helpful for the nurse to put his or her feet on a low stool so that his or her lap is not sloping down. If the nurse is comfortable, the baby will be more settled. Swaddling may also be used as a way of providing support to the head and trunk during feeding.

As preterm babies often have low muscle tone, the best position for feeding is one that gives good support to the trunk and head, with the baby's shoulder girdle also well supported in a slightly protracted position. This gives a firm base of support from which the action of sucking and swallowing can take place. In general, the natural position to provide this support is against the carer's body (Fig. 37.19). Elevated side lying on the carer's lap may sometimes be useful when introducing oral feeding (Fig. 37.20). The advantage of this position is that it is possible to give good support in a symmetrical posture with the arms forwards. Then the baby may be able to control the milk in the mouth more easily and develop a more active swallow, as the milk does not fall straight back into the throat.

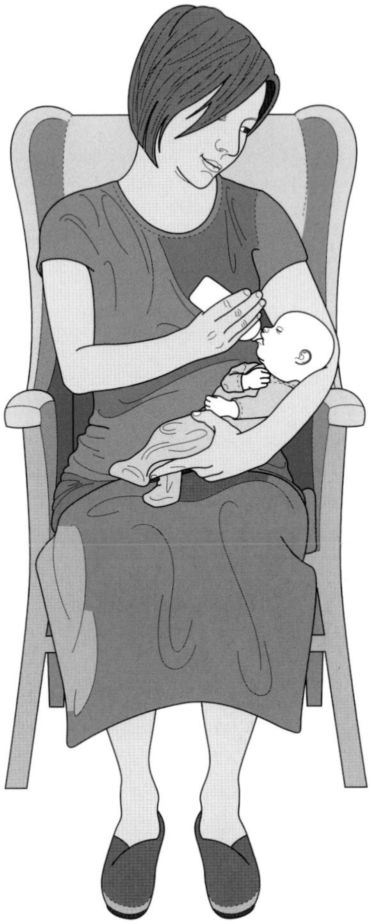

Fig. 37.19 • Bottle feeding: support the body and head and encourage arms forward.

Common difficulties

Babies who have needed a longer period of ventilation, continuous positive airway pressure or longer term oxygen sometimes develop the habit of having a slightly extended neck, as this helps them to breathe. However, learning to tuck in the chin and lengthen the back of the neck is something that babies usually learn by the age of 3 months (corrected age). When handling preterm babies it is important to minimise neck extension and prevent a habit pattern of extension developing. This can be dangerous later when oral feeding starts, particularly with babies who do have neurological problems, as a slightly extended neck opens the airway and aspiration can occur, as mentioned above (Fig. 37.21).

Summary

The most important thing during handling and positioning is to hold in mind the experience of the baby, given each baby's particular history, and to respond to the baby's cues. There may be certain medical constraints on the choice of

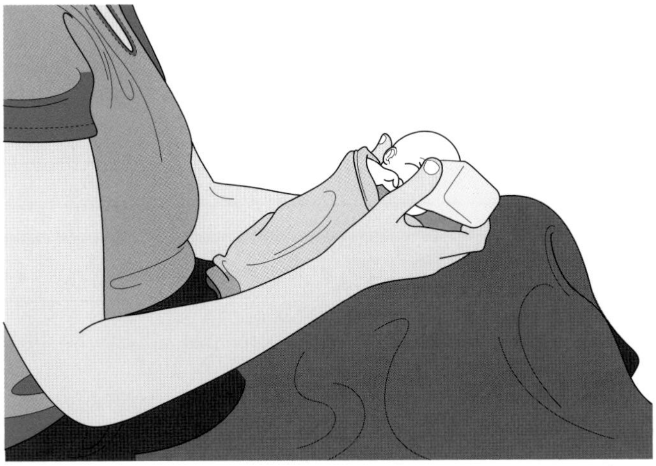

Fig. 37.20 • Feeding in elevated side lying. (Courtesy of Katy Thompson.) Note: ensure the head is well supported

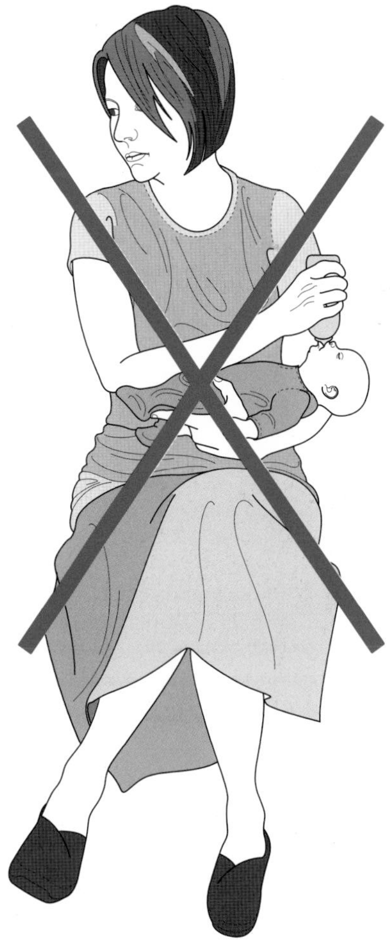

Fig. 37.21 • Incorrect position for bottle feeding.

Procedures Box 37.1 Developmentally supportive positioning and handling of neonates

1

Throughout all procedures

Actions
Keep in mind how the procedure might feel to the baby and how it may affect the various systems (autonomic, nervous, motor, sleep, interaction).

Respond empathically to baby's cues.

Reason *This is crucial to the stability of the baby (blood pressure, respiration, etc.) and also to optimal brain development!*

2

Moving the baby

Action
Prepare the baby by gently but firmly placing your hands on the baby and telling the baby what you are about to do.

Reasons *Prepares the baby and eliminates the surprise element (which can cause sudden extension movement patterns). Starts to promote a trusting relationship.*

Action
Move the baby slowly.

Reason *The baby has an immature vestibular system, so fast movement will create disorientation and increase cortisol levels.*

Action
Tuck in the limbs when lifting the baby.

Reason *Maintains physical containment, prevents flailing limbs and keeps the baby more settled.*

3

General positioning

Action
Position preterm babies in a flexed position.

Reasons *Replicates the intrauterine environment and discourages the habit pattern of arching back. Self-comfort is facilitated.*

Action
Position the limbs to avoid excessive abduction and external rotation and to keep good alignment of the limbs and head on the body.

Reason *Prevents the abnormal postural habits and shortening of soft tissues that could contribute to motor delay.*

Action
Position so that the baby can see and touch her or his own body.

Reason *Facilitates self-comfort and contributes to learning of motor skills.*

Action
Provide firm boundaries to push against.

Reason *Allows exercise of muscles as in utero and contributes to a feeling of security.*

4

Specific positions

Side lying is the position of choice but the baby's condition may sometimes require a different position.

Action
Side lying.

Reason *Facilitates motor development because:*
- *it allows hand-to-hand and foot-to-foot contact*
- *it encourages hand to mouth*
- *the baby has the best chance of seeing the rest of the body.*

Action
Left side lying.

Reason *Discourages reflux.*

Action
Prone lying.

Reason *Enables better oxygenation but more asymmetry of the body; it is also harder to nest well.*

Action
Supine lying.

Reason *May be necessary after abdominal surgery but:*
- *it encourages abduction and extension*
- *it is hard to see the rest of the body*
- *it is more difficult to self-comfort.*

5

During uncomfortable or frightening procedures

Action
Pace the intervention to the baby's cues as much as possible.

Reason *Minimises adverse affects on the baby's autonomic and neurological systems.*

Action
Prior to starting the procedure and during the procedure, talk to the baby and comfort as necessary.

Reasons *Prepares the baby and eliminates the surprise element. Starts to promote a trusting relationship.*

Action
Have the baby in side-lying position when possible.

Reason *It is easier to 'contain' the baby with the hands and prevent uncontrolled extension of the limbs.*

Action
Enlist the help of parents if appropriate.

Reason *Facilitates parents' positive relationship with the baby.*

Action
Consider the use of non-nutritive sucking.

Reason *Limits distress.*

Action
Use containment hold or swaddling, or offer a finger for the baby to grasp, whichever is most appropriate and effective in preventing adverse reaction during this procedure.

Reason *Limits distress and prevents the baby arching his or her back.*

position, but apart from this, side lying is the position of choice. Although commercially made positioning equipment is very useful, it is not absolutely essential. The baby can be positioned well using rolled towels, sheets and nappies. Whatever equipment is used for nesting, the baby should be well flexed with the limbs and body well aligned. Firm boundaries should be provided so that the baby has a feeling of secure containment and a surface to push against similar to the uterine walls.

References

Als H, Duffy F, McAnulty G et al (2004) Early experience alters brain function and structure. Pediatrics 113:846–857

Bhat R, Leipala J, Singh N et al (2003) Effect of posture on oxygenation, lung volume, and respiratory mechanics in premature infants studied before discharge. Pediatrics 112(1):29–32

Bion W (1962) Learning from experience. Heinemann, London

Bower E, McLellan D, Arney J et al (1996) A randomised controlled trial of different intensities of physiotherapy and different goal setting procedures in 44 children with cerebral palsy. Developmental Medicine and Child Neurology 38:226–237

Cicchetti D, Tucker D (1994) Development and self-regulatory structures of the mind. Development and Psychopathology 6:533–549, cited in Schore 2003a, op. cit.

Dobbing J, Sands J (1973) Quantitative growth and development of human brain. Archives of Diseases in Childhood 48:757–767, cited in Schore 2003a, op. cit.

Ehrsson H, Fagergren A, Jonsson T et al (2000) Cortical activity in precision versus power grip tasks: MRI study. Journal of Neurophysiology 83:528–536

Ewer A, James M, Tobin J (1999) Prone and left side lying position reduce gastro-oesophageal reflux in preterm infants. Archives of Diseases in Childhood: Fetal and Neonatal Edition 81:201–205

Lewis D, Douglas L (1998) Dynamic systems approach. In Mascolo M, Griffiths S (eds) What develops in emotional development? Plenum Press, New York

NIDCAP Federation International (2007) Online. Available:http://www.NIDCAP.org

Norman J (2001) The psychoanalyst and the baby: a new look at work with infants. International Journal of Psychoanalysis 82:83–100

Perry B, Pollard R, Blakely T et al (1995) Childhood trauma, the neurobiology of adaptation, and 'use dependent' development of the brain: how 'states' become 'traits'. Infant Mental Health Journal 16:4

Peters K (1998) Neonatal stress reactivity and cortisol. Journal of Perinatal and Neonatal Nursing 11(4):45–60

Prechtl H, Einspieler C, Cioni G et al (1997) An early marker for neurological deficits after perinatal brain lesions. Lancet 349:1361–1363

Robertson J (2005) A psychoanalytic perspective on the work of a physiotherapist with infants at risk of neurological problems: comparing the theoretical background of physiotherapy and psychoanalysis. Infant Observation 8(3):259–278

Sahni R, Schulze K, Kashyap S (2005) Sleeping position and electrocortical activity in low birthweight infants. Archives of Diseases in Childhood: Fetal and Neonatal Edition 90(4):311–315

Schore A (2003a) Affect dysregulation and disorders of the self. WW Norton, New York

Schore A (2003b) The human unconscious: the development of the right brain and its role in early emotional life. In Green V (ed) Emotional development in psychoanalysis, attachment theory and neuroscience. Brunner-Routledge, London

Symington A, Pinelli J (2003) Developmental care for promoting development and preventing morbidity in preterm infants. Cochrane Database of Systematic Reviews 4, CD001814

Warren I (2000) (ed.) Guidelines for infant development in the neonatal nursery. St Mary's Hospital, London

Winnicott D (1960) The theory of the parent–infant relationship. In Winnicott D 1990 The maturational process and the facilitating environment. Karnac, London

38 Caring for the child requiring lumbar puncture

Alison Hough • Jackie Gekas

The term *lumbar puncture* refers to a procedure whereby a specially designed needle is inserted into the lower back between the spinal processes, usually between L5–4, L4–3 or L3–2, in order to access the cerebral spinal space and the fluid that is contained there (Figs 38.1 and 38.2).

In children and babies this procedure is most commonly performed for diagnostic purposes, usually when there is a suspicion of meningitis (Holdgate & Cuthbert 2001). If the infant or child is acutely unwell the lumbar puncture may be postponed until his or her general condition has improved, as there is some evidence to suggest that lumbar puncture may be associated with brain herniation (Grande 2005; see *Complications and Side Effects of Lumbar Puncture*, below). With the emergence of the polymerase chain reaction (PCR) test, which examines a blood specimen for DNA evidence of pathogens, it could be argued that it is no longer necessary to perform lumbar punctures in order to identify the causative organism. The PCR test has the advantage over blood culture of being able to detect traces of pathogens such as *Neisseria meningitidis* even if antibiotics have already been given (Carrol et al 2000). However, PCR testing is not routinely available at many hospital laboratories, and there is a delay involved in obtaining the results of this investigation. The laboratory services of most hospitals can identify pathogens in cerebrospinal fluid (CSF) by microscopy in a very short time, thereby providing a rapid diagnosis.

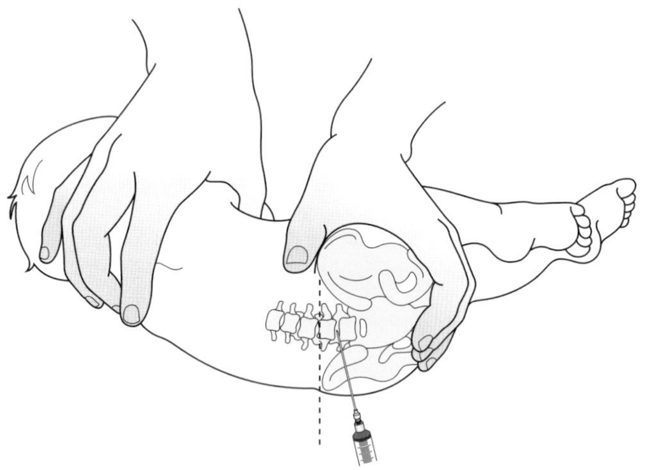

Fig. 38.1 • Area of spine where cerebral spinal space and CSF might be accessed. (Reproduced by kind permission of the Children's Hospital at Westmead © New South Wales Health Department 2007)

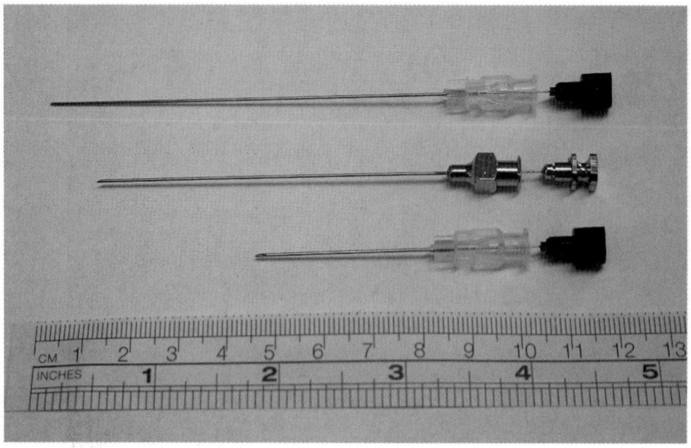

Fig. 38.2 • Commonly used sizes of spinal needle for lumbar puncture.

Another reason for performing lumbar puncture is to measure the pressure of the CSF by attaching a manometer to the spinal needle. This may be done for children who have conditions that cause an over-production of CSF or blockage of its normal drainage pathways, such as may occur in the presence of some types of brain tumours, or who have low CSF pressure caused by conditions such as chronic occult leakage of CSF (Lindsay & Bone 2004).

Lumbar puncture is commonly performed as part of an infection screen in sick neonates, although it has been questioned whether this practice is routinely necessary (Joshi & Barr 1998). Although subarachnoid haemorrhage is rare in children a lumbar puncture may be performed as part of the diagnostic process for this condition. Lumbar puncture is also sometimes used to establish disease stage in retinoblastoma (Azar et al 2003).

A further indication for lumbar puncture is for giving intrathecal chemotherapy, which forms part of the treatment protocols for conditions such as childhood leukaemia. During the procedure CSF is withdrawn prior to giving treatment so that can be examined for the presence of malignant cells. Although the procerdure is carried out in exactly the same way, most centres anaesthetise children who will require multiple lumbar punctures as part of their treatment and so preparation will be different.

Special note

Because of the occurrence of several fatal accidents when patients have mistakenly been given neurotoxic vinca alkaloids via the intrathecal route, there are very strict national protocols that must be followed regarding the storage, prescribing, checking and administration of intrathecal drugs (Department of Health 2003).

Complications and side effects of lumbar puncture

Herniation of the brainstem

When there is acutely raised intracranial pressure, such as is caused by infection of the meninges, the pressure release created by lumbar puncture and loss of CSF may cause the brain to herniate through the foramen magnum at the base of the skull, causing catastrophic and invariably fatal damage (Grande 2005). However, it has been suggested that the cerebral oedema resulting from meningitis causes brainstem compression and that in some cases herniation would occur even if lumbar puncture was avoided (Holdgate & Cuthbert 2001).

Headache and backache

Less serious but much more common side effects of lumbar puncture are headache and backache, long thought to be caused by pressure changes but the exact mechanism is not well understood. It is an interesting observation that children appear to be less troubled by post-lumbar puncture headache and backache than are adults, but this may reflect the paucity of research in this area (Ebinger et al 2004). It remains common practice to recommend that patients remain in bed following the procedure despite some evidence to suggest that bed rest following lumbar puncture does not prevent or alleviate headache (Thornberry & Thomas 1988, Vilming et al 1988).

Leakage of CSF from puncture site

Recovery from lumbar puncture may be hindered by persistent leakage of CSF from the puncture site, and there is evidence to support this as a cause of unresolving postprocedure headache. (Grande 2005).

Pain and discomfort during the procedure

Pain and discomfort during the procedure performed when the child is awake will be minimised with adequate preparation and explanation (see Ch. 2). Local anaesthesia to the puncture site may be injected to numb the area, and for a planned procedure a local anaesthetic preparation such as Ametop™ may be used.

Infection

An entirely avoidable consequence of lumbar puncture is the introduction of infection, and this should not occur if the procedure is carried out using an aseptic technique.

Currently, lumbar puncture is one of the most common invasive diagnostic procedures carried out on children and adolescents (Ebinger at al 2004). Essentially this is a procedure that is carried out safely in the majority of children (Cunningham et al 2003). As an invasive procedure a lumbar puncture must be performed aseptically (Gough 2006). Broadly, the key components to a successful lumbar puncture procedure are preparation, positioning, technique, and procedural and post procedural care.

Preparation

Kneen et al (2002) advise that a lumbar puncture is not undertaken if one of the following is present:

- Indicators of raised intracranial pressure, such as papilloedema, altered pupillary responses, absent doll's eye reflex, decerebrate or decorticate posturing, abnormal respiratory pattern, hypertension and bradycardia
- A recent or prolonged fit
- A focal or tonic fit
- Other focal neurological signs, such as a paralysis affecting one side of the body, paralysis affecting a single part of the body, extensor plantar responses and eye palsies
- Altered neurological status
- Evidence of meningococcal infection
- Shock
- Topical infection at the lumbar puncture area
- Clotting disorder.

Informed consent must be obtained by the person carrying out the procedure prior to commencement of this invasive procedure (Department of Health 2001). A written information sheet can support the full verbal explanation (Great Ormond Street Hospital for Children NHS Trust Patient Information Group 2002).

If this is a planned procedure, i.e. general anaesthetic for intrathecal chemotherapy, then ongoing therapeutic play combined with the use of a general anaesthetic plays a fundamental role in minimising distress and anxiety to the child and family (Crock et al 2003, Moules & Ramsay 1998). Children having multiple lumbar punctures for intrathecal chemotherapy, who have a general anaesthetic administered via a face mask, demonstrate lower levels of pain, distress and the need for restraint in order to accomplish the procedure when contrasted with sedation (Crock et al 2003). Equally, healthcare professionals need to be aware that the child in this situation may prefer not to have a general anaesthetic but a combination of all or any of the following: sedation, topical and local anaesthesia, and non-pharmacological therapies such as play (Crock et al 2003, Harvey & Morton 2007).

Children should not be subjected to avoidable distress during a procedure, not only because of long-term effects but because the procedure may be difficult or unsafe in an uncooperative child (Krauss & Green 2006, Murphy 1997). Effective preparation enables the procedure to be carried out safely within a minimum time frame and empowers the child and family to play a meaningful role.

In the acute situation it may not be appropriate to administer sedation or have sufficient time to apply topical anaesthetic, but that does not preclude their use being considered and the parents or primary caregivers being given the option of staying with their child and being supported through the procedure. Often, lumbar punctures are performed once the acute phase has stabilised and therefore this can then become in essence a planned procedure (Advanced Life Support Group 2005). In short, there is no 'one size fits all' way of preparing the child and family for this procedure.

Krauss & Green (2006) regard topical anaesthetic agents as an important preference for instrument-related procedures such as a lumbar puncture. The most commonly used topical local anaesthetic agents are Ametop™ gel and EMLA™; EMLA™ is an abbreviation of eutectic mixture of local anaesthetics and is a 1:1 oil-in-water emulsion of low-concentration lidocaine and prilocaine hydrochloride, and Ametop™ contains 4% tetracaine (*British National Formulary for Children* 2006, Harvey & Morton 2007). EMLA™ needs to be applied 60 min prior to the lumbar puncture and after removal from skin remains active for 1–2 h; Ametop™ needs to be applied 45 min prior to the lumbar puncture and after removal from skin remains active for approximately 4–6 h (*British National Formulary for Children* 2006, Harvey & Morton 2007). Nevertheless, topical local anaesthetic agents must be administered as per local protocols. Oral sucrose is a useful adjunct given, as per local guidelines, usually 2 min prior to the procedure and reduces the term or preterm baby's response to pain (Stevens et al 2004). Local anaesthetic agents such as lidocaine need to be given intradermally, which in itself is painful, therefore a topical local anaesthetic will need to be used as well (Harvey & Morton 2007).

To identify the area to place the local anaesthetic gel or cream, draw a pretend line from the top of the posterior iliac crest across the spine to the opposite iliac crest. Then place the local anaesthetic gel or cream over the spine at approximately the midpoint of the pretend line at L4 (Hockenberry et al 2003). Drawing around the area at the time of application will ensure that the area can be identified after the Ametop™ or EMLA™ has been removed.

If sedation is used then a multifaceted process of decision-making must be utilised to identify the type of sedation required to sefely accomplish the procedure. The most commonly used are sedative-hypnotics, for example, midazolam and other drugs in a pharmacological class of their own such as chloral hydrate (Krauss & Green 2006). Two other sedation techniques could include inhalation sedation via the use of nitrous oxide or dissociative sedation such as ketamine (Krauss & Green 2006). Midazolam and ketamine have the advantage of being administered via different routes; however, ketamine can cause hallucinations and nightmares (Harvey & Morton 2007).

Positioning

Correct and supportive positioning is a vital factor to ensure a successful and safe outcome of the procedure (Gough 2006, Hockenberry et al 2003). Prior to supportive holding for this procedure, ensure that all the required equipment is present and that the medical practitioner is ready to proceed.

Haslem (2004) maintains that an acutely unwell neonate can be placed in the upright position because respiratory and circulation anomalies leading to respiratory arrest are more common in the recumbent position. However, Speidel et al (1998) suggest that the neonate is positioned on their side, held at the shoulders and buttocks with their neck straight to prevent airway obstruction and to keep the spine horizontal. Therefore it is important that the neonate is assessed by the medical practitioner prior to the commencement of the procedure to ascertain the safest supportive holding position.

The baby or child needs to be supportively held in the knee-to-chest position with the neck flexed towards the knees either in the side-lying or sitting position to provide maximum separation of the vertebral bodies, thus enabling optimal alignment to complete the procedure safely (Hockenberry et al 2003).

The parent or primary caregivers can supportively hold during a lumbar puncture procedure; the child is held upright against their chest and the child's legs wrapped around the adult with a small pillow placed between the child's abdomen and the adult to arch the child's back (Hockenberry et al 2003). However, this positioning would require the parent or primary caregiver to be standing in order for the medical practitioner to carry out the procedure.

Equally important to supporting the baby or child through this procedure are the healthcare professionals involved. Sales & Utting (2002) maintain that poor posture results when the neutral position of the spine is disrupted and the spine's natural curves are displaced. Therefore the aim of the healthcare professional involved in this procedure is to keep the spine in as neutral a position as possible and to maintain balance with the centre of gravity over the base of support (Sales & Utting 2002).

Technique

An important issue when a lumbar puncture is performed is safe and accurate positioning of the lumbar puncture needle. Similarly, it is fundamental to be aware that the lumbar puncture needle does not enter the spinal cord, because the lumbar puncture is carried out at L3–4 or L4–5 below the level to which the spinal cord extends (Haslam 2004). However, Milner & Hull (1998) suggest that in an infant the spinal cord may continue to the third lumbar spine.

The most commonly used size of lumbar puncture needle is 22 French gauge with a length of 1–1½ inches under 1 year of age; over 1 year, 2½ inches; and over 40 kg in weight, 2½–3 inches (Gough 2006). Liaison with the medical practitioner will determine the size required.

The lumbar puncture needle is inserted into the mid-sagittal plane and directed slightly in the cephalad direction (Haslam 2004). The medical practitioner carrying out the procedure will often feel a characteristic pop as the needle penetrates the dura and enters the subarachnoid space; the lumbar puncture needle stylet is removed and the needle is gently rotated to check the CSF flow (Speidel et al 1998). Once it is established that CSF is present then samples are obtained into the three sample pots; typically 5–10 drops will be required for each labelled sample pot.

The usual colour of CSF is that of water; cloudy CSF results from a raised white or red cell count (Haslam 2004). A cloudy CSF is indicative of infection, and the presence of red blood cells can be indicative of a traumatic tap (which may be visible at removal of the lumbar puncture needle stylet but should subsequently be clear) or a subarachnoid haemorrhage (Rudolf & Levene 1999).

The measuring of CSF pressure is via a manometer. The normal neonatal CSF pressure is in a range of 0–8 cm of H_2O, with a mean of 3 cm of H_2O; in older children the upper limit of CSF pressure is similar to an adult value of 19 cm of H_2O (Milner & Hull 1998).

If the purpose of this procedure is to administer intrathecal cytotoxic medication then it must be administered only by a suitably trained medical practitioner (Department of Health 2003). Equally, intrathecal chemotherapy is administered according to national guidelines on the safe administration of intrathecal chemotherapy (Department of Health 2003).

Historically, lumbar punctures have been carried out by doctors; however, the advent of the advanced neonatal nurse practitioner has changed this perspective. The *Scope of Professional Practice* (UK Central Council for Nursing, Midwifery and Health Visiting 1992) enables a flexible and professionally challenging way to develop practice. The seminal documents *Making a Difference* (Department of Health 1999), *The Report of the Higher Level of Practice Pilot and Project* (UK Central Council for Nursing, Midwifery and Health Visiting 2002), *A Health Service of All Talents* (Department of Health 2000) and the *National Framework for Children* (Department of Health & Department for Education and Skills 2004) have help create a competency-based framework that facilitates procedures such as a lumbar puncture to be carried out by advanced neonatal nurse practitioners.

Procedural care

The procedure must be carried out in a suitably safe environment with appropriate emergency equipment and trained healthcare professionals to carry out resuscitation if required (Advanced Life Support Group 2005).

Baseline vital signs should be measured at the outset, with continuous monitoring and regular recording throughout the procedure (Krauss & Green 2006). Early detection of potential procedural complications, particularly respiratory compromise in babies who desaturate more rapidly, is paramount (advanced life support group 2005).

The use of mechanical monitoring combined with continuous visualisation of the baby or child will identify any procedural complications. If any of the following occur during the procedure then the procedure must be stopped for appropriate intervention to occur (Advanced Life Support Group 2005):

- Abnormal breathing pattern
- Tachycardia
- Bradycardia
- Decreased responsiveness
- Abnormal posture
- Dilated pupils
- Leg pain
- Bruising
- Herniation of the brainstem.

Gough (2006) rightly maintains that this procedure should be carried out with two children's nurses present as well as the medical practitioner. Nurse 1 can assist the medical practitioner and nurse 2 can visually monitor the baby or child throughout the procedure while supportively holding and providing explanations to the parent or primary caregiver (Hazinski 1992). Concomitant to this, nurse 2 can provide an age-appropriate description to the child as to what is happening and how the child can help (Gough 2006).

Post procedural care

Once the procedure is completed monitoring of the baby or child needs to be continued; however, local recommendations may vary, not least if the baby or child has had a general anaesthetic or sedation.

In principle, monitoring should continue until the baby or child is alert and has an age-appropriate level of consciousness, stable vital signs and age-appropriate language and activity (Krauss & Green 2006). The lumbar puncture site needs to be observed during this period for any signs of CSF leakage, haematoma and infection and subsequently to 24 h post procedure when the skin occlusion agent can be removed (Gough 2006).

If the baby or child is experiencing any postprocedure pain then appropriate and adequate analgesia should be given (Harvey & Morton 2007).

The equipment used throughout the procedure must be cleared away according to the hospital disposal of waste policy and hands washed likewise to ensure a safe environment. If the parents or primary caregivers have not been present during the procedure then they should be invited to return and updated as to how the procedure progressed. At this juncture it could be appropriate to continue the use of therapeutic play.

The lumbar puncture procedure must be documented to provide an accurate record of what has occurred (Nursing and Midwifery Council 2005). Also, if intrathecal chemotherapy has been administered then the baby's or child's prescription chart must be completed to ensure that the medication is not administered twice (Nursing and Midwifery Council 2004, 2005).

If the procedure is carried out as a day case then the child will be discharged home according to local policy and with appropriate written advice.

Procedures Box 38.1 Lumbar puncture

Action
Collect the required equipment:

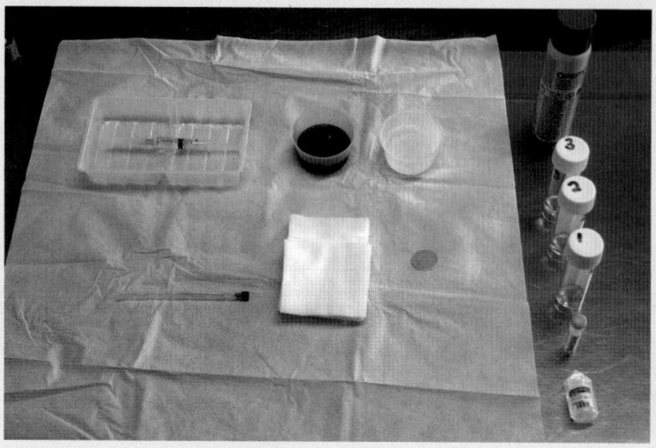

- Lumbar puncture needle
- Three fluid collection pots labelled 1, 2 and 3
- One sample pot for CSF glucose
- One sterile dressing pack
- Sterile gauze squares
- Alcohol-based skin-cleaning fluid
- Waterproof skin occlusion agent
- Sterile towel
- Sterile gloves (size appropriate to the procedure operative)
- Sterile gown
- Two sterile drapes
- Three-way tap, if required
- Spinal fluid pressure manometer, if required
- Therapeutic medication, if required
- Ampoule of 1% lidocaine or equivalent, if required
- 23-French gauge needle
- 25-French gauge needle
- 5-mL syringe
- Two plastic aprons
- Topical local anaesthetic gel or cream
- Oral sucrose, if appropriate
- Sedation, if appropriate.

Action
Explain the procedure to the family and child.
Reason *Promotes psychological support.*

Action
If a general anaesthetic is to be administered then the baby or child must be starved as per hospital policy.
Reason *Maintains the baby's or child's safety and minimises the risk of aspiration of gastric contents (Great Ormond Street Hospital for Children NHS Trust 2004).*

Action
If appropriate, administer oral sucrose as prescribed.
Reason *Reduces the baby's response to pain, maintains comfort and reduces anxiety (Stevens et al 2004).*

Action
If sedation is appropriate give it as prescribed (*British National Formulary for Children* 2006).
Reason *Reduces the child's anxiety.*

Action
Apply topical local anaesthetic to intact skin over the appropriate area.
Reasons *Provides local anaesthetic over the lumbar puncture site. Maintains comfort and reduces anxiety.*

Action
Document the time of application.
Reason *To remove local anaesthetic gel or cream at the appropriate time.*

Action
Mark the area with a marker pen.
Reason *Identifies the area once the local anaesthetic gel or cream has been removed.*

Action
Wash your hands according to hospital policy and put on a plastic apron.
Reason *Prevents cross-infection.*

Action
Clean the trolley with an antiseptic cleaning agent prior to placing equipment on the trolley.
Reason *Lumbar puncture is an aseptic procedure.*

Action
Remove and dispose of the plastic apron.
Reason *Prevents cross-infection.*

Action
Wash your hands according to hospital policy and put on a new plastic apron

Action
The medical practitioner will wash her or his hands and dry them with a sterile towel.
Reason *Lumbar puncture is an aseptic procedure.*

Action
Assist the medical practitioner to gown up and assemble the required equipment.

Action
Remove topical local anaesthetic at the appropriate time.

Procedures Box 38.1 Lumbar puncture—cont'd

Reason *Ensures maximum benefit from topical local anaesthetic.*

Action
Document the time of removal and the state of the skin.

Reason *Ensures no adverse reaction from topical local anaesthetic.*

Action
Change the nappy.

Reason *Prevents cross-infection.*

Action
Invite the child to go to the lavatory.

Reason *Promotes psychological support and prevents cross-infection.*

Action
Parents or primary caregivers should be given the option of staying or not staying with their child during the procedure.

Reason *Promotes psychological support and family-centred care.*

Action
In general, the nurse places and supportively holds the baby or child in the knee-to-chest position, either seated or side lying; the baby's or child's neck needs to be flexed towards the knees.

Reason *Supportive holding prevents sudden movement during the procedure, maximises separation of the vertebral bodies and enables the procedure to be completed as safely as possible.*

Actions
A baby is supportively held in the side-lying position by the nurse, flexing the baby's thighs on the abdomen and then holding the baby's elbows and knees with both hands.

The baby's neck is flexed towards his or her knees.

In a child, the side-lying position requires the nurse to hold the child in a flexed position, enabling access to the spine and preventing sudden movement, which may be harmful to the child.

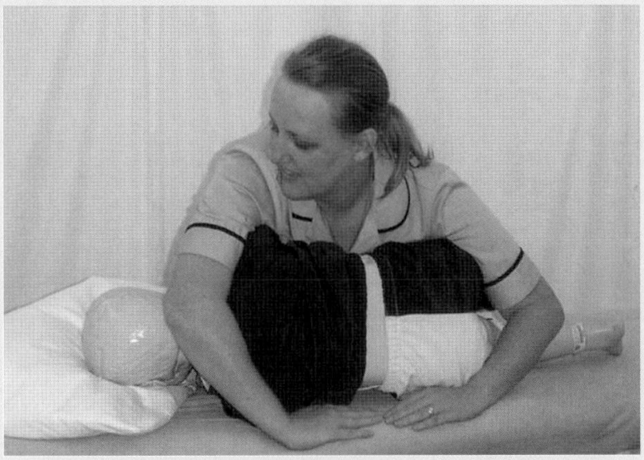

Care should be taken not to lean on the child but to support the flexed position.

Action
The sitting position is an option for the older child, with her or his elbows resting on the knees and the back arched.

Reason *This supportive holding technique gives the older child some choice, input and control to this procedure.*

Action
Hockenberry et al (2003) suggest that a parent or primary caregiver could supportively hold the child up against the standing adult.

Reason *Promotes psychological support and family-centred care.*

Action
The procedure should take place in a setting with appropriate emergency equipment (Advanced Life Support Group 2005, Krauss & Green 2006).

Reason *Ensures the baby's or child's safety.*

Action
Therapeutic play is an appropriate means of supporting the child and family before, during and after the procedure.

Reasons *Enables the child's cooperation with the procedure and empowers the child.*
Minimises the effects of the procedure in both the immediate and long term.

Action
The medical practitioner will identify the lumbar puncture site once the baby or child is positioned.

Reason *Confirms the gap in the vertebral bodies through which the lumbar puncture needle will be advanced.*

Action
The skin is cleaned with an alcohol-based fluid.

Reason *Prevents the baby or child acquiring an infection either at or via the lumbar puncture site.*

Action
Sterile drapes are placed around the identified lumbar area.

Reason *Prevents cross-infection.*

Action
If 1% lidocaine or equivalent is used then the medical practitioner will infiltrate lidocaine or equivalent intradermally around the area to be punctured.

Reasons *Provides subcutaneous local anaesthesia to the site. Promotes minimal discomfort to the child.*

Action
The lumbar puncture needle is inserted into the subarachnoid space by the medical practitioner.

Reason *To access the CSF.*

Action
The lumbar puncture needle stylet is removed by the medical practitioner.

Reason *Enables CSF to free drip externally.*

Action
Samples are collected for laboratory analysis.

Reason *To identify any infection or abnormalities in CSF composition.*

Action
If no CSF freely drips then the spinal needle will require repositioning.

Reason *To locate the subarachnoid space and access the CSF.*

Procedures Box 38.1 Lumbar puncture—cont'd

Action
If repositioning is unsuccessful then the procedure will move to reintroducing the stylet and removal.

Reason *Lessens the discomfort and anxiety of the baby or child and the parent or primary caregiver.*

Action
If measurement of CSF pressure is required the manometer is attached to the needle hub via the three-way tap.

Reason *CSF is allowed to fill the manometer and is measured on a scale and documented.*

Action
Chemotherapy is administered if that is the purpose of the lumbar puncture.

Reason *Chemotherapy is to be administered safely as per national guidelines and current policies (Department of Health 2003, Nursing and Midwifery Council 2004).*

Action
The stylet is reintroduced to the lumbar puncture needle and then removed by the medical practitioner while at the point of removal applying a gauze pad to the exit site.

Reasons *Prevents leakage of CSF.*
Prevents leakage of chemotherapy if that has been administered.

Action
Apply pressure with a gauze pad.

Action
If CSF continues to leak, affix the gauze pad with tape (Great Ormond Street Hospital for Children NHS Trust 2004).

Reason *Prevents leakage of CSF and/or chemotherapy.*

Action
When CSF has stopped leaking dressing can be removed then or within 24 hours post procedure (Great Ormond Street Hospital for Children NHS Trust 2004).

Reason *Prevents baby or child acquiring an infection via the site.*

Action
If waterproof skin occlusion agent is used this too can be removed within 24 hours post procedure (Great Ormond Street Hospital for Children NHS Trust 2004).

Reason *Reduces the risk of infection.*

Action
If the parents or primary caregivers are not present during the procedure then notify them at the earliest opportunity on completion of the procedure.

Reason *Promotes psychological support.*

Action
Throughout the procedure the baby or child must be monitored for any potential complications, such as (Advanced Life Support Group 2005):

- abnormal breathing pattern
- tachycardia or bradycardia
- decreased responsiveness
- abnormal posture
- dilated pupils
- leg pain
- bruising
- herniation of the brainstem.

Reason *Maintains the baby's or child's safety throughout the procedure.*

ALERT
If at any time during the procedure the baby's or child's condition deteriorates then the procedure must be stopped immediately.

Action
If the procedure is carried out under general anaesthetic or sedation, vital signs need to be monitored and recorded until the baby or child is fully awake.

Reason *Ensures the baby's or child's safe recovery.*

Action
After the procedure is completed, remove the equipment and dispose of it as per hospital policy.

Reason *Prevents the spread of infection and needlestick injuries.*

Action
Wash your hands according to hospital policy.

Reason *Minimises the risk of infection.*

Action
After the procedure the baby or child and the lumbar puncture site must be monitored; record and document your observations for any potential problems.

Reason *To observe for signs of potential problems.*

Action
Inform medical staff if any of the following occur:

- Leakage of CSF
- Infection
- Haematoma
- Change in neurological status.

Action
CSF is sent for laboratory analysis.

Action
Notify parents or primary caregivers as soon as any results are available.

Reason *Promotes psychological support and maintains family-centred care.*

Action
Document the procedure.

Reason *To maintain accurate documentation of the events and individual roles during the procedure (Nursing and Midwifery Council 2005).*

Now test your knowledge

- Critically evaluate how you would prepare an 8-year-old for a lumbar puncture. What information would be required for this child's parents or carers to give consent for this procedure? How would you support this child and family before, during and after a planned and non-planned lumbar puncture procedure?
- What factors need to be considered when supportively holding a baby for a lumbar puncture?
- Why would a lumbar puncture be carried out?

References

Advanced Life Support Group (2005) Advanced Paediatric Life Support: the practical approach, 4th edn. BMJ Publishing, London

Azar D, Donaldson C, Dalla-Pozza L (2003) Questioning the need for routine bone marrow aspiration and lumbar puncture in patients with retinoblastoma. Clinical and Experimental Ophthalmology 31:57–60

British National Formulary for Children (2006) British National Formulary for children 2006. BMJ Publishing Group, London

Carrol ED, Thomson APJ, Riordan FAI et al (2000) Increasing microbiological confirmation and changing epidemiology of meningococcal disease on Merseyside, England. Clinical Microbiology and Infection 6(5):259–262

Crock C, Olsson C, Phillips R et al (2003) General anaesthesia or conscious sedation for painful procedures in childhood cancer: the family's perspective. Archives of Diseases in Childhood 88(3):253–257

Cunningham S, Rose M, Laing IA (2003) Understanding and explaining practical procedures and their management. In McIntosh N, Helms P, Smyth R (eds) Forfar and Arneil's textbook of pediatrics, 6th edn. Churchill Livingstone, Edinburgh

Department of Health (1999) Making a difference: strengthening the nursing, midwifery and health visiting contribution to health and healthcare. Department of Health, London

Department of Health (2000) A health service of all the talents: developing the NHS workforce. Consultation document on the review of workforce planning. Department of Health, London

Department of Health (2001) 12 key points on consent: the law in England. Department of Heatlh, London

Department of Health (2003) Updated national guidance on the safe administration of intrathecal chemotherapy. Health Service Circular 2003/010. Department of Health, London

Department of Health, Department for Education and Skills (2004) National Service Framework for Children, Young People and Maternity Services. Department of Health, Department for Education and Skills, London

Ebinger F, Kosel K, Pietz J, Rating D (2004) Headache and backache after lumbar puncture in children and adolescents: a prospective study. Pediatrics 113(6):1588–1592

Gough L (2006) Lumbar puncture. In Trigg E, Mohammed TA (eds) Practices in children's nursing: guidelines for hospital and community, 2nd edn. Churchill Livingstone, Edinburgh

Grande P (2005) Mechanisms behind postspinal headache and brainstem compression following lumbar dural puncture – a physiological approach. Acta Anaesthesiologica Scandinavica 49:619–626

Great Ormond Street Hospital for Children NHS Trust Patient Information Group (2002) Lumbar puncture: information for families. Great Ormond Street Trust Patient Information Group

Great Ormond Street Hospital for Children NHS Trust (2004) Clinical Procedure Guidelines. Intrathecal Cytotoxic Chemotherapy: Administration via a Lumbar Puncture or Ommaya Reservoir, Version 1. London: Great Ormond Street Hospital for Children NHS Trust.

Harvey AJ, Morton NS (2007) Management of procedural pain in children. Archives of Disease in Childhood – Education and Practice 92(1):20–26

Haslam RHA (2004) The nervous system. In Behrman RE, Kliegman RM, Jenson HB (eds) Nelson textbook of pediatrics, 17th edn. Saunders, Philadelphia

Hazinski MF (1992) Nursing care of the critically ill child, 2nd edn. Mosby-Year Book, St Louis

Hockenberry MJ, Wilson D, Winkelstein ML, Kline NE (2003) Wong's nursing care of infants and children, 7th edn. Mosby, Philadelphia

Holdgate A, Cuthbert K (2001) Perils and pitfalls of lumbar puncture in the emergency department. Emergency Medicine 13:351–358

Joshi P, Barr P (1998) The use of lumbar puncture and laboratory tests for sepsis by Australian neonatologists. Journal of Paediatrics and Child Health 34:74–78

Kneen R, Solomon T, Appleton R (2002) The role of lumbar puncture in suspected CNS infection – a disappearing skill? Archives of Disease in Childhood 87(3):181–183

Krauss B, Green SM (2006) Procedural sedation and analgesia in children. Lancet 367(9512):766–780

Lindsay KW, Bone I (2004) Neurology and neurosurgery illustrated, 4th edn. Churchill Livingstone, Edinburgh

Milner AD, Hull D (1998) Hospital paediatrics, 3rd edn. Churchill Livingstone, Edinburgh

Moules T, Ramsay J (1998) The textbook of children's nursing. Stanley Thornes, Cheltenham

Murphy MS (1997) Sedation for invasive procedures. Archives of Disease in Childhood 77(4):281–284

Nursing and Midwifery Council (2004) Guidelines for the administration of medicines. NMC, London

Nursing and Midwifery Council (2005) Guidelines for record and record keeping. NMC, London

Rudolf MCJ, Levene MI (1999) Paediatrics and child health. Blackwell Science, Oxford

Sales R, Utting J (2002) Manual handling and nursing children. Paediatric Nursing 14(2):36–42

Speidel B, Fleming P, Henderson J et al (eds) (1998) A neonatal vade mecum, 3rd edn. Arnold, London

Stevens B, Yamada J, Ohlsson A (2004) Sucrose for analgesia in newborn infants undergoing painful procedures. Cochrane Library, issue 3. John Wiley, Chichester

Thornberry EA, Thomas TA (1988) Posture and post spinal headache. A controlled trial in 80 obstetric patients. British Journal of Anaesthetics 60:195–197

UK Central Council for Nursing, Midwifery and Health Visiting (1992) The scope of professional practice. UKCC, London

UK Central Council for Nursing, Midwifery and Health Visiting (2002) The report of the Higher Level of Practice pilot and project. Online. Available:http://www.nmc-uk.org/aFrameDisplay.aspDocumentID=686 6 May 2007

Vilming ST, Schrader H, Monstad I (1988) Post-lumbar puncture headache: the significance of body posture. A controlled study of 300 patients. Cephalgia 8:75–78

39 Electrocardiography monitoring and interpretation

Marie Elen

The aetiology of cardiorespiratory arrest in children is normally associated with respiratory insufficiency when the heart stops due to ischaemia or hypoxia secondary to another condition (Resuscitation Council UK 2004). Primary cardiac disease in the paediatric population is rare: fewer than 10% of children present in cardiopulmonary arrest (Brennan et al 2003).

The arrest rhythm is usually bradycardia due to severe hypoxia, progressing to asystole if hypoxia is not treated with immediate high-flow oxygen, therefore successful outcome depends on prevention or prompt resuscitation. The airway should be assessed and secured, then the efficacy of breathing must be evaluated and treated, when necessary, before advancing to the assessment and treatment of circulation.

Electrocardiography (ECG) monitoring, along with a basic knowledge and understanding of the principles of ECG recognition, is imperative in advanced life support. This enables a rapid diagnosis of the rhythm, evaluation of cardiac function, implementation of the correct treatment algorithm and finally an evaluation of the response from any intervention (Jevon 2004).

The utmost care must be taken to treat the patient and not the monitor through accurate evaluation of patient status prior to the implementation of treatment (Resuscitation Council UK 2004). However, ECG demonstrates only the movement of the electrical impulse through the heart; it does not indicate the efficacy of myocardial function, the effectiveness of perfusion to the tissues or the general health of the child (Resuscitation Council UK 2004).

The indications for ECG monitoring in children have to be considered, which is a fundamental part of cardiovascular assessment in paediatric emergency management. There are various occasions when a monitor should be attached to a child, which include loss of consciousness, clinical dehydration and electrolyte imbalance, ingestion of toxic substances, major trauma and respiratory distress. This list is by no means exhaustive; however, the optimum standard should be that when a child's condition is causing concern an ECG monitor should be attached immediately.

To interpret normal sinus rhythm on lead II requires correct placement of the electrodes and knowledge of how the ECG machine functions. Lead II measures the voltage between the right shoulder and the left lower chest and consequently produces the configuration that commonly displays the most prominent P wave and QRS amplitude (Fig. 39.1), providing that atrial activity is present (Meek & Morris 2002).

To simplify the application of the electrodes to the chest in cardiac monitoring the ECG cables are usually colour-coded. The red lead is attached to the electrode on the right shoulder (red to right), the yellow lead is attached to the electrode on the left shoulder (lemon to left), and finally the green or ground lead is normally placed on the upper abdominal wall (green to spleen) (Fig. 39.2). To minimise electronic interference the electrodes are best placed situated over bone rather than muscle.

An understanding of the electrical pathway of the heart must be present to allow identification of the waves and what they represent. The term *cardiac cycle* refers to the pumping action of the heart, during which two phases occur: systole when the heart is contracting and diastole when the heart is relaxing and refilling with blood, preparing for the next phase of systole (Fig. 39.3). This contraction and relaxation occurs due to depolarisation and repolarisation of the myocardial cells. These changes within the heart manifest themselves to produce the ECG recording on the monitor via electrodes attached to the chest (Mattson Porth 2002).

Atrial contraction can be referred to as the first stage of the cardiac cycle. It corresponds with the P wave on the ECG recording, which represents atrial depolarisation causing contraction of the muscle in the atria wall. As the atria contract there is an increase in the pressure within the atria, which opens the atrioventricular valves allowing the ventricle to fill with blood (Gracia & Holtz 2003).

The next stage of the cardiac cycle represents ventricular depolarisation; this ventricular depolarisation is reflected in the QRS complex on the ECG recording. The impulse spreads via the atrioventricular node and Purkinje system, causing the ventricles to contract.

The T wave that follows represents ventricular repolarisation, which is the relaxation period prior to the next cardiac cycle commencing (Boudreau Canover 2003).

There are three classes of rhythm disturbances associated with circulatory failure, which are the absent pulses (cardiac arrest rhythms), slow pulses (bradycardias) and fast pulses (tachycardias) (Campbell & Glasper 2001).

An absent pulse is associated with the cardiac arrest rhythms such as asystole, pulseless electrical activity and ventricular fibrillation (VF), which require immediate intervention with advanced life support.

The following structured approach will assist in the analysis of the rhythm strip and determine appropriate management of a child presenting with an arrhythmia (Resuscitation Council

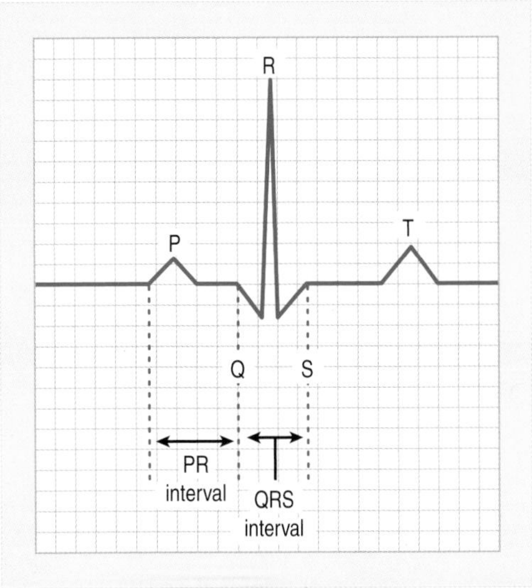

Fig. 39.1 • ECG recording demonstrating electrical activity of the heart.

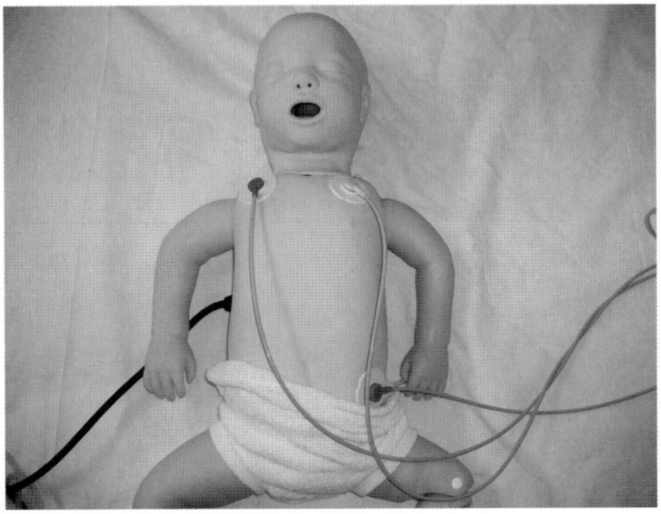

Fig. 39.2 • Application of electrodes.

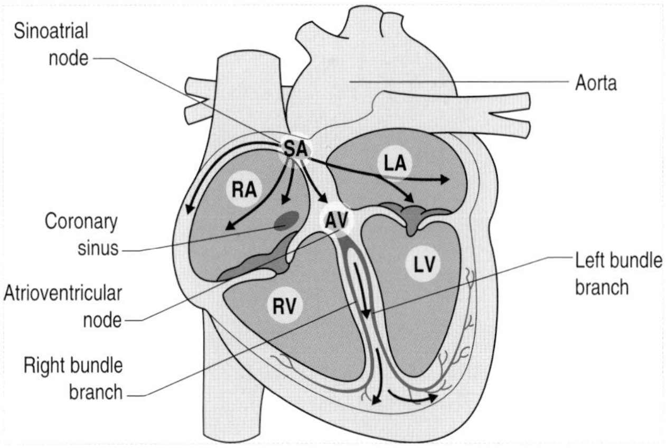

Fig. 39.3 • The conduction system of the heart. LA, left atrium; LV, left ventricle; RA, right atrium; RV, right ventricle.

UK 2004). An *arrhythmia* is a term associated with an irregular rhythm more commonly due to a defect in electrical activity of the heart (Tortora & Derrickson 2006).

1. What is the ventricular rate?

   Is the heart rate fast or slow? The normal range of the heart rate depends on the child's age (Neill & Knowles 2004). An assessment of the adequacy of the circulation and cardiovascular status is imperative. The presence or absence of a pulse will influence the effects of circulatory inadequacy on the other organs.

2. Is the QRS complex regular or irregular?

   This can be established by measuring the distance between two R waves on an ECG rhythm strip. If this distance is equal this represents a regular rhythm, and if the distance is variable it represents an irregular rhythm.

3. Are the P waves visible?

   This will determine whether there is atrial activity when the atria are contracting. If the P waves are upright on lead II they have originated from the sinoatrial node.

4. Is atrial activity related to ventricular activity?

   This will confirm normal cardiac function when contraction and relaxation occur due to depolarisation and repolarisation of the myocardial cells. Normally there will be one P wave per QRS complex; any change in this ratio indicates a blockage in the conduction pathway.

5. Is the QRS complex narrow or broad?

   Arrhythmias may be divided into narrow complexes and broad complexes for the purpose of rapid recognition. Because the ventricles depolarise via the Purkinje system the QRS complexes are of normal width and are termed *narrow complex rhythms*. Arrhythmias arising from the ventricles will be broad complex rhythms.

Atrial and ventricular asystole usually coexist so that the ECG recording is a line with no deflections.

Asystole

In cases of suspected asystole (Fig. 39.4) there are essential checks that should be implemented to confirm asystole prior to commencing treatment. The ECG gain should be increased to maximum, the clinical state of the patient should be assessed and the leads should be checked to ensure optimal contact.

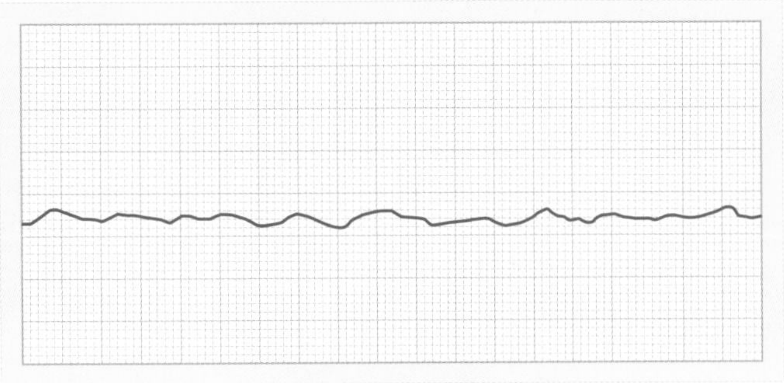

Fig. 39.4 • Asystole.

Box 39.1. The causes of pulseless electrical activity: the four *H*'s and the four *T*'s

The four *H*'s

1. Hypoxia
2. Hypovolaemia
3. Hyper- or hypokalaemia
4. Hypothermia

The four *T*'s

1. Tension pneumothorax
2. (Cardiac) tamponade
3. Toxins
4. Thromboemboli

This is to confirm the diagnosis of asystole and prevent a differential diagnosis of fine VF being attributed in error.

Asystole is the most common arrest arrhythmia in paediatrics due to the response of an immature heart to prolonged hypoxia producing bradycardia, which will progress to asystole if not treated effectively (Jevon 2004).

The term *pulseless electrical activity* can also be referred to as electrical mechanical dissociation, which means that the electrical activity is normal and present; however, there is no cardiac output and the patient presents in cardiac arrest.

Pulseless electrical activity

The diagnosis is made clinically by the absence of a pulse when there is electrical activity that would allude to cardiac activity (Fig. 39.5). Pulseless electrical activity can occur due to various reversible causes (Box 39.1) that must be considered and treated effectively to reverse the cardiac arrest state (Curley & Moloney-Harmon 2001).

Ventricular fibrillation

In VF the ventricles contract in a chaotic disorganised rapid irregular fashion when all coordination of electrical activity is lost (Fig. 39.6), leading to ineffective ventricular contraction and death.

The incidence of VF in the paediatric population in the past has been reported as extremely rare; however, more recent evidence suggests that VF as the primary arrhythmia occurs more frequently with increasing age (Samson et al 2003).

In the paediatric casualty, basic life support with airway adjuncts is normally established before placement of a cardiac monitor to determine the rhythm, which may account for primary VF not being identified. If early recognition and defibrillation in adult victims improves outcome, one could assume that early defibrillation in paediatric patients presenting in VF has the potential to improve outcome (Samson et al 2003).

Bradycardia

Bradycardia is the term used to define a heart rate lower than that of the child's normal rate for his or her age (Table 39.1). It is a preterminal sign more commonly associated with abnormal cardiac function as a consequence of hypoxia, acidosis and profound hypovolaemia.

The immediate administration of high-flow oxygen, with or without ventilation, and the implementation of cardiac compressions if the heart rate is equal to or below 60 beats/min should precede the administration of any medication (Tortora & Derrickson 2006). The routine use of an alkalising agent has not been shown to be beneficial. Sodium bicarbonate increases intracellular carbon dioxide levels, therefore administration, if used at all, should follow assisted ventilation with oxygen and effective basic life support (Resuscitation Council UK 2005).

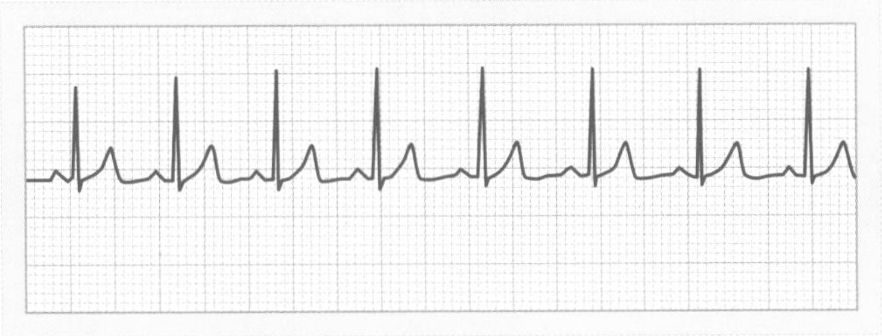

Fig. 39.5 • Pulseless electrical activity.

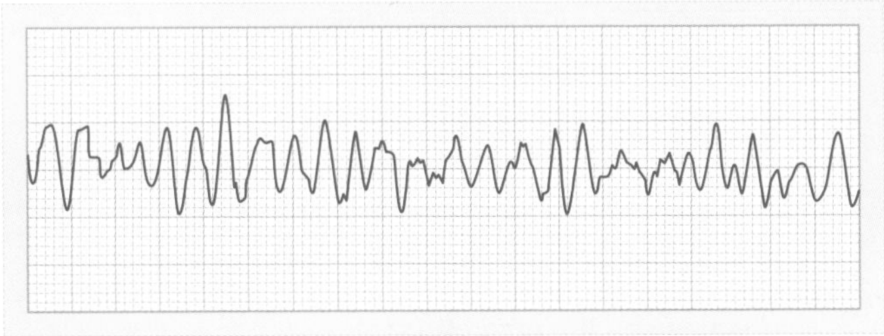

Fig. 39.6 • VF.

Table 39.1. Normal range of heart rates in children at rest

Age (years)	Pulse (beats/min)
< 1	100–160
2–5	95–140
5–12	80–120
> 12	60–100

(After Neill & Knowles 2004, with permission.)

Tachycardia

Tachycardia is the term used to define a heart rate higher than that of the child's normal rate for his or her age (Table 39.1). A tachycardia may be due to the normal body response to infection, pain and exercise, which normally produces a sinus tachycardia (Tortora & Derrickson 2006).

An abnormal rhythm such as a supraventricular tachycardia (SVT) may require immediate intervention.

The differential diagnosis of SVT from sinus tachycardia is determined by the rate of the heart. In an infant below 1 year of age, if the heart rate is faster than 220 beats/min this can be diagnosed as SVT. In the older child more than 1 year of age, if the heart rate is over 180 beats/min this can be diagnosed as SVT (Resuscitation Council UK 2004). Differential diagnosis can also be confirmed by performing a 12-lead ECG recording.

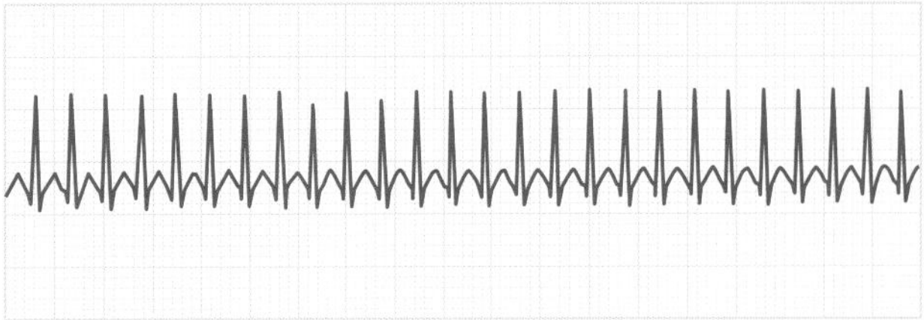

Fig. 39.7 • SVT.

In sinus tachycardia, P waves are present, whereas P waves are not visible in SVT.

Supraventricular tachycardia

Supraventricular tachycardia (Fig. 39.7) is a common arrhythmia in the paediatric population. There is no definite aetiology but it can be a consequence of a viral illness without underlying cardiac defects. SVT occurs due to a re-entry mechanism of the impulse via the atrioventricular node. If the period of SVT is prolonged the child may become compromised, requiring immediate intervention.

Summary

In summary, life-threatening cardiac arrhythmias in children are usually the result rather than the cause of acute illness. The most common pattern of cardiorespiratory arrest is bradycardia that progresses to asystole if not recognised and treated immediately.

Procedures Box 39.1 Applying the electrodes and using the monitor

1

Action
Collect the required equipment:

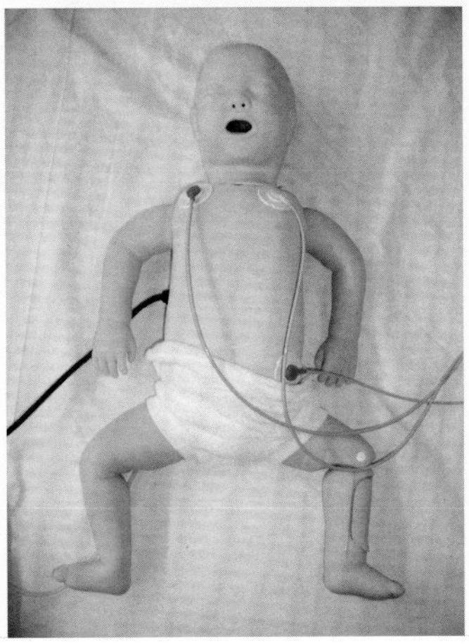

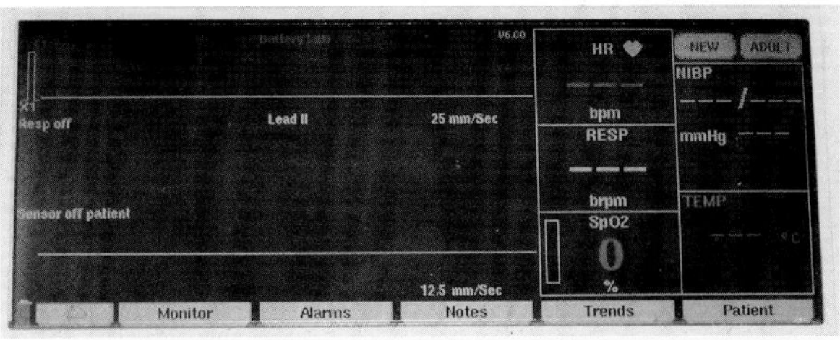

- cardiac monitor
- cardiac electrodes.

2

Action
Wash and dry your hands.

Reason *Prevents cross-infection.*

Procedures Box 39.1 Applying the electrodes and using the monitor—cont'd

3

Action
Explain to the child and parent that you are going apply cardiac electrodes and the reason for doing so.

Reason *Promotes psychological support.*

4

Action
Place the electrodes in the correct positions.

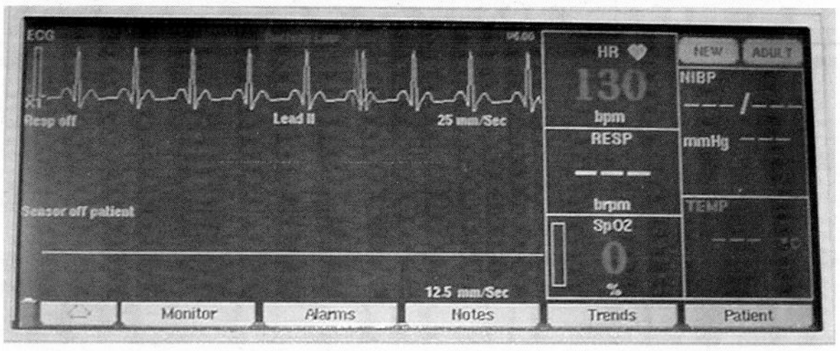

Reasons *To interpret normal sinus rhythm on lead II requires the correct placement of electrodes and knowledge about how the ECG machine functions.*
To simplify the application of the electrodes to the chest in cardiac monitoring the ECG cables are usually colour-coded:

- *the red lead is attached to the electrode on the right*
- *the yellow lead is attached to the electrode on the left shoulder*
- *the green lead is normally placed on the upper abdominal wall.*

5

Action
Turn on the monitor and place on lead II.

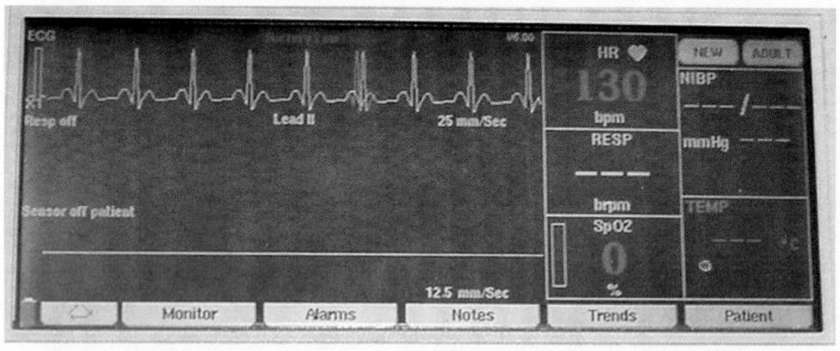

Reason *Lead II measures the voltage between the right shoulder and the left lower chest and consequently produces the configuration that commonly displays the most prominent P wave and QRS amplitude, providing that atrial activity is present.*

6

Action
Normal sinus rhythm seen.

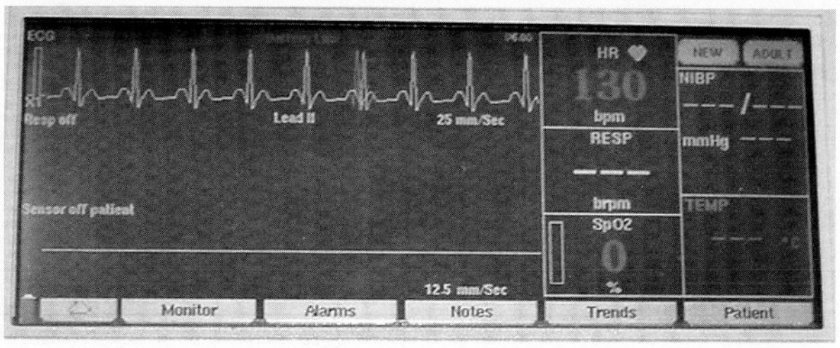

7

Action
Asystole seen.

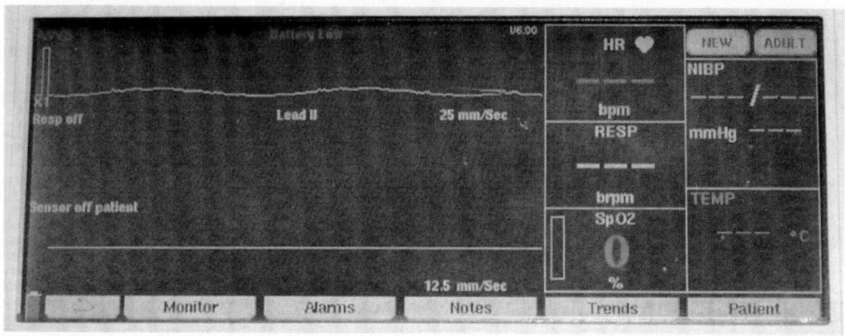

Reason *Atrial and ventricular asystole usually coexist so that the ECG recording is a line with no deflections, a wandering baseline.*

8

Action
Ventricular fibrillation seen.

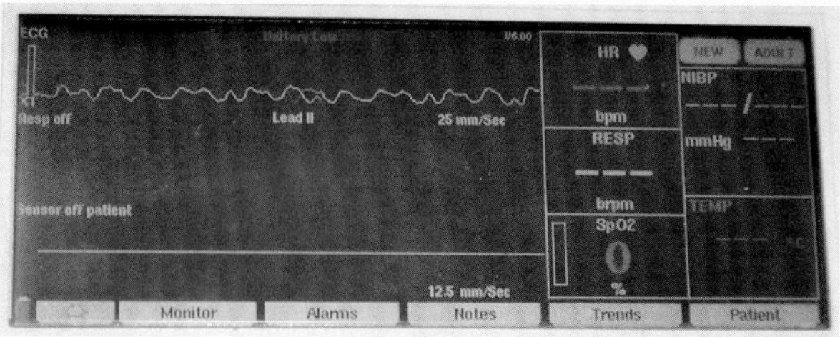

Reason *The ventricles contract in a chaotic disorganised rapid irregular fashion when all coordination of electrical activity is lost, leading to ineffective ventricular contraction.*

Procedures Box 39.1 Applying the electrodes and using the monitor—cont'd

9

Action
Sinus tachycardia seen.

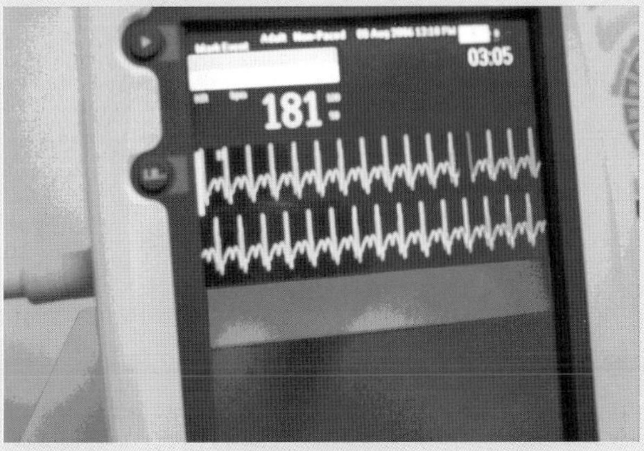

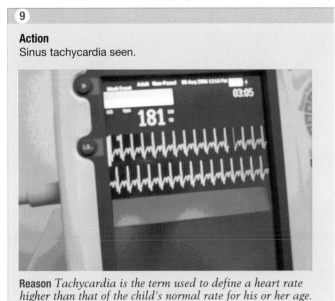

Reason *Tachycardia is the term used to define a heart rate higher than that of the child's normal rate for his or her age.*

10

Action
Sinus bradycardia seen.

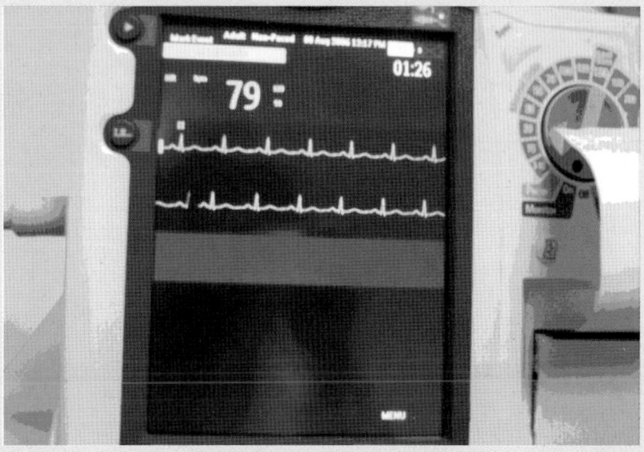

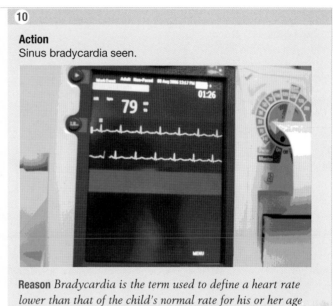

Reason *Bradycardia is the term used to define a heart rate lower than that of the child's normal rate for his or her age*

Now test your knowledge

Question 1

Describe the most frequent arrhythmia in paediatrics and discuss the aetiology of this rhythm.

Question 2

What is the commonest cause of collapse in the paediatric population?

Question 3

Outline the indications for the use of ECG and the rationale for its use.

Question 4

Provide the rationale for the use of lead II when monitoring and interpreting an ECG recording.

Question 5

In relation to physiology discuss what the P, QRS and T waves represent.

Question 6

List the common or more frequent cardiac arrest arrhythmias in paediatrics.

Question 7

Discuss the structured approach to rhythm strip analysis.

Question 8

Outline the essential checks that must be made when asystole is suspected and provide a rationale.

Question 9

Define the term *bradycardia* and discuss the most common aetiology.

Question 10

Define the term *tachycardia* and discuss the aetiology.

References

Boudreau Canover M (2003) Understanding electrocardiography, 8th edn. Mosby, St Louis

Brennan PO, Berry K, Powell C (2003) Handbook of pediatric emergency medicine. Bios Scientific Publishers, Abingdon

Campbell S, Glasper EA (2001) Whaley and Wong's children's nursing. Mosby, St Louis

Curley MAQ, Moloney-Harmon PA (2001) Critical care nursing of infants and children, 2nd edn. Saunders, Edinburgh

Garcia T, Holtz N (2003) Introduction to 12 lead ECG. The art of interpretation. Jones and Bartlett Publishers, Boston

Jevon P (2004) Paediatric advanced life support – a practical guide. Butterworth Heinemann, Edinburgh

Mattson Porth C (2002) Essentials of pathophysiology: concepts of altered health states. Lippincott Williams&Wilkins, Philadelphia

Meek S, Morris F (2002) ABC of clinical electrocardiography. Introduction. I-Leads, rate, rhythm, and cardiac axis. British Medical Journal 324:415–418

Neill S, Knowles H (2004) The biology of child health. Reader in development and assessment. Palgrave MacMillan, Basingstoke

Resuscitation Council UK (2004) European Paediatric Life Support course manual. Resuscitation Council, London

Resuscitation Council UK (2005) Online. Available: http://www.resus.org.uk

Samson R, Berg B, Bingham R (2003) Use of automated external defibrillators for children: an update. An advisory statement from the Paediatric Advanced Life Support Task Force, International Liaison Committee on Resuscitation. Resuscitation 57(3):237–243

Seeley RR, Stephens TD, Tate P (2005) Essentials of anatomy and physiology, 5th edn. McGraw-Hill, New York

Tortora GJ, Derrickson B (2006) Principles of anatomy and physiology, 11th edn. Wiley, Chichester

40 Application and care of traction

Julia Judd

'Orthopaedic traction occurs when a pulling force is exerted on a part or parts of the body' (Davis 1989, Davis & Barr 1999; Fig. 40.1). Traction can be manual, for example when a pull is exerted on a limb to reduce a fracture prior to the application of plaster, or weights and pulleys may be attached to a limb to maintain the pull (Makins 1992). Counter-traction is 'when a pulling force is exerted that opposes the direct pull of the traction' (Davis & Barr 1999).

Traction can be either fixed or balanced in its nature and either skin or skeletal:

- *Fixed* traction is when there is a pull between two fixed points. An example is in the treatment of a fractured femur when the skin extension cords are tied to the end of the splint. Counter-pressure is exerted by the ring of the splint up against the ischial tuberosity of the pelvis.
- *Balanced* traction is a pull between weights attached to skin extension cords with counter-traction provided by the patients' weight.

Traction may be via the skin or directly via the bony skeleton:

- *Skin* traction may be either adhesive or non-adhesive. The choice is normally dependent on the length of treatment. Skin traction is applied with skin extension cords attached to the limb and held in place with bandages. The traction force is exerted through the skin to the bone, either fixing the traction or balancing it. The normal recommended maximum pull is 4.5–6.7 kg (10–15 lbs) (Davis & Barr 1999).
- *Skeletal* traction is used when a stronger force is required, commonly in the treatment of fractures when pulling and maintaining the fractured bone ends into position and alignment. The pull is transmitted via a metal pin inserted through the distal part of the fracture.

Note that 'Traction must always be opposed by counter traction or the pull exerted against a fixed object' (Flinders University School of Medicine).

Rationale for the use of traction

Traction can be used to:

- reduce, correct and maintain position (e.g. a fracture)
- immobilise a limb (e.g. osteomyelitis – bone infection)
- reduce muscle spasm (e.g. Legg–Calvé–Perthes disease – avascular necrosis of the femoral head, or post hip surgery)
- prevent contraction of soft tissues following surgery
- rest a limb to minimise pain (e.g fracture, transient synovitis of the hip).

Types of traction

Skin traction

This was devised by Gordon Buck in 1840 as a method to treat a fractured femur. Lengths of adhesive plaster strips are applied longitudinally to the sides of the legs and secured with bandages. Cords attached to ends of the adhesive plaster are tied to a weight holder that is suspended over a pulley system at the end of the bed. Counter-traction is supplied by the patient's body weight with the end of the bed tilted up. This traction is alternatively called Pugh's traction, when the traction cords are tied directly to the bed without a weight system (Flinders University School of Medicine).

Bryant or gallows traction

Bryant described this traction in 1873. It is the application of skin traction to the legs. The hips are flexed to 90° and the legs are vertically extended so that the traction cords can be secured to either an overhead bar above the cot, or a pulley-and-weight system. The child's sacrum is elevated so that it is lifted just off the bed, enabling the nurse to pass a flat hand underneath (Judd & Wright 2005). It is the child's body weight that provides the counter-traction (Davis & Barr 1999). Bryant or Gallows traction can be used in the treatment of femoral fractures in children up to the approximate age of 18 months and under the weight of 16 kg (Davis & Barr 1999). In some centres prereduction traction is used prior to surgery for a closed or an open reduction of the hip in the treatment of developmental dysplasia. The rationale is to gently stretch the blood supply to the femoral head to reduce the incidence of avascular necrosis, which is reported in approximately 15–20% of cases (Gage & Winter 1973, Judd & Wright 2005, PatientPlus 2007). Although studies suggest the positive outcomes of prereduction traction in reducing the risk of avascular necrosis, Weinstein (1997) argues that with the absence of specific clinical or experimental studies on the direct effect of traction 'as a single variable' (Weinstein 1997: 1) these outcomes cannot be proven.

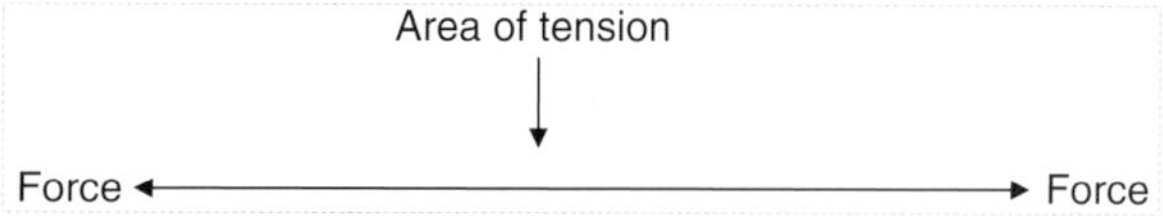

Fig. 40.1 • Traction is the action of pulling involving the opposition of forces of equal strength.

Thomas splint traction

Thomas splint traction was designed by Hugh Owen Thomas in 1870 (Davis & Barr 1999). It was first known as the knee splint and initially used to treat patients with tuberculosis. It was later adapted for use in the First and Second World Wars to transport soldiers with a femoral fracture from the battlefield. Today the Thomas splint is one treatment option in the management of femoral shaft fractures. High-impact incidents such as road traffic accidents and falls (Cusick et al 2005, Parsch 2002) are a frequent cause of this common injury in children (Stanitski 1998). Nursing staff, however, should always be alerted to the possibility of child abuse, especially in the non-ambulant child. The Thomas splint can be used as a method of treatment either for the duration of fracture healing or in some centres as a temporary measure until surgical intervention.

Rationale for thomas splint traction for fractured femur

- To relieve pain due to muscle spasm and maintain the limb in a position of rest and comfort.
- To restore and maintain the alignment of the fracture.
- To allow the child to be moved comfortably.

The Thomas splint can be applied so that the traction is either fixed or balanced (Judd & Wright 2005).

Fixed thomas splint traction

Hugh Owen Thomas' method was to use fixed traction, when the pull is exerted against two points:

- Point 1: the skin traction tapes are secured to the cross-piece at the end of the Thomas splint.
- Point 2: the ring of the splint that abuts against the top of the limb; the counter-traction is therefore being applied against the ischial tuberosity by the ring of the splint.

Balanced traction

The Thomas splint can also be used for balanced traction, when the leg rests on the splint and the pull is exerted against the opposing force provided by the child's body weight. The weights are attached directly to the skin extension tapes, and the foot of the bed is raised, providing counter-traction.

There are five issues to be considered in the application of Thomas splint traction:

1. The expertise of the staff
2. Child and family needs
3. Choice of equipment
4. Principles of safe application
5. Principles of care.

Expertise of the staff

Application of Thomas splint traction requires two staff members, both trained and deemed competent in the procedure. Ideally an expert orthopaedic nurse, with the underlying knowledge pertinent to the anatomy and physiology of fracture reduction and its aftercare, leads the procedure, with help from an assistant.

LINK CHAPTER **2**

Child and family needs

Preparation of the child and family is paramount. A clear explanation outlining the procedure is given to alleviate the child's fears and reduce the parents' anxiety (Judd & Wright 2005). It is important to keep them informed of every stage throughout the procedure and to allow the parents to comfort their child.

LINK CHAPTER **3**

Analgesia needs to be effective. Evidence suggests that a femoral nerve block is effective in reducing the pain of femoral shaft fractures in children (McGlone et al 1987, Ronchi et al 1989, Tondare & Nadkarni 1982). However, a femoral nerve block, although safe, does not always give complete pain relief (Tondare & Nadkarni 1982). It is therefore best supported with morphine and ketamine. Morphine will minimise the child's pain while ketamine as a dissociative anaesthetic has the potential for amnesia relating to the procedure (Ng & Ang 2002).

LINK CHAPTER **18**

For the older child, Entonox (self-administered nitrous oxide) has been shown to be an effective short-term analgesic that works well in conjunction with a femoral nerve block or an opiate. Bruce & Franck (2000) highlight studies that have demonstrated the value of Entonox in the reduction of children's fractures (Hennrikus et al 1995, Wattenmaker et al 1990).

Choice of equipment

The splint must be the correct size in both its length and its size of ring to ensure a good fit that will maintain the reduction of the fracture and reduce the potential for pressure sores.

A list of the equipment for setting up a traction bed (Balkan beam) and how to measure for correct fit is given in Boxes 40.1 and 40.2.

Box 40.1. Traction bed

Balkan beam

- Four end posts connected with crossbars at the ends of the bed
- Middle bar to connect between both ends
- Extension bars for the end of the bed
- Five pulleys
- Three weight hangers
- Assorted weights

Box 40.2. Thomas splint

- Adhesive skin extension set
- Four to six crepe bandages (10 cm)
- Adhesive tape
- Scissors
- Correct size Thomas splint and ring (see *Application of Thomas splint traction* procedure box)
- Velcro slings to make up the splint
- Gamgee
- Two tongue depressors (windlass)
- Traction cord

Principles of safe application

Have the equipment ready (Fig. 40.2) and the bed frame assembled as shown (Fig. 40.3).

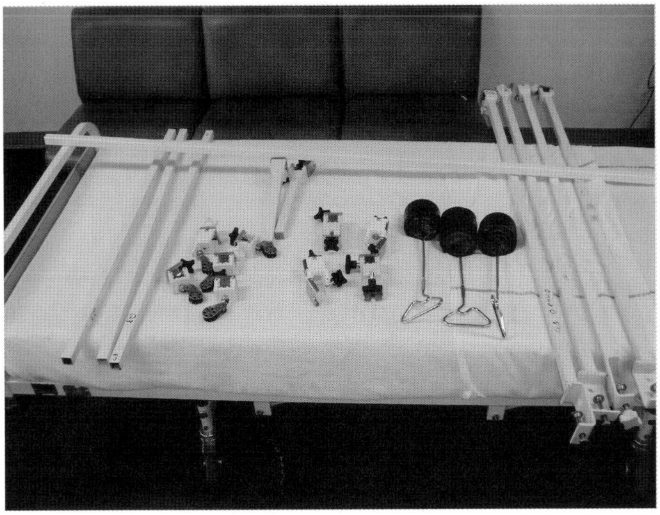

Fig. 40.2 • Traction equipment.

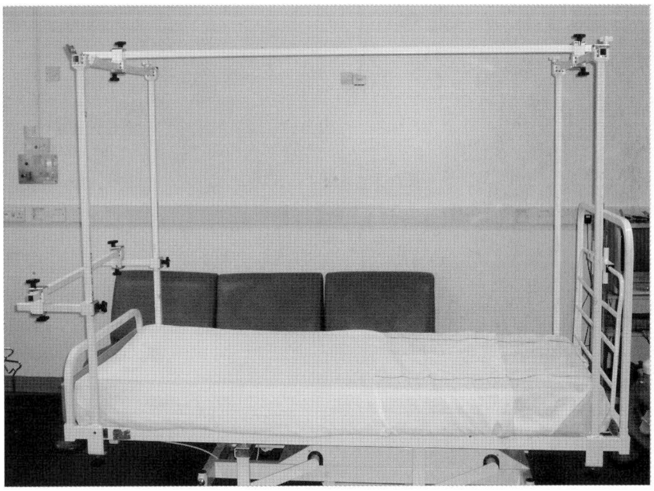

Fig. 40.3 • The bed frame.

Procedures Box 40.1 Application of thomas splint traction

Action
Ensure that the bed is assembled, with frame, prior to application of the splint.

Reason *So the bed is ready for transfer of the patient from the emergency department trolley following application of the splint.*

Actions
Meet with the child and family in the emergency department.

Explain the procedure for reduction of the fractured femur and application of the splint.

Reason *Psychological preparation of child and family.*

Action
Measure the unaffected limb.

Note: check the equipment that your centre uses; some companies provide specific instructions that are pertinent to the set-up of their splints.

Reason *Prevents unnecessary discomfit.*

Action
Carry out the splint measurements.

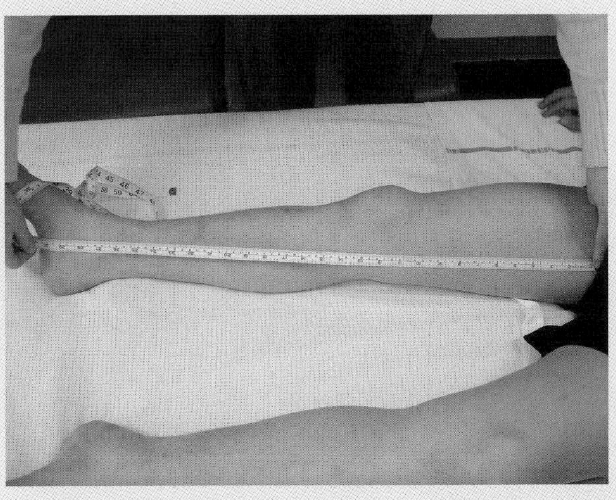

Length: measure the inside of the unaffected leg down to the heel.

Procedures Box 40.1 Application of thomas splint traction—cont'd

Ring: measure the circumference of the good thigh at its widest part (obliquely, circle at top of leg) and add several centimetres (approximately 5 cm).

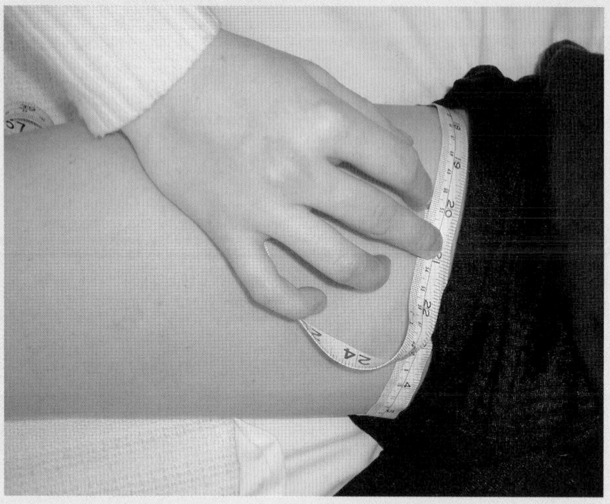

Allow for swelling (caused by the haematoma in association with the fractured femur).

Action

Select the ring that corresponds to the thigh circumference and the appropriate splint (i.e. paediatric or adult).

Attach the ring and splint together.

Adjust the length of the Thomas splint so that it is 15 cm longer than the child's leg length.

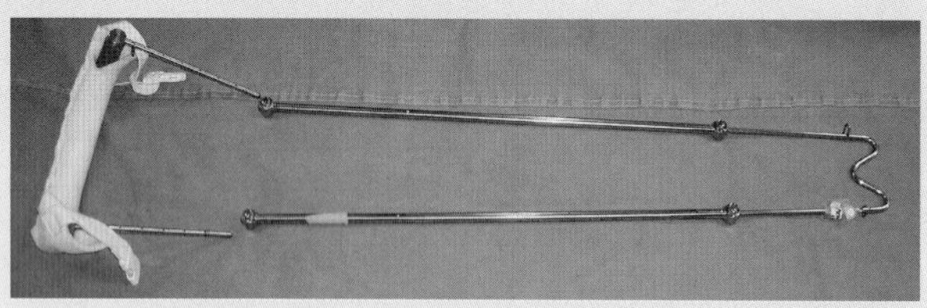

Obliquely position the ring so that it corresponds to the angle of the child's groin on the affected side.

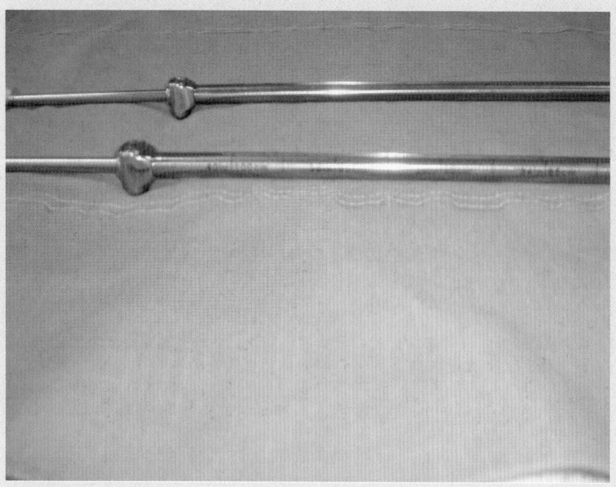

Actions

Attach slings along the splint as shown and secure together with Velcro strips; they should sag slightly and the distal sling should end before the heel.

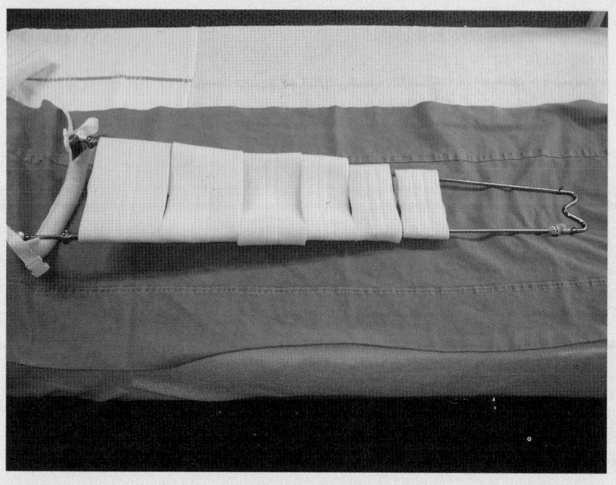

Reason *To accommodate the natural shape of the leg. The heel should not be resting on a sling, as this would cause a pressure sore.*

Action

Layer Gamgee (soft cotton padding) on top of the slings (two layers).

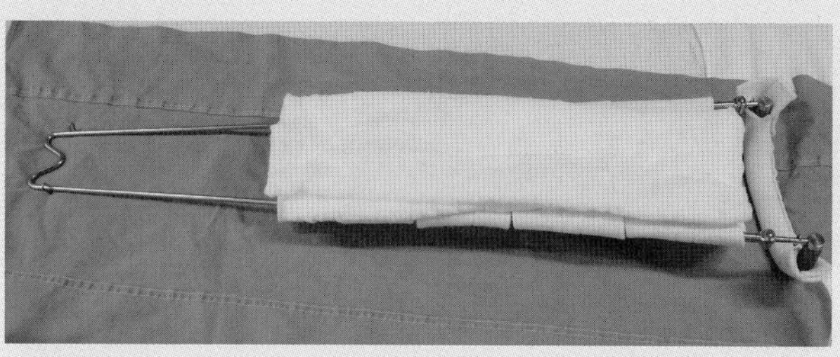

Action

An extra pad may be placed under the knee.

Reason *To allow for 5° knee flexion to maintain femur alignment.*

Action

Ask the family if the child has any known allergies to tape.

ALERT

When applying skin traction ensure that the child has no known allergy to adhesive tape; if so, non-adhesive may have to be used.

Action

The extension set can be cut to the required length and the ends rounded.

Reasons *Provides the correct length to fit the child's leg. Rounded corners help to prevent the edges peeling down.*

Procedures Box 40.1 Application of thomas splint traction—cont'd

Action
Perform a neurovascular assessment of the affected limb (Pieper 1994, Tucker 1998).

Reason *To record baseline observations and ensure normal circulation, sensation and movement.*

Action
Ensure that appropriate analgesia has been administered prior to application of the splint.

Reason *Reduces pain.*

Actions
Manual traction is applied by the hands gripping and holding at the ankle, keeping the leg in alignment.

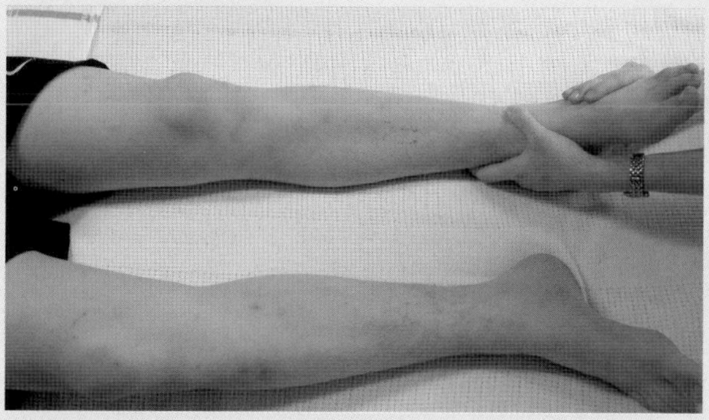

Maintain checks on the dorsalis pedis pulse.

Reasons *Straightens the limb and reduces fracture.*
Aids the application of traction tapes.
Checks the neurovascular status of the limb and ensures that the foot pulse is not lost when the fracture is reduced.

Action
Place traction tapes to the medial and lateral aspects of the limb with foam padding protecting the malleoli.

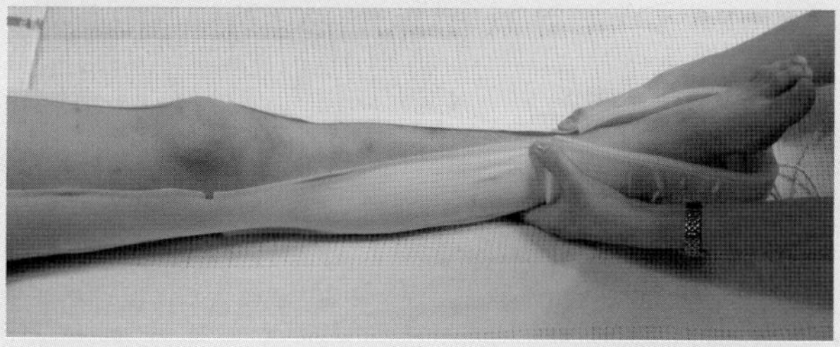

Reason *Protects bony prominences against pressure sores.*

Actions
Check that there are no creases in the skin extension tape.

Cut nicks in the extension tape over the knee area to improve conformity.

Reason *Prevents potential blister formation.*

Action
Leave enough room at the sole of the foot to allow for plantar flexion and dorsiflexion of the foot.

Reason *Facilitates normal ankle movement, preventing potential foot drop.*

Action
Secure the traction tapes with crepe bandages in figure-of-eight style (Love 2000), starting just above the malleoli up to the upper thigh; leave the knee area exposed.

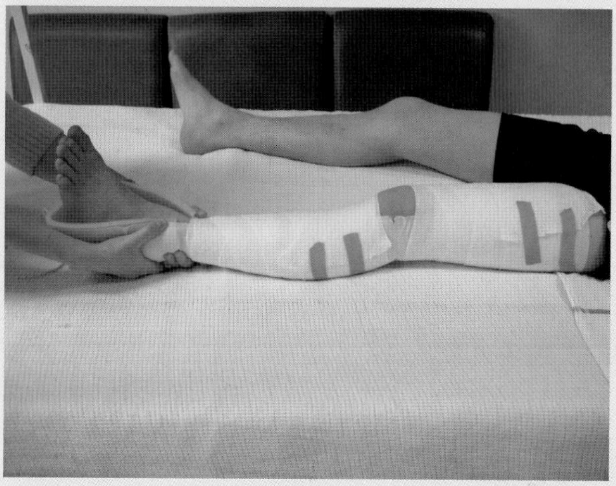

Reasons *Keeps traction tapes in place.*
Note: tight bandaging over the fibula head at the knee can cause peroneal nerve compression (foot drop).
Leaving the knee exposed also allows for checking of leg alignment.

Action
The bandages should avoid the malleoli, Achilles tendon and peroneal nerve (Draper & Scott 1996).

Reason *Avoids pressure over at-risk areas.*
Pressure over the peroneal nerve, which runs around the proximal fibula, has the potential to cause foot drop (Love 2000).

Actions
While manual traction is maintained the Thomas splint is positioned underneath the limb, sliding it under at the side of the leg.

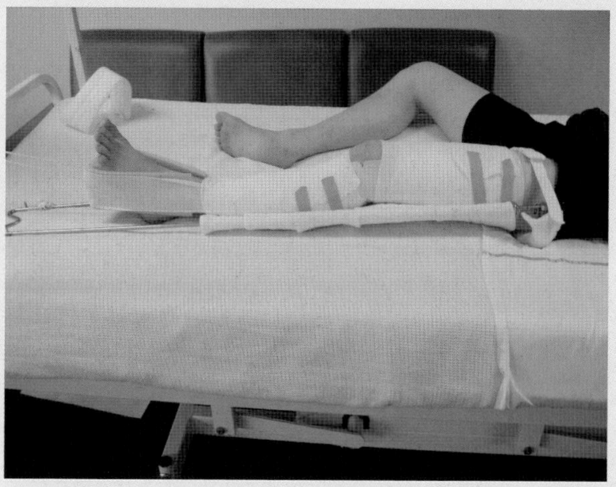

Procedures Box 40.1 Application of thomas splint traction—cont'd

Action
The ring fits into the groin.

Reason *It rests against the ischial tuberosity – one point of fixed traction.*

Actions
Fixed traction: extension tape cords are secured, placing the outer cord over the lateral bar of the splint and the inner cord under the medial bar.

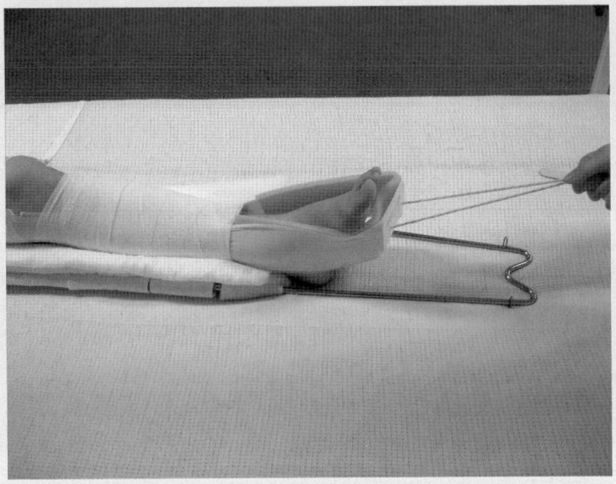

Traction is achieved through the ring abutting against the ischial tuberosity and fixation of the extension tapes to the end of the splint.

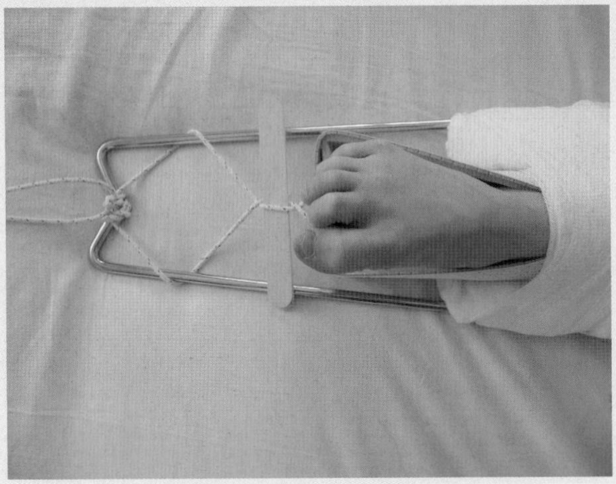

Reason *Helps to prevent rotation of the limb.*

Action
Windlass: two tongue depressors are inserted in between the tied extension tapes and rotated laterally.

Reason *To exert stronger traction pull on the fracture.*

Action
The child can be comfortably transferred to the X-ray department.

Reasons *The fracture is immobilised.*
An X-ray will confirm the reduction of the fracture and its alignment.

Action
Transfer the child to the ward and on to a traction bed.

Actions
Suspend the splint so that it is not resting on the bed, using traction cord and weights.

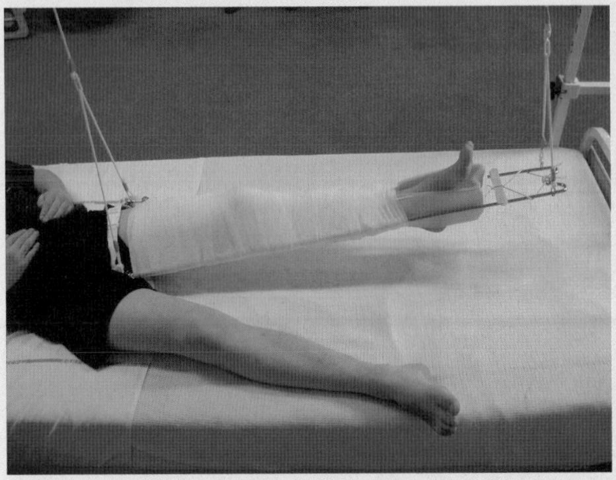

Keep the ends of the traction cord short and secure them with adhesive tape; do not cover the actual knots with tape, only the tape ends.

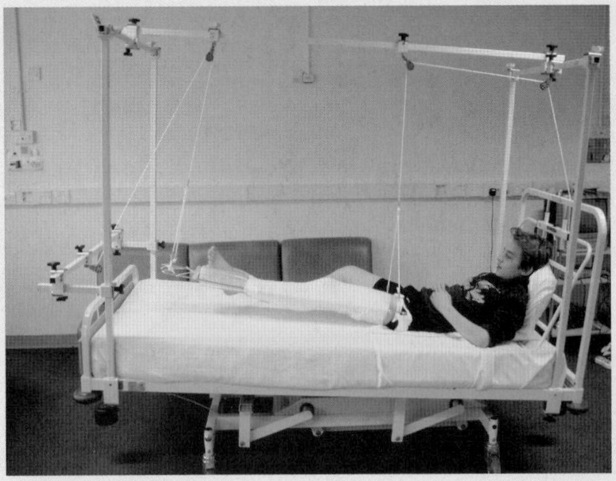

Reasons *Enables patient mobility in the bed and reduces the potential for pressure sores.*
Traction cord is non-stretchable and strong (Davis & Barr 1999).
To prevent from fraying, the knot should be secure without additional tape; leaving them free of tape allows for adjustments to be made.

Action
With *fixed traction*, weights can be attached to the end of the splint if the splint is causing pressure problems in the groin (Nichol 1995).

Reason *This does not affect the pull on the fracture; the weights are used to pull the ring out of the groin if it is uncomfortable and causing pressure problems in the perineum.*

Principles of care

The principles of caring for a child on traction are as below:

- Mechanical principles
- Physical needs
- Psychosocial needs.

Procedures Box 40.2 Principles of care

1 Mechanical principles

Action
Check daily the free running of the traction cord over the pulleys.

Reason *Ensures that there is no evidence of the cord fraying; this would hinder the traction pull should the cord break or become caught in the pulley.*

Action
Check daily the security of the knots, clamps and pulleys.

Reason *Ensures their security.*

Action
Check daily that the overall alignment of the limb, splint and traction pull is straight.

Reason *Maintains the optimum position of the fracture.*

Action
Check daily to ensure that weights (if used) are secure and do not get caught on the bed end as the patient moves around the bed.

Reason *Allows free movement of the patient in the bed and maintains traction pull.*

2 Physical needs

Actions
Pain levels should be assessed frequently, especially in the first 48 h.

Pain scoring tools appropriate for the child's age should be used to obtain an accurate assessment (Gregory 2005).

To keep the child comfortable anticipate the potential for pain and intervene early with appropriate analgesia.

Reason *A fractured femur causes pain and muscle spasm.*

Action
Neurovascular assessment of the fractured limb should be maintained hourly for the first 12 h, observing for neurovascular impairment and the potential for compartment syndrome (Judd & Wright 2005); thereafter the regularity of observations can be reviewed.

Reasons *Neurovascular impairment can result from an injury (Maher et al 1994, Tucker 1998) such as a fractured femur, caused by the haematoma compressing the nerve or blood supply to the limb (Altizer 2002).*
The affected limb is assessed for normal colour, sensation, capillary refill time, the presence of distal pulses, swelling and normal movement of the distal limb. Concern is raised if pain is increased on passive and active movement (Grippen Bryant 1998).

Action
Consider administering muscle relaxants if the child is experiencing muscle spasm.

Reason *Large muscle attachments to the femur (quadriceps) are interrupted when it is fractured, causing painful spasms.*

Actions
Check daily the integrity of the skin.

Regular ring care should be performed: the nurse's fingers are passed under the ring so that the child's skin is moved away from the pressure of the ring; the fingers can be lightly covered with talcum powder to facilitate this.

If the child or parent wants to do this themselves, the nurse needs to ensure that it is performed correctly.

Reason *Prevents the complication of ring sores developing under the buttock or in the groin.*

Action
Check daily the security of the bandages.

Reason *To check that they are in position and have not rugged up or are too tight or loose.*

Action
Check daily the child's general health.

Reason *To regularly review the potential for complications of bed rest (e.g. pressure sores, constipation and chest infection).*

Action
Observe for complaints of itching under the skin traction.

Reason *This could be an early sign of a blister developing and needs prompt investigation.*

Actions
Instruct the child in the importance of maintaining mobility in the bed within the constraints of the Thomas splint.

Provide a monkey pole to facilitate movement.

Take care when handling the fractured limb when assisting patient movement.

Reason *Maintains the normal range of movement of unaffected joints.*
Prevents the potential for pressure sores.

Action
Support the splint and limb with flat hands underneath.

Reason *Prevents uneven pressure on the fracture.*

Action
Explain the procedure for using a bed pan and/or urinal and ensure that the child's privacy and dignity is maintained.

Reason *Alleviates the child's anxieties.*

Procedures Box 40.2 Principles of care—cont'd

Actions
Ensure that the child receives a nutritious diet while immobilised.

Explain to the parents and child that the aim is to promote bone healing and prevent constipation.

3

Psychosocial needs

Action
Throughout any interaction, investigation and treatment the nurse's prime importance is to alleviate both the child's and the parents' fears.

Reasons *The child with a fractured femur has suffered a traumatic injury that subsequently involves an emergency admission, the nature of which incurs potentially frightening and new experiences.*

Action
Prior to applying Thomas splint traction, provide clear communication supported with pictorial material.

Reason *Enables the parents and child to have a better understanding of what is to be achieved.*

Actions
In some centres traction is the mainstay of treatment for a fractured femur, necessitating a prolonged stay in hospital; Pieper (1994) noted the impact of this on the child's behaviour.

The nurse or play specialist can assist the parents by finding ways of providing entertainment and occupation.

Reasons *Meets the interactive needs of the child and ensures that the child's education needs are met by involving the hospital school.*

(Davis & Barr 1999, Judd & Wright 2005, Royal College of Nursing & Society of Orthopaedic and Trauma Nursing 2002).

LINK CHAPTER **1**

Now test your knowledge

A 6-year-old boy is admitted to the emergency department with a fractured femur:

- What type of traction would you recommend for a femoral fracture in this age group?
- What equipment do you need to prepare for application of the traction?
- Consider what pain relief you could administer.

A child of 9 months is admitted with a femoral fracture. The child is non-ambulant and the history of the injury is unclear. There is concern regarding the cause of the injury:

- Discuss your role as the admitting nurse in relation to a potential child protection procedure, as well as (a) how you would support the family and (b) the type of traction you would use to treat the child's fracture.

You are caring for a child with a femoral fracture who is being nursed on Thomas splint traction:

- Describe the principles of the care you would provide during your shift, including the care of the child's needs and why, and the checks you would make on the traction apparatus.

References

Altizer L (2002) Neurovascular assessment. Orthopaedic Essentials 21(4):48–50

Bruce E, Franck L (2000) Self-administered nitrous oxide (Entonox) for the management of procedural pain. Paediatric Nursing 12(7):15–19

Cusick L, Thompson NW, Taylor TC, Cowie GH (2005) Paediatric femoral fractures – the Royal Belfast Hospital for Sick Children experience. Ulster Medical Journal 74(2):98–104

Davis P (1989) The principles of traction. Journal of Clinical Practice, Education and Management 3(4):5–8

Davis P, Barr L (1999) Principles of traction. Journal of Orthopaedic Nursing 3(4):222–227

Draper J, Scott F (1996) An investigation into the application and maintenance of Hamilton Russell traction on three orthopaedic wards. Journal of Advanced Nursing 23(3):536–541

Flinders University School of Medicine Online. Available: http://som.flinders.edu.au/FUSA/ORTHOWEB/notebook/trauma/traction.html

Gage JR, Winter RB (1973) Avascular necrosis of the capital femoral epiphysis as a complication of closed reduction of congenital dislocation of the hip. Journal of Bone and Joint Surgery 54A:373–388

Gregory J (2005) Pain management and orthopaedic care. In Kneale J, Davis P (eds) Orthopaedic and trauma nursing. Churchill Livingstone, London, p 140–163

Grippen Bryant G (1998) Modalities for immobilisation. In Maher AB, Salmond SW, Pellino TA (eds) Orthopaedic nursing, 2nd edn. Saunders, Philadelphia

Hennrikus WL, Shin AY, Klingelberger CE (1995) Self-administered nitrous oxide and a hematoma block for analgesia in the outpatient reduction of fractures in children. Journal of Bone and Joint Surgery 77:335–339

Judd J, Wright E (2005) Joint and limb problems in children. In Kneale J, Davis P (eds) Orthopaedic and trauma nursing. Churchill Livingstone, London, p 257–264

Love C (2000) Bandaging skills for orthopaedic nurses. Journal of Orthopaedic Nursing 4(2):84–91

McGlone R, Sadhra K, Hamer DW, Pritty PE (1987) Femoral nerve block in the initial management of femoral shaft fractures. Archives of Emergency Medicine 4(3):163–168

Maher AB, Salmond SW, Pellino TA (1994) Orthopaedic nursing. Saunders, St Louis

Makins M (ed.) (1992) Collins concise English dictionary, 3rd edn. Harper Collins, London

Ng KC, Ang SY (2002) Sedation with ketamine for paediatric procedures in the emergency department – a review of 500 cases. Singapore Medical Journal 43(6):300–304

Nichol D (1995) Understanding the principles of traction. Nursing Standard 9(6):25–28

Parsch K (2002) Femoral shaft fractures. In Benson M, Fixsen J, Macnicol M, Parsch K (eds) Children's orthopaedics and fractures, 2nd edn. Churchill Livingstone, London, p 640–645

PatientPlus (2007) Online. Available: http://www.patient.co.uk/showdoc/40024965/

Pieper P (1994) Pediatric trauma. Nursing Clinics of North America 29(4):563–584

Ronchi L, Rosenbaum D, Athouel A et al (1989) Femoral nerve blockade in children using bupivacaine. Anesthesiology 70(4):622–624

Royal College of Nursing, Society of Orthopaedic and Trauma Nursing (2002) Traction Working Party. A traction manual. RCN Publishing, London

Stanitski D (1998) Femur fractures. In Staheli L (ed.) Pediatric orthopedic secrets. Hanley and Belfus, Philadelphia, p 127–129

Tondare AS, Nadkarni AV (1982) Femoral nerve block for fractured shaft of femur. Canadian Anaesthesiology Society Journal 29(3):270

Tucker KR (1998) Compartment syndrome: the orthopaedic nurse's vital role. Journal of Orthopaedic Nursing 2(1):33–36

Wattenmaker I, Kasser JR, McGravey A (1990) Self-administered nitrous oxide for fracture reduction in children in an emergency room setting. Journal of Orthopaedic Trauma 4(1):35–38

Weinstein SL (1997) Traction in developmental dislocation of the hip: is its use justified? A Tribute to Dr. Paul Griffin. Clinical Orthopaedics and Related Research 338:79–85.

41 Application of plaster and observation for neurovascular deficit

Elizabeth Wright

In orthopaedic nursing it is often necessary to immobilise children's bones or joints using plaster- or resin-based casts. The purpose of casting is to maintain bone alignment for fracture healing or to maintain surgical correction until healed. Casting also promotes pain relief by resting the affected limb or joint and can assist with correcting deformities by plaster wedging or serial casting (Prior & Miles 1999).

Casting techniques vary slightly but usually three layers are applied: stockinette (Fig. 41.1), wool padding (Fig. 41.2) then plaster- or resin-based cast (Fig. 41.3). Often a plaster cast is applied, and this is then strengthened with a resin-based cast. In many centres the child can choose the colour of the resin cast. This helps to engage the child in the process and generate acceptance of the plaster.

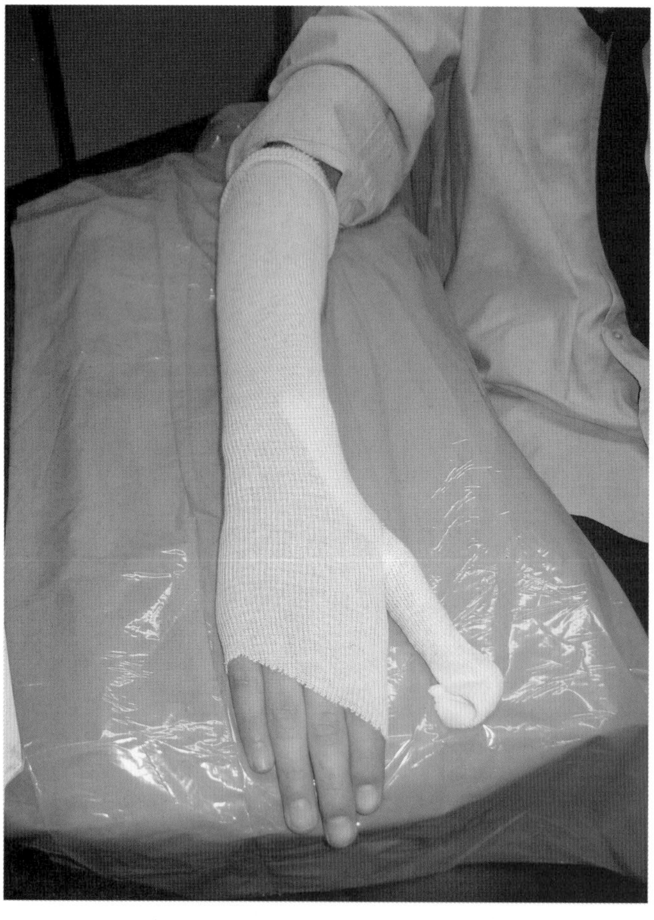

Fig. 41.1 • Application of stockinette.

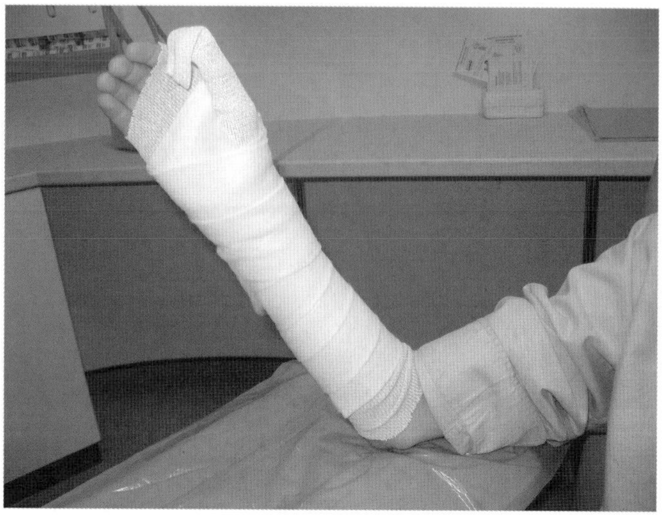

Fig. 41.2 • Application of wool padding.

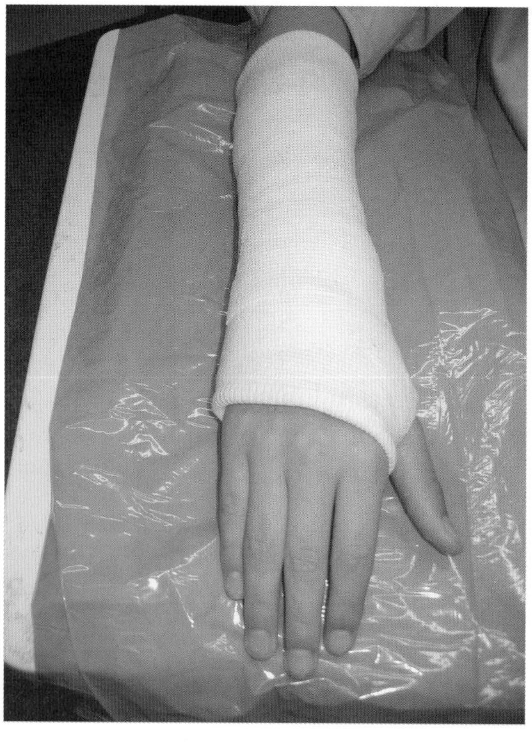

Fig. 41.3 • Completed resin cast.

For the child, application of a plaster can be a frightening experience. For many children it is a new experience and the plaster room can seem a very clinical and alien environment. The noise of the plaster saw can heighten the child's anxiety, particularly if it is being used in the next cubicle and the child cannot see what is happening. Healthcare professionals must be aware of these factors and try to alleviate the child's anxiety. The environment should be made more welcoming by the provision of appropriate pictures on the walls, soft music and toys. The environment should be bright and as far as possible child-oriented.

LINK CHAPTER **1**

The procedure should always be fully explained to the child and parent or carer first. Pictures of the process are useful. Any abnormal sounds should be explained and the child reassured, without breaking confidentiality.

LINK CHAPTERS **2 and 3**

It must also be recognised that applying plaster to a new fracture or post recent surgery can be painful. A pain assessment should be completed prior to the procedure using a recognised tool and, with explanation, appropriate analgesia given. Entonox is particularly useful for painful procedures of short duration.

Procedures Box 41.1 Initial nursing care of the child post plaster application

Action
Regular neurovascular assessment of plastered limb(s) (see *Neurovascular assessment* procedure box).

Reasons *For the early identification of neurovascular impairment or compartment syndrome.*
To check if medical advice is needed and prevent limb amputation.

Action
Advise the child and carer that the cast will feel warm for a few hours.

Reason *The chemical reaction to set the cast produces heat.*

Action
Handle the wet cast with the palm of your hand.

Reason *Prevents denting.*

Action
Expose the cast to the air.

Reason *Facilitates drying.*

Action
Do not use a hairdryer.

Reason *Plaster conducts heat, and the patient could experience a burn.*

Action
Elevate the limb with a cast.

Reason *Prevents or reduces oedema.*

Action
Rest and elevate the affected limb on pillows with a towel.

Reason *The towel absorbs excess moisture and assists drying.*

Action
For children in large body casts, turn 2-hourly.

Reason *Facilitates drying of the plaster.*

Action
Observe the cast for dents, cracks or skin rubbing.

Reasons *Dents or cracks could mean that the plaster is weakened and therefore not achieving its clinical objective, i.e. maintaining fracture alignment.*
Also, dents, cracks or skin rubbing can indicate a poor-fitting plaster that can lead to plaster sores and skin infection.

Action
Report to a senior nurse or medical staff.

Reason *The plaster may need to be removed or modified.*

LINK CHAPTER **18**

All children who have had an orthopaedic injury or treatment necessitating immobilisation of a limb in plaster must have regular neurovascular assessments of the affected limb. This is essential, as early identification of neurovascular deficit or compartment syndrome will allow prompt treatment and so prevent limb amputation (Table 41.1). Initially the cast will feel warm because a chemical reaction occurs as the cast sets. The child and her or his parent or carer should be forewarned of this. The wet cast should be handled using the palm of the hand to prevent denting. This is especially important, as dents in plaster will rub the skin, causing irritation at best and severe pressure sores at worst.

LINK CHAPTER **12**

Newly applied casts should be left to dry naturally by exposure to the air. Hairdryers or other devices must never be used. Plaster conducts heat, and use of a hairdryer or resting the limb on a hot radiator may result in a burn. Children in large body casts should be turned two-hourly to facilitate drying of the plaster. It is recommended that the affected limb should be rested on pillows with a towel. The towel absorbs excess moisture and assists drying.

Following orthopaedic injury or surgery the limb is likely to swell. Therefore the newly plastered limb should be elevated to reduce swelling or oedema (Fig. 41.4). This is important, as swelling can cause neurovascular compromise and/or compartment syndrome.

Table 41.1. Neurovascular assessment

Sign or symptom	Nursing action(s)
Increasing *pain* out of proportion to the injury or surgical intervention – the first most reliable sign (Wright & Bogoch 1992)	• Regular pain assessments using an age-appropriate pain tool. • Give all prescribed analgesia.
Pallor	• Observe perfusion of digits on the affected limb. • Assess that capillary refill time is less than 1 s.
Paraesthesia	• Ask if the child can feel pins and needles in the digits. • Lightly touch all digits, asking the child to confirm that he or she can feel the touch and that the feeling is normal or the same as in the non-affected hand.
Paralysis	• Ask the child to move the affected digits; the child may be reluctant to move the digits because of pain but should be able to do so.
Pulselessness – the last sign; if pulselessness occurs then the compartment syndrome is well established and amputation is likely	• Record the pulse distal to the site of injury; it may be necessary to make a hole in the plaster to access the pulse.
Coldness	• Feel the digits for warmth and compare with the other limb.

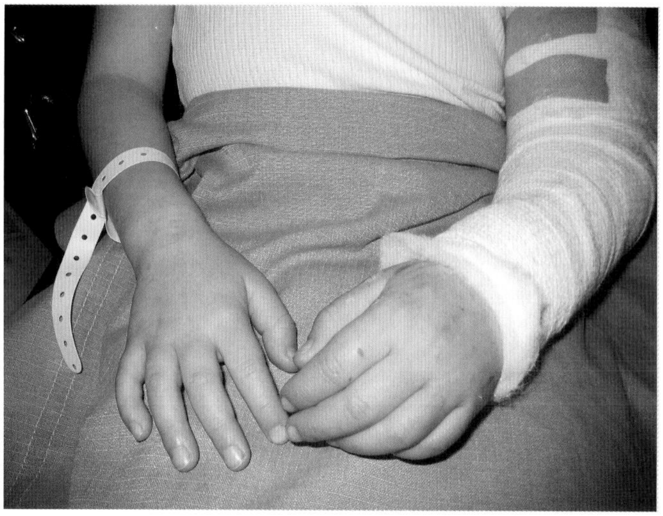

Fig. 41.4 • Swelling of fractured limb due to lack of elevation.

Finally the nurse should observe the cast for dents, cracks or skin rubbing. Dents or cracks could mean that the plaster is weakened and therefore not achieving its clinical objective, i.e. maintaining fracture alignment.

Also, dents, cracks or skin rubbing can indicate a poor-fitting plaster that can lead to plaster sores and skin infection. Any concerns with regard to a child with a plaster must be reported to a senior nurse or medical staff, as it may be necessary to remove or modify the plaster.

The cast should be kept dry at all times, as moisture will soften the cast and it will cease to achieve its clinical objective, i.e. maintaining fracture alignment. Wet plasters have to be removed. Removing a wet cast and applying a new cast is not desirable, because there is a grave risk that the fracture alignment or surgical correction will be lost. If this occurs then further surgical intervention may be necessary.

Casts should not be covered with plastic for showering or bathing, because condensation forms under the plastic and

Procedures Box 41.2 Ongoing nursing care of a child in plaster

Action
Keep the cast dry.

Reasons *Moisture will soften the cast and it will cease to achieve its clinical objective, i.e. maintaining fracture alignment.*
Wet plasters have to be removed, risking loss of fracture alignment or surgical correction; further surgical intervention may be necessary.

Action
Do not cover the cast with plastic for showering or bathing.

Reason *Condensation can form under the plastic and make the cast wet.*

Action
Do not put anything down the cast.

Reason *Small objects may not be retrieved and will cause a pressure sore.*

Action
Do not use objects to scratch the skin under the cast, for example knitting needles.

Reason *This may cause a skin laceration or traumatise the skin, making it more susceptible to sores.*

Action
Avoid beaches and sandpits.

Procedures Box 41.2 Ongoing nursing care of a child in plaster—cont'd

Reason *Sand under a plaster can cause skin abrasions.*

Action
Give the following discharge advice to the child and carers.

Seek medical advice if:

- the toes or fingers become blue, swollen and painful to move
- the limb becomes more painful
- pins and needles are felt in the digits or they feel numb
- the cast feels uncomfortable or rubbing is noticed
- an unpleasant smell is noticed from the cast and/or a discharge is seen on the plaster (Lucus & Davis 2005).

Reasons *For ongoing observation for neurovascular impairment or compartment syndrome.*
For ongoing observation of the cast functionality.
For ongoing observation for plaster sores and/or wound infection.

this results in making the cast wet. Children and their families should be advised to wrap the plaster with a towel to protect the plaster from splashes while conducting hygiene activities.

Do not put anything down the cast, as small objects may not be retrieved and will cause a pressure sore. Equally, objects should not be used to scratch the skin under the cast, for example knitting needles. This may cause a skin laceration or traumatise the skin, making it more susceptible to sores. Children and their families should be advised to avoid beaches and/or sand play because if sand gets under a plaster then it acts like sandpaper and makes the skin sore.

Before discharge from hospital the following discharge advice should be given to the child and his or her parents or carers.

ALERT
Medical advice should be sought immediately if the digits become blue, swollen and painful to move, or if the limb becomes more painful, pins and needles are felt in the digits or they become numb. All these signs are indicators of neurovascular deficit and potential compartment syndrome. Medical advice should also be sought if the cast feels uncomfortable or if rubbing is noticed. This indicates a functional problem with the cast. Also, an unpleasant smell from the cast and/or a discharge on the plaster may indicate a wound infection or infected plaster sore (Lucus & Davis 2005). This clearly needs further medical management.

Assessment of neurovascular status

Any child is at risk of neurovascular deficit or compartment syndrome following orthopaedic injury or trauma. A plaster cast can either initiate or compound neurovascular deficit and/or compartment syndrome. Therefore all children with a new cast applied must have regular neurovascular assessment.

Neurovascular deficit is the interruption, partial or complete, of the nerve or blood supply to a limb (Altizer 2002, Foley 1988). It may occur as a result of the injury or from treatment of the injury or orthopaedic condition (Maher et al 1994), and if left untreated it may precede to compartment syndrome. Commonly, neurovascular deficit results from a restricting plaster, bandage or traction. The blood vessels and nerves that supply the limb are compressed, resulting in diminished blood and nerve supply to the distal limb. If the external pressure is not relieved it may lead to compartment syndrome.

Compartment syndrome occurs because there is 'high pressure within the muscle compartment in the closed fascial space' (Pellino & Polacek 1994), which 'reduces capillary blood flow below a level necessary for tissue viability' (Scott & Mubarak 1995). Commonly after an injury or surgery a haematoma develops within the muscle or swelling occurs from an inflammatory response. The muscle is encased by the fascia, which does not have the capacity to expand. Therefore the pressure internalises on the blood vessels and nerves that permeate the muscle compartment, ultimately impinging the blood and nerve supply and resulting in muscle necrosis. If left untreated this may lead to amputation of the limb (Whitesides et al 1975) or even death of the patient due to renal failure (Love 1998).

Signs and symptoms of neurovascular impairment or compartment syndrome, and nursing observations

Dykes (1993) lists the signs and symptoms of compartment syndrome as the five *P*'s: pain, pallor, paraesthesia, paralysis and pulselessness (Table 41.1). An additional indicator is coldness.

Nursing observations for neurovascular impairment should occur at least hourly, and more frequently if there is clinical concern.

Procedures Box 41.3 Neurovascular assessment

Actions
Carry out regular pain assessments using an age-appropriate pain tool.

Give all prescribed analgesia.

Reason *Increasing pain out of proportion to the injury or surgical intervention is the first most reliable sign (Wright & Bogoch 1992).*

Actions
Observe perfusion of digits on the affected limb.

Assess capillary refill time to check whether it is less than 1 s.

Reason *Pallor: if there is compartmental pressure then the blood vessels will be partially or completely occluded, reducing blood flow.*

Actions
Ask if the child can feel pins and needles in the digits.

Lightly touch all digits, asking the child to confirm that she or he can feel the touch and that the feeling is normal or the same as in the non-affected hand.

Reason *Paraesthesia: if there is compartmental pressure then the nerves will be partially or completely occluded, reducing nerve conduction.*

Action
Ask the child to move the affected digits; the child may be reluctant to move the digits because of pain but should be able to do so.

Reason *Paralysis will occur if the blood and nerve supply to a muscle is occluded.*

Action
Record the pulse distal to the site of injury. It may be necessary to make a hole in the plaster to access the pulse.

Reason *Pulselessness: the last sign; if pulselessness occurs then the compartment syndrome is well established and amputation is likely, as the blood supply has been completely occluded.*

Action
Feel the digits for warmth and compare with the other limb.

Reason *Coldness will result if the blood supply is reduced or occluded.*

Now test your knowledge

- How long does it take for plaster of Paris to dry?
- How long does it take for a resin-based cast to dry?
- How should a plaster be dried?
- How should you handle a plaster and why?
- When should a patient and/or parent or carer seek further medical advice?
- List the signs and symptoms of compartment syndrome.
- What could be the outcome if compartment syndrome is left untreated?

References

Altizer L (2002) Neurovascular assessment. Orthopaedic Essentials 21(4):48–50

Dykes PC (1993) Minding the five Ps of neurovascular assessment. American Journal of Nursing 93(6):38–39

Foley J (1988) Pinch and squeeze: neurovascular assessment in extremity injuries. Emergency Medical Services 17(5):73–83

Love C (1998) A discussion and analysis of nurse led pain assessment for the early detection of compartment syndrome. Journal of Orthopaedic Nursing 2(3):160–167

Lucus B, Davis P (2005) Why restricting movement is important. In Kneale J, Davis P (eds) Orthopaedic and trauma nursing. Churchill Livingstone, London, p 105–139

Maher AB, Salmond SW, Pellino TA (eds) (1994) Orthopaedic nursing. Saunders, Philadelphia

Pellino T, Polacek L (1994) Complications of orthopaedic disorders and orthopaedic surgery. In Maher A, Salmond S, Pellino T (eds) Orthopaedic nursing. Saunders, Philadelphia, p 196–238

Prior M, Miles S (1999) Principles of casting. Journal of Orthopaedic Nursing 3(3):162–170

Scott J, Mubarak MD (1995) Technique of diagnosis and treatment of the lower extremity compartment syndromes in children. Operative Techniques in Orthopaedics 5(2):178–189

Whitesides TE, Haney TC, Morimoto K, Harada H (1975) Tissue pressure measurements as a determinant for the need of fasciotomy. Clinical Orthopaedics and Related Research 113:43–51

Wright J, Bogoch ER (1992) Compartment syndrome: a diagnostic dilemma. Journal of the American Academy of Physician Assistants 5(2):94–98

42

Skeletal pin site care

Sonya Clarke • Olga Richardson

Today the orthopaedic treatment of children reflects innovative multiprofessional practice that has embraced significant developments such as the use of external fixation devices. These devices, whether monolateral, multiplanar or hybrid (Gugenheim 2004), with their multiple pins and wires, offer treatment options for a number of conditions such as the management of fractures, correction of limb length discrepancy and conditions such as Perthes' disease (Caterall 2006). Orthopaedic pins and wires have been used in practice for many years to apply skeletal traction; however, the use of external fixation devices (Maiocchi 1998) such as the monolateral external fixator (Fi g. 42.1), with the pins penetrating just into the bone, and the multiplanar Ilizarov frame (Fig. 42.2), with the pins penetrating through the bone and exiting on the other side, have increased their use.

This use of multiple pins has increased the risk of complications such as intractable pain, tethering and tenting of the surrounding skin, muscle spasm, swelling and soft tissue tension, and infection at the pin site, which is the main concern and can result in loosening of the pin, loss of fixation and osteomyelitis (Patterson 2005). Pin site care, which is identified by Santy (2000a) as requiring specialised nursing care, is a psychomotor skill initially undertaken by the nurse and then executed by either the child or the parent following appropriate education and a period of supervised practice. This chapter addresses the evidence on how best to manage and care for pins and wires, which fundamentally aims to reduce or prevent the aforementioned complications.

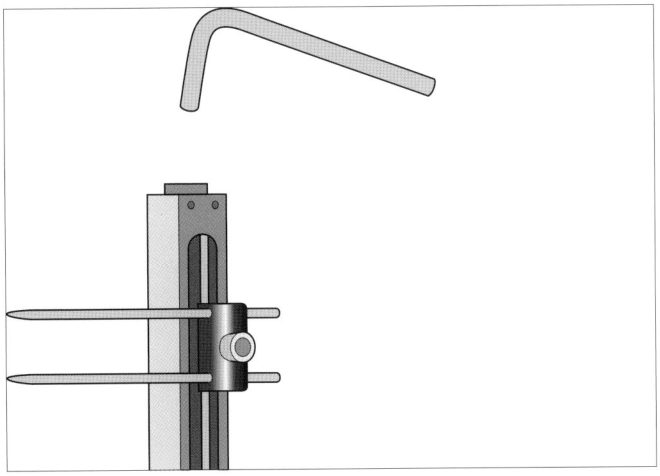

Fig. 42.1 • A monolateral external fixator.

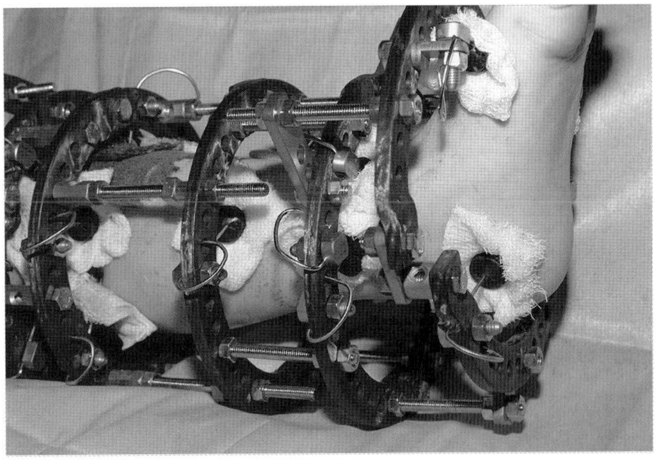

Fig. 42.2 • A multiplanar Ilizarov frame.

Definitions of infection

Patterson (2005) in the USA highlights that the terms *reaction* and *infection* have been interchangeably used in the literature, describing Jones-Walton's (1988: 30) definition of pin site reaction as 'adverse tissue response to the presence of skeletal pins 72 hours after insertion that either resolves spontaneously, requires lancing of the skin around the pin (incision and drainage) or necessitated removal of the pins'. In the UK the expert British nursing consensus group on pin site care (Lee-Smith et al 2001) differentiate clearly between the terms *reaction*, *colonisation* and *infection* when discussing pin site care. Definitions developed from the consensus group are as follows.

- *Reaction.* Reaction refers to the normal changes that occur at the pin site interface following insertion of the pin and include changes in normal skin tone, increased warmth and serous or bloody ooze at the pin site.
- *Colonisation.* Colonisation is present when the skin around the pin site is red and warm with increased drainage, associated pain at the pin site and microbes present in cultures.
- *Infection.* Infection includes all signs outlined above, with visible drainage of pus, pin loosening and increased microbial growth.

Various classifications have been outlined that grade the level of infection (Checketts 2000, Saleh & Scott 1992, Ward 1998).

Table 42.1. Stages of pin site reaction

Stage	Clinical finding	Treatment
1	Copious serous drainage in the first 72 h	Absorbent dressing
2	Superficial cellulites: erythema, tenderness, swelling around the pin	Oral antibiotics
3	Deep infection: purulent drainage, swelling erythema over several pins, loose pins	Intravenous antibiotics or pin removal
4	Osteomyelitis: loose pin, radiological ring sequestrum, persistent drainage	Surgical debridement, intravenous antibiotics (long term)

Rockwood et al (1996) outlined stages representing the severity of infection and definitive treatment, which correspond to Sims & Saleh's (1996) classification adapted by Patterson (2005) in Table 42.1.

Factors contributing to reaction and infection have been identified as skeletal pin type, pin size and location, surgical technique of insertion, length of time in situ, pin care protocol, skin tension and motion (Gordon et al 2000, Hutson & Zych 1998, Teebagy 1996), while Marsh (2004) has highlighted the issue of the mechanical integrity of the pin–bone interface or pin stability.

Evidence indicates that infection rates vary widely because of the different ways of defining infection, different research methods utilised and differing populations studied (Gordon et al 2000, Hay et al 1997, Henry 1996, Sims & Saleh 2000). It is important that hospital trusts and agencies use a standardised way of defining pin site infection in order to assist internal monitoring.

Management of skeletal pin site care

Issues to be addressed include method and frequency of cleansing, choice of dressing, management of crusts, skin adherence to the pin, general care of the patient, risk assessment in pin site care and education of the patient and family.

Method of cleansing

There is much debate regarding the choice of cleansing solutions and little research evidence to support their use. In 1996 Sims & Saleh carried out a survey on pin site care in 68 hospitals in the UK, which demonstrated the use of normal saline 0.9% (70%), povidone–iodine (12%), chlorhexidine (12%), surgical spirits (alcohol, 6%), and hydrogen peroxide (6%). The survey reported the use of 54 pin site care protocols based on doctor or nurse preference.

Wound research has reported that hydrogen peroxide and the use of Betadine (povidone–iodine) at certain concentrations may be cytotoxic to osteoblasts and damaging to healthy tissues (Kaysinger et al 1995, Rabenberg et al 2002). In addition, hydrogen peroxide at 1:10 and 1:5 concentrations may not be bactericidal (Rabenberg et al 2002). Hydrogen peroxide is used more frequently in the USA, and recently Patterson (2005) in a small study demonstrated that cleaning with half-strength hydrogen peroxide and applying Xeroform dressings had the best outcome of the seven protocols she examined. However, the generalisability of the findings is limited by the small sample size, therefore necessitating further study.

A recent prospective study by Davies et al (2005) compared two protocols of operative technique and pin site care in 120 patients with external fixation. Group A (46 patients) had care of the pin sites using saline (Sims & Saleh 1996), and group B (74 patients) were treated with the technique used by the Russian Ilizarov Scientific Centre for Restorative Traumatology and Orthopaedics. The Russian method uses a strong antiseptic solution (chlorhexidine), which imparts a drying effect to the skin, and bulky pressure dressings to restrict movement between the skin and pin. Results showed that in group B a lower proportion of infected pin sites were reported and the time to the first episode of infection was longer, with a 50% incidence of an infected pin after 24 days in group A (traditional method) but only after 90 days in group B. However, in group B prolonged skin contact with a strong antiseptic solution produced hypersensitivity reactions in 13 (17.6%) patients (Davies et al 2005). The substitution of alcoholic chlorhexidine with normal saline in these patients resolved the hypersensitivity issue but resulted in the development of pin site infection in 12 patients. More recently, Holmes & Brown (2005) reported on a non-experimental study by W-Dahl & Toksvig-Larsen (2004), who compared the use of chlorhexidine 2 mg/mL with normal saline 0.9% as a cleansing agent. There were fewer positive cultures, a lower frequency of *Staphylococcus aureus* and fewer days' use of antibiotics. Also, lower rates of grade 2 infections were found with chlorhexidine using the Checketts et al (1993) classification system. More randomised controlled trials are required, but these findings would appear to support Davies et al (2005) and Henry (1996) regarding the higher incidence of infection with saline.

Previously, in 1996, Henry's randomised controlled trial compared the use of normal saline 0.9% with 70% alcohol and a no solution group (dry gauze removal of crusting) to cleanse the skin around the pin sites. The findings indicated that the lowest rate of pin site infection was 7.5% in the no solution group, with a 25% infection rate in the group using normal saline 0.9% and a 17.5% infection rate in the 70% alcohol group. These findings appeared to indicate that the use of alcohol results in a lower infection rate than the use of normal saline; however, Kerstein (1997) reminds us that alcohol evaporates and is toxic to healthy tissue.

A high rate of infection has also been reported with soap-and-water protocols (Hutson & Zych 1998, Sproles 1985). Recently, Gordon et al (2000) in a study on children compared a nihilistic approach of no care versus showering using soap and water, and noted that all the children who showered required oral antibiotics on several occasions. The authors suggested that the outcome was due to the soap residue that remained and irritated the tissues.

The British consensus group of expert orthopaedic nurses on pin site care (Lee-Smith et al 2001) in the UK suggested that because of the limited research studies available, sterile normal saline or water should be used to clean the area around the pin sites. Although the research is limited, it must be said that the studies of Henry (1996) and more recently of Davies et al (2005) and W-Dahl & Toksvig-Larsen (2004) appear to indicate a higher infection rate with the use of normal saline in comparison with chlorhexidine or alcohol, and that there is a better outcome with chlorhexidine (Davies et al 2005, W-Dahl & Toksvig-Larsen 2004).

Frequency of pin site care

To ensure patient comfort and early detection of potential complications the wound should be inspected within 24h (Blaisier et al 1992). All pin sites should be dressed after 24h, as there is likely to be exudate. However, no solution should be used on the immediate postoperative dressing (Henry 1996, Lee-Smith et al 2001) except to clean exudate and blood away from the surrounding area using aseptic technique. One randomised study of adults who were operated on for knee deformities found equivalent infection rates with daily and weekly pin site care using 0.9% normal saline solution (W-Dahl et al 2003). Marsh (2004), citing Moroni et al (2002), offered the opinion that 'the development and severity of pin-site infection is probably associated more with the mechanical integrity of the pin–bone interface or pin stability than with the technique of caring for the pin-sites'. Holmes & Brown (2005) recommend weekly pin site care for pins that are considered to be problematic but indicated that in all other papers reviewed pin site care was undertaken daily. Pin site care should, however, be increased if mechanical signs of looseness or early signs of infection are present. The British consensus group (Lee-Smith et al 2001) indicate that pin sites should be cleaned only if exudate is present, otherwise do not clean. Therefore we would recommend cleaning only if there is exudate present.

Showering

General hygiene needs may be met by showering providing there are no contraindications by the manufacturer of the external fixator. According to Holmes & Brown (2005), a review of pin site care webpages revealed that there are quite a few practices in the USA and Europe that allow showering after 5–10 days. Gordon et al's (2000) study examined children with tibial fixators with the pins open to water flow after postoperative day 5. No major infections occurred in the 212 pin sites. This practice is supported by the Sheffield protocol (Sims & Saleh 2000). In addition, the consensus group of orthopaedic nurse experts on pin site care (Lee-Smith et al 2001) in the UK recommend showering and drying the fixator with a clean towel afterwards. They state that there is little support for sterile cleansing after showering. In contrast, the W-Dahl studies (W-Dahl & Toksvig-Larsen 2004, W-Dahl et al 2003) required covering of the fixator during showering. This would support the British consensus group for pin site care and recommends showering.

Dressings

The use of dressings is another issue for which there is no research and considerable variation in practice. Dressing type may or may not include the use of antibiotic agents (dry gauze versus antibiotic-impregnated gauze or application of antibiotic ointment). Betadine was used quite frequently before 1996 but caused skin staining and allergic reactions (Bernardo 2001, Santy 2000b, Teebagy 1996). Sims & Saleh's survey in 1996 found great variation in practice regarding the type of dressing; 29% used dressings all the time whereas 71% used dressings only when pins were draining. Dressing type (stable versus loose or no dressing) may also affect infection rates because the dressing type may influence the degree of movement at the tissue–pin interface, which has been associated with increased infection (Hutson & Zych 1998, Mahan et al 1991). Davies et al (2005) report the use of bulky pressure dressings to restrict movement between the skin and pin in the Russian method, which may have influenced the outcome in their study. More research is needed.

All pin sites should be redressed after 24h. Dressings should be absorbent, non-stick, easy to remove and inexpensive (Lee-Smith et al 2001), and they should be of a non-shredding material such as gauze (Rowe 1997). Sims & Saleh (1996) highlighted the importance of applying a little pressure with the dressing to prevent tenting of the skin along the pin, and more recently Sims & Saleh (2000) suggest using a rolled gauze dressing only if there is exudate during the first 48h, when there is often drainage. Patterson (2005) demonstrated the effectiveness of a non-stick dressing, and in the W-Dahl studies (W-Dahl & Toksvig-Larsen 2004, W-Dahl et al 2003) a non-stick absorbent dressing was held in place with a soft roll dressing. Tape should not be used to hold the soft roll dressing to the skin or pin. This supports the use of non-stick absorbent dressing if there is exudate.

Management of crusts

There is no agreement regarding the management of crusts. Crusts may form at the pin site interface (Ward 1998). Henry (1996) and Lee-Smith et al (2001) require crust removal, whereas W-Dahl & Toksvig-Larsen (2004) specified no crust removal unless signs of infection were present. Crusts are considered by some to be a normal protective mechanism, and removing them could disturb healthy tissue, increasing the risk of infection. However, the British expert panel on pin site care (Lee-Smith et al 2001) specify that if exudate remains after showering it should be removed using normal saline or boiled water. Scab or crust removal has been indicated to allow drainage of exudate that could be a refuge for infection (Hay et al 1997,

Hutson & Zych 1998, Santy 2000b, Sims & Saleh 1996). We would recommend crust removal.

Skin adherence to the pin

The Sheffield protocol (Sims & Saleh 2000) and Henry (1996) recommend massage to release skin that adheres to the pin. The term *massage* simply means the freeing of skin from the pin to allow free drainage. Cleaning or rubbing with dry gauze is considered sufficient to prevent skin adherence and allow free drainage (Lee-Smith et al 2001). Less movement at the pin and bone interface is preferable, as movement will predispose to infection (Lee-Smith et al 2001, Marsh 2004).

General care of the patient

General care of the patient should include regular observation of the pin sites and circulation of the limb. The practitioner should note any pain or tenderness reported at the pin site, along with evidence of increased exudate, pus, odour and signs of inflammation. According to Hutson & Zych (1998) the skin should not be taut or tenting along the pin. Monitoring of infection and any other pathology should be ongoing.

Risk assessment

It is important to consider risk assessment in patient care, and Lee-Smith et al (2001) identified the physical, social and psychological factors that may have an adverse effect on patient care and outcome and that require discussion regarding treatment options between the patient and healthcare professionals (Box 42.1).

Patient and family information and teaching

The education and support of patients and their family is important, as for many patients the external fixation devices are applied following trauma with little or no time for preoperative information.

LINK CHAPTER 2

Children especially need time spent in explaining and helping them to understand the need for the device.

LINK CHAPTER 3

Information needs to be available in written, oral and visual format. A combination of written material, illustrations, oral presentations and practice sessions enhances the amount of information the individual retains (Beare 1999, Phillips 1999). The use of clear simple language free of jargon and medical terminology will enhance verbal instructions (Phillips 1999). The image of an external fixator can have considerable impact on patients and their body image and in some instances can lead to non-compliance regarding care. Patient compliance is fundamental to a successful outcome, and poor compliance with educational programmes often occurs because of the patient's inability to understand instructions. Having the patient and carer repeat instructions as the nurse writes them down in familiar terms improves the patient's comprehension of material (Phillips 1999). The use of the specialist Ilizarov nurse, meeting other patients with a device in situ and information regarding the Ilizarov wearers support group are also very helpful. Regular contact with healthcare personnel assists in maintaining compliance and provides a point of contact.

Patients and families who are taught how to care for their device in hospital should be reassured about their competence once discharged home. The specialist nurse should liaise with general practitioners and community nurses to give them consistent support and up-to-date advice regarding evidence-based care regimens. It is important that the care is maintained at home.

Box 42.1. The presence of underlying pathological changes, including the effects of ageing or medications

- Poor nutritional status
- Smoking
- Compromised capillary blood flow
- Depressed or immature immune system and immune response
- The presence of other infections
- Social environment; level of personal hygiene; or activities such as being outdoors, in playgrounds or in dirt
- Poor patient understanding and compliance with regimens
- The effects of trauma: high-impact injury, excess skin loss or dirty wound
- Inappropriate surgical technique, insertion during night hours
- Pins being sited too close to joints (Hutson & Zych 1998)
- Inappropriate or inadequate pin site care
- Loosening or motion between the pin and the surrounding tissues (Mahan et al 1991)

(From Lee-Smith et al 2001.)

Clinical guidelines

Clinical protocols and guidelines act as a framework to assist healthcare personnel with clinical decision making in practice. As Holmes & Brown (2005) highlight, they reflect the current evidence-based knowledge from the literature regarding the effectiveness and appropriateness of procedures and practices culled from critical reviews of research literature and expert opinion. A review of the literature confirms that opinion differs on the most appropriate management of skeletal pin sites and that protocols are often based on doctor or nurse preference (Sims & Saleh 1996). There is little scientific evidence to support one technique over another (Gordon et al 2000), and indeed the literature highlights the dearth of actual completed research studies on skeletal pin site care. The guidelines in this chapter are offered as recommendations demonstrating only the traditional and Russian methods, and they should be used in conjunction with local guidelines for wound care and infection control and following discussion and agreement with other relevant members of the healthcare team and reviewed on an ongoing basis.

Procedures Box 42.1 Traditional method for cleaning pin sites (wires and pins)

Action
Prepare the patient:

- seek verbal consent
- check the patient's position or alternatively check if the shower room is vacant.

Actions
Record the patient's pain score.

Offer analgesia, if appropriate.

Reason *There is potential pain during pin site dressings.*

Actions
Collect the required equipment:

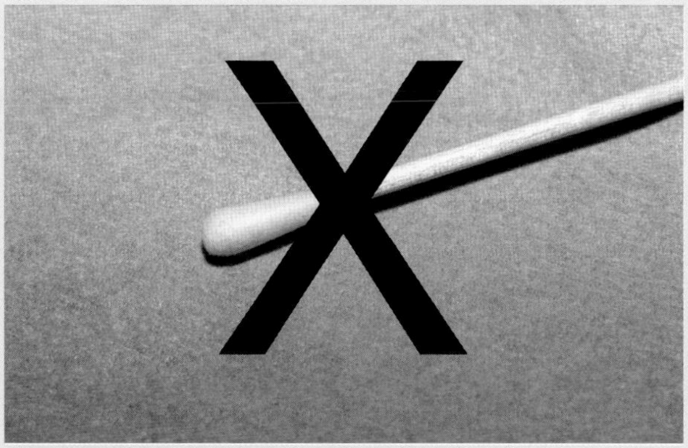

- dressing pack
- apron
- sterile scissors
- sterile gloves
- non-sterile gloves
- forceps (optional)
- cleaning solution
- tape
- non-woven gauze and *not* Q-tips (long cotton buds).

On day 1 or 2 post surgery, reduce and renew dressings at the bedside using aseptic technique (no shower).

Leave no fibres at the pin site.

Action
Wash and dry your hands and put on a plastic apron.

Reason *Prevents cross-infection.*

Action
Apply non-sterile gloves.

Action
Remove existing dressings and discard them in a yellow clinical waste bag.

Reason *Exposes pin sites.*

Action
Inspect all pin sites.

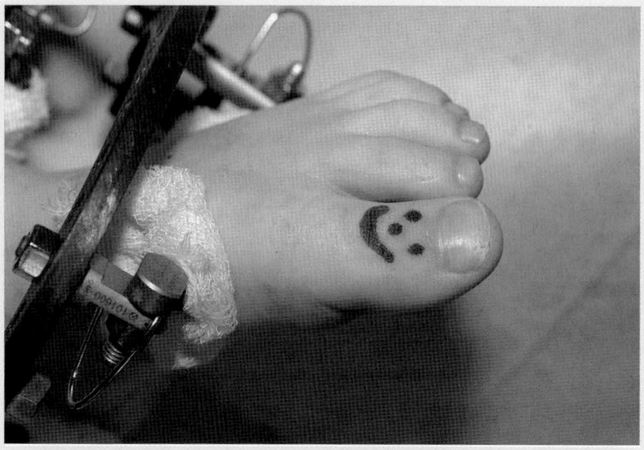

Reason *To observe for signs of pin site reaction or infection.*

Action
Wash your hands.

Reason *Prevents cross-infection.*

Action
Open all sterile dressings and equipment to be used.

Reason *Prepares for aseptic technique.*

Action
Using a separate piece of non-woven gauze (gloved finger or forceps), clean each individual pin site using a sweeping action.

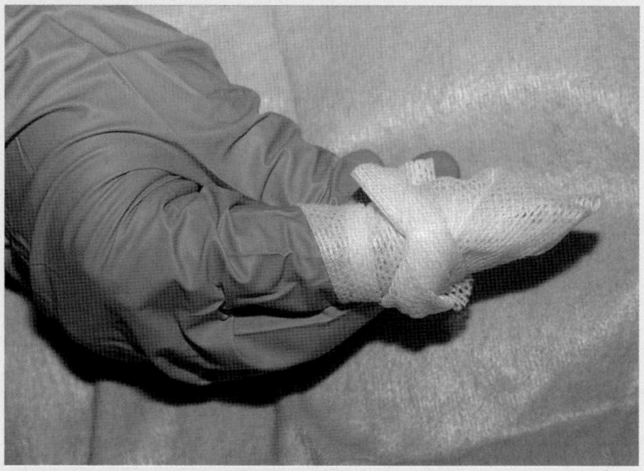

Reasons *Attempts to prevent infection at the pin site. Non-woven gauze will not shed; Q-tips produce shedding fibres.*

Actions
Following 24–48 h, postoperative reduction and redressing of pin sites at the bedside.

Procedures Box 42.1 Traditional method for cleaning pin sites (wires and pins)—cont'd

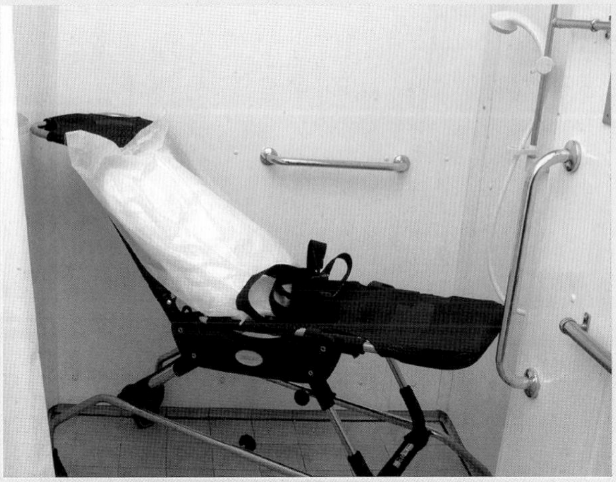

Commence daily showering of pin sites: clean away exudate or dried blood from skin using normal saline or chlorohexidine 2 mg/mL and attach required gauze rolls, otherwise do not clean.

A shower chair (as shown) can be used to assist in the cleaning of pin sites.

Actions
Keep metalwork socially clean.

Gently remove scabs and crusts around the pin site.

Reason *Attempts to prevent infection at the pin site.*

Actions
Clean or dry rub the surrounding skin with gauze.

Do not massage.

Reason *Prevents skin tenting or tethering.*

Action
Expose pin sites if non-symptomatic.

Reason *Prevents infection.*

Action
Re-dress red or oozing pin sites with gauze roll and secure with tape (alternatively at the bedside on return from the shower room).

Reason *Soaks up exudate.*

Actions
Place solutions in a secure cupboard.

Discard all dressings, gloves and the apron in a clinical waste bag.

Reason *For health and safety.*
Prevents cross-infection.

Action
Wash your hands.

Reason *Prevents cross-infection.*

Action
Reassess the patient's pain score.

Reason *To review analgesia.*

Actions
Teach the patient to shower at home and dry the fixator with a clean towel used only for this purpose.

Actively clean pin sites only if exudate is present.

Keep the regimen simple and provide instruction.

Expect poor or non compliance.

Reason *Tampering with pin sites excessively can lead to infection.*

Action
Educate the patient, family and community staff to look for signs of pin infection.

Reason *Identifies problems early.*

Actions
Provide as much written and verbal information as possible, with contact numbers.

Provide opportunities to contact other patients and support groups.

Reason *Reduces anxiety, increases compliance and provides support.*

Action
Provide psychosocial support.

Reason *Pins and wires amount to a major insult to self-image.*

(After Lee Smith et al 2001.)

Procedures Box 42.2 Russian method for cleaning pin sites (wires and pins)

Actions
Prepare the patient:

- seek verbal consent
- check the patient's position.

Collect the required equipment:

- dressing pack
- sterile scissors
- sterile gloves
- bandages
- non-sterile gloves
- forceps (optional)
- Hydrex (pink chlorhexidine gluconate 0.5% w/v, 70% v/v)
- non-woven gauze squares.

Actions
Record the patient's pain score.

Offer analgesia, if appropriate.

Reason *There is potential pain during pin site dressings.*

Actions
On day 2 post surgery, reduce and renew dressings.

Procedures Box 42.2 Russian method for cleaning pin sites (wires and pins)—cont'd

Thereafter dressings will be changed at 7-day intervals (a shower can be taken prior to pin site care).

Leave no fibres at the pin site.

Action
Wash and dry your hands and put on a plastic apron.

Reason *Prevents cross-infection.*

Action
Pull back the black rubber bungs.

Reason *Provides access to existing dressings.*

Action
Apply non-sterile gloves.

Action
Remove existing bandages and dressings and discard them in a yellow clinical waste bag.

Reason *Exposes pin sites.*

Action
Inspect all pin sites.

Reason *To observe for signs of infection etc.*

Action
Wash your hands.

Reason *Prevents cross-infection.*

Action
Open all sterile dressings and equipment to be used.

Reason *Prepares for aseptic technique.*

Action
Apply sterile gloves.

Reason *Prevents cross-infection.*

Action
Prepare gauze squares by making a slit in the gauze (keyhole dressing).

Reason *Allows the gauze to fit over the wire at the pin site.*

Action
Using a separate piece of gauze (gloved finger or forceps), clean each individual pin site with Hydrex 0.5% w/v 70% v/v alcohol solution using a sweeping action.

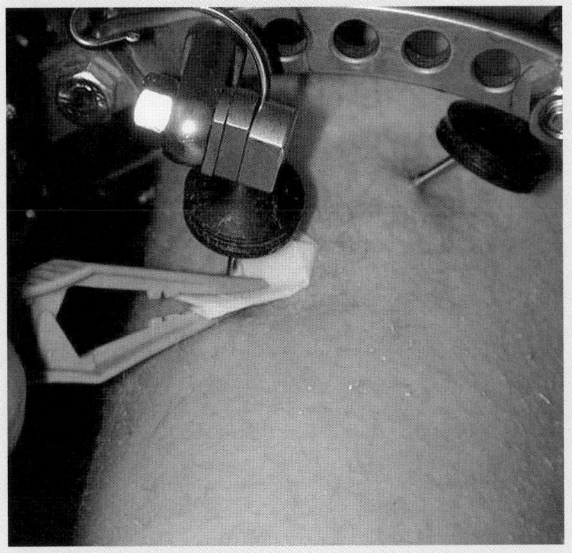

Reason *Attempts to prevent infection at the pin site.*

Actions
Do not remove crusts or scabs.

Keep metalwork socially clean.

Reason *Attempts to prevent infection at the pin site.*

Action
Moisten all required gauze squares in Hydrex 0.5% w/v 70% v/v alcohol solution and remove excess liquid from each gauze square.

Reason *Attempts to prevent infection at the pin site and reduce skin irritation.*

Actions
Apply the moistened keyhole gauze square dressing to each pin site.

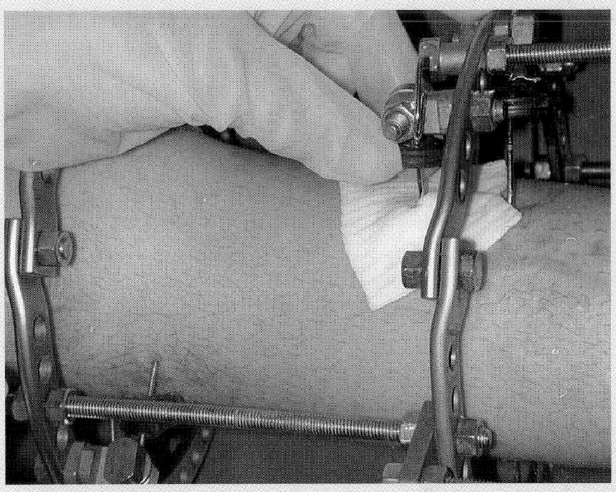

Use keyhole dressings of gauze, two or three layers thick and moistened with Hydrex solution–alcoholic chlorhexidine, with excess liquid removed.

Reason *Prevents infection and skin irritation.*

Action
Position the rubber bung on to each presoaked gauze square at each pin site.

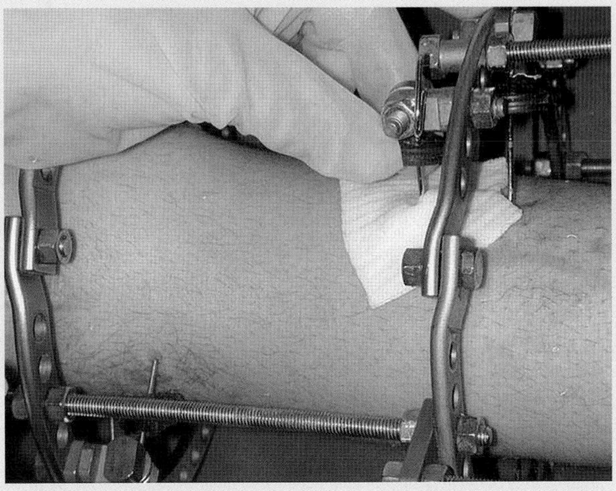

Procedures Box 42.2 Russian method for cleaning pin sites (wires and pins)—cont'd

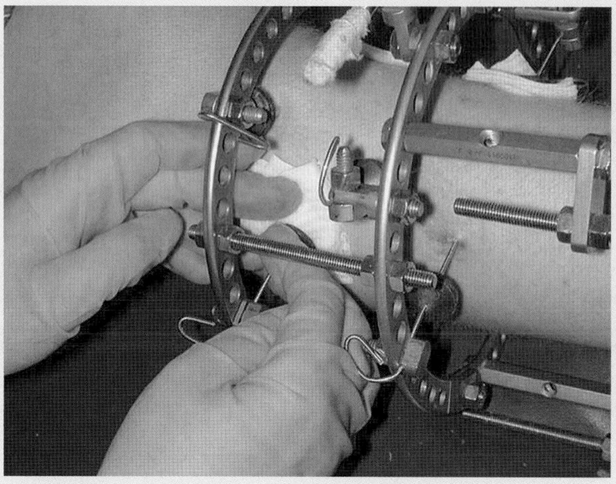

Reason *Secures gauze stays in position at the pin site.*

Actions
Bandage each pin site.

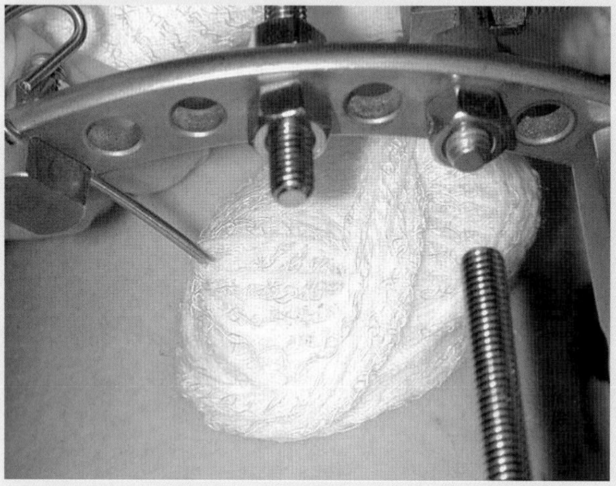

Bandage in a figure of eight to secure dressings and ensure that the bungs do not lift.

Action
Place solutions in a secure cupboard and discard all dressings, gloves and the apron in a clinical waste bag.

Reasons *For health and safety.*
Prevents cross-infection.

Action
Wash your hands.

Reason *Prevents cross-infection.*

Action
Reassess the patient's pain score.

Reason *To review analgesia.*

Actions
Teach the patient and family a similar regimen.

Keep the regimen simple and provide instruction.

Expect poor or non-compliance.

Reason *Tampering with pin sites excessively can lead to infection.*

Actions
Educate the patient, family and community staff to look for signs of pin infection.

In some cases arrangements can be made to have the dressings completed by the Ilizarov nurse specialist.

Reason *Identifies problems early.*

Actions
Provide as much written and verbal information as possible, with contact numbers.

Provide opportunities to contact other patients and support groups.

Reason *Reduces anxiety, increases compliance and provides support.*

Action
Provide psychosocial support.

Reason *Pins and wires amount to a major insult to self-image.*

(After Davies et al 2005 and Lee Smith et al 2001.)

Now test your knowledge

- How would you educate the child and parent about the care of pin sites?
- What would you be advising and checking when supervising the child and parent carrying out pin site care?
- Consider the impact of having an external fixator in situ on the child and family.

References

Beare PG (1999) Health teaching and compliance. In Stanley M, Beare PG (eds) Gerontological nursing: a health promotion/protection approach, 2nd edn. FA Davis, Philadelphia, p 55–63

Bernardo JM (2001) Evidence-based practice for pin-site care in injured children. Orthopaedic Nursing 20(5):29–34

Blaisier RD, Aronson J, Turskey EA (1992) External fixation of paediatric femur fractures. Journal of Paediatric Orthopaedics 17(3):342–346

Caterall A (2006) Reading list: Perthes' disease. Online. Available: http://www.jbjs.org.uk/misc/RLperthesdisease,dtl

Checketts RG (2000) Pin track infection and the principles of pin site care. In De Bastiani A, Apley AG, Goldberg DE (eds) Orthofix external fixation in trauma and orthopaedics. Springer, Berlin, p 97–103

Checketts RG, Otterburn M, MacEachern G (1993) Pin track infection: definition, incidence and prevention. Journal of Orthopaedic Trauma 3(suppl.):16–18

Davies R, Holt N, Nayagam S (2005) The care of pin sites with external fixation. Journal of Bone and Joint Surgery 87B:5716–5719

Gordon JE, Kelly-Hahn J, Carpenter CJ, Schoenecker PL (2000) Pin site care during external fixation in children: results of a nihilistic approach. Journal of Paediatric Orthopaedics 20:163–165

Gugenheim JJ (2004) External fixation in orthopaedics. JAMA 291:2122–2124

Hay SM, Rickman M, Saleh M (1997) Fracture of the tibial diaphysis treated by external fixation and the axial alignment grid: a single surgeon's experience. Injury 28(7):437–443

Henry C (1996) Pin sites: do we need to clean them? Practice Nursing 7(4):12–17

Holmes S, Brown S (2005) Skeletal pin site care: National Association of Orthopaedic Nurses guidelines for orthopaedic nursing. Orthopaedic Nursing 24(2):99–107

Hutson J, Zych G (1998) Infections in periarticular fractures of the lower extremity treated with tensioned wire hybrid fixators. Journal of Orthopaedic Trauma 12(3):214–218

Jones-Walton P (1988) Effects of pin care on pin reactions in adults with extremity fracture treated with skeletal traction and external fixation. Orthopaedic Nursing 7(4):29–33

Kaysinger KK, Nicholson NC, Ramp WK, Kellman JF (1995) Toxic effects of wound irrigation solutions on cultured tibiae and osteoblasts. Journal of Orthopaedic Trauma 9(4):303–311

Kerstein M (1997) The scientific basis of healing. Advances in Wound Care 10(3):30–36

Lee-Smith J, Santy J, Davis P, Jester R, Kneale J (2001) Pin site management. Towards a consensus: part 1. Journal of Orthopaedic Nursing 5:37–42

Mahan J, Seligson D, Henry S, Hynes P, Dobbins J (1991) Factors in pin tract infection. Orthopaedics 14(3):305–308

Maiocchi A (1998) General principles of the Ilizarov external fixation. In Maiocchi A (ed.) Treatment of fractures, non unions and bone loss of the tibia with the Ilizarov method. Smith & Nephew, Memphis

Marsh JL (2004) Commentary on W-Dahl et al 2003. Journal of Bone and Joint Surgery 86A(8):1835.

Moroni A, Vannini F, Mosca M, Giannini S (2002) State of the art review: techniques to avoid pin loosening and infection in external fixation. Journal of Orthopaedic Trauma 16(3):189–195

Patterson M (2005) Multicentre pin site care study. Orthopaedic Nursing 24(5):349–359

Phillips LD (1999) Patient education: understanding the process to maximise time and outcomes. Journal of Intravenous Nursing 22(1):19–35

Rabenberg VS, Ingersoll CD, Sandrey MA, Johnson MT (2002) The bactericidal and toxic effects of antimicrobial wound cleansers. Journal of Athletic Training 37(1):51–54

Rockwood CA, Green DP, BuchHolz RW, Heekrian JD (1996) Rockwood and Green's fractures in adults, vol. 1, 4th edn. Lippincott-Raven, Philadelphia

Rowe S (1997) A review of the literature on the nursing care of skeletal pins in the paediatric and adolescent setting. Journal of Orthopaedic Nursing 1:26–29

Saleh M, Scott BW (1992) Pitfalls and complications in leg lengthening: the Sheffield experience. Seminsrs in Orthoapedics 7(3):207–222

Santy J (2000a) Nursing the patient with an external fixator. Nursing Standard 14(31):47–52

Santy J (2000b) Conference reports. Pin Sites Consensus Conference, 17 April 2000, Birmingham, UK. Journal of Orthopaedic Nursing 4:145–146

Sims M, Saleh M (1996) Protocols for the care of external fixator pinsites. Professional Nurse 11:261–264

Sims M, Saleh M (2000) External fixation – the incidence of pin site infection: a prospective audit. Journal of Orthopaedic Nursing 4(2):59–63

Sproles K (1985) Nursing care of skeletal pins: a closer look. Orthoapedic Nursing 4(1):11–19

Teebagy A (1996) Orthopaedic quality improvement plan: pin care study. University of Massachusetts, Worchester

Ward P (1998) Care of skeletal pins: a literature review. Nursing Standard 12:34–38

W-Dahl A, Toksvig-Larsen S (2004) Pin site care in external fixation: sodium chloride or chlorhexidine solution as a cleansing agent. Archives of Orthopaedic Trauma Surgery. Online. Available: http://www.springerlink.com/meche/BAGMPLRQMLJ&(DYVNYD9L/contributors/H/Q/H9Q

W-Dahl A, Toksvig-Larsen S, Lindstrand A (2003) No difference between daily and weekly pin site care: a randomised study of 50 patients with external fixation. Acta Orthopaedica Scandinavica 74(6):704–708

43

Breaking bad news to parents

Jayne Price • Patricia McNeilly

Breaking bad news is undoubtedly an extremely difficult and challenging process for any healthcare professional (Gregg & Vandekieft 2001, Smyth 2004, Wakefield 2000). The children's nurse is a key member of the multiprofessional team caring for the child and family, and as such is central to this complex communication process (Price et al 2006). In this chapter we specifically examine the multifaceted role of the children's nurse in the procedure of breaking bad news to parents.

Many definitions exist in the literature as to what constitutes bad news; it is essential to take cognizance of the fact that bad news can mean different things to different people. Bad news is any news that alters a patient's view of his or her future (Buckman, 1984). Arber & Gallagher (2003) identify bad news as any information that is not welcome. Another definition by Farrell (1999) discusses bad news as 'news of life-threatening illness, disability or impending or actual death'.

Bad news for parents within the child healthcare arena encompasses a variety of issues, which may include a congenital abnormality at birth (Bloom 2001, Robb 1999), diagnosis of a life-threatening or life-limiting illness (Association for Children with Life-threatening or Terminal Conditions & Royal College of Paediatrics and Child Health 2003, Department of Health, Social Services and Public Safety & Northern Ireland Group of the National Council for Hospice and Specialist Palliative Care 2003) or disability, the death of a child following an accident, or the fact that disease has reoccurred and that death is imminent. Given the range of situations in which bad news may need to be broken to parents, the children's nurse working in any area within the hospital or community setting may at some stage be involved in this challenging process and also in supporting families at this time. It is imperative to remember that there is no script for breaking bad news, with every situation being unique and each individual family being armed with their own values, beliefs, knowledge and experiences (Price et al 2006).

In a study examining general practitioners' experiences of breaking bad news, management of their own emotional responses was identified as the most difficult aspect of the process (Vegni et al 2001). Despite this, evidence suggests that there is little training for those involved in delivering bad news (Rabow & McPhee 2000, Smyth 2004). Wakefield et al (2003) suggest the value of giving nurses and doctors the opportunity of learning the skills necessary to engage in joint consultations when breaking bad news, as a means of enhancing practice. Indeed, there is much scope for the development of interprofessional education and training within this arena, particularly because two-thirds of parents of children with a severe disability have indicated their dissatisfaction in relation to how bad news was delivered (Quine & Pahl 1987).

Buckman (1992) highlights that when news is broken badly a detrimental and harmful effect can be experienced by those receiving the news. Other studies have also indicated that the way families were informed of the bad news was remembered in detail for a long time (Dear 1995, Department of Health 2003, Fallowfield 1993, Martin 1995). It is essential that the children's nurse recognises that communicating bad news well is not viewed as an optional skill but as a fundamental element of professional practice (Department of Health, Social Services and Public Safety & Northern Ireland Group of the National Council for Hospice and Specialist Palliative Care 2003).

A number of frameworks have been devised, although they do not provide a blueprint for the process but rather offer guidelines for directing thought processes and practice (Baile et al 2000, Department of Health, Social Services and Public Safety & Northern Ireland Group of the National Council for Hospice and Specialist Palliative Care 2003, Kaye 1996, Rabow & Mc Phee 2000). Many of the frameworks and the literature existing around this process are primarily focusing on the role of the medical staff, with little reference to the role of the nurse when the bad news is being broken.

Because of the lack of clarity about the role of the nurse, the expansion of nursing roles and the development of evidence-based practice within nursing, there has been some examination of the nurse's role in the process of breaking bad news (Arber & Gallagher 2003). A framework for the children's nurse's role in supporting parents who are hearing bad news has also been developed (Price et al 2006; Fig. 43.1), and although initially primarily designed for use with children's palliative care it can be applied to other areas within child healthcare practice.

In the medical literature, Rabow & McPhee (2000) discuss the importance of building a therapeutic environment and relationship with the person or people being told the bad news. They further suggest that providing a private area with adequate seating is important, as is the practice of using touch and empathy to create this therapeutic relationship. Peel (2003) feels very strongly that it would be unwise to presume that the doctor is the best person to break bad news. Buckman (1992) regards the responsibility of breaking bad news as that of the healthcare professional who has continuity of care and commitment to the patient. It is important to remember that relatives often expect to receive such news from a doctor, who

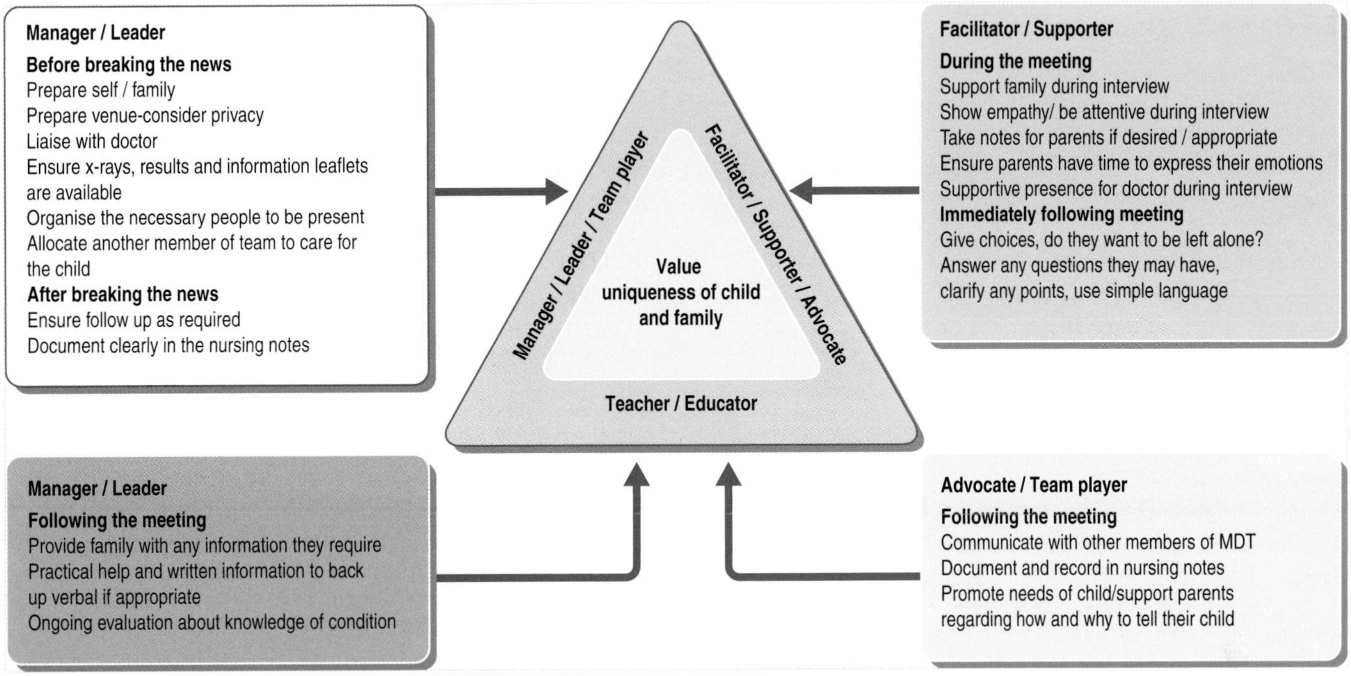
Manager / Leader
Before breaking the news
Prepare self / family
Prepare venue-consider privacy
Liaise with doctor
Ensure x-rays, results and information leaflets are available
Organise the necessary people to be present
Allocate another member of team to care for the child
After breaking the news
Ensure follow up as required
Document clearly in the nursing notes
Manager / Leader / Team player
Facilitator / Supporter / Advocate
Value uniqueness of child and family
Teacher / Educator
Facilitator / Supporter
During the meeting
Support family during interview
Show empathy/ be attentive during interview
Take notes for parents if desired / appropriate
Ensure parents have time to express their emotions
Supportive presence for doctor during interview
Immediately following meeting
Give choices, do they want to be left alone?
Answer any questions they may have, clarify any points, use simple language
Manager / Leader
Following the meeting
Provide family with any information they require
Practical help and written information to back up verbal if appropriate
Ongoing evaluation about knowledge of condition
Advocate / Team player
Following the meeting
Communicate with other members of MDT
Document and record in nursing notes
Promote needs of child/support parents regarding how and why to tell their child

Fig. 43.1 • A framework for supporting parents hearing bad news. (After Price et al 2006, International Journal of Palliative Nursing, reproduced with permission of MA Healthcare Ltd.)

they may see as having access to more information than other professionals (Cooley 2000). The Royal College of Nursing (1999) published guidance for nurses, midwives and health visitors supporting parents when they are told of their child's health disorder or disability. This guidance is described as a starting point, designed with the hope that it would stimulate the development of more detailed nursing policies at a local level (Royal College of Nursing 1999). The fact that this paper is entitled *Supporting Parents* would indicate that the nurse has a pivotal role in offering and facilitating support for the parents rather than actually breaking the news. This would be consistent with other literature, for example May (1993), who describes the nurse as the practical manager following disclosure and also an interpreter of medical information following the event (Department of Health, Social Services and Public Safety & Northern Ireland Group of the National Council for Hospice and Specialist Palliative Care 2003).

In order to ensure that nurses can interpret this information, if required, for the parents, it is essential that they are present to ensure that they know exactly what the parents have been told. In addition to the nurse's role post disclosure the nurse has a role prior to and during the meeting, organising, managing and offering a supportive presence to the family and also to the medical practitioner as required. Although it has been recognised that nurses and midwives may on occasions be involved in directly breaking bad news to parents (Bloom 2001, Reynolds 2003, Robb 1999), it is possibly more usual for the nurse to be present in a supportive role.

The process of breaking bad news

Regardless of who actually carries out the procedure, the breaking of bad news must be carried out within a partnership approach to caring, with the children's nurse having a key role to play (Casey 1988). The healthcare professional must use a broad perspective in order to address the holistic needs of the child and his or her family. In addition to physical needs, the psychological, social and spiritual needs of the child and family must therefore be pivotal in care packages, and when parents are being told of their child's health disorder this holistic approach is no exception (Price et al 2006). The child's and parents' cultural beliefs need to be considered; advice on supporting families of different cultures can be found at a number of websites (Child Bereavement Trust 2007, Department of Health 2007, Royal College of Nursing 2007).

The children's nurse has a multidimensional role, which includes that of facilitator, supporter, counsellor, educator, teacher, advocate for the child and key member of the multidisciplinary team (Graham & Price 2005). Baile et al (2000) describe the process of breaking bad news as attempting to address four essential goals (Box 43.1).

It may be suggested that two additional goals may be required: first, the need to foster realistic hope, if appropriate, for example in relation to the quality of life and symptom management; and furthermore, to outline specific support mechanisms available to the family within the hospital, community or hospice setting.

Box 43.1. Breaking bad news: the goals

1. Gather information from the patient and family.
2. Provide intelligible information in accordance with the patient's and family's needs and desires.
3. Support the patient and family by employing skills to reduce the emotional impact and isolation experienced by the recipient.
4. Develop a strategy, a plan of action, with input and cooperation from the patient and family.

(After Baile et al 2000, with permission.)

Medical models in existence provide organised recommendations in the form of the SPIKES mnemonic (Box 43.2). The aim of this model is to aid professionals breaking bad news in an empathic and straightforward manner.

The SPIKES model and other models (Department of Health, Social Services and Public Safety & Northern Ireland Group of the National Council for Hospice and Specialist Palliative Care 2003, Rabow & McPhee 2000) all highlight that the planning and preparatory stage is imperative and should centre on the individual child and the unique needs of the family (Gregg & Vandekieft 2001). Cognizance of specific cultural needs (Arber & Gallagher 2003) is fundamental, and these cultural needs may indicate that an interpreter may be required. Again, nurses should liaise with the consultant and utilise their organisational skills in ensuring that an interpreter is available (Mowatt & Dowes 2001). The preparation is extremely important, and the nurse's leadership skills play a fundamental part in this; Dear (1995) suggests that the most ideal situation to break bad news is in a planned interview, in which the environment can be prearranged. However, it is essential to recognise also that there are certain circumstances that do not permit this (Bloom 2001), for example following the sudden death of a child or young person.

When possible, the nurse present should be the child's named nurse or the nurse looking after the child on that particular shift (Mowatt & Dowes 2001). It is important that the nurse ensures that she or he delegates the care of the child to another nurse during her or his absence. It is important for the child but also for the parents, as they may be less distracted if they know who is looking after their child. Parents report that they prefer not being told when they are alone (Royal College of Nursing 1999), therefore it is important to ensure that if both parents are not present the support of a friend or relative is available (Royal College of Nursing 1999). It is important to discuss with the parents who they would wish to have present; the nurse will organise the attendance of those required (Butow et al 1996). The number of professionals present should be limited in terms of respecting parents' vulnerability and privacy (Royal College of Nursing 1999).

The role of any staff present should be made clear to the parents (Butow et al 1996) at the commencement of the meeting. Although the lead in breaking the news is usually taken by the consultant or other medical officer, the nurse plays the role of supporter at this time. Support is highlighted as one of the most important factors that help caregivers of children cope during difficult periods (Baxandall & Reddy 1993, cited in McGrath 2001), and the breaking of bad news is no exception. It is well documented that support has three dimensions: emotional support, instrumental support and informational support (Kirk & Glendinning 2002). These dimensions are also applicable in this instance. The nurse must have a supportive presence, showing consideration and respect for the child and family. It is important that a direct caring and sensitive approach is used in order to communicate the news well; the avoidance of medical terms and jargon is also essential (Rabow & McPhee 2000). The nurse may take notes for the parents (Royal College of Nursing 1999).

LINK CHAPTER **2**

It is essential to recognise that non-verbal communication is also extremely pertinent in this process (Price et al 2006). Posture and facial expression have been identified as major communication messages (Ray 1996). The nurse also needs to employ attentive listening skills and use skilled observation to assess parental reactions (Royal College of Nursing 1999) in order to provide appropriate support to the parents afterwards as required. Parents' reactions can vary greatly, and the children's nurse should have knowledge of their possible responses, although specific individual reactions are impossible to anticipate. Denial, anger, bargaining, depression and acceptance (Kubler-Ross 1969) may be some initial feelings expressed by parents; acute shock may also be apparent (Greenswag 1983). The children's nurse must be responsive to all these reactions.

It is important to convey kindness and compassion during the meeting (Fogarty et al 1999, Salander 2002), and the nurse can demonstrate these through the use of touch (Rabow & McPhee 2000) and general demeanour. Within the role of facilitator and supporter, the nurse may play a part interpreting for parents, listening and asking questions (Dunneice & Slevin 2002, May 1993). Time should be given for the opportunity to ask questions about what the parents have been told (Department of Health 2003).

The children's nurse's role as supporter and facilitator continues following the interview, in addition to the role of teacher and educator for the family. The nurse's role as

Box 43.2. Approach for breaking bad news

- Setting up
- Perception
- Invitation
- Knowledge
- Emotions
- Strategy and summary

(After Baile et al 2000, with permission.)

practical manager (May 1993) and the interpreter of medical information following the event (Department of Health, Social Services and Public Safety & Northern Ireland Group of the National Council for Hospice and Specialist Palliative Care 2003) will become apparent at this stage. Again, as in the previous phases the uniqueness of the individual parent dictates the type of support required. The parents may want time to be on their own before returning to the child, or they may want to leave the hospital for a period. The nurse can meet information needs by using a range of strategies for both child and family (Price 2003). Information is a prerequisite to education and teaching, and the nurse may have to educate the family or further develop the information the family have been already given about a condition or a treatment modality. It is not uncommon for the nurse to be asked to revise and reiterate what has been said during the meeting, as parents frequently find it hard to internalise all the information. This teaching role may commence following the meeting; however, it must be staged and built on (Kennedy 2001). Following the meeting the nurse may simply sit with the family if this is what they desire; it is essential for the healthcare professional to recognise that silence is also an important communication tool (Price et al 2006).

LINK CHAPTER **1**

Once the parents have assimilated the information received, it is important to consider what and how to tell the child (if appropriate); as the advocate of the child the nurse may need to guide and support the parents with this undertaking. The breaking of bad news to children is beyond the remit of this chapter; however, some useful guidance is offered by Hindmarch (1999: Ch. 14).

As a key member of the multiprofessional team caring for the child and family, the nurse should liaise with other team members, ensuring that they know that the interview has taken place and the outcomes. It may be useful for the nurse to communicate and liaise with the doctor or other professionals present at the interview to debrief (Price et al 2006). An interprofessional debriefing session may be useful following the meeting to reflect on the breaking of bad news, in order to ensure that high standards of care are met in this challenging aspect of care and to identify the need for change or practice development. The nurse should ensure that the interview is documented in the child's nursing notes following the Nursing Midwifery Council's guidelines for record keeping (Nursing and Midwifery Council 2004).

Procedures Box 43.1 Breaking bad news to parents

Action
Select the place where the bad news is to be broken carefully.

Reason *The maintenance of privacy and confidentiality is paramount.*

Actions
If the doctor is breaking the bad news a nurse should be present in a supportive capacity.

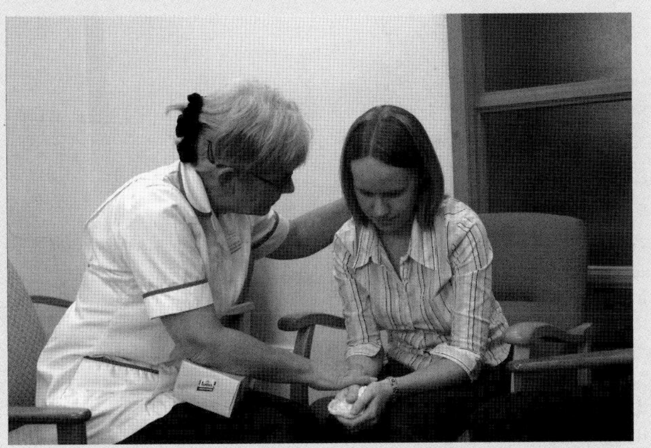

When possible this should be the child's named nurse or a nurse who has built up a therapeutic relationship with the child and family.

It is also important that the nurse is aware of the information imparted in order to provide adequate and knowledgeable support afterwards.

Actions
The nurse and doctor should ensure that adequate planning and preparation are undertaken.

The nurse should ensure that all notes, blood results or X-rays are at hand.

Reason *Ensures that all information is available, causing minimum disruption.*

Action
The nurse should also liaise with the doctor beforehand.

Reason *So that the nurse is aware of what information is to be imparted, which will aid in the preparation of self.*

Action
Any information leaflets that may be useful should be collected for the parents beforehand when possible (e.g. information on the death of a child or any specific condition the child may be diagnosed with).

Reason *Ensures that verbal information is backed up with written information that parents can refer to as required.*

Action
A 'Do not disturb' sign should be displayed, if possible.

Reason *Ensures that interruptions are minimised.*

Action
The role of any staff present should be made clear to the parents and they should be seated at the same level.

Reason *The doctor and parents should be made to feel as comfortable as possible in the environment.*

Action
Notes could be taken by the nurse if desired by the parents.

Procedures Box 43.1 Breaking bad news to parents—cont'd

Reason *To be used as aide-memoires for the parents afterwards.*

Action
The person breaking the bad news should use honest yet simple language and avoid the use of jargon or medical language and terminology.

Reason *Ensures that the news is easily understood.*

Action
The procedure, regardless of the circumstances, should not be hurried.

Reason *Permits some time for the parents to assimilate the information.*

Action
The parents should be given time – time to ask questions and to voice concerns.

Reason *To clarify understanding and to gain further knowledge.*

Action
There should be encouragement regarding the venting of emotions and feelings.

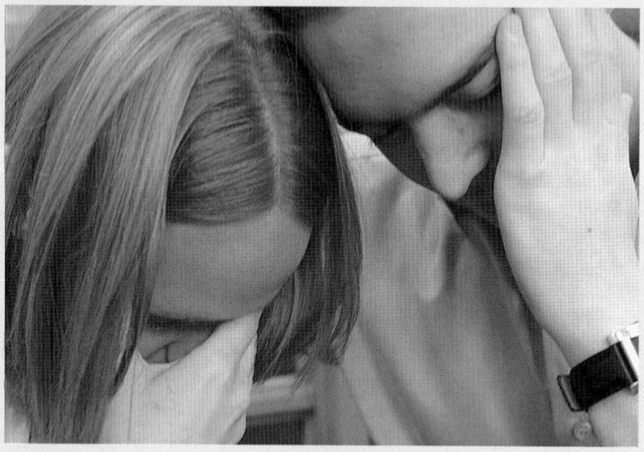

Reason *To permit a response.*

Action
It is important to be aware of non-verbal as well as verbal communication.

Reason *Non-verbal responses by parents and healthcare professionals can be extremely powerful communication tools.*

Action
Parents should be given the choice at the end of the interview to be left alone or have someone stay with them if need be.

Reason *This is directed by individual need.*

Action
The nurse should ensure that the interview is documented in the child's nursing notes following the Nursing and Midwifery Council's guidelines for record keeping.

Reason *Ensures that all team members are aware of what has taken place and the information imparted.*

Action
The nurse should return to the parents a short time after the interview.

Reason *To offer ongoing support, clarify any points and check understanding.*

Now test your knowledge

- Consider the factors that can affect the psychological response to bad news.
- Reflect on an incident from practice in which you were involved when parents were told bad news. What would you do differently in a similar situation in the future? A model of reflection such as McNeilly et al (2006) may assist you.
- Jake is a 4-year-old boy admitted to hospital with bruising, lethargy and bony pain. The consultant is to meet with his parents to confirm a diagnosis of acute lymphoblastic leukaemia. You are Jake's nurse and are to be present at the interview. Discuss your role before, during and after the breaking of the bad news.

References

Arber A, Gallagher A (2003) Breaking bad news revisited: the push for negotiated disclosure and changing practice implications. International Journal of Palliative Nursing 9(4):166–172

Association for Children with Life-threatening or Terminal Conditions, Royal College of Paediatrics and Child Health (2003) A guide to the development of children's paediatric services, 2nd edn. ACT, Bristol

Baile W, Buckman R, Lenzi R, Glober G, Beale E, Kudleka A (2000) SPIKES – A six-step protocol for delivering bad news: application to the patient with cancer. Oncologist 5:302–311

Baxandall S, Reddy P (1993) The courage to care: the impact of cancer on the family. David Lovell Publishing, Melbourne. Cited in McGrath P 2001 Identifying support issues of parents of children with leukemia. Cancer Practice 9(4):198–205

Bloom M (2001) Breaking bad news: parents' perspectives. Paediatric Nursing 13(6):16–20

Buckman R (1984) How to break bad news: Why is it still so difficult? British Medical Journal, 288, 1597–9

Buckman R (1992) How to break bad news: Papermac, London

Butow PN, Kazenu JN, Beeney IJ, Griffin AM, Dunn SM, Tattersall MHN (1996) When the diagnosis is cancer: patient communication and preferences. Cancer 77(12):2630–2637

Casey A (1988) A partnership with child and family. Senior Nursing 8(4):8–9

Child Bereavement Trust (2007) Online. Available: http://www.childbereavement.org.uk/professionals/supportingfamilies_beliefs.php

Cooley C (2000) Communication skills in palliative care. Professional Nurse 15:603–605
Dear S (1995) Breaking bad news: caring for the family. Nursing Standard 10(11):31–33
Department of Health (2003) Getting the right start: National Service Framework for Children, Young People and Maternity Services. Department of Health, London, p 17
Department of Health (2007) Online. Available: http://www.dh.gov.uk/.../Bereavement/BereavementUsefulLinks
Department of Health, Social Services and Public Safety, Northern Ireland Group of the National Council for Hospice and Specialist Palliative Care (2003) Breaking bad news: regional guidelines DHSSPS, Belfast
Dunneice U, Slevin E (2002) Nurses' experiences of being present with a patient receiving a diagnosis of cancer. Journal of Advanced Nursing 32(3):611–618
Fallowfield L (1993) Giving sad and bad news. Lancet 341:477–478
Farrell M (1999) The challenge of breaking bad news. Intensive Critical Care Nursing 15:101–110
Fogarty LA, Curbow BA, Wingard JR et al (1999) Can 40 seconds of compassion reduce patient anxiety? Journal Clinical Oncology 17(1):371–379
Graham M, Price J (2005) Chemotherapy-induced nausea and vomiting in the young person with cancer. Cancer Nursing Practice 4(8):29–34
Greenswag LR (1983) Coping with birth defects: how to help. Occupational Health Nursing 3(10):21–23
Gregg K, Vandekieft MD (2001) Breaking bad news. American Family Physician 64:1975–1978
Hindmarch C (1999) On the death of a child. Radcliffe Medical Press, London
Kaye P (1996) Breaking bad news: a 10 step approach. EPL Publications, Northampton
Kennedy I (2001) The inquiry into the management of children receiving complex heart surgery at Bristol Royal Infirmary. Stationery Office, London
Kirk S, Glendinning C (2002) Supporting 'expert' parents – professional support and families caring for a child with complex health care and families caring for a child with complex health care needs in the community. International Journal of Nursing Studies 39:625–635
Kubler-Ross E (1969) On death and dying. Macmillan, New York
McNeilly P, Price J, McCloskey S (2006) A model for reflection in paediatric palliative care. European Journal of Palliative Care 13(1):31–34
Martin V (1995) Helping parents cope. Nursing Times 91(31):38–40
May C (1993) Disclosure of terminal prognoses in a general hospital – a nurse's view. Journal of Advanced Nursing 18:1362–1368
Mowatt P, Dowes K (2001) Breaking bad news protocol and benchmarking. Bradford Hospitals NHS Trust, Bradford
Nursing and Midwifery Council (2004) Guidelines for records and record keeping. NMC, London
Peel N (2003) The role of the critical care nurse in the delivery of bad news. British Journal of Nursing 12(16):966–971
Price J (2003) Information needs of the child with cancer and their family. Cancer Nursing Practice 2(7):35–37
Price J, McNeilly P, Surgenor M (2006) Breaking bad news to parents: the children's nurse's role. International Journal of Palliative Nursing 12(3):115–120
Quine L, Pahl J 1987 Cited in Robb F (1999) Congenital malformations: breaking bad news. British Journal of Midwifery 7(1):26–31
Rabow M, McPhee S (2000) Beyond breaking bad news: helping patients who suffer. Student BMJ March:45–88
Ray MC (1996) Seven ways to empower dying patients. American Journal of Nursing 96(5):56–57
Reynolds S (2003) Down's syndrome: breaking bad news. British Journal of Midwifery 11(12):722–724
Robb F (1999) Congenital malformations: breaking bad news. British Journal of Midwifery 7(1):26–31
Royal College of Nursing (1999) Supporting parents when they are told of their child's health disorder or disability – guidance for nurses, midwives and health visitors. RCN, London
Royal College of Nursing (2007) Online. Available: http://www.rcn.org.uk/resources/transcultural/childhealth
Salander P (2002) Bad news from a patient's perspective: an analysis of the written narratives of newly diagnosed cancer patients. Social Science Medicine 55(5):721–732
Smyth D (2004) Breaking bad news: part 1. International Journal of Palliative Nursing 10(2):610
Vegni E, Zannini L, Visoli S, Moga EA (2001) Giving bad news: a GP's narrative perspective. Supportive Care in Cancer 9(5):390–396
Wakefield AB (2000) Nurses' responses to death and dying: a need for relentless self care. International Journal of Palliative Nursing 6(5):245–251
Wakefield A, Cooke S, Boggis C (2003) Learning together: use of simulated patients with nursing and medical students for breaking bad news. International Journal of Palliative Nursing 9:132–138

44 Care of the child after death

Patricia McNeilly • Jayne Price

The death of a child, whether sudden or anticipated, causes a devastating loss to families (Price & McFarlane 2006) and is a particularly challenging time for the children's nurse and the wider interdisciplinary team. The recent proliferation of services that provide care for children with life-limiting, life-threatening and terminal conditions (Price et al 2005) has afforded families the choice of home, hospital or hospice care at the time of death, and it is imperative that such choices and options are discussed at an early stage. Evidence suggests that when death is expected, early preparation and planning can have a positive and lasting effect on the experience of the family at the time of death and during the bereavement process (Davies 1997).

Care of the child at the time of death

A sensitive and caring approach towards the parents and wider family is particularly important at this time. One of the most important aspects of care immediately following death is the provision of time and privacy. Indeed, previous research suggests that time spent with the child after death can have a lasting effect on parental grief (Davies 2005). It is imperative therefore that the parents do not feel rushed in the hours and days following the death of their child. Parents should be encouraged to hold and caress their child.

Written and verbal information at this time is paramount in order to facilitate informed decision making. In the case of a planned or an expected death, parents should be informed of their choices regarding taking their child home (Whittle & Cutts 2002). Parents may choose to take their child home or arrange for a funeral director to collect them from the ward. In some circumstances it may still be necessary for the child to be transferred to the hospital mortuary. Should parents want to take their child home via private transport, then this should be facilitated, and this is often the case. An explanatory letter should be provided and the local police service informed in case of any potential eventualities on the way home.

Washing the child

Parents or other close family members may request assistance or support to wash their child, while others may wish to perform this task themselves. Much consideration is frequently given to how children are dressed for burial or cremation, and this is a sensitive and personal decision taken usually by the parents. Parents should be warned about the noises that may be emitted by the body following death, in order to avoid confusion about signs of life (Trigg & Mohammed 2006), and the change in appearance of the child following death. If a post-mortem is not required then items such as cannulas and tracheostomy or percutaneous endoscopic gastrostomy tubes can be removed from the child and covered with a dressing to prevent leakage (McGarry 2006). However, the removal of such items should be first discussed with the child's parents. Some authors suggest that it may be necessary to place a pillow under the child's chin if the mouth is gaping or place dampened cotton wool on the eyelids to keep them closed, although these issues are commonly addressed by the funeral director (Dominica 2006, Trigg & Mohammed 2006). The decision to undertake these procedures should be discussed with and explained to the parents in a very sensitive manner. Most families choose a variety of the child's possessions, for example a favourite cuddly toy or blanket, to remain with them up to and during the burial or cremation.

ALERT
Medical devices such as cannulas and tracheostomy or percutaneous endoscopic gastrostomy tubes should not be removed if a post-mortem is required.

Keepsakes

A range of strategies may be used to provide keepsakes as a lasting memory of the child, in keeping with the wishes of the family. Evidence suggests that such mementoes are a precious and final way of remembering the child (Osborne 2000), and the children's nurse is instrumental in facilitating this. Photographs are commonly taken, with appropriate consent. Family members may wish to take their own photographs and will have some idea about the format of these. However, given the emotionality and uniqueness of the situation, some guidance may be required in relation to taking multiple pictures from a variety of perspectives in order to ensure an optimal outcome that may provide comfort and lasting memories for years to come. Digital photography is now frequently used and has the advantage of immediate viewing (Dent & Stewart 2004).

Locks of hair and hand- or footprints or moulds are also commonly offered to the family at this time (see the procedure box).

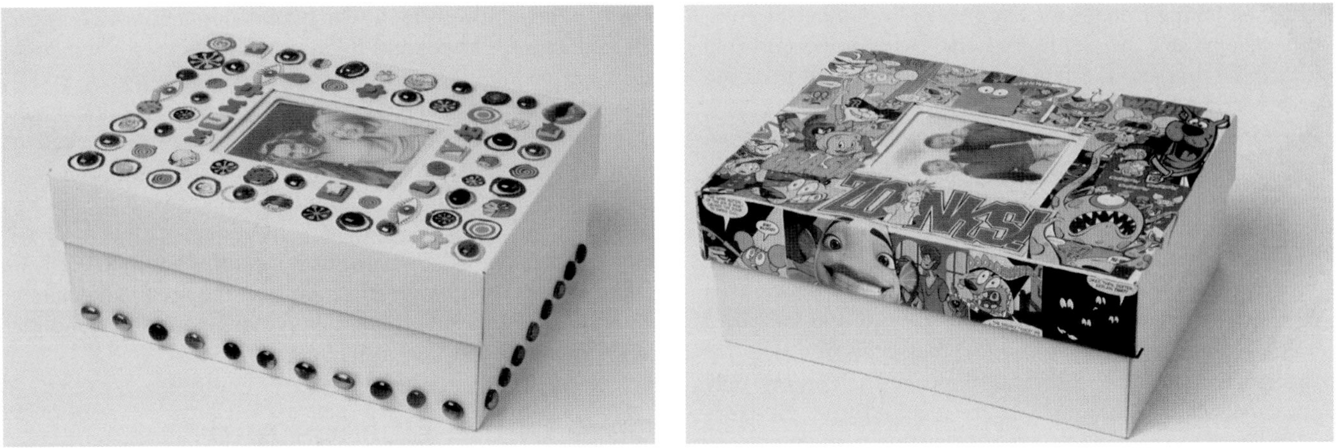

Fig. 44.1 • Examples of memory boxes available from Winston's Wish (2007).

Should the family initially decline the offer of such mementoes, the healthcare professional can, with the parents' consent, offer to keep these in the child's file should the family alter their decision at a later date. Over time, parents, siblings or close family members may wish to put together a memory box in order to collect special memories of the child. Winston's Wish provides a number of different designs to suit individual needs (Fig. 44.1).

Practical issues to be addressed following the death

A number of practical issues require consideration following the death of the child. These issues may be addressed by the parents themselves or by other family members. However, some parents who have not experienced a previous bereavement may require guidance from the children's nurse.

The death must be verified and the medical certificate of the cause of death issued by a registered medical practitioner (Dimond 2004), and this normally occurs at the time of death (Cook 2000). In some cases, for example when the death has been referred to the coroner for post-mortem and/or public enquiry (see examples, Box 44.1), this process may be delayed, and it is imperative that the family is given clear instructions as to how and where to obtain the death certificate so that the funeral arrangements can go ahead as planned. This medical certificate is required by the registrar for births, deaths and marriages in order to register the death within the required 5 days (Dimond 2004). The death may be registered either in the district where the child lived or the district where the child died. This certificate is also required by the funeral director prior to burial or cremation. Written information booklets are beneficial for parents to refer to later (Davey 1995), because they can find it difficult to retain information at this time.

The parents may or may not have a preferred family funeral director. Some funeral directors provide a free service in the case of a child's death or have particular expertise in this area and are therefore frequently recommended in this situation. Sensitivity is paramount when informing parents of this. In any case, funeral directors should be members of the National Association of Funeral Directors or the Society of Allied and Independent Funeral Directors. Both these organisations have codes of practice to ensure high standards of service provision. Funeral costs can be a major issue for some families (Joseph Rowntree Foundation 2001), and assistance may be available from local social services or charitable organisations such as Rapid Effective Assistance for Children with Potentially Terminal Illness.

Box 44.1. Main reasons for referral to the coroner

- Accidental or sudden, unexplained death
- Death occurring in suspicious circumstances
- Death during an operation
- Death following anaesthesia or surgical procedures
- When the death may have been related to a medical procedure or treatment

(After National Health Service 2006.)

Post-mortems and retention of organs

The issue of post-mortem and retention of organs is an emotive subject and one that the children's nurse needs to be familiar with. Following the events at Alder Hey and the subsequent Redfern Report (Redfern 2001) there has been greater emphasis on the information needs of the family in relation to the post-mortem examination and the retention of organs for education or research purposes. Although obtaining consent for post-mortem is primarily the responsibility of medical staff, the children's nurse has a vital part to play as part of the interdisciplinary team in terms of acting as an advocate for the child and family (Royal College of Nursing

2001). The issue of post-mortem involves a number of complex decisions, and the children's nurse has an important role to play in supporting the family and reinforcing information provided by medical staff.

In essence there are two types of post-mortem examination: a hospital post-mortem that can be carried out only with parental consent, and a coroner's post-mortem that is required by law and therefore does not legally require the consent of the parents (National Health Service 2003a). In the event of either type of post-mortem, parents must give written consent for the retention of whole organs, blocks or slides containing small amounts of tissue that may be used for further investigation or educational purposes. Parents may request that all organs and tissue are reunited with the body prior to burial or cremation. If this is the case the funeral may be significantly delayed until the post-mortem investigation is complete, and it is imperative that this is discussed with the parents. Alternatively, parents may decide to proceed with the burial or cremation and arrange the collection and burial or cremation of any remaining organs or tissue at a later date (National Health Service Retained Organs Commission 2002). This can be arranged by the family or via the family's funeral director. Receiving an organ or tissue at a later date can be very poignant, and it is imperative that the family have an identified support system to use at this time, if desired. Numerous resources relating to post-mortems and retention of organs have been produced to provide information for both bereaved parents and relatives (Department of Health 2003, National Health Service 2003a,b). Making such decisions is fraught with difficulty at an already stressful emotional time, and the children's nurse can provide much support in order to guide the family through this decision-making process.

The funeral

The format of the funeral service is again a matter of personal preference, and these preferences range from a very traditional service to a much-personalised one as a means of reflecting on the life of the particular child. Favourite songs, poems and stories may be used by some families in addition to themed flower arrangements or balloon releases at the end of the service (Dent & Stewart 2004). In the case of a planned death, families often give consideration to the funeral prior to the actual death and may wish to discuss their wishes with nursing and other staff. Evidence suggests that careful forward planning is important in ensuring that the wishes of the family and child, if appropriate, are addressed. Close family members or healthcare professionals may be asked to contribute to the service as a final tribute to the child and family.

Burial or cremation

This is a personal decision for the parents and close family and may be governed to some extent by traditional, cultural and religious influences. Cremation is forbidden by Orthodox Jews and Muslims. However, all Christian denominations permit it. Sikhs, Hindus, Parsees and Buddhists normally use cremation, although young children may be buried (Hindmarch 2000). A number of additional requirements need to be fulfilled should the family decide on cremation, for example two independent medical practitioners must complete the necessary statutory cremation forms (unless the coroner has been involved) and the fittings of the coffin must be made from combustible material. However, individual crematoriums can offer additional practical advice and support to the family if required. The funeral director can also advise the family of the practicalities of burial or cremation.

Care of the siblings and wider family

The death of a child has a profound effect on his or her siblings, grandparents and wider family circle. Siblings may experience a confusing myriad of emotions from resentment (and associated guilt) about the continued focus on their brother or sister to a sense of sadness and loss. Although some parents may think it better to protect the siblings in the time leading to and after the death, in fact children are highly perceptive and tend to fabricate and fill in the gaps in their knowledge, which can lead to unnecessary anxiety. A number of resources are available for use with young children to prompt discussion prior to and after the death (see Fig. 44.2 and Box 44.2). It is important for parents to have an understanding of children's perceptions of death in order to support them fully. A number of practical issues need to be addressed, for example whether or not siblings will be present at the time of death, view the child after death and attend or participate in the funeral. Families often struggle with these issues, and the experienced children's nurse who knows the family well is in a good position to listen and provide advice and support as necessary. Dent & Stewart (2004) provide a comprehensive summary of the support that siblings may require following the death of a child (Box 44.3).

Grandparents also need much support, as they are grieving for the loss of their grandchild but also have added anxiety around the well-being of their own child (Association for Children with Life-limiting, Life-threatening and Terminal Conditions 2004). The knowledge that the death of a child defies the normal order of events may have particular implications for some grandparents, who feel that they have lived their life and therefore it is they who should have died instead of the child.

Spiritual and cultural issues

A growing number of spiritual and cultural practices exist in the UK, and given this increasing diversity of our society children's nurses have a duty to update their knowledge in order to fully respect individual beliefs and rituals surrounding the death of a child. An in-depth discussion of these practices is beyond the scope of this chapter. However, a particularly

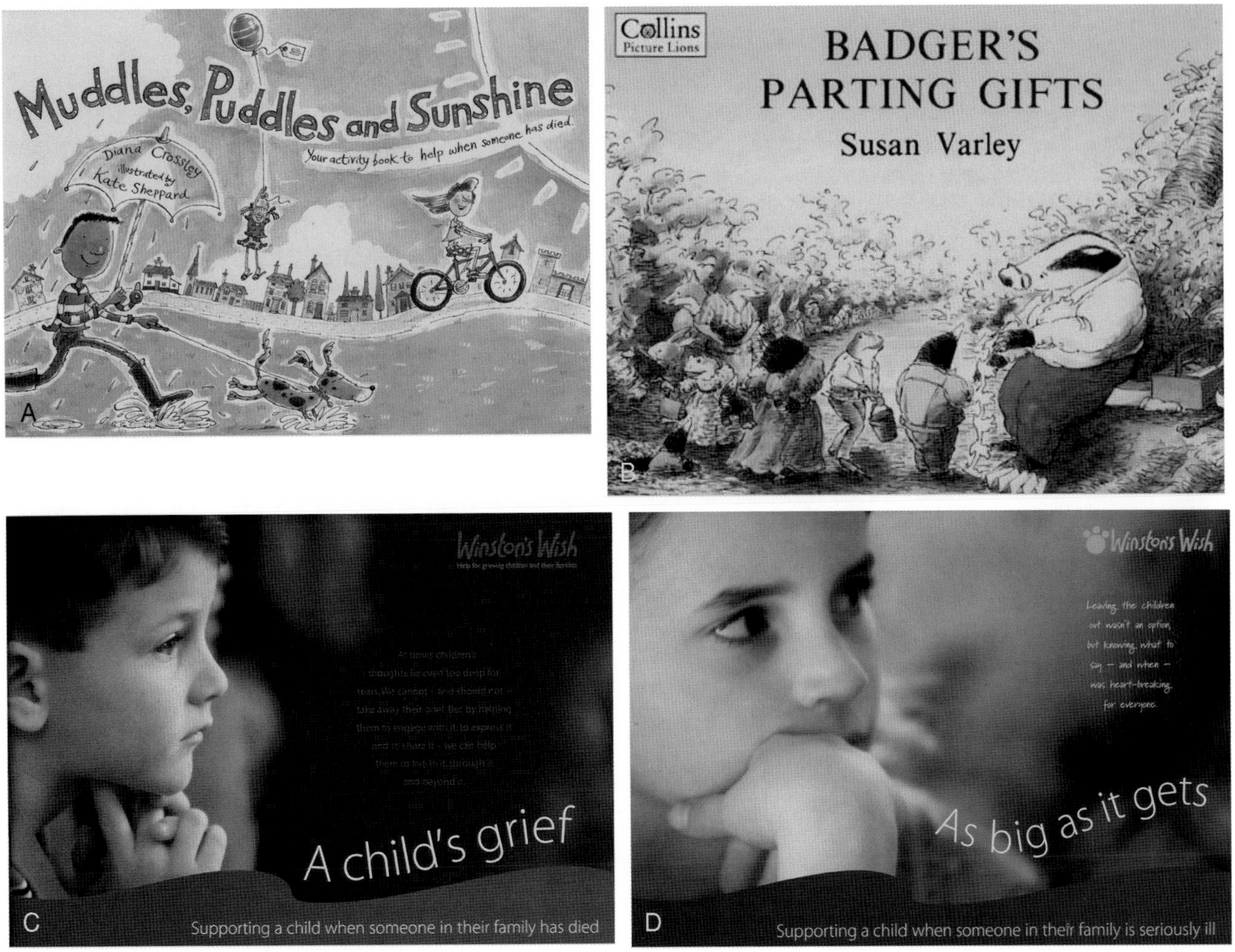

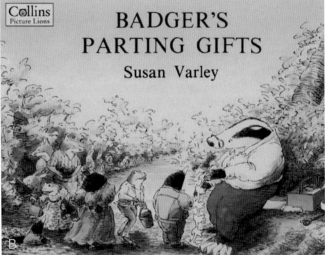

Fig. 44.2 • Resources that may be of benefit for siblings (all available from Winston's Wish). (Reproduced by kind permission of Winston's Wish; B. reproduced with permission of Collins Publishers Ltd.)

Box 44.2. Further resources that may help parents talk to children about death

- *Water Bugs and Dragonflies* by Doris Stickney
- *The Huge Bag of Worries* by Virginia Ironside
- *Badger's Parting Gifts* by Susan Varley
- *When Someone Very Special Dies* by Marge Heegaard
- *A Child's Grief*, available from Winston's Wish (2007)
- *As Big as It Gets*, available from Winston's Wish (2007)
- *Muddles, Puddles and Sunshine*, available from Winston's Wish (2007)

A variety of further resources are available from:

- the Child Bereavement Trust (2007)
- Cruse Bereavement Care (2007)
- Hospice Net (2007)

Box 44.3. Helping parents support their surviving children

- Supply information about the death as soon as possible
- Understand that they grieve in their own way
- Provide careful and sensitive listening if at all possible
- Preserve routine activities and boundaries
- Offer choices after explanations (e.g. seeing the body, going to the funeral)
- Reassure that they are not to blame
- Talk through their fears and anxieties
- Involve and include whenever possible
- Nurture and share moments together; parents can provide a grieving model (e.g. crying together is OK)
- Give opportunities to remember the dead person

(From Dent & Stewart 2004: 212.)

valuable practical resource is *Caring for People of Different Faiths* (Neuberger 2004). Nurses should be aware of those religions that do not permit them to touch the dead child or leave her or him alone, for example the Jewish, Hindu, Islamic and Sikh faiths (Ethnicity Online 2006). It is vital that the children's nurse takes advice from the family about spiritual and religious rituals, and indeed this is invariably the case.

Follow-up care

The provision of follow-up care varies with each particular situation. For example, research shows that parents whose child has experienced a sudden death often receive the least support when compared with parents whose child had a chronic illness (Nussbaumer & Russell 2003). Regardless of circumstances, follow-up care should be individualised and negotiated with each particular family by someone who knows the family well. Effective communication, not only with the family but also between members of the interdisciplinary team, is of the essence.

Frameworks such as the Association for Children with Life-limiting, Life-threatening and Terminal Conditions (2004) care pathway for the dying child may be utilised to facilitate communication and a seamless approach to the follow-up process. Trusts commonly use a checklist following the death of a child, and this can provide a useful means of communicating details of follow-up care to relevant healthcare professionals including community staff and voluntary organisations, as appropriate. The family may choose to consult with one of the many voluntary agencies that provide bereavement support, for example Cruse Bereavement Care, Compassionate Friends or the Child Death Helpline.

Procedures Box 44.1 Care of the child after death

Actions
Approach the family in a calm, sensitive and caring manner at the time of death and afterwards.

Explain to the parents that you will need to contact the doctor.

Reason *The care received by the family can leave a lasting impression on their bereavement experience and memories for years to come.*

Action
Contact a medical practitioner (preferably an experienced one who knows the family well) to verify the death.

Reason *This is required by law.*

Action
Ensure that events immediately following the death are not hurried.

Reason *It is imperative that parents feel that they have been given time to hold, caress and spend time with their child.*

Action
Ask the family if they would like assistance to contact family members or friends, their minister of religion or a funeral director, if desired.

Action
Provide a quiet and private environment for parents and family to make phone calls, if desired.

Reason *So that there are no interruptions or distractions.*

Action
Discuss with the family the usual procedure that follows, while ensuring that their individual needs and wishes are facilitated; verbal information should be supported by written information.

Reason *Some parents may not have experienced a family death before and so may require guidance about the practical arrangements.*

Actions
Collect all the necessary equipment to wash the child:

- basin of water
- soap
- child's own towel and facecloths, if available
- chosen clothes
- clean linen
- linen skip
- dressings to cover intravenous sites etc. if no post-mortem is required
- brush
- any equipment required to obtain mementoes (e.g. scissors, equipment to obtain a handprint)
- digital camera, if desired by the parents
- written information, usually in the form of a booklet for the family.

Assist the parents and family (if desired) to wash their child, dress her or him in the clothes selected (if available) and change the bed linen; note that some parents may prefer the nurse to do this or they may want to do it entirely themselves.

Action
Remove any cannulas, catheters, tubes or other equipment if a post-mortem is not required, if this is in accordance with the parents' wishes; a dressing may be applied to prevent leakage.

If a post-mortem is required await instructions from medical staff.

ALERT
Medical devices such as cannulas and tracheostomy or percutaneous endoscopic gastrostomy tubes should not be removed if a post-mortem is required.

Reason *Such items may not be removed prior to post-mortem.*

Action
Offer to obtain a lock of hair (from the back of the child's head), a hand- or footprint, or other mementoes for the parents.

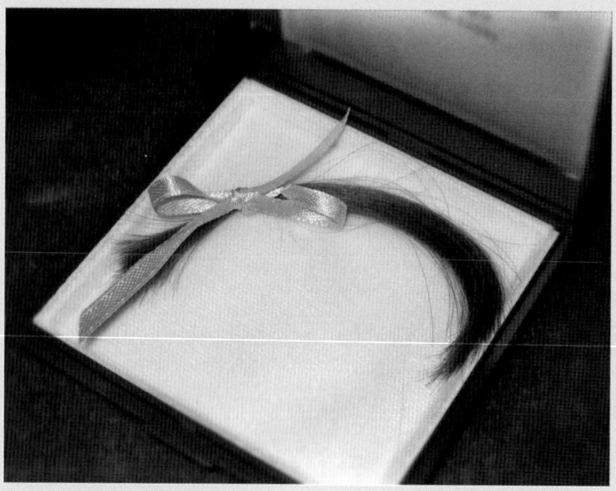

Procedures Box 44.1 Care of the child after death—cont'd

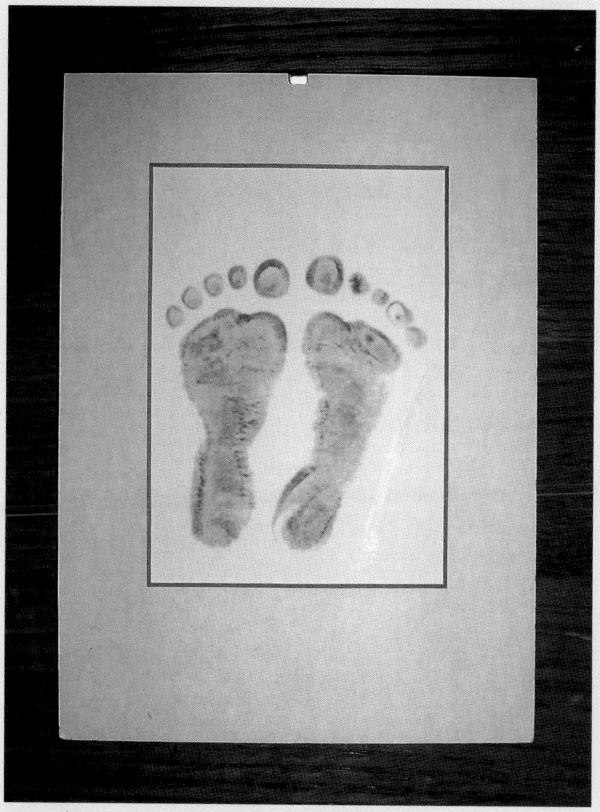

Reason *Many parents treasure such mementoes as a lasting memory of their child.*

Action
Assist the family to take photographs of their child if desired; a digital camera should be available for this purpose.

Reason *The use of a digital camera facilitates checking of the images to ensure the desired outcome.*

Actions
Lay the child's body out with the eyes and mouth closed.

Note: be aware of any cultural variations.

Provide support and advice to the parents in relation to telling the child's siblings about the death, supporting the siblings (if present) or facilitating a visit by the siblings (if appropriate).

Action
Provide information regarding the family's options around taking the child home, and support the family in making the decision about where to care for the child prior to burial or cremation.

Reason *Parents may not be aware of their options and have lasting memories of the time between the death and the child's funeral or cremation.*

Action
Communicate with the family in a sensitive manner regarding requirements about taking the child home by car, arranging collection of the child's body by a funeral director or transfer to a hospital mortuary.

Action
Offer to stay with the child if the family need to leave the room for any reason.

Reason *The parents and family may not wish the child to be alone.*

Actions
Complete relevant documentation, care plans or checklists used by the trust.

Place a sticker on the outside of the child's chart so that it is apparent to healthcare and administrative staff that the child has died.

Reason *To adhere to local policy, to ensure optimal communication and to make certain that no further appointments or 'Did not attend' letters are sent out to the family.*

Action
Arrange a follow-up appointment with the paediatrician at the end of a clinic when there will be no interruptions and plenty of time for the parents to express their feelings and ask any questions they may have.

Reason *To maintain communication, answer any questions the parents and family may have and continue to provide support in the period after the death.*

Action
Communicate with the child's general practitioner and wider interdisciplinary team and voluntary agencies, as appropriate.

Reason *So that all concerned are aware of the death and to provide them with the opportunity to contact the family and attend the funeral, if appropriate.*

Actions
Ensure that the child's health visitor cancels all immunisation and other routine appointments (if applicable).

Ensure that all current appointments are cancelled, including those for hospital and community clinics.

Reason *So that the parents do not receive an appointment for the child or a 'Did not attend' notification.*

Action
Identify nursing staff who wish to attend the funeral on behalf of the ward or community nursing team, if appropriate.

Action
Facilitate continuing open lines of communication with the family and ensure that they know that they can ring and speak to staff at any time.

Reason *To offer a continuing support mechanism for the parents and family, if so desired.*

Action
Provide written information (usually in the form of a booklet) about the weeks and months that may follow, and recommended contact numbers of local practitioners and bereavement organisations that the family may want to access at a later date.

Reason *To provide information about what the family may expect in the weeks and months to follow and where they may obtain support, if desired.*

Now test your knowledge

- Reflect on the death of a child you have cared for and identify from a practical perspective what went well and what could have been improved. Using a model of reflection may assist you to do this; see for example McNeilly et al (2006) .
- Review the resources available in your trust to both parents and the interdisciplinary team around this area of practice and update or improve as necessary. Consider the possibility of developing a number of resource boxes for use in your place of work.
- Consider the role of the nurse in relation to the process of gaining consent for a post-mortem after the death of a child.

References

Association for Children with Life-limiting, Life-threatening and Terminal Conditions (2004) Integrated multi-agency care pathway for children with life-threatening and life-limiting conditions. ACT, Bristol

Child Bereavement Trust (2007) Online. Available: http://www.childbereavement.org.uk/resources/

Cook P (2000) Supporting sick children and their families. Baillière Tindall, London

Cruse Bereavement Care (2007) Online. Available: http://www.crusebereavementcare.org.uk/pdf/publications%20c&%2006.06.pdf

Davey N (1995) Paediatric bereavement care. Paediatric Nursing 7(9):24

Davies C (1997) When a baby dies. Nursing Times 93(8):28–29

Davies R (2005) Mothers' stories of loss: their need to be with their dying child and their child's body after death. Journal of Child Health Care 9(4):288–300

Dent A, Stewart A (2004) Sudden death in childhood – support for the bereaved family. Butterworth-Heinemann, London

Department of Health (2003) Families and post mortems. A code of practice. Online. Available: http://www.dh.gov.assetRoot/04/05/43/12/04054312.pdf 23 Jun 2006

Dimond B (2004) The law and the certification, verification and registration of death. British Journal of Nursing 13(8):480–481

Dominica F (2006) After the child's death: family care. In Goldman A, Hain R, Liben S (eds) Oxford textbook of palliative care for children. Oxford University Press, Oxford

Ethnicity Online (2006) Cultural awareness in health-care. Online. Available: http://www.ethnicityonline.net

Hindmarch C (2000) On the death of a child, 2nd edn. Radcliffe Medical Press, Oxford

Hospice Net (2007) Online. Available: http://www.hospicenet.org/html/child.html

Joseph Rowntree Foundation (2001) The financial implications for parents of the death of a child. Online. Available: http://www.jrf.org.uk/knowledge/findings/socialcare/pdf/231.pdf 31 Jul 2006

McGarry B (2006) Bereavement care. In Trigg E, Mohammed TA (eds) Practices in children's nursing: guidelines for hospital and community. Churchill Livingstone, London

McNeilly P, Price J, McCloskey S (2006) A model of reflection in children's palliative care. European Journal of Palliative Care 13(1):31–34

National Health Service (2003a) A guide to the post mortem examination procedure involving a baby or child. Online. Available: http://www.dh.gov.uk/assetRoot/04/08/39/60/04083960.pdf 23 Jun 2006

National Health Service (2003b) A simple guide to the post mortem examination procedure. Online. Available: http://www.dh.gov/assetRoot/04/05/47/50/04054750.pdf 23 Jun 2006

National Health Service (2006) NHS Direct online health encyclopaedia. Inquest – when should it be done? Online. Available: http://www.nhsdirect.nhs.uk/articles/article.aspx?articleId=489&sectionId=11017 20 Jul 2006

National Health Service Retained Organs Commission (2002) Return of organs and tissue direct to families – an information leaflet for parents and relatives. Department of Health, London

Neuberger J (2004) Caring for people of different faiths, 3rd edn. Radcliffe Medical, Abingdon

Nussbaumer A, Russell RLR (2003) Bereavement support following sudden and unexpected death in children. Current Paediatrics 13:555–559

Osborne M (2000) Photographs and mementos – the emergency nurse's role following infant death. Emergency Nurse 7(9):23–25

Price J, McFarlane M (2006) Care of the child requiring palliative care. In Glasper A, Richardson J (eds) A textbook of children's and young people's nursing. Elsevier, London

Price J, McNeilly P, McFarlane M (2005) Paediatric palliative care in the UK: past, present and future. International Journal of Palliative Nursing 11(3):124–126

Redfern M (2001) The report of the Royal Liverpool Children's Inquiry. Stationary Office, London. Online. Available: http://www.rlcinquiry.org.uk 30 Jul 2006

Royal College of Nursing (2001) Retention of organs and tissues following post mortem examination: RCN recommendations. Paediatric Nursing 13(1):12–13

Trigg E, Mohammed TA (2006) Practices in children's nursing: guidelines for hospital and community. Churchill Livingstone, London

Whittle M, Cutts S (2002) Time to go home: assisting families to take their child home following a planned hospital or hospice death. Paediatric Nursing 14(10):24–28

Winston's Wish (2007) Online. Available: http://www.winstonswish.org.uk

Appendix Answers to questions

Chapter 9

Assessment of blood pressure

Question 1

The most accurate non-invasive method to obtain a BP in children is by:
b sphygmomanometer (manual)

Question 2

The most preferable method to obtain a systolic BP using a sphygmomanometer in the under fives is:
b Doppler

Question 3

To choose the most accurate cuff size to use in measuring BP in any age group:
b measure the size using the cuff that covers 90–100% of the arm circumference

Question 4

Using a cuff that incorporates a bladder that is too small (too short, too narrow or both) is likely to result in:
b an overestimation of BP

Question 5

You would expect the difference in sleeping and waking BP to be:
d 10% difference

Question 6

If the BP measurement needs to be retaken, the following time should elapse before the second measurement:
c 1 min

Question 7

When using any form of BP-measuring equipment, the five most important principles for measuring BP accurately are:

- correct cuff size
- correct positioning of the cuff
- appropriate relaxed and friendly environment
- the child remains still while the BP is being measured
- well-maintained equipment

Chapter 10

Neurological assessment

Question 1

Other situations in which you may undertake a period of neurological assessment are as follows.

- In a child with unconsciousness of unknown cause
- Road traffic accident
- Unwitnessed fall or trauma in which head injury may have occurred but may not be the primary injury
- Illnesses affecting cerebral function, such as meningitis and encephalitis
- Accidental or deliberate ingestion of noxious substances
- Alcoholic intoxication
- Following a convulsion
- Shock
- Post resuscitation
- Diabetic ketoacidosis to detect potential risk of cerebral oedema
- Severe fluid or electrolyte imbalance
- Metabolic or respiratory acidosis or alkalosis
- Hemiparesis or limb weakening of unknown cause
- Severe headaches
- Postoperative: neurological surgery
- Postoperative: ventricular shunt surgery
- Any other situation in which the child's conscious level appears to be impaired

Question 2

An extremely rapid assessment of conscious level during the initial, critical stage of assessing the child's illness or injury can be achieved using the AVPU scale, which assigns the child to one of four categories.

1. A: *alert*
2. V: responds to *voice*
3. P: responds only to *pain*
4. U: *unresponsive* to all stimuli.

Question 3

The responses that the GCS assesses and scores assigned to each category are as follows.

- Eye opening: 4
- Verbal response: 5
- Motor response: 6

Question 4

The following may lead you to suspect that a child or young person is developing signs of raised intracranial pressure.

- Deteriorating level of consciousness
- Headache, nausea or vomiting
- Confusion, agitation, drowsiness
- Bulging or tense fontanelle
- Response only to pain
- Pupil reaction: unequal, sluggish, unreactive, dilated
- Abnormal motor activity, reflexes or posture (decorticate or decerebrate)
- Decreasing oxygen saturation levels
- Altered temperatures

LATE SIGNS include:

- decreasing heart rate
- increasing blood pressure
- decreasing respiratory rate with altered breathing pattern
- Cushing's triad (late and preterminal sign).

Question 5

Gently shake the child prior to applying the chosen painful stimulus to confirm a deeper level of consciousness and avoid unnecessary distress to the child. Explain to the parent or carer and child what you are going to do to gain the parent's or carer's consent and prepare the child even if she or he appears deeply unconscious.

You may consider pulling the frontal hair but often there is limited hair growth in this age group. If this is the case a sternal rub may be more appropriate. Trapezius squeeze is ineffective in children under 5 years of age, and supraorbital ridge pressure should be applied only by a trained practitioner in a deeply unconscious child.

ALERT
A child who responds only to pain or who is unresponsive has a significant and concerning altered level of consciousness. Senior, experienced medical assistance should be summoned immediately, as intubation to secure the airway may be necessary.

Question 6

If a child or young person has left-sided weakness and a sluggish and dilated right pupil, the *right* side of the brain is affected.

Question 7

The grimace score can be used to assess verbal response in a preverbal or intubated child or young person. Responses and scores are as follows.

- Spontaneous normal facial or oromotor activity: 5
- Less than usual spontaneous ability or only response to touch stimuli: 4
- Vigorous grimace to pain: 3
- Mild grimace to pain: 2
- No response to pain: 1

Question 8

Request a medical review. Undertake a set of neurological observations immediately. Revert to half-hourly observations for at least 2 h. If the GCS score is consistently 15, reduce to hourly observations for 4 h and then two-hourly observations.

Question 9

Dimming the overhead lighting will make it easier for you to see a reaction. Ensure that you use only a thin beam of light and shine this from the outer aspect to the centre of the eye. If you remain unsure of the reaction ask for senior experienced assistance immediately.

Chapter 11

Personal hygiene

Question 1

You should clean a child's teeth at least twice a day, ideally after each meal as well.

Question 2

You should change your toothbrush every 3 months.

Question 3

Indications of a healthy mouth include:

- pink moist tongue
- teeth clean and free from debris
- adequate salivation
- smooth moist lips
- no eating or chewing problems.

Question 4

Predisposing factors contributing to an unhealthy mouth include:

- nausea
- vomiting
- anorexia
- dysphagia
- dehydration
- oral tumour
- chemotherapy

- debility
- radiotherapy
- poor fluid intake
- poor saliva production
- surgery to the mouth.

Question 5

Regular flossing is important to remove debris and plaque between teeth.

Question 6

Moisten dry lips with Vaseline, white soft paraffin or proprietary lip balm.

Chapter 16

Administration of medicines

Question 1

Prior to administering medication:

- ask the patient to tell you her or his name and date of birth
- check that the details on her or his wristband match those on the prescription chart.

Question 2

Rectal administration may be appropriate when administration via the oral route results in nausea, vomiting or gastric pain; patients are uncooperative or have decreased consciousness; or access to the intravenous route is difficult.

Question 3

To reduce the discomfort caused by injection, nursing staff can use age-appropriate preparation; topical anaesthetic cream; ethyl chloride spray; ice packs; pressing on the skin for 10s prior to inserting the needle; distraction and relaxation techniques during the procedure, such as singing, blowing bubbles and guided imagery; self-administration of inhaled nitrous oxide (in school age children and young people); and giving sucrose solution (to reduce discomfort in infants). (Discomfort in infants can also be reduced by asking the mother to breastfeed immediately before injection.)

Question 4

Actions to prevent mechanical backlash or mechanical slack include fitting the syringe tightly into the pump; using the prime facility on the syringe pump, if this is available; and using a smaller sized syringe, if available and appropriate.

Question 5

Advantages of using the intravenous route are that it ensures rapid and predictable delivery of the medicine and can be used if the patient is unconscious or uncooperative. Disadvantages include a higher risk of anaphylaxis than with other routes; risk of speed shock if the medicine is administered too rapidly; and risk of extravasation or infiltration, infection and phlebitis.

Question 6

Possible complications of an intramuscular injection are nerve injury, septic or sterile abscesses, muscle fibrosis and contracture, gangrene and intramuscular haemorrhage.

Question 7

Absorption of medication via subcutaneous injection is fastest from the abdomen, next from the upper arm, then from the thighs, and slowest from the hips and buttocks.

Question 8

From a pressurised metered dose inhaler the drug is emitted at high speed and is mostly deposited in the oropharynx. Use of a spacer (valved holding chamber) with the inhaler allows the patient to breathe tidally from a reservoir of the drug so that more of the drug reaches the lungs.

Question 9

After inhalation of corticosteroids, children should rinse their mouth or clean their teeth to prevent oral thrush.

Question 10

The three methods of nasal administration are drops, pumped aqueous sprays and powered nasal sprays.

Question 11

Drops and ointments should be placed on to the conjunctival sac behind the eyelid to reduce pain and trauma to the eye.

Question 12

The patient should leave his or her ear facing up for 5 min after the ear drops have been given to allow the solution to come into contact with the affected area.

Chapter 17

The use of calculations in the administration of medicines

Question 1

1. Two capsules
2. 1 mL
3. 3 mL
4. 3.5 mL

Question 2

1. 25.4 kg
2. 9.5 kg
3. 3.8 kg
4. 3.2 kg

Question 3

1. 750 mg
2. 50 mg
3. 25.4 kg, 508 mg
4. 60 micrograms

Question 4

1. 500 mg
2. 2500 micrograms
3. 6250 micrograms
4. 45 000 nanograms

Question 5

1. 500 mL
2. 0.45 L
3. 2 mL
4. 1300 mL

Question 6

1. 10 g
2. 100 mg
3. 0.8 mL
4. 0.4 mL

Question 7

1. 40 mL
2. 30 mL
3. 1:6
4. 1:40

Question 8

1. 83.3 mL/h
2. 675 mL
3. 240 mL
4. 22.5 mL

Chapter 18

The management of procedural pain in children using self-administered Entonox (50% nitrous oxide, 50% oxygen)

Question 1

Entonox is 50% nitrous oxide and 50% oxygen.

Question 2

The Entonox cylinder should be stored horizontal and above −6°C, with the demand system stored in a separate place to the cylinder.

Question 3

To use Entonox, children must be old enough:

- to hold the mask or mouthpiece by themselves
- to trigger the demand valve and inhale the gas
- to understand the concepts of Entonox.

Question 4

Entonox could be used for:

- changing dressings
- removal of sutures from painful areas
- removal of drains or wires
- short-term dental work
- cannulation or venepuncture
- application of traction
- physiotherapy
- acute trauma.

Question 5

Interventions that could be considered before using Entonox are:

- distraction
- guided imagery
- local anaesthetic creams
- psychological intervention.

Question 6

Possible adverse effects when breathing Entonox are:

- nausea and dry mouth
- dizziness
- drowsiness
- loss of inhibitions, becoming verbally abusive or giggly
- euphoria.

Question 7

Entonox becomes fully effective in six to eight breaths.

Question 8

If a child starts to complain of pain:

- ask the person carrying out the procedure to stop for a while
- encourage the child to take deeper breaths of the Entonox
- encourage the child to relax
- continue with the procedure, but if the child continues to complain halt the procedure and administer alternative sedation and analgesia.

Question 9

The effects of Entonox wear off in 10–20 min.

Question 10

Measures to minimise infection during Entonox administration are:

- use of a single-patient use filter and mouthpiece
- use of clean masks

- use of clean equipment
- appropriate cleaning of all working parts after use with soap and water and alcohol-based wipes according to organisational policy.

Chapter 19

Peak flow monitoring

Question 1

- Poor technique; this requires more effort when blowing.
- A different make of peak flow meter to the one used at home.
- Is he using a low-flow peak flow meter or a standard adult peak flow meter at home?
- Worsening asthma.
- Time of day: early morning readings are often lower.
- He does not want to have to take more asthma medication.

Question 2

- Yes, these are all symptoms of uncontrolled asthma.
- Peak flow measurements taken morning and evening for a fortnight can be recorded in a diary to help diagnose asthma.

Question 3

- A personal best peak flow can be a baseline measurement against which children can judge if their asthma is good or worsening.
- It may be used in an asthma action plan to direct self-management.

Chapter 20

Oxygen therapy

Question 1

Oxygen is a clear and colourless gas and constitutes approximately 21% of the air that we breathe.

Tissues require oxygen for survival, and delivery depends on adequate ventilation, gas exchange and circulatory distribution. Failure of any of these processes will result in tissue hypoxia. Therefore the early identification of tissue hypoxia is crucial.

Oxygen is necessary for the functioning of all body cells. Glucose and oxygen are used by the cells to create ATP; this molecule in turn provides energy for most cell activities.

Question 2

Oxygen should be regarded as a drug and as such it is found in the *British National Formulary for Children*. It is often given without careful evaluation of its potential benefits and side effects. As with any drug, nurses need to fully aware of when to give oxygen, the benefits of doing so and the potential side effects.

Inappropriate concentrations may have serious effects and high concentrations can cause convulsions and retinal damage, especially in preterm neonates.

Question 3

One of the most informative skills that nurses have is observation. Therefore initial assessment of the need for oxygen is based on looking at the child.

Initially, looking at the child's demeanour will be informative. If the child is restless, confused or lethargic then hypoxia could be present.

Observing the respiratory rate, depth and any respiratory noises will indicate the level of compensation. Additionally, the child, depending on age, may show other signs of respiratory distress, for example recession and nasal flaring. If an older child shows signs of recession then the practitioner should be aware of its seriousness.

Cyanosis is a severe indication of hypoxia. This happens when a large amount of haemoglobin in the blood is poorly saturated. The result is a blue–purple colour being visible in the nail beds, mucosal membranes and skin.

Question 4

Methods of oxygen administration:

- oxygen masks
- non-rebreathing masks
- nasal cannulae
- head box.

Other methods are wafting oxygen and self-inflating bags.

Question 5

The pulse oximeter evaluates the oxygen status of a patient. Their use should, however, be in conjunction with sufficient knowledge of the physiology of oxygen transportation.

The information provided by a pulse oximeter tells the user how much oxygen is being carried by individual haemoglobin molecules, i.e. how saturated the molecules are with oxygen. It does *not* inform the user as to how much haemoglobin is present or how well the oxygen is being transported around the body to the tissues and cells.

Question 6

Pulse oximeters give a falsely high reading in the presence of carbon monoxide. Carbon monoxide has a greater ability to bind to haemoglobin molecules, and once in place it prevents the binding of oxygen molecules. It also turns haemoglobin red, so the pulse oximeter is unable to distinguish between carbon monoxide molecules and oxygen.

Chapter 30

Blood gas sampling and analysis

Question 1
Acidosis

Question 2
Alkalosis

Question 3
Respiratory acidosis

Question 4
Metabolic acidosis

Question 5
Metabolic alkalosis

Question 6
Metabolic acidosis with renal compensation

Question 7
Respiratory acidosis with metabolic compensation

Question 8
Metabolic alkalosis with respiratory compensation

Question 9
Mixed metabolic and respiratory alkalosis

Question 10
Mixed metabolic acidosis and respiratory acidosis

Question 11
Mixed metabolic acidosis and respiratory acidosis

Question 12
Respiratory alkalosis with renal compensation

Chapter 36

Neonatal jaundice and phototherapy

Question 1
In the unconjugated form bilirubin is fat-soluble and must become water-soluble before being excreted.

Question 2
Two processes that result in neonatal jaundice are:

1. bilirubin production elevation due to red blood cell destruction
2. hepatic function being inadequate in the newborn to conjugate effectively.

Question 3
Physiological jaundice usually appears between days 3 and 5.

Question 4
Phototherapy is a treatment using lights to alter the unconjugated bilirubin under the skin and begins the process of conjugation before it reaches the liver.

Question 5
Types of phototherapy include:

- overhead lamps
- spotlights
- blankets
- mattresses
- Babygro.

Question 6
Factors that can affect the efficacy of phototherapy include:

- dirty Plexiglass
- the distance of the baby from the lamp
- the surface area of the baby's skin exposed to the lamp
- the brightness of the light tubes
- other light sources being blocked to allow maximum exposure.

Question 7
An oxygen saturation monitor is sometimes required when using blue lamps because the blue lights can mask cyanosis.

Question 8
Babies pass loose stools as part of the excretion process; the stools have a high content of bile salts, which are very acidic and can burn the skin.

Question 9
Eye pads should be changed at least every 4 h to prevent drying and infection.

Question 10
An overheated baby appears flushed, may lie in an extended posture and may have an increased heart rate and respiratory rate.

Question 11
A baby having phototherapy should receive approximately 10–20% extra fluid. Some units give 10% extra per phototherapy lamp.

Question 12
Bottle- or tube-fed babies require extra fluids, so they should be fed three-hourly when possible.

Question 13
Transepidermal water loss occurs when fluid is lost via the skin and results in dehydration and fluid and electrolyte imbalance.

Question 14

Side effects of phototherapy include:

- temperature instability
- excessive transepidermal water loss
- eye damage
- eye infections
- skin rashes
- DNA damage
- sterility or DNA damage of sperm.

Chapter 39

Electrocardiography monitoring and interpretation

Question 1

The most common arrhythmia in the paediatric population is a bradycardia normally associated with severe hypoxia; the bradycardia will progress to asystole if left untreated.

Question 2

The commonest cause of collapse in paediatrics is normally associated with respiratory insufficiency when the hearts stops due to ischaemia or hypoxia secondary to another condition. Primary cardiac arrest in paediatrics is rare.

Question 3

An ECG recording is a fundamental part of cardiovascular assessment in paediatric emergency management. There are various occasions when a monitor should be attached to a child, for example respiratory distress, major trauma and electrolyte imbalance; however, the optimum standard would be when a child's condition is causing concern.

Question 4

Lead II measures the voltage between the right shoulder and the left lower chest, which consequently produces the configuration that commonly displays the most prominent P wave and QRS amplitude, providing that atrial activity is present. In the normal heart an ECG recording on lead II will produce a classic textbook PQRS complex.

Question 5

Atrial contraction can be referred to as the first stage of the cardiac cycle. It corresponds with the P wave on the ECG recording, which represents atrial depolarisation causing contraction of the muscle in the atria wall. As the atria contract there is an increase in the pressure within the atria, which opens the atrioventricular valves allowing the ventricle to fill with blood.

The next stage of the cardiac cycle represents ventricular depolarisation; this ventricular depolarisation is reflected in the QRS complex on the ECG recording. The impulse spreads via the atrioventricular node and Purkinje system, causing the ventricles to contract.

The T wave that follows represents ventricular repolarisation, which is the relaxation period prior to the next cardiac cycle commencing.

Question 6

The common or more frequent cardiac arrest arrhythmias in paediatrics are:

- asystole
- VF
- pulseless electrical activity.

Question 7

The following structured approach will assist in the analysis of the rhythm strip and determine appropriate management of a child presenting with an arrhythmia.

1. What is the ventricular rate?
2. Is the QRS complex regular or irregular?
3. Are the P waves visible?
4. Is atrial activity related to ventricular activity?
5. Is the QRS complex narrow or broad?

Question 8

In cases of suspected asystole there are essential checks that should be implemented to confirm asystole prior to commencing treatment. The ECG gain should be increased to maximum, the clinical state of the patient should be assessed and the leads should be checked to ensure optimal contact. This is to confirm the diagnosis of asystole and prevent a differential diagnosis of fine VF being attributed in error.

Question 9

Bradycardia is the term used to define a heart rate lower than that of the child's normal rate for his or her age. It is a preterminal sign more commonly associated with abnormal cardiac function as a consequence of hypoxia, acidosis and profound hypovolaemia. The response of an immature heart to prolonged hypoxia produces bradycardia.

Question 10

Tachycardia is the term used to define a heart rate higher than that of the child's normal rate for his or her age. A tachycardia may be due to the normal body response to infection, pain and exercise, which normally produces a sinus tachycardia.

Index

Note: Page numbers in **bold** refer to boxes/tables and page numbers in *italics* refer to figures.

A

B

C

D

E

F

G

H

I

Q

R

S

V

W

X

Y

Z